SURGICAL RECONSTRUCTION OF THE DIABETIC FOOT AND ANKLE

SURGICAL RECONSTRUCTION OF THE DIABETIC FOOT AND ANKLE

Second Edition

Editor

THOMAS ZGONIS, DPM, FACFAS

Professor and Director
Externship and Reconstructive Foot and Ankle Fellowship Programs
Division of Podiatric Medicine and Surgery
Department of Orthopaedics
UT Health San Antonio Long School of Medicine
San Antonio, Texas

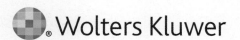 Wolters Kluwer

Philadelphia • Baltimore • New York • London
Buenos Aires • Hong Kong • Sydney • Tokyo

Acquisitions Editor: Brian Brown
Editorial Coordinator: Dave Murphy
Marketing Manager: Dan Dressler
Production Project Manager: Joan Sinclair
Design Coordinator: Holly McLaughlin
Manufacturing Coordinator: Beth Welsh
Prepress Vendor: Absolute Service, Inc.

Second Edition

9 8 7 6 5 4 3 2 1

Printed in China

Library of Congress Cataloging-in-Publication Data

Names: Zgonis, Thomas, editor.
Title: Surgical reconstruction of the diabetic foot and ankle / editor,
  Thomas Zgonis.
Description: Second edition. | Philadelphia : Wolters Kluwer, [2018] |
  Includes bibliographical references and index.
Identifiers: LCCN 2017040604 | ISBN 9781496330079
Subjects: | MESH: Diabetic Foot--surgery | Limb Salvage--methods |
  Ankle--surgery
Classification: LCC RD563 | NLM WK 835 | DDC 617.5/85059--dc23 LC record available at https://lccn.loc.gov/2017040604

I want to thank my beautiful wife, Kristen,
adorable daughters, Labrini and Ioanna, and entire family
for their continuous love, patience, and understanding
throughout all these years
as well as my mentors and teachers
for guiding me in academic medicine.

With love

Preface

It is with great honor, respect, and appreciation that I am able to share with you my ambition of producing the second edition of *Surgical Reconstruction of the Diabetic Foot and Ankle*. I am also humbled and thankful to all of my students, residents, national and international fellows, and colleagues as well as contributing authors for making this textbook a reality. It is because of your continuous motivation of learning and commitment to patient care excellence, education, and service that I am capable of providing this second edition in its most updated version with the latest surgical techniques in diabetic lower extremity reconstruction.

Diabetic foot and ankle surgery has become a surgical subspecialty, and extensive surgical training is required in some of the most challenging clinical scenarios of severe infections, lower extremity deformities, peripheral arterial disease, and soft tissue compromise. A multidisciplinary team consisted of medical and surgical services with an interest in the management of the diabetic patient is a necessity for the patient's successful outcome. In addition, major surgical procedures are best suited and managed in a large academic and/or health care system where multiple services are readily available for any necessary surgical procedure. Patient and family education as well as frequent medical visits are also of equal importance in the prevention of diabetic foot and ankle complications.

Having spent my entire training and career in academic medicine, I can surely attest to the fact that surgical treatment of the diabetic foot and ankle requires a team approach and effort from multiple disciplines with expertise in the treatment of the diabetic patient. This textbook will address topics from the preoperative management of the diabetic patient to surgical reconstruction by various surgical teams and postoperative management with long-term successful outcomes. Elective, reconstructive, traumatic, and revisional diabetic foot and ankle surgery is well-covered by national and international authors with great knowledge and experience in treating diabetic patients. Great emphasis is given to the surgical reconstruction of osseous and soft tissue defects by providing a stepwise approach for the treatment of diabetic foot infections, osteomyelitis, nonhealing wounds, and Charcot neuroarthropathy.

As I am finishing this *Preface*, my whole family is also getting ready to visit Greece. This year is very special to me because I will have the opportunity to share with them my childhood years and visit the places of where my values and work ethic were built in an era of poverty, hard work, and lack of education. Keeping in mind the powerful words that were taught to me by my grandfather—*faith*, *family*, and *education*, I have always strived for the patient's successful recovery by empowering the need of teamwork in the management of diabetic foot and ankle complications.

In conclusion, I hope that the second edition of the *Surgical Reconstruction of the Diabetic Foot and Ankle* will provide you with the most comprehensive reference when dealing with reconstruction of the diabetic lower extremity and also help raise awareness to the public and health care systems for the subspecialty of diabetic foot and ankle surgery.

TZ

Acknowledgment

I would like to thank the Acquisitions Editor, Brian Brown; Editorial Coordinator, Dave Murphy; Marketing Manager, Dan Dressler; Production Project Manager, Joan Sinclair; Design Coordinator, Holly McLaughlin; and all the members of the production services group involved with this text for their great support and guidance throughout the project.

Contributors

John Joseph Anderson, DPM, FACFAS
Director, American Foundation of Lower Extremity Surgery
and Research Fellowship
Foot, Ankle, and Leg Reconstructive Surgery
Alamogordo, Las Cruces, and Ruidoso, New Mexico
New Mexico Bone & Joint Institute
Alamogordo, New Mexico

Javier Aragón-Sánchez, MD, PhD
Head of Department of Surgery and Diabetic Foot Unit
La Paloma Hospital
Las Palmas de Gran Canaria, Spain

David G. Armstrong, DPM, MD, PhD
University Distinguished Outreach Professor of Surgery
Director, Southern Arizona Limb Salvage Alliance
University of Arizona College of Medicine
Tucson, Arizona

Christopher E. Attinger, MD
Professor, Georgetown University School of Medicine
Co-Director, Center for Wound Healing & Hyperbaric Medicine
MedStar Georgetown University Hospital
Department of Plastic Surgery
Washington, DC

Hani M. Badahdah, DPM, MD, MS
Associate Consultant of Foot and Ankle Surgery
Department of Surgery
King Faisal Specialist Hospital & Research Center
Jeddah, Saudi Arabia

Neal R. Barshes, MD, MPH
Associate Professor of Surgery
Division of Vascular and Endovascular Surgery
Michael E. DeBakey Department of Surgery
Baylor College of Medicine
Michael E. DeBakey Veterans Affairs Medical Center
Houston, Texas

Devin Bland, DPM
Associate, American Foundation of Lower Extremity Surgery
and Research
Foot, Ankle, and Leg Reconstructive Surgery
Alamogordo, Las Cruces, and Ruidoso, New Mexico
New Mexico Bone & Joint Institute
Alamogordo, New Mexico

Peter A. Blume, DPM, FACFAS
Clinical Assistant Professor of Surgery, Anesthesia, and
Orthopaedics
Yale School of Medicine
New Haven, Connecticut

Troy J. Boffeli, DPM, FACFAS
Director, Foot and Ankle Surgery Residency
Regions Hospital
HealthPartners Institute for Education and Research
Saint Paul, Minnesota

Ashley A. Bruno, DPM
Resident, Podiatric Medicine and Surgery
Yale New Haven Hospital
New Haven, Connecticut

Patrick R. Burns, DPM, FACFAS
Assistant Professor of Orthopaedic Surgery
Division of Foot and Ankle Surgery
University of Pittsburgh School of Medicine
Program Director, Podiatric Surgical Residency
University of Pittsburgh Medical Center at Mercy
Pittsburgh, Pennsylvania

Alan R. Catanzariti, DPM, FACFAS
Director, Residency Training Program
Division of Foot and Ankle Surgery
West Penn Hospital, Allegheny Health Network
Pittsburgh, Pennsylvania

Ketan Dhatariya, MBBS, MSc, MD, MS, FRCP
Consultant in Diabetes, Endocrinology, and General
Medicine
Elsie Bertram Diabetes Center
Norfolk and Norwich University Hospitals NHS
Foundation Trust
Norwich, United Kingdom

Andrew D. Elliott, DPM, JD
Attending, Orthopaedic Center
Gundersen Health System
La Crosse, Wisconsin

Karen K. Evans, MD
Associate Professor, Georgetown University School of
    Medicine
Center for Wound Healing & Hyperbaric Medicine
MedStar Georgetown University Hospital
Department of Plastic Surgery
Washington, DC

Alexandru V. Georgescu, MD, PhD
Professor, Plastic Surgery and Reconstructive Microsurgery
University of Medicine Iuliu Hațieganu
Spitalul Clinic de Recuperare
Cluj-Napoca, Romania

John M. Giurini, DPM, FACFAS
Associate Professor of Surgery
Harvard Medical School
Boston, Massachusetts
Chief, Division of Podiatric Surgery
Department of Surgery
Beth Israel Deaconess Medical Center
Boston, Massachusetts

Mark S. Goss, DPM
Resident, Foot and Ankle Surgery
Regions Hospital
HealthPartners Institute for Education and Research
Saint Paul, Minnesota

Lisa M. Grant-McDonald, DPM
Resident, Foot and Ankle Surgery
Division of Foot and Ankle Surgery
West Penn Hospital, Allegheny Health Network
Pittsburgh, Pennsylvania

David C. Hatch Jr, DPM
Resident, Podiatric Medicine and Surgery
Tucson Medical Center
Tucson, Arizona

Matthew J. Hentges, DPM
Teaching Faculty, Residency Training Program
Division of Foot and Ankle Surgery
West Penn Hospital, Allegheny Health Network
Pittsburgh, Pennsylvania

Paul J. Kim, DPM, MS, FACFAS
Associate Professor, Georgetown University School of
    Medicine
Director of Research, MedStar Georgetown University
    Hospital
Center for Wound Healing & Hyperbaric Medicine
Department of Plastic Surgery
Washington, DC

Armin Koller, MD
Chief, Division of Technical Orthopaedics
Co-Chief, Interdisciplinary Diabetic Foot Center
Mathias Hospital
Rheine, Germany

Chrisovalantis Lakhiani, MD
Resident, Plastic Surgery
Center for Wound Healing & Hyperbaric Medicine
MedStar Georgetown University Hospital
Department of Plastic Surgery
Washington, DC

Bradley M. Lamm, DPM, FACFAS
Director, Foot and Ankle Deformity Center
and Foot and Ankle Deformity Correction Fellowship
Paley Orthopaedic & Spine Institute
Palm Beach Children's Hospital and St. Mary's Medical Center
West Palm Beach, Florida

Manuel Llusá-Pérez, MD, PhD
Professor of Human Anatomy and Embryology
University of Barcelona
Department of Orthopaedic Surgery
Vall d'Hebron University Hospital
Barcelona, Spain

Jeffrey M. Manway, DPM
Clinical Instructor of Orthopaedic Surgery
Division of Foot and Ankle Surgery
University of Pittsburgh School of Medicine
Pittsburgh, Pennsylvania

Ileana R. Matei, MD, PhD
Lecturer, Plastic Surgery and Reconstructive Microsurgery
University of Medicine Iuliu Hațieganu
Spitalul Clinic de Recuperare
Cluj-Napoca, Romania

Spencer J. Monaco, DPM
Attending, Premier Orthopaedics & Sports Medicine
Chester County Orthopaedic Associates Division
West Chester, Pennsylvania

Kyle R. Moore, DPM
Fellow, Foot and Ankle Deformity Correction
Paley Orthopaedic & Spine Institute
Palm Beach Children's Hospital and St. Mary's Medical Center
West Palm Beach, Florida

Amber Rose Morra, DPM
Resident, Podiatric Medicine and Surgery
Yale New Haven Hospital
New Haven, Connecticut

William B. Morrison, MD
Professor of Radiology
Thomas Jefferson University Hospital
Philadelphia, Pennsylvania

Jennifer L. Pappalardo, DPM
Assistant Professor of Surgery
University of Arizona College of Medicine
Tucson, Arizona

Crystal L. Ramanujam, DPM, MSc, FACFAS
Assistant Professor/Clinical and Chief
Division of Podiatric Medicine and Surgery
Department of Orthopaedics
UT Health San Antonio Long School of Medicine
San Antonio, Texas

Barry I. Rosenblum, DPM, FACFAS
Assistant Clinical Professor of Surgery
Harvard Medical School
Boston, Massachusetts
Associate Chief, Division of Podiatric Surgery
Department of Surgery
Beth Israel Deaconess Medical Center
Boston, Massachusetts

Thomas S. Roukis, DPM, PhD, FACFAS
Attending, Orthopaedic Center
Gundersen Health System
La Crosse, Wisconsin

Michel Saint-Cyr, MD
Director, Division of Plastic Surgery
Wigley Professor in Plastic Surgery
Baylor Scott & White Health
Temple, Texas

Vlad Sauciuc, DPM
Resident, Podiatric Medicine and Surgery
Tucson Medical Center
Tucson, Arizona

Daniel J. Short, DPM
Attending, Mid-Atlantic Permanente Medical Group
Springfield Medical Center
Springfield, Virginia

Devin C. Simonson, DPM
Attending, Orthopaedic Center
Gundersen Health System
La Crosse, Wisconsin

John J. Stapleton, DPM, FACFAS
Attending, Foot and Ankle Surgery
Lehigh Valley Physician Group Orthopaedics
Lehigh Valley Hospital
Allentown, Pennsylvania
Clinical Assistant Professor of Surgery
Penn State College of Medicine
Hershey, Pennsylvania

John S. Steinberg, DPM, FACFAS
Professor, Georgetown University School of Medicine
Co-Director, Center for Wound Healing & Hyperbaric Medicine
Program Director, MedStar Washington Hospital Center
Podiatric Surgery Residency
MedStar Georgetown University Hospital
Department of Plastic Surgery
Washington, DC

Drew H. Taft, DPM, FACFAS
Chief of Podiatric Surgery
Winchester Hospital
Winchester, Massachusetts

Caitlin S. Zarick, DPM
Assistant Professor, Georgetown University School of
    Medicine
Center for Wound Healing & Hyperbaric Medicine
MedStar Georgetown University Hospital
Department of Plastic Surgery
Washington, DC

Thomas Zgonis, DPM, FACFAS
Professor and Director
Externship and Reconstructive Foot and Ankle Fellowship
    Programs
Division of Podiatric Medicine and Surgery
Department of Orthopaedics
UT Health San Antonio Long School of Medicine
San Antonio, Texas

Wenchuan Zhang, MD, PhD
Professor and Vice Director
Department of Neurosurgery
Xinhua Hospital
Shanghai Jiao Tong University School of Medicine
Shanghai, China

Contents

Perioperative Management for the Elective Outpatient and Hospitalized Inpatient with Diabetes Mellitus

Ketan Dhatariya

INTRODUCTION

Diabetes mellitus is the most common metabolic disorder. It is estimated that there are currently 415 million people in the world with the condition, of whom over 90% have type 2 diabetes mellitus (29). In North America and the Caribbean, the estimated prevalence of diabetes mellitus in 2014 was 39 million people—12.9% of the adult population (29). Over the next decade, the exponential rise in obesity is predicted to increase the prevalence of diabetes mellitus to almost 650 million by 2040 (29). This has major implications for health care services, with particular impact on hospitalized inpatient care. Data from the United Kingdom in 2015 suggested that 10% of the National Health Service primary care drugs bill for England alone was spent on diabetes mellitus drugs, £868 million ($1.08 billion) annually, up from 6.6% of overall drug expenditure in 2005 to 2006 (25).This is when the prevalence of diabetes mellitus among adults in the United Kingdom is between 6% and 7%. In economies, where the prevalence of diabetes mellitus is higher, this proportion of spending is also likely to have increased. Additional expense comes from looking after the complications of diabetes mellitus, including the diabetic foot. In a detailed economic analysis, it has been estimated that in the United Kingdom, approximately £1 billion or £1 in every £150 spent in the National Health Service is on the "diabetic foot" (31). Because diabetes mellitus–related comorbidities increase the need for surgical and other operative procedures, it is not surprising that at least 10% of patients undergoing surgery have diabetes mellitus, and this percentage is also likely to rise.

Data from the 2016 United Kingdom National Diabetes Inpatient Audit (NaDIA) showed that the prevalence of hospital inpatient population with diabetes mellitus ranged from 2.4% to 40.5% (50). Previous work has shown that people with diabetes mellitus have a longer length of hospital stay and higher mortality rates than those without the condition (26). This is a particular problem in surgical patients with diabetes mellitus

where the excess bed days were recently estimated to be 45% greater than for people with diabetes mellitus admitted to medical wards (43). Data have also shown that patients with diabetes mellitus are often inappropriately denied same-day surgical procedures (42). In particular, patients admitted for general and orthopedic surgery have some of the longest lengths of hospital stay (59). All of these issues lead to an overall rise in costs (32).

The high-risk surgical population is made up of elderly patients with coexisting medical conditions undergoing complex or major surgery, often as an emergency. The most important comorbid diseases include ischemic heart disease, heart failure, respiratory disease, impaired renal function, and diabetes mellitus. There is clear evidence that such diseases are strongly associated with poor outcomes after major surgery (5,6,40,53). The primary aim of perioperative management of the surgical patient with diabetes mellitus is to decrease morbidity and hopefully reduce the duration of hospital stay.

The perioperative mortality rate for people with diabetes mellitus is reported to be up to 50% higher than that of the nondiabetic population (16). The reasons for these adverse outcomes are multifactorial but include the following:

- Hypo- and hyperglycemia
- Multiple medical comorbidities including microvascular and macrovascular complications
- Complex polypharmacy, including misuse of insulin
- Inappropriate use of intravenous insulin infusion
- Management errors when converting from the intravenous insulin infusion to usual medication
- Perioperative infection

The Importance of Perioperative Glycemic Control

Poor perioperative glycemic control in the form of high concentrations of glycated hemoglobin (HbA_{1c}) or glucose has been associated with poor outcomes in several surgical specialities. These include elective or emergency foot and ankle surgery (61), vascular surgery (54), trauma (34), mastectomy (69), spinal surgery (70), cardiac surgery (1,24), colorectal surgery (23), neurosurgery, cholecystectomy, and other hepatobiliary surgery (2,4). "Poor outcomes" may be defined as increased rates of wound infection, urinary tract infections, time spent in intensive care, development of acute kidney injury, acute coronary syndromes, or death.

There is a suggestion from a recent systematic review that preoperative HbA$_{1c}$ has little impact on outcomes (55). However, the authors acknowledged that the studies to date have been of poor quality with small sample sizes and much heterogeneity. Indeed, there are data to show that if a person is known to have diabetes mellitus prior to an operation, then his or her outcomes are better than those people who are hyperglycemic and not previously known to have diabetes mellitus (39). Why this may be is unknown but may be more to do with the increased nursing care given to people with diabetes mellitus (e.g., bedside capillary blood glucose monitoring) that may detect problems earlier. It would be tempting to extrapolate from the data to say that if poor perioperative glucose levels are associated with harm, normalizing glucose levels would improve outcomes. However, to date, there is little data to confirm this (8).

Complications of Diabetes Mellitus

Diabetes mellitus is associated with a two- to fourfold increase in cardiovascular disease including hypertension, coronary artery disease, and stroke (62). The majority of people with diabetes mellitus scheduled for surgery are likely to have one or more of these cardiovascular diseases and a significant number will have microvascular disease (nephropathy or neuropathy). Those with impaired cardiac function and/or nephropathy are at greater risk for fluid overload. Postoperative cardiac arrhythmias are more common in people with diabetes mellitus, particularly in those with autonomic dysfunction or a prolonged QTc interval (14,68). The incidence of postoperative hypotension is increased, related to a combination of autonomic dysfunction, inadequate fluid replacement, and inadequate monitoring of hypotensive therapies.

Peripheral neuropathy affects between 30% and 50% of people with diabetes mellitus and places them at increased risk for heel ulceration, particularly if peripheral arterial disease is also present (22). Care should always be taken to protect the feet and heels in hospitalized patients with diabetes mellitus.

The Foot Protection Team

All patients admitted to the hospital with diabetes mellitus–related foot problems should be seen and assessed by a member of the multidisciplinary foot protection team, ideally within a few hours of acute hospital admission (47). The team should be experienced in dealing with the "diabetic foot"—in particular, able to grade the severity of any infection as well as being able to assess the vascular status of the lower extremities. All members of the team should have urgent access to any other member of the specialist team as necessary. If possible, all inpatients with diabetes mellitus–related foot problems should

TABLE 1.1
Members of the Foot Protection Team (47)

- Diabetologist (± internist/hospitalist) with an interest in the diabetic foot
- Vascular surgeon
- Orthopedic foot and ankle surgeon
- Podiatrist/Podiatric surgeon
- Diabetes mellitus specialist nurse/Diabetes mellitus educator
- Tissue viability nurse
- Casting service
- Plastic/Reconstructive surgeon
- Microbiologist/Infectious disease specialist[a]
- Interventional radiologist[a]
- Biomechanics and orthotists[a]

[a]These members of the team should be available for consultation and may not necessarily be part of the immediate foot protection team. Other teams that should be available to give advice include rehabilitation services, psychological services, and nutritional services.

be seen and assessed regularly by the foot protection team. Table 1.1 shows the inpatient diabetic foot protection team.

There is evidence to show that the foot protection team reduces the incidence of major amputations in an outpatient clinical setting (35,57). For patients who are hospitalized, however, the priority would be to optimize glycemic control and other comorbidities prior to any planned surgical procedure (72). In addition, the prevention of iatrogenic foot pathology, such as the development of pressure-related heel ulcers, should be paramount.

Patients with diabetes mellitus admitted with foot problems frequently have several other comorbidities (e.g., cardiac and renal). Previous myocardial infarction, atrial fibrillation, respiratory disease, and a history of congestive cardiac failure all increase the risk of postoperative complications after noncardiac surgery (38). There is clear evidence that such diseases are strongly associated with poor outcomes after major surgery (5). It is likely that the incidence of perioperative morbidity and mortality among patients with diabetes mellitus could be reduced with better preoperative assessment and optimization of blood pressure, cardiovascular, and renal reserve.

FACTORS LEADING TO ADVERSE OUTCOMES

Failure to Identify Patients with Diabetes Mellitus

If diabetes mellitus is not identified before admission, there will be no opportunity for preadmission planning. This increases the risk of management errors during the admission (41). United States and United Kingdom guidelines recommend an identifier in the medical record for all patients with diabetes mellitus admitted to a hospital (9,43).

Lack of Institutional Guidelines for Management of Diabetes Mellitus

Data suggest that not all hospitals have comprehensive guidelines for management of dysglycemia in inpatients, and many lack a strategy for achieving good glycemic control (58). An analysis of 44 United States hospitals revealed shortcomings in diabetes mellitus management including persistent hyperglycemia (71). In the United Kingdom, there are specific national guidelines for the perioperative management of adult patients undergoing surgery, which have been widely adopted or adapted (9). They have recently been updated, and there is data emerging to show that by adopting these guidelines, variations in practice are minimized and thus improve the standard of patient care.

Poor Knowledge of Diabetes Mellitus among Staff Delivering Care

Understanding of diabetes mellitus and its management is poor among both medical and nursing staff (21). Undergraduate and postgraduate medical training often has little or no focus on the practical aspects of delivery of diabetes mellitus care. Although their own knowledge and experience is limited, hospital ward staff is frequently reluctant to allow the patients to make their own decisions about the management of their diabetes mellitus. The problem is compounded by uncertainty about the legal aspects of inpatient self-medication.

Complex Polypharmacy and Insulin Prescribing Errors

Patients with diabetes mellitus frequently require complex drug regimens with high potential for error that may include, but not limited, to the following:

- Incorrect prescription
- Omitted in error or judiciously stopped and never restarted
- Continued inappropriately (e.g., in presence of renal impairment)
- Drug-drug interaction

PREOPERATIVE AND PERIOPERATIVE MANAGEMENT OF THE ELECTIVE SURGICAL PATIENT WITH DIABETES MELLITUS

All institutions should initiate a pathway of care for patients with diabetes mellitus undergoing elective or emergency surgery. For this pathway of care to work effectively, complete and accurate information should be communicated by staff at each stage to staff at the next stage. Wherever possible, the person with diabetes mellitus should be included in all communications, and the management plan should be devised in agreement with the patient.

The multidisciplinary team responsible for the patients' usual, ongoing diabetes care—that is, primary or secondary care—should aim to optimize glycemic control (HbA$_{1c}$ of less than 69 mmol/mol, 8.5%) prior to their surgical referral and if it is felt that further optimization is safely achievable. They should be able to postpone any elective procedure to facilitate this optimization. The reason for this pragmatic approach is that high preoperative HbA$_{1c}$ has been shown to be associated with poorer outcomes (65), and that in a population more likely to be elderly with longstanding diabetes mellitus, there is little data to show that more aggressive glycemic control is beneficial, but there is data to show that there is a greater risk of immediate harm in the form of severe hypoglycemia (i.e., requiring help from a third party). Thus, 69 mmol/mol is a target that can usually be achieved in many people with diabetes mellitus given sufficient time, such as those being referred for elective surgery.

Glycemic Targets

This is often a controversial area. The physiologic stress of acute illness is associated with production of several counter-regulatory hormones (catecholamines, growth hormone, and cortisol) that raise blood glucose levels, so called "stress hyperglycemia" (11). For many years, the fear of undetected hypoglycemia during general anesthesia was the major influence in determining blood glucose concentrations. High glucose values were tolerated on the basis that "permissive hyperglycemia" was safer than rigorous blood glucose control with the associated risk of hypoglycemia. A number of studies have looked at the impact of tight blood glucose control on postoperative outcomes, with varying conclusions. However, the results from these studies have been inconsistent, with some studies showing benefit (17,67) and other showing potential harm (20,52). For these reasons, the target blood glucose in the preoperative anesthetized or sedated patient has been advocated to be 6.0 to 10.0 mmol/L (108 to 180 mg/dL), with up to 12 mmol/L (216 mg/dL) being acceptable (36). For the awake postoperative patient not on a variable rate intravenous insulin infusion (VRIII), a range of 4.0 to 12.0 mmol/L (72 to 216 mg/dL) may be acceptable. This is because anesthesiologists who feel that in the sedated or sleeping patients who are unable to make others aware if they are hypoglycemic, aiming for close to 4.0 mmol/L (72 mg/dL) puts them at risk for developing hypoglycemia.

In addition, the Normoglycemia in Intensive Care Evaluation-Survival Using Glucose Algorithm Regulation (NICE-SUGAR) study of 6,024 Intensive Care Unit (ICU) patients (who aimed for 4.5 to 6.0 mmol/L [81 to 108 mg/dL] in the intensive treatment arm) found that 82.4% of all moderate hypoglycemic episodes (that occurred in 45% of the entire cohort) occurred in the intensive treatment arm, and 93.3% of all severe hypoglycemic episodes (that were experienced by 3.7% of the entire cohort) occurred in the intensive treatment arm (51). This recommendation would be approximately concordant with the position statement of the American Association of Clinical Endocrinologists and American Diabetes Association and minimizes the risks of hyperglycemia and hypoglycemia (43). It also reduces the risk of variability in blood glucose, which is more likely to occur if the target is <6.1 mmol/L (110 mg/dL) and has been associated with worse outcomes (44).

THE PATIENT WITH DIABETES MELLITUS JOURNEY TO SURGERY

For elective surgical procedures in patients with diabetes mellitus, the journey can be divided into 7 stages, depending on the health system. These are primary care referral to the surgeons, surgical outpatients, preoperative assessment clinic, admission to the emergency room, hospital admission, operative room and recovery, and postoperative care and hospital discharge. At each stage, the themes are communication from one team to another, and that glycemic control is optimized wherever possible, aiming for HbA_{1c} of less than 69 mmol/mol (8.5%).

Primary Care Team

The aims of primary care in the management of patients with diabetes mellitus undergoing surgery are the following:

- Ensure that the potential effects of diabetes mellitus and associated comorbidities on the outcome of surgery are considered before referral for elective procedures.
- Ensure that the relevant medical information is communicated fully at the time of referral.
- Ensure that diabetes mellitus and comorbidities are optimally managed before the surgical procedure.

To achieve these aims, primary care teams should optimize glycemic control, aiming for HbA_{1c} of less than 69 mmol/mol (8.5%) before referral if possible and if it is safe to do so. A referral to a specialist diabetes mellitus team may be necessary. However, because it will take a minimum of 3 months to know if the glycemic optimization has affected the HbA_{1c}, if the surgery is deemed more urgent, referral should not be delayed. All referral letters to the surgeons should contain the relevant information for the surgeons to make informed decisions about prioritization. This information is listed in Table 1.2.

Surgical Outpatient Procedures

The aim of the surgical outpatient consultation is to arrange a preoperative assessment as soon as possible after the decision is taken to proceed with surgery to allow optimization of care. Wherever possible, day of surgery admission should be the "default" position.

To achieve these aims, systems should be in place to allow early preoperative assessment to identify people with suboptimal diabetes mellitus control. In addition, each institution should have plans in place to facilitate day of surgery admission and prevent unnecessary overnight preoperative admission. Furthermore, hospital patient administration systems should be able to identify all patients with diabetes mellitus so they can be prioritized on the operating list, thus avoiding prolonged starvation periods.

At the time of the surgical outpatient procedures, once a decision has been made to admit the patient with diabetes mellitus for elective surgery requiring a period of starvation, patients should be provided with written information about diabetes mellitus management. Finally, surgeons in the outpatient clinical setting should ensure that patients with diabetes mellitus are not scheduled for an evening procedure. This avoids prolonged

TABLE 1.2
Minimum Data Required from Primary Care Team When Referring a Patient with Diabetes Mellitus for Surgery

- Duration and type of diabetes mellitus
- Place of usual diabetes mellitus care (primary or secondary)
- Other medical comorbidities
- Treatment
  - For diabetes mellitus oral agents/insulin doses and frequency
  - For other medical comorbidities
- Complications
  - At-risk foot
  - Renal impairment
  - Cardiac disease
- Relevant measures (measured within the previous 3 months)
  - Body mass index
  - Blood pressure
  - Hemoglobin A_{1c}
  - Estimated glomerular filtration rate

starvation times, the use of a VRIII, and a potentially unnecessary overnight stay.

Preoperative Assessment

The aims here are multiple. The preoperative assessment team should ensure that the HbA_{1c} is less than 69 mmol/mol (8.5%)—if it is safe and appropriate to do so. Advice from the diabetes mellitus team may need to be sought. An individualized diabetes mellitus management plan should be agreed with the patients and written advice given as to how to manipulate their diabetes mellitus medication on the day prior to and on the day of admission. Medical comorbidities should be recognized and optimized. Advice from other medical teams may need to be sought, especially if bridging therapies need to be considered during admission (e.g., anticoagulation or renal replacement therapy).

To achieve these aims, several issues need to be addressed. Once a decision has been made that the patient needs surgery, they should be seen in the preassessment clinic as soon as possible to allow for the diabetes mellitus and any medical comorbidities to be optimized, referring to other specialties where necessary. As previously stated, the risk of delaying surgery should be balanced against the risks of poor glycemic control. The following are some of the issues that may need to be addressed in the preoperative assessment:

- The inpatient stay should be planned if feasible.
- The timing of surgery is paramount.
- Preadmission management of medications
- Availability of the patients' usual medication
- Plans for enhanced recovery partnership program in the context of diabetes mellitus

At all times, the patient should be fully consulted and engaged in the proposed plan of management. At the time of the preassessment clinic, plans about the duration of stay and preliminary discharge arrangements should be discussed with the patient. The hospital admission ward staff should be appraised of any plans and should be able to activate them on the day of admission. Lastly, the need for home support following hospital discharge should be considered, with the primary care team being involved in the discharge planning discussions.

Case Order for Surgical Procedures in Patients with Diabetes Mellitus

Although many considerations determine the case order for surgical procedures, for people with diabetes mellitus, one of the most important goals is to minimize the starvation time to allow early resumption of their normal diet and to take their usual medication at the normal time. Thus, it is recommended that the elective surgical patient with diabetes mellitus is prioritized on the case order for a surgical procedure.

Hospital Admission

The aims during the admission process are to ensure that the plan that was formulated in the preoperative assessment clinic is put in place and that there is adequate and appropriate communication between everyone concerned, including the patient. In addition, appropriate glycemic control is maintained throughout the hospital stay. Achieving good glycemic control may involve allowing the patients to self-manage their diabetes mellitus if they are able to do so, and the institution has processes in place allowing them to do so. Insulin, which is one of the highest risk drugs, should be prescribed correctly—that is, using the brand name and ensuring the word "unit" is written out (not using the abbreviation "u"). Electronic prescribing may reduce some of these risks.

To achieve these aims, the hospital should have written guidelines for hospital staff and patients to allow the modification of commonly used diabetes mellitus treatment regimens on the day prior to and day of surgery. The type and length of surgery should help determine whether the patients will miss more than one meal, and if so, they will need to manage their diabetes mellitus according to local protocols, for example, using a VRIII or a basal bolus regimen (64).

The capillary blood glucose concentrations should be monitored regularly (at least hourly—more frequently if readings are outside the target range). The target blood glucose in the preoperative, anesthetized, or sedated patient should be 6.0 to 10.0 mmol/L (108 to 180 mg/dL) (up to 12.0 mmol/L [216 mg/dL] may be acceptable). The target of 6.0 to 10.0 mmol/L (108 to 180 mg/dL) is for those who are treated with glucose-lowering agents—that is, insulin, (either subcutaneously or via an insulin infusion) or sulphonylurea therapy. In the awake patient on agents that do not produce hypoglycemia, provided they have not been given insulin, lower blood glucose values down to 3.5 mmol/L (63 mg/dL) are safe and do not require intravenous glucose or other rescue treatment.

Hypoglycemia sometimes manifests as drowsiness, which may be wrongly attributed to sedation. Furthermore, for patients requiring a VRIII, the long-acting analogue should be continued alongside the intravenous insulin infusion during the perioperative period. Evidence has suggested that this reduces the risk of rebound hyperglycemia when the VRIII is discontinued (28). However, the dose of long-acting insulin that the patient takes when he or she is well should be reduced by 20% while he or she is in the hospital (56).

Operating Room and Recovery Time

The aim of management while the patient undergoes the operation is that glycemic control and electrolyte concentrations should be maintained at all times. The target blood glucose in the preoperative, anesthetized, or sedated patient should be 6.0 to 10.0 mmol/L (108 to 180 mg/dL) (up to 12.0 mmol/L [216 mg/dL] may be acceptable). In addition, the anesthesiologist should provide multimodal analgesia with appropriate antiemetics to enable an early return to a normal diet and usual diabetes mellitus regimen postoperatively.

The individualized care plan should be adhered to where appropriate, and in the same fashion as during the initial hospital admission, the target of 6.0 to 10.0 mmol/L (108 to 180 mg/dL) is for those who are treated with glucose-lowering agents—that is, insulin (either subcutaneously or via an insulin infusion) or sulphonylurea therapy. In the awake patient on agents that do not produce hypoglycemia, provided they have not been given insulin, lower blood glucose values down to 3.5 mmol/L (63 mg/dL) are safe and do not require intravenous glucose or other rescue treatment.

Use of VRIIIs should be avoided if possible, in particular for short starvation times (one missed meal), but never stop an insulin infusion in someone with type 1 diabetes mellitus unless subcutaneous insulin has been given; otherwise, they risk developing diabetic ketoacidosis very swiftly.

Postoperative Care

This is a potentially dangerous time for patients with diabetes mellitus due to the physiologic trespass of surgery, the stress hyperglycemia, the change in insulin sensitivity associated with surgery, and the interruption in oral intake. Glucose control may be unpredictable and requires skill and experience on the part of the clinicians (60). The diabetes mellitus specialist team should be involved promptly if good glycemic control cannot be maintained (15).

The aims of good management during this time are to encourage the patient an early return to normal eating and drinking and, at the same time, to facilitate return to usual diabetes mellitus regimen. There may be some glycemic variability around this time, but the ideal situation would be to maintain glucose concentrations in the awake patient not on a VRIII between 4.0 and 12.0 mmol/L (72 to 216 mg/dL), however, for the time until the patient is eating and drinking normally, and if the patient is on an intravenous insulin infusion, then the acceptable range remains 6.0 to 12.0 mmol/L (108 to 216 mg/dL).

Hospital Discharge

Hospital discharge planning should be built into the preoperative assessment process in collaboration with the patient and should look beyond the inpatient period of care. This is to ensure patient safety after discharge and reduce the risk of readmission (12). The diabetes mellitus specialist team can play a pivotal role in this process. Hospital ward staff should be provided with clearly defined discharge criteria to prevent unnecessary delays when the patient is ready to leave the hospital. Multidisciplinary teamwork is required to manage all aspects of the discharge process (3,7).

The diabetes mellitus specialist team should be involved at an early stage if the blood glucose is not well controlled (15). The diabetes mellitus inpatient specialist nurse and/or diabetes mellitus educator, with the support of generalist nurses, can provide the patient education that is an essential part of discharge planning. Inpatient education can allow earlier discharge and improved postdischarge outcomes (49).

Because the metabolic and endocrine effects of surgery may last for several days, patients and/or carers should be advised about blood glucose management during this period. In particular, patients who normally self-monitor their blood glucose concentrations may need to do so more frequently. Clear blood glucose targets should be documented as part of the discharge care plan, and patients should be able to access specialist advice if they are concerned about their blood glucose levels. In addition, written guidance on management of blood glucose during illness should be provided at the preoperative assessment clinic and should be reinforced on hospital discharge.

EMERGENCY SURGERY IN PATIENTS WITH DIABETES MELLITUS

By definition, there may be no opportunity for preadmission planning. The release of high levels of catabolic hormones in response to the crisis is certain to lead to hyperglycemia. Many emergencies result from infection which will add further to the hyperglycemia. Prompt action should be taken to control the blood glucose, and generally, the emergency patient will require a VRIII. In the postoperative period, catabolic stress and infection predispose to hyperglycemia and ketogenesis, and it is crucial to maintain glycemic control to optimize the outcome. However, there are certain circumstances where patients may be suitable for manipulation of their normal diabetes mellitus medications, thus avoiding the need for intravenous insulin (e.g., those requiring minor peripheral orthopedic procedures) (Tables 1.3 and 1.4).

The blood glucose should be closely monitored, and if it rises above 10.0 mmol/L (180 mg/dL), a VRIII should be commenced and continued until the patient is eating and drinking. The HbA$_{1c}$ should be measured to assess the level of preadmission blood glucose control because this may influence subsequent diabetes mellitus management. Early involvement of the critical care and diabetes mellitus specialist teams is recommended in the management of any high-risk surgical patient with diabetes mellitus.

At the preoperative assessment clinic, all patients should have an emergency treatment plan for hypoglycemia written on their drug chart (i.e., GlucoGel and 20% dextrose). Rapid-acting insulin should also be prescribed. The patients should also be warned that their blood glucose control may be erratic for a few days after the procedure.

Continuous Subcutaneous Insulin Infusion Pump

There are very few data on the use of continuous subcutaneous insulin infusions (CSII) in the management of people with diabetes mellitus undergoing surgery. If the starvation period is short, CSII pump therapy should be continued, and patients should remain on their basal rate until they are eating and drinking normally. Generally, patients on a CSII are very well educated and will be able to self-manage their diabetes mellitus appropriately if given the opportunity to do so. It is likely that they will be able to adjust their insulin rates to achieve glucose levels of 6.0 to 10 mmol/L (108 to 180 mg/dL). The anesthesiologist should not give bolus insulin doses via the CSII. If hypoglycemia occurs while on the CSII, then it should be treated according to local guidance. Regular capillary blood glucose testing will be necessary, with electrolyte measurements, if the pump is stopped for any length of time. If more than 1 meal is to be missed, the pump should be removed, and a VRIII or a basal bolus insulin regimen should be used.

Perioperative hypotension can decrease skin perfusion and reduce insulin absorption; therefore, normal hydration and blood pressure must be maintained. The stress of surgery and perioperative complications such as infection is likely to change the insulin requirement, and close liaison with the diabetes mellitus specialist team is advised. If the blood glucose cannot be maintained in the target range in the intraoperative or immediate postoperative period, a VRII or basal bolus insulin regimen should be initiated unless the patient is well enough to self-manage with bolus corrections. Advice should be sought from the diabetes mellitus specialist team.

If a CSII has been continued throughout the perioperative period, mealtime boluses should be recommended once the patient is eating and drinking normally. The patient needs to be warned that his or her blood glucose may vary for a few days postoperatively and that corrections in his or her doses may need to be made. If the insulin pump has been discontinued and replaced with a VRIII, the CSII should be restarted (including the usual mealtime boluses) once the patient is eating and drinking, and the VRIII should be discontinued 30 minutes after the first mealtime bolus.

MANAGING OF MEDICAL COMORBIDITIES

Cardiac Disease, Lipids, and Blood Pressure

Foot problems in people with diabetes mellitus such as ulcers (many of which will be infected) or deformity are usually a culmination of several factors taking their toll over a number

TABLE 1.3	Guidelines for Perioperative Adjustment of Insulin			
		Day of Surgery/While on a VRIII		
Insulins	Day Prior to Admission	Patient for AM Surgery	Patient for PM Surgery	If a VRIII Is Being Used[a]
Once daily (evening) (e.g., Lantus or Levemir, Tresiba, Insulatard, Humulin I, Insuman Basal)	Reduce dose by 20%.	Check blood glucose on admission and hourly until eating and drinking normally.	Check blood glucose on admission and hourly until eating and drinking normally.	Continue at 80% of the usual dose.
Once daily (morning) (e.g., Lantus or Levemir, Tresiba, Insulatard, Humulin I, Insuman Basal)	Reduce dose by 20%.	Reduce dose by 20% Check blood glucose on admission and hourly until eating and drinking normally.	Reduce dose by 20% Check blood glucose on admission and hourly until eating and drinking normally.	Continue at 80% of the usual dose.
Twice daily (e.g., NovoMix 30, Humulin M3, Humalog Mix 25, Humalog Mix 50, Insuman Comb 25, Insuman Comb 50, Levemir or Lantus)	No dose change for the morning insulin, but the evening dose will need to be reduced by 20%	Halve the usual morning dose. Check blood glucose on admission and hourly until eating and drinking normally. Leave the evening meal dose unchanged.	Halve the usual morning dose. Check blood glucose on admission and hourly until eating and drinking normally. Leave the evening meal dose unchanged.	Stop until eating and drinking normally.
Twice daily—separate injections of short-acting (e.g., animal neutral, NovoRapid, Humulin S, Apidra) and intermediate-acting (e.g., animal isophane Insulatard, Humulin I, Insuman)	The morning and doses should remain unchanged. The evening meal short-acting insulin dose should remain unchanged, but the evening dose of background insulin will need to be reduced by 20%.	Calculate the total dose of both morning insulins and give half as intermediate acting only in the morning. Check blood glucose on admission and hourly until eating and drinking normally. Leave the evening meal dose unchanged	Calculate the total dose of both morning insulins and give half as intermediate-acting only in the morning. Check blood glucose on admission and hourly until eating and drinking normally. Leave the evening meal dose unchanged.	Stop until eating and drinking normally.
Three, four, or five injections daily (e.g., an injection of mixed insulin three times a day or three mealtime injections of short-acting insulin and once or twice daily background)	The morning and lunchtime doses should remain unchanged. The evening meal short-acting insulin dose should remain unchanged, but the evening or night time dose of background insulin will need to be reduced by 20%	**Basal bolus regimens:** omit the morning and lunchtime short-acting insulins. If the dose of long-acting basal insulin is usually taken in the morning then the dose should be reduced by 20%.[a] **Premixed AM insulin:** halve the morning dose and omit lunchtime dose. Check blood glucose on admission and hourly until eating and drinking normally.	Take usual morning insulin dose(s). Omit lunchtime dose. Check blood glucose on admission.	Stop until eating and drinking normally.

[a]If the patient requires an ongoing VRIII, then the long-acting background insulin should be continued but at 80% of the dose the patient usually takes when he or she is well. Normal insulin doses should be recommenced when the patient is eating and drinking normally.

AM, morning; PM, afternoon; VRIII, variable rate intravenous insulin infusion.

of years. The vascular disease and peripheral neuropathy does not limit itself to the feet. Ideally, the management of people with diabetes mellitus in primary and secondary care should begin at the time of diagnosis, in particular aggressively addressing the multiple cardiovascular risk factors that people with diabetes mellitus have (48). This aggressive multiple risk factor intervention has been shown to have cardiovascular benefits in terms of reduction in premature mortality (27,46). However, these data are extrapolated from population-based studies, and individual risks are more difficult to define. Thus, by the time someone presents with established diabetic foot disease, it is often a manifestation of generalized atherosclerosis, peripheral neuropathy, or both. The evidence for this is that people with diabetic foot disease have a significantly

TABLE 1.4	Guidelines for Perioperative Adjustment of Noninsulin Medication			
		Day of Surgery/While on a VRIII		
Tablets	Day Prior to Admission	Patient for AM Surgery	Patient for PM Surgery	If a VRIII Is Being Used[a]
Acarbose	Take as normal.	Omit morning dose if NPO.	Give morning dose if eating.	Stop once VRIII commenced; do not recommence until eating and drinking normally.
Meglitinide (e.g., repaglinide or nateglinide)	Take as normal.	Omit morning dose if NPO.	Give morning dose if eating.	Stop once VRIII commenced; do not recommence until eating and drinking normally.
Metformin (eGFR is greater than 60 mL/min/1.73 m² and procedure not requiring use of contrast media[b])	Take as normal.	If taken once or twice a day—take as normal. If taken three times per day, omit lunchtime dose.	If taken once or twice a day—take as normal. If taken three times per day, omit lunchtime dose.	Stop once VRIII commenced; do not recommence until eating and drinking normally.
Sulphonylurea (e.g., glibenclamide, gliclazide, glipizide, glimepiride)	Take as normal.	If taken once daily in the morning—omit the dose that day. If taken twice daily—omit the morning dose that day.	If taken once daily in the morning—omit the dose that day. If taken twice daily—omit both doses that day.	Stop once VRIII commenced; do not recommence until eating and drinking normally.
Pioglitazone	Take as normal.	Take as normal.	Take as normal.	Stop once VRIII commenced; do not recommence until eating and drinking normally.
Dipeptidyl peptidase-4 (DDP-4) inhibitor (e.g., sitagliptin, vildagliptin, saxagliptin, alogliptin, linagliptin)	Take as normal.	Take as normal.	Take as normal.	Stop once VRIII commenced; do not recommence until eating and drinking normally.
Glucagon-like peptide 1 (GLP-1) analogue (e.g., exenatide, liraglutide, lixisenatide, dulaglutide)	Take as normal.	Take as normal.	Take as normal.	Take as normal.
Sodium-glucose cotransporter 2 (SGLT-2) inhibitors (e.g., dapagliflozin, canagliflozin, empagliflozin)	Take as normal.	Omit on day of surgery.	Omit on day of surgery.	Omit until eating and drinking normally.

[a]If the patient requires an ongoing variable rate intravenous insulin infusion, then the long-acting background insulin should be continued, but at 80% of the dose the patient usually takes when he or she is well. Normal insulin doses should be recommenced when the patient is eating and drinking normally.
[b]If contrast medium is to be used and eGFR less than 60 ml/min/1.73 m², metformin should be omitted on the day of the procedure and for the following 48 hours.
AM, morning; eGFR, estimated glomerular filtration rate; NPO, nil per os (nothing by mouth); PM, afternoon; VRIII, variable rate intravenous insulin infusion.

higher rate of cardiovascular abnormality, resulting in premature cardiovascular morbidity and mortality when compared to people without diabetic foot disease (13,45,66). Previous work from a multidisciplinary foot clinic in Edinburgh showed that a cohort treated between 1995 and 1999 had a 5-year mortality of 48% (73). The team then instituted a management plan of aggressively addressing cardiovascular risk factors using a combination of statins, antiplatelet agents, angiotensin-converting enzyme inhibitors, and beta-blockade. They then looked at the 5-year mortality for the next 5 years, between 2001 and 2004, and found that they had significantly reduced 5-year mortality to 26.8% (73).

Data from these intervention studies suggest that people with diabetes mellitus with any other additional cardiovascular risk factors should be started on a statin, regardless of their starting cholesterol levels, and should be on an antihypertensive regimen that includes an angiotensin-converting enzyme inhibitor to get their blood pressure to <140/80 mmHg (18). In individuals with proven atherosclerotic disease, for example, previous cardiovascular event (e.g., stroke, acute coronary syndrome) or symptomatic disease (e.g., angina, intermittent claudication, or evidence of compromised peripheral circulation), should also be on an antiplatelet agent. In addition, a cardiology consultation may need to be sought in patients who have diabetic foot disease and electrocardiogram abnormalities (e.g., QTc interval prolongation) because this may be a manifestation of underlying silent coronary heart disease (13). This may need to be done at the time of preoperative assessment, or in the case of emergency admission, prior to any planned surgical procedure, if feasible.

Renal Disease

Chronic kidney disease is also common, and the presence of renal disease increases the risk of diabetic foot disease, major amputation, and premature mortality. Data from the United Kingdom suggest that 5-year survival for individuals with diabetes mellitus starting renal replacement therapy is 70% for 18 to 44 year olds, but only 48% for individuals in the 45 to 64 years age group (63). There is also a strong temporal relationship between starting renal replacement therapy and the development of diabetes mellitus–related foot disease (19). Once again, managing the kidney disease starts in the diabetes mellitus clinic, with multiple risk factor intervention, aggressively managing the glycemic control, the blood pressure, and the lipids. Once the chronic kidney disease is established, then the object would be to prevent progression. However, during an acute hospital admission secondarily to sepsis, the use of intravenous contrast for imaging studies, or potentially nephrotoxic antibiotics and other drugs, could significantly worsen renal function, and therefore, early assessment by the renal team would be valuable.

Anticoagulation

Lower limb surgery is associated with an increased risk of postoperative venous thromboembolic disease, in particular if there has been a history of previous deep vein thrombosis or pulmonary embolism. Several studies from general orthopaedic patients have reported that the use of low molecular weight heparin reduces the incidence for deep vein thrombosis but not pulmonary embolism, with no increase in major bleeding (30,33,37). For patients already on warfarin, coumarin or other oral anticoagulants, local policies should be followed for elective surgery. This would usually involve stopping the anticoagulant several days in advance of the surgery. If continuous anticoagulation is required (e.g., for a prosthetic heart value), the use of low-dose low molecular weight heparin or an intravenous infusion of unfractionated heparin may be necessary.

The need for bridging anticoagulation in patients with atrial fibrillation, however, has recently been questioned (10). When necessary, hematology consultation should be sought.

Conclusion

In summary, diabetes mellitus–related foot disease is often a manifestation of longstanding macro-and microvascular disease occurring in particular as a result of poor glycemic control, hypertension, and dyslipidemia. Aggressive management of these cardiovascular risk factors should have been started at the time of diagnosis of diabetes mellitus, but if they had not been, they should be initiated at the initial presentation to foot clinic. Aggressive risk factor management has been shown to reduce the risk of premature mortality that patients with diabetes mellitus are subject to.

For patients undergoing elective foot surgery, the key for the patient's successful outcome is good communication at all stages of the patient's surgical journey. Good planning of medications used to treat the diabetes mellitus helps to avoid unnecessary admission and iatrogenic harm and to prevent prolonged length of hospital stay. With the increasing prevalence of diabetes mellitus across the world, the numbers of patients developing complications and being admitted to the hospital will also inevitably rise; thus, educating everyone who cares for patients with diabetes mellitus should remain a priority for all health care systems.

References

1. Alserius T, Anderson RE, Hammar N, et al. Elevated glycosylated haemoglobin (HbA$_{1c}$) is a risk marker in coronary artery bypass surgery. Scand Cardiovasc J 2008;42:392–398.
2. Ambiru S, Kato A, Kimura F, et al. Poor postoperative blood glucose control increases surgical site infections after surgery for hepato-biliary-pancreatic cancer: a prospective study in a high-volume institute in Japan. J Hosp Infect 2008;68:230–233.
3. Borrill C, Shapiro D, Garrod S, et al. Team working and effectiveness in health care. Aston Centre for Health Service Organization Research. Available at: http://www.itslifejimbutnotasweknowit.org.uk/files/Team_effectiveness.pdf. Published 2001. Accessed July 26, 2017.
4. Chuang SC, Lee KT, Chang WT, et al. Risk factors for wound infection after cholecystectomy. J Formos Med Assoc 2004;103:607–612.
5. Cullinane M, Gray AJ, Hargraves CM, et al. Who operates when? II. The 2003 report of the National Confidential Enquiry into Perioperative Deaths. Available at: https://www.ncepod.org.uk/2003report/Downloads/03intro.pdf. Published November 20, 2003. Accessed July 26, 2017.
6. Cuthbertson BH, Amiri AR, Croal BL, et al. Utility of B-type natriuretic peptide in predicting medium-term mortality in patients undergoing major non-cardiac surgery. Am J Cardiol 2007;100:1310–1313.
7. Department of Health. National Service Framework for Diabetes. Available at: http://webarchive.nationalarchives.gov.uk/+/http://www.dh.gov.uk/en/Publicationsandstatistics/Publications/PublicationsPolicyAndGuidance/Browsable/DH_4096591. Published 2003. Accessed July 26, 2017.

8. Dhatariya K. Should inpatient hyperglycaemia be treated? BMJ 2013;346:f134.

9. Dhatariya K, Levy N, Kilvert A, et al. NHS diabetes guideline for the perioperative management of the adult patient with diabetes. Diabet Med 2012;29:420–433.

10. Douketis JD, Spyropoulos AC, Kaatz S, et al. Perioperative bridging anticoagulation in patients with atrial fibrillation. N Eng J Med 2015;373:823–833.

11. Dungan KM, Braithwaite SS, Preiser JC. Stress hyperglycaemia. Lancet 2009;373:1798–1807.

12. Dunning T. Care of people with diabetes: a manual of nursing practice. 2nd ed. Oxford (United Kingdom): Blackwell Publishing, 2003.

13. Fagher K, Löndahl M. The impact of metabolic control and QTc prolongation on all-cause mortality in patients with type 2 diabetes and foot ulcers. Diabetologia 2013;56:1140–1147.

14. Fagher K, Nilsson A, Löndahl M. Heart rate-corrected QT interval prolongation as a prognostic marker for 3-year survival in people with type 2 diabetes undergoing above-ankle amputation. Diabetic Med 2015;32(5):679–685.

15. Flanagan D, Ellis J, Baggott A, et al. Diabetes management of elective hospital admissions. Diabet Med 2010;27:1289–1294.

16. Frisch A, Chandra P, Smiley D, et al. Prevalence and clinical outcome of hyperglycemia in the perioperative period in noncardiac surgery. Diabetes Care 2010;33:1783–1788.

17. Furnary AP, Zerr KJ, Grunkemeier GL, et al. Continuous intravenous insulin infusion reduces the incidence of deep sternal wound infection in diabetic patients after cardiac surgical procedures. Ann Thorac Surg 1999;67:352–362.

18. Gaede P, Lund-Andersen H, Parving HH, et al. Effect of a multifactorial intervention on mortality in type 2 diabetes. N Eng J Med 2008;358:580–591.

19. Game FL, Chipchase SY, Hubbard R, et al. Temporal association between the incidence of foot ulceration and the start of dialysis in diabetes mellitus. Nephrol Dial Transplant 2006;21:3207–3210.

20. Gandhi GY, Nuttall GA, Abel MD, et al. Intensive intraoperative insulin therapy versus conventional glucose management during cardiac surgery: a randomized trial. Ann Intern Med 2007;146:233–243.

21. George JT, Warriner D, McGrane DJ, et al. Lack of confidence among trainee doctors in the management of diabetes: the Trainees Own Perception of Delivery of Care (TOPDOC) Diabetes Study. QJM 2011;104:761–766.

22. Gordois A, Scuffham P, Shearer A, et al. The health care costs of diabetic peripheral neuropathy in the US. Diabetes Care 2003;26:1790–1795.

23. Gustafsson UO, Thorell A, Soop M, et al. Haemoglobin A1c as a predictor of postoperative hyperglycaemia and complications after major colorectal surgery. Br J Surg 2009;96:1358–1364.

24. Halkos ME, Lattouf OM, Puskas JD, et al. Elevated preoperative hemoglobin A1c level is associated with reduced long-term survival after coronary artery bypass surgery. Ann Thorac Surg 2008;86:1431–1437.

25. Health and Social Care Information Centre. Prescribing for diabetes, England - 2005/06 to 2014/15. Available at: http://content.digital.nhs.uk/catalogue/PUB18032. Published August 12, 2015. Accessed July 26, 2017.

26. Holman N, Hillson R, Young RJ. Excess mortality during hospital stays among patients with recorded diabetes compared with those without diabetes. Diabet Med 2013;30(12):1393–1402.

27. Holman RR, Paul SK, Bethel MA, et al. 10-Year follow-up of intensive glucose control in type 2 diabetes. N Eng J Med 2008;359:1577–1589.

28. Hsia E, Seggelke S, Gibbs J, et al. Subcutaneous administration of glargine to diabetic patients receiving insulin infusion prevents rebound hyperglycemia. J Clin Endocrinol Metab 2012;97:3132–3137.

29. International Diabetes Federation. IDF diabetes atlas. 7th ed. Available at http://www.idf.org/diabetesatlas. Published 2015. Accessed July 26, 2017.

30. Jørgensen PS, Warming T, Hansen K, et al. Low molecular weight heparin (Innohep) as thromboprophylaxis in outpatients with a plaster cast: a venografic controlled study. Thromb Res 2002;105:477–480.

31. Kerr M. Diabetic foot care in England: An economic study. Available at: https://www.diabetes.org.uk/Upload/Shared practice/Diabetic footcare in England, An economic case study (January 2017).pdf. Published January 2017. Accessed July 26, 2017.

32. Kerr M. Inpatient care for people with diabetes: the economic case for change. Available at: https://www.diabetes.org.uk/upload/News/Inpatient Care for People with Diabetes The Economic Case for Change Nov 2011.pdf. Published November 2011. Accessed July 26, 2017.

33. Kock HJ, Schmit-Neuerburg KP, Hanke J, et al. Thromboprophylaxis with low-molecular-weight heparin in outpatients with plaster-cast immobilisation of the leg. Lancet 1995;346:459–461.

34. Kreutziger J, Schlaepfer J, Wenzel V, et al. The role of admission blood glucose in outcome prediction of surviving patients with multiple injuries. J Trauma 2009;67:704–708.

35. Krishnan S, Nash F, Baker N, et al. Reduction in diabetic amputations over 11 years in a defined U.K. population: benefits of multidisciplinary team work and continuous prospective audit. Diabetes Care 2008;31:99–101.

36. Kristensen SD, Knuuti J, Saraste A, et al. 2014 ESC/ESA guidelines on non-cardiac surgery: cardiovascular assessment and management: the Joint Task Force on non-cardiac surgery: cardiovascular assessment and management of the European Society of Cardiology (ESC) and the European Society of Anaesthesiology (ESA). Eur J Anaesthesiol 2014;31:517–573.

37. Kujath P, Spannagel U, Habscheid W. Incidence and prophylaxis of deep venous thrombosis in outpatients with injury of the lower limb. Haemostasis 1993;23(suppl 1):20–26.

38. Kumar R, McKinney WP, Raj G, et al. Adverse cardiac events after surgery: assessing risk in a veteran population. J Gen Intern Med 2001;16:507–518.

39. Kwon S, Thompson R, Dellinger P, et al. Importance of perioperative glycemic control in general surgery: a report from the Surgical Care and Outcomes Assessment Program. Ann Surg 2013;257:8–14.

40. Lee TH, Marcantonia ER, Mangione EJ, et al. Derivation and prospective validation of a simple index for prediction of cardiac risk of major noncardiac surgery. Circulation 1999;100:1043–1049.

41. Levetan CS, Passaro M, Jablonski K, et al. Unrecognized diabetes among hospitalized patients. Diabetes Care 1998;21:246–249.

42. Modi A, Levy N, Lipp A. A national survey on the perioperative management of diabetes in day case surgery units. J One Day Surg 2012;22(3 suppl):P15.

43. Moghissi ES, Korytkowski MT, DiNardo MM, et al. American Association of Clinical Endocrinologists and American Diabetes Association consensus statement on inpatient glycemic control. Diabetes Care 2009;32:1119–1131.

44. Monnier L, Mas E, Ginet C, et al. Activation of oxidative stress by acute glucose fluctuations compared with sustained chronic hyperglycemia in patients with type 2 diabetes. JAMA 2006;295: 1681–1687.

45. Moulik PK, Mtonga R, Gill GV. Amputation and mortality in new-onset diabetic foot ulcers stratified by etiology. Diabetes Care 2003;26:491–494.

46. Nathan DM, Cleary PA, Backlund JY, et al. Intensive diabetes treatment and cardiovascular disease in patients with type 1 diabetes. N Eng J Med 2005;353:2643–2653.

47. National Institute for Clinical and Healthcare Excellence. Diabetic foot problems: prevention and management. Available at: http://www.nice.org.uk/guidance/ng19. Published January 2016. Accessed July 26, 2017.

48. National Institute for Clinical and Healthcare Excellence. Type 2 diabetes in adults: management (NG 28). Available at: http://www.nice.org.uk/guidance/cg87/resources/guidance -type-2-diabetes-pdf. Published May 2017. Accessed July 26, 2017.

49. Nettles AT. Patient education in the hospital. Diabetes Spectr 2005;18:44–48.

50. NHS Digital. National Diabetes Inpatient Audit (NaDIA) - 2016. Available at: http://www.content.digital.nhs.uk/catalogue/PUB23539. Published March 8, 2017. Accessed July 26, 2017.

51. NICE-SUGAR Study Investigators. Hypoglycemia and risk of death in critically ill patients. N Eng J Med 2012;367:1108–1118.

52. NICE-SUGAR Study Investigators. Intensive versus conventional glucose control in critically ill patients. N Eng J Med 2009;360:1283–1297.

53. O'Brien MM, Gonzales R, Shroyer AL, et al. Modest serum creatinine elevation affects adverse outcome after general surgery. Kidney Int 2002;62:585–592.

54. O'Sullivan CJ, Hynes N, Mahendran B, et al. Haemoglobin A1c (HbA1C) in non-diabetic and diabetic vascular patients. Is HbA1C an independent risk factor and predictor of adverse outcome? Eur J Vasc Endovasc Surg 2006;32:188–197.

55. Rollins KE, Varadhan KK, Dhatariya K, et al. Systematic review of the impact of HbA1c on outcomes following surgery in patients with diabetes mellitus. Clin Nutr 2016;35(2):308–316.

56. Rosenblatt SI, Dukatz T, Jahn R, et al. Insulin glargine dosing before next-day surgery: comparing three strategies. J Clin Anesth 2012;24:610–617.

57. Rubio JA, Aragón-Sánchez J, Jiménez S, et al. Reducing major lower extremity amputations after the introduction of a multidisciplinary team for the diabetic foot. Int J Low Extrem Wounds 2014;13:22–26.

58. Sampson MJ, Brennan C, Dhatariya K, et al. A national survey of in-patient diabetes services in the United Kingdom. Diabet Med 2007;24:643–649.

59. Sampson MJ, Dozio N, Ferguson B, et al. Total and excess bed occupancy by age, speciality and insulin use for nearly one million diabetes patients discharged from all English acute hospitals. Diabetes Res Clin Pract 2007;77:92–98.

60. Sato H, Carvalho G, Sato T, et al. The association of preoperative glycemic control, intraoperative insulin sensitivity, and outcomes after cardiac surgery. J Clin Endocrinol Metab 2010;95: 4338–4344.

61. Shibuya N, Humphers JM, Fluhman BL, et al. Factors associated with nonunion, delayed union, and malunion in foot and ankle surgery in diabetic patients. J Foot Ankle Surg 2013;52:207–211.

62. Stamler J, Vaccaro O, Neaton JD, et al. Diabetes, other risk factors, and 12-yr cardiovascular mortality for men screened in the Multiple Risk Factor Intervention Trial. Diabetes Care 1993;16:434–444.

63. Steenkamp R, Sham C, Feest T. UK Renal Registry 15th Annual Report: chapter 5 survival and causes of death of UK adult patients on renal replacement therapy in 2011: national and centre-specific analyses. Available at: https://www.renalreg.org /wp-content/uploads/2014/09/Chapter_5.pdf. Published 2012. Accessed July 26, 2017.

64. Umpierrez GE, Smiley D, Jacobs S, et al. Randomized study of basal-bolus insulin therapy in the inpatient management of patients with type 2 diabetes undergoing general surgery (RABBIT 2 Surgery). Diabetes Care 2011;34:256–261.

65. Underwood P, Askari R, Hurwitz S, et al. Preoperative A1C and clinical outcomes in patients with diabetes undergoing major noncardiac surgical procedures. Diabetes Care 2014;37:611–616.

66. van Baal J, Hubbard R, Game F, et al. Mortality associated with acute Charcot foot and neuropathic foot ulceration. Diabetes Care 2010;33:1086–1089.

67. van den Berghe G, Wouters P, Weekers F, et al. Intensive insulin therapy in critically ill patients. N Eng J Med 2001;345:1359–1367.

68. Veglio M, Chinaglia A, Cavallo-Perin P. QT interval, cardiovascular risk factors and risk of death in diabetes. J Endocrinol Invest 2004;27:175–181.

69. Vilar-Compte D, Alvarez de Iturbe I, Martín-Onraet A, et al. Hyperglycemia as a risk factor for surgical site infections in patients undergoing mastectomy. Am J Infect Control 2008;36:192–198.

70. Walid MS, Newman BF, Yelverton JC, et al. Prevalence of previously unknown elevation of glycosylated hemoglobin in spine surgery patients and impact on length of stay and total cost. J Hosp Med 2010;5:E10–E14.

71. Wexler DJ, Meigs JB, Cagliero E, et al. Prevalence of hyper- and hypoglycemia among inpatients with diabetes: a national survey of 44 U.S. hospitals. Diabetes Care 2007;30:367–369.

72. Wukich DK, Armstrong DG, Attinger CE, et al. Inpatient management of diabetic foot disorders: a clinical guide. Diabetes Care 2013;36:2862–2871.

73. Young MJ, McCardle JE, Randall LE, et al. Improved survival of diabetic foot ulcer patients 1995-2008: possible impact of aggressive cardiovascular risk management. Diabetes Care 2008;31: 2143–2147.

CHAPTER 2

Medical Imaging for Diabetic Foot Infections and Charcot Neuroarthropathy

William B. Morrison

INTRODUCTION

Diagnosis of neuropathic osteoarthropathy and diabetic pedal infection can be challenging. Radiologic examinations can improve patient care if applied appropriately early in the disease process. However, misdiagnosis or delayed diagnosis can lead to poor outcomes. This chapter discusses the advantages and disadvantages of imaging modalities, the imaging appearance of Charcot neuroarthropathy (CN) and pedal infection, as well as complicating factors and pitfalls.

PATHOETIOLOGY AND RELEVANCE TO IMAGING EXAMS

Although hematogenous spread is the most common cause of osteomyelitis in most other areas of the body, contiguous spread and direct implantation is the most common route for osteomyelitis in the foot and ankle (15). Direct implantation can occur from puncture wounds or deep lacerations, open fractures, and surgery or injection procedures. The vast majority of osteomyelitis involving the foot and ankle in diabetic patients, however, occurs through contiguous spread from adjacent ulceration and subsequent soft tissue infection (4,5,6,13,15). This concept is important when interpreting imaging exams, especially when a bone marrow finding is present and infection is questioned. If a marrow finding is adjacent to an ulcer, it is more likely to represent bone infection, whereas a marrow finding without associated ulceration may be related to fracture, CN, or other conditions.

Sensory neuropathy in diabetic patients leads to diminished perception of minor foot trauma, including cuts, ulcers, blisters, friction-related skin breakdown, tendon and ligament injury, joint injury, and fractures (5,6,13). This can result in CN, and the imaging findings mirror its underlying nature as an aggressive, deforming degenerative arthritis. Collapse of the longitudinal arch results in a rocker bottom deformity of the foot with plantar callus formation and ulceration. Peripheral neuropathy causes diffuse muscle atrophy and imbalance that contributes to the CN deformity. Autonomic dysfunction also occurs and, when combined with vascular fragility, ischemia, and reduced muscular activity, results in deposition of fluid in the soft tissues. On magnetic resonance imaging (MRI), it is common to observe diffuse soft tissue edema and muscle atrophy reflecting this pathology. Meanwhile, unrecognized fractures can induce a tremendous hyperemic response with swelling and erythema simulating infection.

Atherosclerotic disease associated with diabetes mellitus results in baseline ischemia, creating a setting in which cuts or other minor injuries heal poorly and calluses tend to undergo ulceration. Diabetic immunopathy, coupled with vascular disease and diminished sensation, leads to multiorganism wound infection (8,10,17,18). If not treated, infected ulcers lead to soft tissue abscess formation, sinus tracts, septic tenosynovitis, and eventually septic arthritis and osteomyelitis. The extent of spread of infection in the bone and soft tissues is best evaluated using MRI (2,7). More advanced ischemia may cause gangrene, particularly at the toes and forefoot. Severe chronic ischemia may result in bone marrow infarction. Imaging modalities depending on vascular flow (i.e., nuclear medicine exams) are potentially limited in this setting and can result in false-negative results (9,16). Each imaging modality has advantages and disadvantages; it is very helpful for the practitioner caring for diabetic patients to know the basics of each and optimal utilization (Table 2.1).

RADIOGRAPHY

For patients with clinical suspicion of pedal infection, radiographs are the most appropriate screening examination (2). Although most findings associated with infection are nonspecific and others are not observed in the early stages, ease of availability and low expense make radiography an excellent test for initial evaluation. Early infection is seen as soft tissue swelling; skin ulceration is common, with interruption

TABLE 2.1	Advantages and Disadvantages of Imaging Modalities		
Modality	Advantages	Disadvantages	Comments
Radiography	Inexpensive; widely available	Poor sensitivity	Initial study
Computed Tomography	Tarsal anatomy; fractures	Limited bone marrow evaluation; poor sensitivity	Limited utility in diabetic pedal disease
Ultrasound	Problem solving; identification of fluid collections, tendon pathology	Limited visualization of anatomy; bones	Best reserved for answering specific questions regarding soft tissue pathology
Magnetic Resonance Imaging	Best depiction of anatomy, extent of disease; highly sensitive and specific	Expensive; contraindicated in patients with some implanted devices such as pacemakers	Best overall test for evaluation of infection and Charcot neuroarthropathy
Nuclear Medicine	High sensitivity for infection	Limited sensitivity in setting of vascular disease; poor anatomic definition	Best reserved for patients who cannot undergo magnetic resonance imaging

of the skin margin that may be apparent if imaged tangential to the ulcer. Soft tissue air or gas may be present, characterized by foci of soft tissue lucency, typically adjacent to a skin ulcer (Fig. 2.1). This may represent communication of open air through an ulcer, or gangrenous transformation superinfected with a gas-forming organism. Septic arthritis is characterized in the early stages by a joint effusion which may be difficult to identify. Joint effusion presents in the interphalangeal joints as fusiform swelling. In later stages, septic arthritis can be indistinguishable from other inflammatory arthropathies such as rheumatoid arthritis and gout, with marginal erosions and diffuse joint space narrowing. Early osteomyelitis present with focal rarefaction, or decreased density of bone, followed by periostitis and erosion leading to bone destruction. Findings in osteomyelitis can be delayed as much as 2 weeks after infection is established; sensitivity of radiographs is well known to be poor. Therefore, whether negative or positive, additional imaging is often necessary. Despite these limitations, the overview of anatomy makes radiography excellent for follow-up; evaluation

of postoperative changes; identification of soft tissue calcification, gas, and foreign bodies; and characterization of the pattern and distribution of arthritis, including CN.

COMPUTED TOMOGRAPHY

Computed tomography (CT) provides similar information as radiographs but with cross-sectional and reconstruction capabilities (Fig. 2.2). If intravenous contrast medium is administered, soft tissue enhancement reflecting cellulitis and rim-enhancing fluid collections indicating abscess formation can be detected. In early osteomyelitis, periostitis and rarefaction of bone will be seen. Eventually, frank bone destruction ensues. Effusion, joint space narrowing, and marginal erosions indicate septic arthritis; cross-sectional capabilities of CT make detection of these findings easier. However, the capability of CT in determining the extent of infection is poor. Therefore, use of CT as a clinical tool is limited in the algorithm for diabetic pedal disease. However, if anatomic information

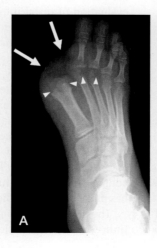 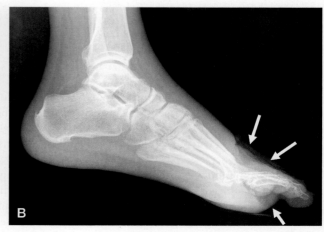

FIGURE 2.1 Radiographic findings associated with pedal infection. Oblique **(A)** and lateral **(B)** radiographic views of the foot in a patient with prior great toe amputation show soft tissue swelling and a defect *(arrows)* representing plantar and dorsal ulceration. Bone erosion is present at the residual first metatarsal head as well as the second and third metatarsophalangeal joints *(arrowheads)* consistent with osteomyelitis and septic arthritis.

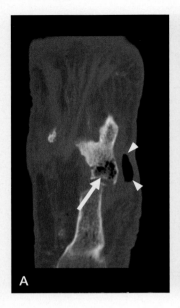
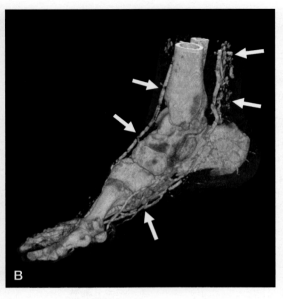

FIGURE 2.2 Computed tomography (CT) findings of infection of the foot. **A.** Axial CT image of the foot in a patient with osteomyelitis shows gas in the lateral subcutaneous tissues *(arrowheads)* adjacent to an ulcer (not pictured); frank bone destruction is present with gas in the medullary space *(arrow)*. **B.** CT provides three-dimensional (3D) information and can be reconstructed in any plane or reformatted to show surface rendering of the bony architecture for surgical planning. Linear densities *(arrows)* represent calcified blood vessels.

specific to bone architecture is needed, CT may be useful; for example, CT can be used for characterization of deformities related to CN and associated fractures.

ULTRASONOGRAPHY

Ultrasound offers excellent depiction of soft tissue anatomic detail and can be useful for answering specific questions, such as whether there is a fluid collection in the subcutaneous tissues (Fig. 2.3). Abscesses and effusions are seen as focal regions of hypoechogenicity often with complex internal characteristics. Joint effusions and tendon sheath fluid can be detected, but these findings are common and nonspecific for infection. Power Doppler can demonstrate hyperemia of the synovium and surrounding tissues, suggestive of inflammation. Although ultrasonography cannot visualize the marrow compartment, a focused examination can demonstrate cortical breakthrough and periosteal elevation. Owing to availability of other modalities that offer a more comprehensive evaluation, use of ultrasonography for pedal infection is limited to problem solving, that is, identification of a suspected abscess.

NUCLEAR MEDICINE VERSUS MAGNETIC RESONANCE IMAGING

The relative utility of bone scintigraphy and MRI for evaluation of diabetic pedal disease is a controversial topic in the literature (9,11,12,16,19,20,24). Both modalities are excellent for diagnosis of osteomyelitis, and both have limitations. Three-phase bone scintigraphy is sensitive for osseous involvement but exhibits lower specificity in complicated settings such as neuropathic disease, trauma, and postoperative conditions. Labeled white blood cell imaging lacks anatomic detail, but correlation with three-phase bone scintigraphy increases

specificity (12). However, this involves acquiring 2 exams over a period of days; in addition, ischemia is commonly present in the diabetic population and can prevent radiotracer uptake leading to a false-negative exam (9).

MRI provides excellent anatomic depiction of disease and is highly sensitive for the diagnosis of osteomyelitis (Fig. 2.4). Unlike scintigraphic methods, MRI enables a detailed evaluation of anatomy and soft tissue pathology, visualizing ulcers, sinus tracts, abscesses, as well as extent of disease (7,19,22,23) (Fig. 2.5). MRI can also help characterize neuropathic disease (1,21). Tissue characterization and global multiplanar capability have made MRI the test of choice in most situations, unless the patient has a contraindication (2). MRI is especially useful as a surgical planning tool to determine the extent of soft tissue and bone pathology and to characterize soft tissue structures involved by infection and necrosis (14,16).

Nuclear Medicine

Three-phase bone scintigraphy and labeled leukocyte imaging are the most commonly performed radionuclide tests in the evaluation of pedal infection (20). Although the three-phase bone scan is sensitive for detecting osteomyelitis, many conditions in the diabetic foot demonstrate focal hyperemia and increased bone turnover resulting in uptake mimicking infection; consequently, specificity is low (9). When there is no increased uptake, the test is excellent for excluding the presence of osteomyelitis, except in the setting of severe vascular disease; radiotracer may not collect in the ischemic tissues. Labeled white blood cell examination has higher specificity but lower resolution; it can be difficult to differentiate bone and soft tissue uptake. Therefore, it is generally interpreted in conjunction with the three-phase bone scan, comparing areas of uptake on the 2 studies (Fig. 2.6).

The uptake in three-phase bone scintigraphy using technetium-99m (^{99m}Tc)-labeled methylene diphosphonate is related

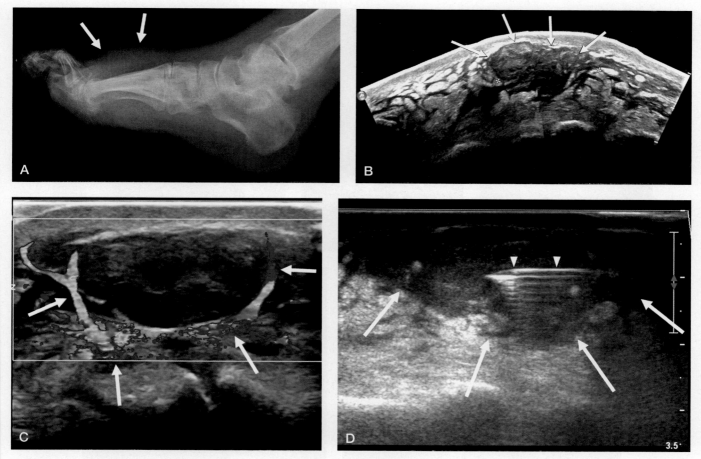

FIGURE 2.3 Ultrasound evaluation of soft tissue infection. **A.** Lateral radiograph of the foot in a diabetic patient shows soft tissue swelling *(arrows)* at the dorsal aspect of the forefoot. Transverse sonographic image of this region **(B)** demonstrates a focal region of heterogeneous, complex hypoechogenic fluid *(arrows)* with power Doppler image **(C)** showing increased blood flow *(arrows)* representing surrounding hyperemia, consistent with an abscess. Ultrasound can be useful for problem solving, identifying soft tissue findings such as abscesses as well as septic arthritis and tenosynovitis. This modality is also useful as a guidance tool for aspiration **(D)**; *arrowheads* show needle entering abscess *(arrows)*.

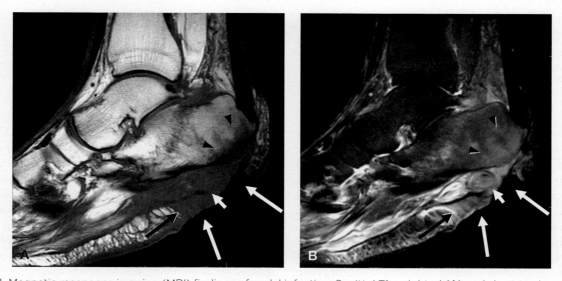

FIGURE 2.4 Magnetic resonance imaging (MRI) findings of pedal infection. Sagittal T1-weighted **(A)** and short tau inversion recovery (STIR) **(B)** images of the ankle show ulceration at the heel *(long white arrows)* with surrounding cellulitis, seen as replacement of the normal subcutaneous fat signal on T1-weighted images and edema on fluid sensitive images *(black arrows)*. Signal abnormality is seen in the adjacent calcaneus *(arrowheads)*, confirming presence of osteomyelitis. Note involvement of the plantar fascia with disruption at the origin *(short white arrow)*.

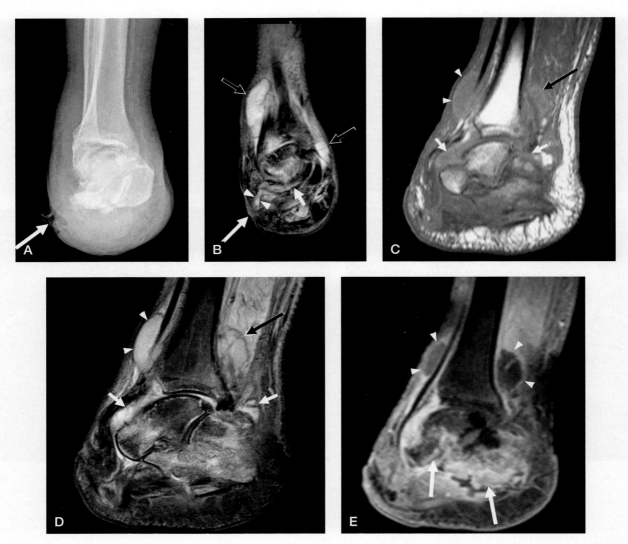

FIGURE 2.5 Extent of infection demonstrated on magnetic resonance imaging (MRI). A diabetic patient with prior amputation at the hindfoot presented with a draining ulcer. **A.** Anteroposterior radiograph of the ankle shows diffuse soft tissue swelling with ulceration at the lateral aspect *(arrow)*. MRI **(B–D)** was acquired. Coronal T2-weighted fat suppressed image **(B)** shows fluid within a sinus tract *(arrowheads)* connecting the subtalar joint *(short arrow)* and the ulcer *(long arrow)*. Note fluid collections in the lower leg *(black arrows)*. Sagittal T1-weighted **(C)** and short tau inversion recovery (STIR) **(D)** images show ankle and subtalar joint effusions *(short arrows)* representing septic arthritis with marrow abnormalities throughout the ankle and hindfoot representing osteomyelitis. Note a fluid collection surrounding the anterior tibialis tendon *(arrowheads)* consistent with septic tenosynovitis and a complex collection in the posterior soft tissues *(long arrow)* representing abscess formation. **E.** A postcontrast sagittal image shows rim enhancement of the collections *(arrowheads)* as well as the infected talus and calcaneus *(arrows)*.

to blood flow and osteoblastic activity. Localized bone uptake on the delayed third phase is nonspecific, but if all 3 phases are positive with clinical suspicion of infection, the test is highly sensitive for diagnosis of osteomyelitis. Cellulitis, abscess, and other soft tissue infections show increased uptake on the initial blood flow and second blood pool phases that fails to concentrate in bone on the third phase. Occasionally, and especially in ischemic feet, there is persistent blood pool activity; ischemia can be suspected if there is poorly defined tracer distribution. Residual bony uptake on a delayed fourth phase, acquired after 24 hours, can help distinguish osteomyelitis from overlying cellulitis in this situation. In addition to ischemia, chronic osteomyelitis or partially treated infection

may not show characteristic uptake on the first 2 phases, resulting in a false-negative examination. Persistent radiotracer uptake may be seen with treated osteomyelitis, resulting in a false-positive exam. Bone turnover and hyperemia caused by CN, trauma, recent surgery, or inflammatory arthropathy can also appear similar to infection. Specificity is lower as a result of vascular insufficiency and complicating CN. In the setting of underlying complicating conditions, where there is nonspecific uptake on the delayed phase, corresponding uptake on a labeled white blood cell scan increases specificity.

White blood cell scanning is based on migration of leukocytes labeled with radiotracer into infected tissue; reported sensitivity and specificity ranges from 75% to 100%

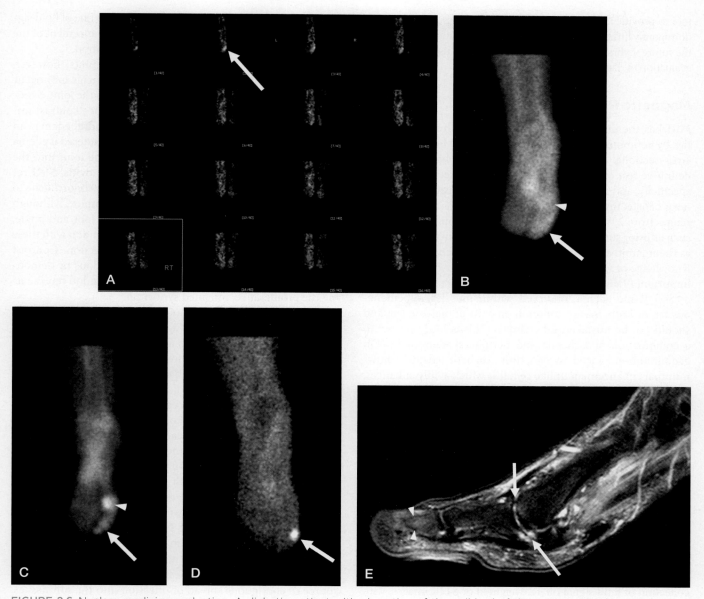

FIGURE 2.6 Nuclear medicine evaluation. A diabetic patient with ulceration of the nail bed of the great toe underwent a three-phase bone scan using technetium-99m (^{99m}Tc)-labeled methyl diphosphonate **(A–C)**. Initial vascular phase **(A)** shows rapid uptake in the toe *(arrow)*. There is concentration of radiotracer in the distal toe *(arrow)* as well as the metatarsophalangeal joint region *(arrowhead)* on blood pool phase **(B)** and delayed phase **(C)**. **D.** A ^{99m}Tc Ceretec–labeled white blood cell scan shows uptake exclusively in the distal toe *(arrow)* representing osteomyelitis in this location only. Subsequent magnetic resonance imaging (MRI) shows the reason for uptake on bone scan in the metatarsophalangeal joint: Sagittal short tau inversion recovery (STIR) image **(E)** shows osteoarthritis of the metatarsophalangeal joint *(arrows)* with marrow edema in the distal phalanx *(arrowheads)* representing osteomyelitis as suggested on the ^{99m}Tc Ceretec–labeled white blood cell scan.

and 69% to 100%, respectively. Combined with three-phase bone scintigraphy, specificity increases to 90% to 100% (20). Focal uptake in the foot, without appreciable amounts of red marrow, is generally indicative of infection. As mentioned earlier, low resolution can make it difficult to separate soft tissue from bone infection. An identical pattern of uptake on a delayed three-phase bone scan can establish the diagnosis of osteomyelitis. False negatives may be seen with prior antibiotic treatment and ischemia. Noninfectious inflammatory conditions such as rheumatoid arthritis and hyperemic

conditions such as acute neuropathic disease can occasionally show increased leukocyte accumulation, resulting in a false-positive exam (9).

18F-fluorodeoxyglucose (18F-FDG) positron emission tomography (PET) combined with CT (PET/CT) has shown promise for imaging infection, related to increased metabolism of glucose in areas of inflammation. Co-registration of anatomic and metabolic information makes PET/CT an attractive option. However, to date, limited data exist to test its efficacy in the diabetic foot. Hybridization of PET with MRI (PET/MRI) is emerging as a new tool to provide important diagnostic information, with data predominantly limited as of yet, to oncologic applications. Perhaps, in the future, hybridization techniques may play a useful role in the evaluation of diabetic foot infection.

Magnetic Resonance Imaging

MRI has the distinct advantage over other imaging modalities by combining tissue characterization and high-resolution cross-sectional capabilities (7). Therefore, it has become the definitive test of choice, offering a high degree of sensitivity, specificity, and anatomic information (2). Sensitivity for diagnosis of osteomyelitis ranges from 77% to 100%, and specificity ranges from 79% to 100%. Superimposed complicating factors such as prior surgery, CN, or other inflammatory disease, such as rheumatoid arthritis, may lower the specificity of MRI (19). Knowledge of various MRI findings and their implications is important (Table 2.2).

Soft tissue edema, observed within muscles, subcutaneous fat, or both, is very common on MRI of diabetic feet and should not be mistaken for cellulitis. This is likely related to a combination of ischemia and peripheral neuropathy. On gadolinium-enhanced images, this "diabetic edema" shows minimal enhancement unlike cellulitis which avidly enhances. In advanced diabetes mellitus, the muscles of the foot are typically atrophied, with decreased size and fatty infiltration. The atrophied muscles often appear edematous on T2-weighted images.

On MRI, cellulitis (see Fig. 2.4) is seen as replacement of the normal fat signal in subcutaneous tissues on T1-weighted images, with high signal (although less than fluid) on T2-weighted or short tau inversion recovery (STIR) images (i.e., fluid-sensitive sequences) and diffuse enhancement after contrast administration. The margins are generally poorly defined. Air or gas is seen as small foci of black signal; as mentioned earlier, this can be associated with cellulitis and is particularly common adjacent to ulcers or in devitalized areas. An abscess appears as a focal collection of fluid signal on T2-weighted or STIR images, with thick rim enhancement on postcontrast images (see Fig. 2.5).

Sinus tracts are characterized by a thin, discrete line of fluid signal extending through the soft tissues with enhancement of the hyperemic margins in a "tram-track" configuration.

Joint effusion is usually seen in septic joints; however, when there is communication to the skin, drainage may occur through a sinus tract leaving only trace fluid in the joint. Synovial thickening and enhancement is seen on postcontrast images. Marginal erosions and reactive subchondral edema can also be observed. Osteomyelitis should be considered if edema signal or enhancement extends away from the joint into the medullary bone. In the case of septic tenosynovitis, MRI reveals fluid within the tendon sheath that is disproportionate to that in other sheaths and which is usually complex. Although mechanical tenosynovitis is common in the foot and ankle, septic tenosynovitis should be suspected if a tendon with these findings traverses a region of soft tissue infection. Contrast enhancement may help identify involved tendons by demonstrating thick rim enhancement around the tendon representing the proliferative, inflamed synovium.

Ulcers and skin breaks should be sought on MRI of the foot in diabetic patients (see Figs. 2.4 and 2.5) because this is the main mode of inoculation and spread of infection in this population. The skin signal should be followed on all images, with interruption of the signal suggesting a skin break, a "dip" and skin signal loss indicating an ulcer. Certain areas of the foot and ankle are susceptible to ulceration. These include areas overlying bony prominences such as the medial and lateral malleolus, the calcaneus (especially in bedridden patients), and over the first and fifth metatarsal heads. Foot deformities lead to ulceration in different areas; posterior tibial tendon dysfunction with spring ligament laxity or CN can result in a rocker bottom deformity with collapse of the longitudinal arch; ulceration can then form at the plantar aspect of the midfoot. Diabetic patients can also acquire claw toe deformities with ulceration over the dorsal aspect of the toes. Ulcers may form at the nail beds, arising from friction or cuts from nail clipping. These skin breaks and ulcers are a source of contiguous spread of infection into the soft tissues, joints, and bone. Deep ulceration is especially important to

TABLE 2.2		Common Pathology and Magnetic Resonance Imaging Findings
Pathology	Components	Magnetic Resonance Imaging Findings
Ischemia	Diffuse soft tissue edema	Diffusely increased T2 signal in soft tissues
	Infarction	Sharply defined intraosseous signal abnormality
	Gangrene	Soft tissue loss, low signal, nonenhancement
Neuropathy	Muscle atrophy	Muscle edema on T2, fat replacement on T1
	Ligament tear	Discontinuity; especially plantar extrinsic ligaments of the Lisfranc joint, spring ligament
	Fracture	Linear T1 signal with severe bone marrow edema
	Deformity	Arch collapse on sagittal images; joint subluxation
Infection	Ulceration	Interruption of skin signal
	Cellulitis	Soft tissue low T1 signal; edema on T2, enhancement
	Sinus tract	Linear fluid signal or "tram-track" enhancement
	Abscess	Focal fluid signal with thick rim enhancement
	Septic arthritis	Joint effusion with thick synovial enhancement
	Osteomyelitis	Marrow low on T1, high on T2; enhancement

identify because there is a high association with underlying osteomyelitis. Wound breakdown can also occur in postoperative patients with ischemia.

Osteomyelitis is characterized by alteration of bone marrow signal (see Figs. 2.4 and 2.5), with low signal (replacement of the normal fat signal) on T1-weighted images, high (edema-like) signal on T2-weighted or STIR images, and enhancement on post-gadolinium T1-weighted images. Other MRI findings in cases of osteomyelitis include cortical disruption and periostitis. Periostitis is seen as a linear pattern of edema and enhancement extending along the outer cortical margin.

Recognition of abnormal bone marrow signal in the appropriate clinical setting results in high sensitivity for diagnosis of osteomyelitis. Other entities can mimic this alteration in signal, including fracture, tumor, active inflammatory arthritis or neuropathic disease, infarction, or recent postoperative changes. However, these other processes usually have different morphology than osteomyelitis, and recognition of these patterns often enables differentiation. For example, identification of a fracture line, a discrete lesion, adjacent arthritis, neuropathic disease, or postoperative metal artifact improves specificity. Correlation with radiographs and clinical history is also important. Additionally, osteomyelitis of the foot and ankle is typically the result of contiguous spread through the skin with the majority of cases demonstrating skin ulceration, cellulitis, soft tissue abscess, or a sinus tract. These findings can be thought of as "secondary signs" of osteomyelitis, recognition of which improves specificity.

Regarding use of gadolinium in MRI, some studies recommend intravenous contrast, whereas others believe it to be unnecessary. It remains controversial whether addition of a contrast-enhanced sequence improves the accuracy of MRI for the diagnosis of osteomyelitis. It is generally agreed, however, that contrast enhancement improves detection of soft tissue infection (19). Enhancement differentiates cellulitis from diabetic soft tissue edema and improves evaluation of the extent of soft tissue disease. It helps detect sinus tracts and abscesses, and it is the only way to delineate areas of devitalization or necrosis. Therefore, administration of gadolinium contrast can provide useful information, especially if the patient is being considered for surgical management. Gadolinium-based contrast agents should be administered with caution in patients with renal failure due to the potential risk of nephrogenic systemic fibrosis (3). The American College of Radiology have established guidelines for patients with varying levels of renal failure based on reduced glomerular filtration rates.

Documentation of the presence and extent of ischemic and devitalized areas facilitate surgical planning for débridement and limited, foot-sparing amputations. Precontrast and postcontrast MRI can detect ischemia and devitalization of the foot as focal or regional absence of soft tissue contrast enhancement. Devitalization, or foot "infarction," is seen as a focal area of nonenhancement with a sharp cutoff with increased enhancement in the surrounding reactive, hypervascular tissue. Only contrast-enhanced images allow reliable recognition of gangrenous tissue because T2- and T1-weighted images reveal nonspecific signal alterations.

SPREAD OF INFECTION

In the diabetic foot, infection does not tend to remain confined by fascial planes; instead, it spreads from the inoculation site across fascial compartments, into and across joints, and along tendons (14). Soft tissue involvement is often more extensive than the osseous disease, requiring careful examination of the soft tissues proximal to the source of infection. Tendons and their sheaths are common routes for spread of infection, and spread via this route should be evaluated on cross-sectional imaging studies. Without proper surgical débridement, the patient may fail the foot-sparing procedure and require more extensive amputation. MRI is the test of choice for preoperative evaluation; extent of infection in soft tissue and bone is fairly well delineated, particularly on postcontrast MRI.

CHARCOT NEUROARTHROPATHY: IMAGING FINDINGS AND DIFFERENTIATION FROM INFECTION

Charcot Neuroarthropathy

Acutely, a warm, swollen, erythematous neuropathic foot may clinically mimic infection. Radiographs may demonstrate little or no deformity, with only diffuse soft tissue swelling present (Fig. 2.7). Owing to marked hyperemia, scintigraphic examinations may be falsely positive. Diffuse soft tissue edema will be seen on MRI and joint effusion is common. On postcontrast MRI, the joint capsule and juxtaarticular soft tissues enhance, but the subcutaneous tissues typically show little enhancement. Bone marrow edema and enhancement is typically centered in the subchondral

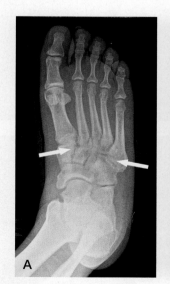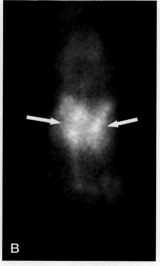

FIGURE 2.7 Early Charcot neuroarthropathy (CN) changes. **A.** An anteroposterior radiograph of the foot shows resorption of the bones around the Lisfranc joint (*arrows*) representing early changes of CN. **B.** Delayed phase of a three-phase bone scan shows intense uptake of radiotracer at the Lisfranc joint and intertarsal joints (*arrows*) compatible with involvement.

bone, reflecting the articular pattern of disease. In more severe cases, prominent edema and enhancement can extend well into the periarticular medullary bone simulating infection. This is especially the case in the setting of neuropathic fracture(s).

MRI can show the anatomic changes associated with this clinical presentation (1,21). Ligament tears are common, especially the spring ligament and the plantar extrinsic ligaments of the midfoot. Interestingly, the Lisfranc ligament tends to be preserved until very late in the disease. At the midfoot, once the plantar capsular ligaments tear, the tarsal bones and metatarsophalangeal joints compress at the dorsal aspect in accordion fashion, resulting in fragmentation of the joint and collapse into the characteristic rocker bottom pattern.

The chronic stage shows more typical imaging characteristics of CN with an overall pattern of disorganization and deformity (Fig. 2.8). Joint deformity with subluxation or dislocation often involves multiple joints. Subchondral cysts and bone proliferation are prominent, with "debris" or intra-articular bodies. Bone density is usually preserved. In later stages of CN, adjacent bones can become necrotic and collapse or resorb. Neuropathic disease of the Lisfranc joint typically results in superolateral subluxation of the metatarsals, leading to a rocker bottom deformity in which the cuboid becomes a weight bearing structure. Imaging findings are characteristic of a chronic, degenerative arthritis, although recurrent episodes of acute disease may result in bone marrow and periarticular edema with enhancement on MRI and uptake on scintigraphic methods.

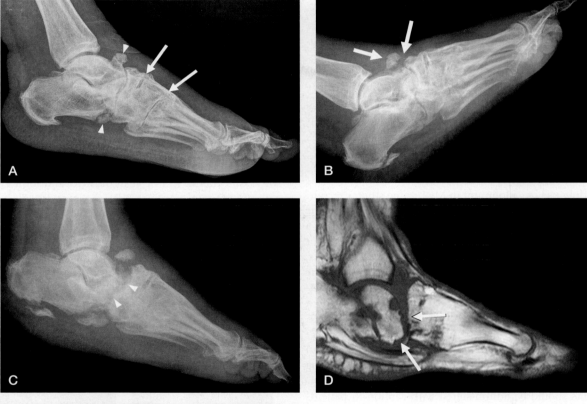

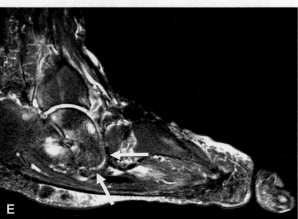

FIGURE 2.8 Late Charcot neuroarthropathy (CN) changes. Progression of CN at the midfoot and hindfoot. **A.** Initial lateral radiograph shows joint space narrowing throughout the intertarsal and tarsometatarsal joints *(arrows)* with early fragmentation at the dorsal and plantar aspects *(arrowheads)*. **B.** Lateral radiograph 2 months later shows soft tissue swelling with increased fragmentation *(arrows)*. **C.** Lateral radiograph an additional 4 months later shows collapse of the hindfoot *(arrowheads)* with dorsal subluxation of the navicular bone relative to the talar head. Fragmentation and soft tissue swelling were further increased. Sagittal T1-weighted **(D)** and short tau inversion recovery (STIR) **(E)** magnetic resonance imaging (MRI) 1-year later shows progressive collapse of the hindfoot with dislocation of the talonavicular joint *(arrows)*.

Differentiation of osteomyelitis and CN can be difficult because both can demonstrate marrow abnormality, joint effusion, and surrounding soft tissue edema. Some rules may be used to help differentiate these entities on MRI. First, the vast majority of cases of osteomyelitis of the foot and ankle are due to contiguous spread. Therefore, a bone marrow abnormality without adjacent skin ulceration, sinus tract, or soft tissue inflammation is less likely to represent infection. This concept is particularly useful when there are extensive bone marrow signal abnormalities and lack of subcutaneous tissue involvement. Second, CN is predominantly an articular process manifesting as instability, often with multiple regional joints involved (e.g., the Lisfranc, Chopart, or multiple adjacent metatarsophalangeal joints). This and other articular manifestations of CN (subluxation, cysts, necrotic debris) are not as common in infection. Associated CN bone marrow changes can be extensive (especially at the midfoot) but tend to be centered equally about a joint and at the subarticular bone. Osteomyelitis shows more diffuse marrow involvement, and unless there is a primary septic arthritis, the marrow changes are generally greater on one side of the joint. Finally, location of disease is important. CN by far is most common at the Lisfranc and Chopart joints. Osteomyelitis occurs predominantly at the metatarsal heads, toes, calcaneus, and malleoli, a distribution that mirrors that of friction, callus, and ulceration. However, contiguous spread of infection can occur at atypical sites if there is a foot deformity (e.g., the cuboid in cases of rocker bottom deformity).

Conclusion

Radiologic examinations play an essential role in diagnosis and management of diabetic patients with pedal disease. The practitioner should maintain up-to-date knowledge regarding advantages and limitations of the different imaging modalities to provide the most efficacious care.

References

1. Ahmadi ME, Morrison WB, Carrino JA, et al. Neuropathic arthropathy of the foot with and without superimposed osteomyelitis: MR imaging characteristics. Radiology 2006;238:622–631.
2. American College of Radiology. ACR appropriateness criteria. Available at: https://acsearch.acr.org/docs/69340/Narrative/. Published 1995. Updated 2012. Accessed February 3, 2016.
3. American College of Radiology Committee on Drugs and Contrast Media. ACR manual on contrast media. Available at: http://www.acr.org/quality-safety/resources/contrast-manual. Published 2015. Accessed February 3, 2016.
4. Baker JC, Demertzis JL, Rhodes NG, et al. Diabetic musculoskeletal complications and their imaging mimics. Radiographics 2012;32:1959–1974.
5. Boulton AJ. The pathway to foot ulceration in diabetes. Med Clin North Am 2013;97:775–790.
6. Chen IW, Yang HM, Chiu CH, et al. Clinical characteristics and risk factor analysis for lower-extremity amputations in diabetic patients with foot ulcer complicated by necrotizing fasciitis. Medicine (Baltimore) 2015;94:e1957.
7. Donovan A, Schweitzer ME. Use of MR imaging in diagnosing diabetes-related pedal osteomyelitis. Radiographics 2010;30:723–736.
8. Game FL. Osteomyelitis in the diabetic foot: diagnosis and management. Med Clin North Am 2013;97:947–956.
9. Glaudemans AW, Israel O, Slart RH. Pitfalls and limitations of radionuclide and hybrid imaging in infection and inflammation. Semin Nucl Med 2015;45:500–512.
10. Hingorani A, LaMuraglia GM, Henke P, et al. The management of diabetic foot: a clinical practice guideline by the Society for Vascular Surgery in collaboration with the American Podiatric Medical Association and the Society for Vascular Medicine. J Vasc Surg 2016;63(2 suppl):3S–21S.
11. Jadvar H, Colletti PM. Competitive advantage of PET/MRI. Eur J Radiol 2014;83:84–94.
12. La Fontaine J, Bhavan K, Lam K, et al. Comparison between Tc-99m WBC SPECT/CT and MRI for the diagnosis of biopsy-proven diabetic foot osteomyelitis. Wounds 2016;28:271–278.
13. Lavery LA, La Fontaine J, Kim PJ. Preventing the first or recurrent ulcers. Med Clin North Am 2013;97:807–820.
14. Ledermann HP, Morrison WB, Schweitzer ME. Is soft-tissue inflammation in pedal infection contained by fascial planes? MR analysis of compartmental involvement in 115 feet. AJR Am J Roentgenol 2002;178:605–612.
15. Ledermann HP, Morrison WB, Schweitzer ME. MR image analysis of pedal osteomyelitis: distribution, patterns of spread, and frequency of associated ulceration and septic arthritis. Radiology 2002;223:747–755.
16. Ledermann HP, Schweitzer ME, Morrison WB. Nonenhancing tissue on MR imaging of pedal infection: characterization of necrotic tissue and associated limitations for diagnosis of osteomyelitis and abscess. AJR Am J Roentgenol 2002;178:215–222.
17. Lipsky BA, Aragón-Sánchez J, Diggle M, et al. IWGDF guidance on the diagnosis and management of foot infections in persons with diabetes. Diabetes Metab Res Rev 2016;32(suppl 1):45–74.
18. Lipsky BA, Berendt AR, Cornia PB, et al. 2012 Infectious Diseases Society of America clinical practice guideline for the diagnosis and treatment of diabetic foot infections. Clin Infect Dis 2012;54:e132–173.
19. Morrison WB, Schweitzer ME, Wapner KL, et al. Osteomyelitis in feet of diabetics: clinical accuracy, surgical utility, and cost-effectiveness of MR imaging. Radiology 1995;196:557–564.
20. Palestro CJ, Love C. Nuclear medicine and diabetic foot infections. Semin Nucl Med 2009;39:52–65.
21. Rogers LC, Frykberg RG, Armstrong DG, et al. The Charcot foot in diabetes. J Am Podiatr Med Assoc 2011;101:437–446.
22. Roug IK, Pierre-Jerome C. MRI spectrum of bone changes in the diabetic foot. Eur J Radiol 2012;81:1625–1629.
23. Toledano TR, Fatone EA, Weis A, et al. MRI evaluation of bone marrow changes in the diabetic foot: a practical approach. Semin Musculoskelet Radiol 2011;15:257–268.
24. Valabhji J, Oliver N, Samarasinghe D, et al. Conservative management of diabetic forefoot ulceration complicated by underlying osteomyelitis: the benefits of magnetic resonance imaging. Diabet Med 2009;26:1127–1134.

CHAPTER 3

Vascular Assessment and Imaging Techniques for Critical Limb Ischemia in Patients with Diabetes Mellitus

Neal R. Barshes

INTRODUCTION

The arterial system delivers oxygen and nutrients to tissue. The arterial circulation of the lower extremity is relevant to those clinicians who manage foot wounds because some minimum level of arterial perfusion is needed for tissue viability and for wound healing. The actual delivery of nutrients to peripheral tissues is difficult to measure in vivo, but the oxygen consumption of oxygen can be estimated by 3 components: (a) amount of blood delivered per unit time (milliliter per minute [mL/min]), (b) oxygen content of blood (milliliter oxygen per liter of blood), and (c) the fraction of oxygen extracted from delivered blood (percentage).

A typical cardiac output for an average-sized man is approximately 5 liter per minute (L/min). The brain receives approximately 10% to 15% of the cardiac output, and the kidneys receive about 20% to 25%. The mean blood flow through the popliteal artery in young, healthy patients at rest is 55 mL/min (22), or approximately 1% of the cardiac output. The amount of oxygen bound to hemoglobin is more than 6,000 higher than that found free in the plasma. As seen in Table 3.1, hemoglobin levels have a relatively higher impact on oxygen content than oxygen saturation. The oxygen extraction fraction of the lower extremity at rest is generally 30% to 45% and may approach 90% or more with activity (23,45). Ischemic limbs can be seen to have lower oxygen partial pressures and lower pH in mixed venous blood than limbs that have undergone revascularization (15). The oxygen consumption of tissues in the foot is much lower than that of other, more active tissue. Myocardium consumes 8 mL O_2/min per 100 mm^3 tissue at rest and 77 mL O_2/min per 100 mm^3 tissue when active. The kidney consumes 5 mL O_2/min per 100 mm^3 tissue. In comparison, gastrocnemius and soleus muscles at rest consume approximately 0.5 mL O_2/min per 100 mm^3 tissue, and skin consumes 0.2 mL O_2/min per 100 mm^3 tissue (25).

WOUND HEALING AND ARTERIAL PERFUSION: THEORETICAL CONCERNS

Wound healing requires anabolic metabolism. Perfusion probably needs to be higher in the setting of wound healing than at steady state. Whole-body caloric requirements increase 20% with mild stress and may increase 60% or more with severe stress or infection (12). It is not known how much regional oxygen/nutrient demand increases with wound healing. Oxygen tension decreases to 50% of normal with bone healing and to 35% of normal with bone healing and infection (2).

Poiseuille law (Fig. 3.1) describes the impact of various variables on flow in the context of nonpulsatile laminar flow. Radius is the major determinant because of the exponential relationship it has with flow; length has an impact as well. When major arteries are occluded, blood flow takes "collateral" pathways to the periphery. As a rule, these collaterals are smaller caliber and increased length (and therefore higher resistance) compared to the primary artery, and this is the reason why blood flow preferentially travels through collateral pathways only when the primary artery is significantly narrowed or occluded. Although the collateral vessels present are numerous, they generally do not provide for as much flow as the primary artery because of their relatively decreased caliber and increased length (Fig. 3.2). Even if making the liberal assumption of collaterals that are 40% of the diameter of the main artery and 30% longer, 51 collaterals of these dimensions would be required to provide the same degree of flow as the primary artery.

$$Q = \frac{\pi \cdot R^4 \cdot (P_1 - P_2)}{8\eta L}$$

FIGURE 3.1 Poiseuille law. η, coefficient of viscosity (expressed in dynes $\times$ sec $\times$ cm^2); L, length; P, pressure; R, radius.

TABLE 3.1	Oxygen Content (in mL Oxygen per L Blood) at Various Levels of Hemoglobin, Oxygen Saturation, and Plasma Oxygen Partial Pressures			
	Hemoglobin 15	Hemoglobin 12	Hemoglobin 10	Hemoglobin 8
$SpO_2 = 99\%$, $PaO_2 = 145$ torr	20.65	16.61	13.91	11.22
$SpO_2 = 97\%$, $PaO_2 = 96$ torr	20.09	16.13	13.49	10.85
$SpO_2 = 95\%$, $PaO_2 = 79$ torr	19.62	15.75	13.16	10.58
$SpO_2 = 92\%$, $PaO_2 = 65$ torr	18.97	15.22	12.71	10.21
$SpO_2 = 88\%$, $PaO_2 = 55$ torr	18.12	14.53	12.14	9.74

PaO_2, partial pressure of oxygen; SpO_2, arterial oxygen saturation.

Pulsatile flow makes things much more complex, and Poiseuille law may greatly underestimate energy losses in pulsatile systems. Turbulence increases energy losses even further still. All this is to say that although 2- or 3-dimensional imaging of atherosclerotic lesions can identify peripheral artery disease and perhaps give some signal of its severity, it cannot quantify its hemodynamic impact.

Normal Arterial Anatomy

Arterial blood ejected from the left ventricle toward the lower extremities passes through the aorta to the lower abdomen and pelvis. The aorta bifurcates into the left and right common iliac arteries, generally at the level of the fourth lumbar vertebra. This vessel becomes the external iliac artery distal to the origin of the internal iliac (also known as hypogastric) artery and the common femoral artery after passing under the inguinal ligament. The common femoral artery is at the level of the femoral head; it can also be found through palpation caudal to a line connecting the anterior superior iliac spine of the ilium and the pubic tubercle of the pubis bone but cephalad to the inguinal crease of the proximal thigh.

The common femoral artery bifurcates into the deep femoral artery (also known as the *profunda femoris* artery)—a lateral branch that distributes throughout the musculature of the thigh—and the superficial femoral artery. The superficial femoral artery spirals through the thigh, from its anterior position in the groin, and then medial in the thigh after passing

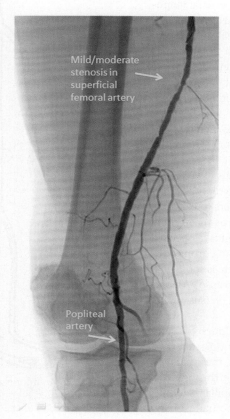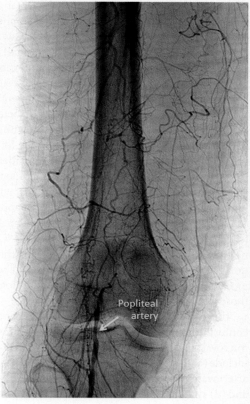

FIGURE 3.2 Angiogram demonstrating blood flow through a normal-caliber superficial femoral and popliteal artery *(left panel)* and through collaterals in the setting of an occluded superficial femoral and proximal popliteal artery *(right panel)*.

under through a hiatus (opening) in the adductor magnus muscle and becoming the popliteal artery, to a position posterior in the leg at the level of the knee. Most people have 2 pairs of bifurcations at the level of the proximal tibia. At the first bifurcation, the popliteal artery divides into the anterior tibial artery and a segment referred to as the tibioperoneal trunk. The tibioperoneal trunk then bifurcates into the posterior tibial and peroneal (fibular) arteries.

The posterior tibial artery divides into the medial and plantar arteries distal to malleoli at the ankle. The anterior tibial artery becomes the dorsalis pedis artery after passing under the extensor retinaculum of the distal ankle. The lateral plantar and dorsalis pedis arteries generally coalesce to form the deep (primary) plantar arch, but many additional communications among the tibial arteries exist (4).

Arterial blood passes through these named arteries and their branches and into arterioles, terminal arterioles, and then capillaries before returning to the venous circulation initially via postcapillary venules. It is these components of the arterial tree that are referred to as the "microcirculation" (<300 μm in diameter) and that are involved in nutrient and gas exchange in soft tissues. Blood supply to the skin is supplied by 3 types of arterioles: direct cutaneous vessels, musculocutaneous perforators, and the fasciocutaneous system (11).

Relationship Between Diabetes Mellitus and Peripheral Arterial Disease

Diabetes mellitus affects the macrovasculature of the lower extremity. Atherosclerotic lesions in patients with diabetes mellitus are generally found in the distal superficial femoral artery, the popliteal artery, and the tibial arteries (18,37) (Fig. 3.3). Many patients presenting with nonhealing ulcers or other tissue loss will be found to have isolated tibial disease (21). Lesions of the aortoiliac (suprainguinal) circulation are generally more often associated with significant smoking history (35). At least 1 pedal vessel is patent and suitable for distal revascularization in the foot in 70% of patients with diabetes mellitus (versus 80% of patients without diabetes mellitus) and only 50% in those with renal insufficiency with or without diabetes mellitus (13). Sparing of vessels in the foot allows for revascularization options in the majority of patients (34).

Primary arterial calcification, including Mönckeberg sclerosis and internal elastic lamina calcification (20), refers to calcification of the media. This finding is present in approximately 60% of patients presenting with acute diabetes mellitus–associated foot problems (1). It has also been associated with chronic kidney disease and other systemic diseases (20). There is some relationship with peripheral arterial disease (PAD) because PAD was present in 60% of those with medial calcification (versus 30% of those without this finding, odds ratio of 4) (1).

The concept of "small vessel disease" continues to cause confusion among physicians. Diabetes mellitus does alter the microvasculature. First recognized in the 1980s, these changes include (a) thickening of the basement membrane, (b) abnormal arteriovenous shunting (8,29), (c) decreased capillary density, and (d) an increased incidence tunica media smooth muscle hy-

perplasia causing occlusion of dermal arterioles (average of 12% in one histologic study) (19), and can result in slower wound healing. These changes, however, do not preclude wound healing if the macrovasculature is intact.

The Identification of Peripheral Arterial Disease Using History and Physical Exam Findings

The clinician should ask about a history of previous revascularization or revascularization attempts (e.g., previous stents in leg arteries, previous leg bypass operations) in either the index or contralateral lower extremity. Unfortunately, little other history and few symptoms have very reliable association with PAD. A history of claudication symptoms does have some association with PAD overall, but most patients presenting with diabetic foot ulcers do not have such a history (perhaps because of the presence of sensory neuropathy or the distribution of atherosclerotic disease in patients with diabetes mellitus) (9,10).

Palpation of peripheral pulses—specifically, the femoral, popliteal, posterior tibial, and dorsalis pedis pulses—constitute the most important exam component when identifying PAD.

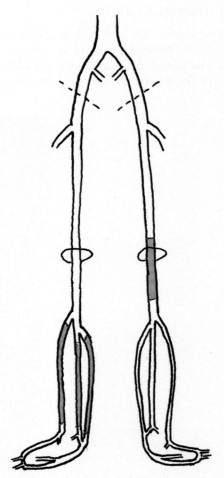

FIGURE 3.3 Anatomic areas in which atherosclerotic lesions commonly occur among patients with diabetes mellitus and peripheral arterial disease.

Palpating a pulse is a simple physical exam maneuver, but results should be interpreted with some degree of caution. This caution is based on the fact that the interrater reliability of a peripheral pulse exam in most studies is lacking quality. Agreement on the presence of peripheral pulses also seemed higher when attempting to categorize as normal, reduced, or absent rather than simply present.

Many clinicians evaluate pedal pulses using a handheld (continuous-wave) Doppler probe. Finding *both* dorsalis pedis *and* posterior tibial artery Doppler signals to be absent or monophasic may signify severe PAD, but the presence of biphasic signals over either or both arteries does *not* rule out hemodynamically significant PAD.

Although many clinicians believe hair loss, atrophic skin, or cool temperature skin are signs of PAD, findings from the Seattle Diabetic Foot Study suggest their diagnostic accuracy is very poor (likelihood ratio of 1.5 when present, 0.81 when absent) (9). The presence of any lower extremity bruit—iliac, femoral, or popliteal location—may be helpful in ruling in PAD, as the absence of a bruit in these 3 locations may decrease the likelihood of PAD (27).

Dependent rubor is a term describing redness present in the periphery of the foot (generally toes and forefoot) when the limb of patients changes to pallor when elevated above the level of the heart. The rubor results from maximal dilation of the microvasculature of the foot in the context of more proximal occlusions. The pallor occurs because the change in elevation further limits marginal perfusion to the foot by eliminating the contribution hydrostatic pressure has in providing arterial perfusion to the limb. Dependent rubor is generally considered a relatively specific sign of severe PAD, although no studies have evaluated its diagnostic accuracy.

QUANTITATIVE NONINVASIVE ARTERIAL TESTING

The theoretical relationship between arterial perfusion to the foot (at least as measured by some of the means described later) and wound healing has been derived empirically by a few studies, and it is thought to be sigmoidal in shape (24). In short, wound healing does not require normal or near-normal levels of arterial perfusion. What we do not know is (a) if there is some minimum level versus variation among patients and wounds and (b) how to best quantify arterial perfusion.

Some have proposed that the concept of "angiosomes" is relevant to the evaluation and management of arterial perfusion of the foot. In general terms, an angiosome is defined as the 3-dimensional volume of tissue that primarily receives blood supply from a particular artery. Attinger and colleagues' (4) cadaver studies have identified 5 angiosomes in the foot: those of the dorsalis pedis artery, the lateral plantar artery, the medial plantar artery, the calcaneal branch of the peroneal artery, and the calcaneal branch of the posterior tibial artery. Several studies have demonstrated that direct revascularization of the artery associated with the angiosome where a foot

ulcer is located (a so-called "direct" revascularization) is associated with higher limb preservation rates than revascularization of an artery that is not associated with the angiosome in which the ulcer is located (a so-called "indirect" revascularization). The concept of angiosomes, however, has been investigated primarily through injection studies in cadavers. The concept assumes that all the main arteries in the foot are end arteries without complementary areas of perfusion. Other studies have suggested that territories of arterial perfusion are much more variable in vivo and that the difference between the outcomes of direct versus indirect revascularization is eliminated if patency of the pedal arch is considered. Nonetheless, the idea that the vascular evaluation of the foot should not be only a global assessment of arterial perfusion but rather specific to the area in which the foot ulcer is located remains important.

Ankle Pressures and the Ankle-Brachial Index

Ankle pressures are the absolute systolic pressure of blood flow detected in the posterior tibial artery or the anterior tibial artery/dorsalis pedis artery. The ankle-brachial index (ABI) is defined as the ratio of the highest ankle pressure to the highest arm pressure. The highest arm pressure is taken as the best representation of central (aortic) pressure because, unlike ankle pressures, arm pressure measurements are rarely falsely elevated by vessel noncompressibility. An interarm systolic blood pressure differential of at least 10 mmHg was present in 9.4% of the Framingham Heart Study population (mean age of 61 years, free of cardiovascular disease at baseline [43], and 26% of a population undergoing vascular surgery operations [14]).

There are 2 methods of obtaining ABI measurements. At the most basic, a manual blood pressure cuff is placed at the level of the ankle. A handheld (continuous-wave) Doppler probe is used to auscultate an arterial signal over the posterior tibial artery at the level of the malleolus. The cuff is manually inflated at least 20 mmHg past the pressure required to extinguish the Doppler signal; 250 mmHg or more pressure may be needed. The cuff is then slowly deflated—rate of 3 to 4 mmHg per second. The pressure at which the Doppler signal over the artery reappears is the ankle pressure for the posterior tibial artery. The process is repeated by holding the Doppler probe over the dorsalis pedis artery in the dorsum of the foot. Blood pressures are obtained in both arms with the pressure detected by either auscultation over the brachial artery (i.e., listening for Korotkoff sounds) near the antecubital fossa or Doppler probe auscultation over the radial artery at the wrist (42). It is worthwhile noting that results represent the systolic pressure at which phasic arterial flow returns at the level of the blood pressure cuff, *not* the level of the Doppler probe.

An appropriately sized cuff is 20% wider than the diameter of the limb. The cuff should go circumferentially around the limb (Fig. 3.4A). Aneroid (manual) blood pressure cuffs (i.e., those with a clock face measuring pressure in the cuff at any

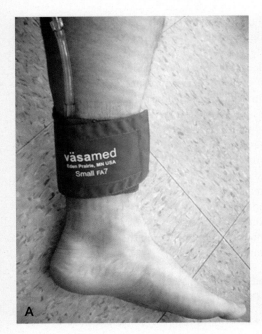 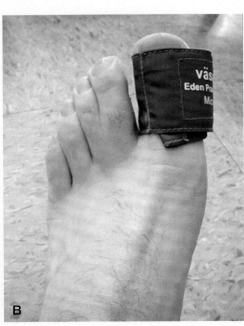

FIGURE 3.4 Ankle **(A)** and toe **(B)** pressure measurements using appropriately sized cuffs.

given time) are very inexpensive and very portable. These features and the fact that they are used for the measurement of arm pressures should make the measurement of ABIs available to clinicians in all but the most severely resource-limited health care environment. Most noninvasive vascular laboratories obtain pressures using automated cuffs. As with aneroid cuffs, these automated cuffs can be the same as those used for the measurement of blood pressure in the arm. These automated devices use oscillations in air pressure within the bladder of the cuff to detect the ankle pressure (or arm pressure). PAD is defined as an ABI ratio less than or equal to 0.9. In the setting of nonhealing ulcers, absolute ankle pressures of less than 70 mmHg are indicative of severely impaired arterial perfusion (32).

As mentioned earlier, ankle pressures and ABIs can be quickly obtained with very inexpensive equipment generally available in most health care settings. The specificity (probability that a normal test result correctly rules out significant PAD) is excellent at 89% (6). There are many important limitations in the use of ankle pressures and ABIs in the setting of diabetic foot wounds. It is widely recognized that falsely elevated pressures (generally ABI >1.3) represent noncompressible vessels and therefore yield no relevant diagnostic information. Less frequently appreciated, however, is the fact that results below this level, including values considered normal or near-normal, can also represent falsely elevated results that erroneously suggest to the clinician that significant PAD is absent. Overall, sensitivity of ABIs is 61% (6) and is lower than that of other diagnostic tests to be discussed later. Use of the *lower* ankle pressure in generating an ankle-brachial ratio may actually improve sensitivity in identifying significant PAD (16) but is not widely done.

Finally, similar pressure measurements at higher levels in the limb (often high thigh, low thigh, and calf) are also often obtained when ankle pressures are obtained in noninvasive

vascular laboratories. A decrease of >10 to 20 mmHg between any 2 consecutive levels may help identify the level of a hemodynamically significant atherosclerotic lesion and therefore may help in case planning prior to revascularization attempts. Still, it is the measurement of ankle pressures and ABIs (or other measures described later) that provides direct information on the overall perfusion to the foot itself.

Toe Pressures

Given that calcification of tibial (including ankle level) arteries is so common among patients with diabetes mellitus, the measurement of toe (digit) pressures developed as a method of measuring blood flow that would not be affected by this process. Measurements are taken with the patient in supine position. Digit cuffs are used on either the first or second toe (Fig. 3.4B); other toes are too small for measurement. As with ankle pressures and ABIs, these can be obtained manually but are most often performed using an automated plethysmography cuff. Whereas automated plethysmography cuffs used for ankle pressures often use air, toe pressure cuffs use photoplethysmography. Toe cuffs emit an infrared light, and the amount of this infrared light reflected by the tissue corresponds to pulsatile blood flow and tissue volume.

A toe-brachial index (TBI) ratio of greater than 0.7 or an absolute toe pressure greater than 60 mmHg should be considered indicative of adequate arterial perfusion to the foot. Toe pressures less than 30 mmHg are generally interpreted as indicating severe PAD, but risk of limb loss may be high only with pressures even lower than this (30). The toe pressure should be interpreted as being the most sensitive indicator of PAD in cases when a discrepancy between toe pressure and ankle pressure exists (e.g., normal ankle pressures, severely impaired toe pressures) (31). Discrepancies are generally due to false-normal ankle pressures

TABLE 3.2	Overall Sensitivity and Specificity of Individual Tests Included among the Diagnostic Testing Strategies			
Variable	Sensitivity	Specificity	PPV	NPV
PE	53.3 (52.1–54.6)	82.6 (82.2–83.1)	42.5 (41.4–43.7)	88.0 (87.6–88.4)
ABI	61.0 (59.7–62.1)	89.1 (88.6–89.6)	74.7 (73.7–75.9)	81.2 (80.6–81.8)
SPP	81.7 (79.9–83.6)	79.3 (77.2–81.1)	81.0 (78.9–83.1)	80.1 (78.2–82.4)
TcPo₂	83.0 (81.8–84.3)	62.8 (61.2–64.4)	66.7 (65.7–68.1)	80.6 (79.1–82.2)
TBI	84.0 (82.8–85.0)	77.8 (76.1–79.5)	86.7 (85.8–87.8)	73.7 (71.9–75.2)

Values in parentheses represent the 25%–75% interquartile range of values.
ABI, ankle-brachial index; NPV, negative predictive value; PE, pulse exam; PPV, positive predictive value; SPP, skin perfusion pressure; TBI, toe-brachial index; TcPo₂, transcutaneous oxygen pressure.

(due to medial calcification) rather than pedal-level atherosclerotic disease (i.e., "small vessel disease").

Toe pressures appear to have excellent sensitivity and specificity (Table 3.2) (6). Measurement is quick and not known to be affected by ambient temperature or other conditions. The first or second toe must be present and without a wound that would preclude measurement, and therefore, toe pressure measurements may not be possible to obtain in all individuals.

Skin Perfusion Pressures

Skin perfusion pressures (SPPs) attempt to directly measure the pressure of skin perfusion in various regions of the foot. These are obtained using a laser Doppler sensor applied to the skin in the area of interest. A cuff is placed around this sensor and inflated. A curve showing the degree of perfusion is generated as the cuff is slowly deflated (Fig. 3.5). The SPP is defined as the point at which skin perfusion increases above the level seen with full inflation. Measurement during slow deflation induces reactive hyperemia, and this is thought to prompt a more sensitive assessment of perfusion.

Similar to toe pressures, SPP measurements less than 30 mmHg should be interpreted as indicating severe PAD (41). SPP measurements between 30 and 60 mmHg suggest mild or moderate impairment, and those over 60 mmHg suggest no significant arterial impairment is present.

Pooled analysis of previously published studies (Table 3.2) (6) suggests that SPPs have excellent sensitivity and specificity

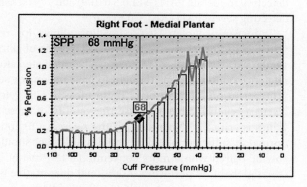
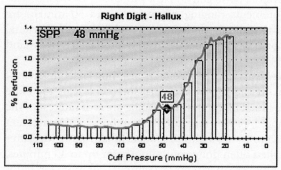
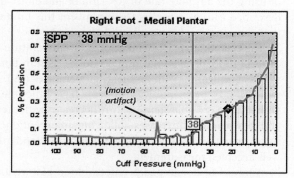
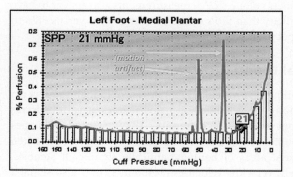

FIGURE 3.5 Skin perfusion pressure (SPP) measurements: normal *(top left)*, mild impairment *(top right)*, moderate impairment *(bottom left)*, and severe impairment *(bottom right)*.

in the detection of significant PAD. The equipment needed for testing is compact and mobile, and obtaining and interpreting requires only limited training. These features make SPPs appealing for point-of-care testing. Unlike toe pressures, SPPs can be obtained anywhere an appropriately sized cuff can be fit. Therefore, measurements specific to the area/angiosome of interest can be obtained, including the lateral forefoot, the midfoot, and the heel. Measurement is done via the laser Doppler sensor and is therefore thought to be somewhat less susceptible to vessel calcification if the cuff is placed below the ankle.

Equipment used to measure SPPs is not as widely available as that needed for TBIs. Measurement may be affected by motion artifacts that occur frequently with involuntary movements of the foot (Fig. 3.5, *lower 2 panels*). Measurement takes 1 to 2 minutes, and pressure applied by the cuff during this duration may be uncomfortable to some patients. Like other modalities, the relationship between various SPP levels and wound healing is incompletely understood.

Transcutaneous Oxygen Pressures

Transcutaneous oxygen pressure (TcPo$_2$) measurements are obtained using a small electrode that is typically placed on a location of the dorsal forefoot away from any bone, hair, hyperkeratotic tissue, or ulcer. Testing must be done with the patient in supine position and in a room with an ambient temperature of 21° to 23°C (70° to 74°F). Testing is often done after a 15- to 20-minute period of acclimatization to these conditions.

TcPo$_2$ measurements have been correlated to clinical outcomes in several studies (17,28,44). Specifically, TcPo$_2$ measurements less than 30 mmHg are considered to indicate severely impaired arterial perfusion and low probability of wound healing. Measurements ranging between 30 and 50 mmHg are considered to indicate moderately or mildly impaired arterial perfusion and a somewhat decreased probability of wound healing (17).

Measurements can be taken in any non-osseous area of intact skin in the foot. TcPo$_2$ measurements can therefore quantify regional blood flow to specific areas of interest in the foot. As noted earlier, measurements require stable ambient conditions and 10 to 15 minutes for acclimatization. Measurements are then often done continuously for up to 30 minutes, so total testing time may require 45 minutes or more for TcPo$_2$ measurements alone. TcPo$_2$ measurements also appear to have less specificity than SPPs or toe pressures (63% versus 78% to 79%, respectively, in a pooled analysis; Table 3.2) (6).

Arterial Blood Flow Velocities

Some noninvasive vascular laboratories obtain and report arterial blood flow velocities of major arteries at various levels throughout the lower extremity. Very elevated velocities (typically 250 centimeter/second [cm/s] or higher) are taken to represent areas of hemodynamically significant stenosis. Conversely, very low velocities (<40 cm/s) may also signal a hemodynamically significant stenosis or occlusion at a more proximal level.

At this time, the use of velocities to evaluate arterial perfusion of the foot is not conventional. Suggested thresholds for velocities representing hemodynamically significant lesions are not universally agreed upon, and there is less data evaluating the diagnostic accuracy of velocities than data evaluating other diagnostic modalities. Measuring native artery velocities throughout the limb is time-consuming, and results can be influenced by the experience and technique of the ultrasound technician more than other testing modalities. Certain arteries or arterial segments can also be difficult to visualize because of their location, especially the peroneal artery (because of its depth).

Adjunctive Vascular Testing Assessments

The use of pulse oximetry as a bedside screening test to identify PAD has previously been described (33). It can be used similar to ABIs, using the return of a pulse oximetry waveform as a substitute for Doppler signal. Similar to ABIs, this can be used to generate an index, referred to as the Lanarkshire oximetry index. These values appear to correlate with ABIs (7).

One group of investigators studied 84 patients. They considered abnormal any of the following results: (a) toe pulse oximetry 2% or more lower than finger oximetry and (b) a decrease of 2% or more when elevating the leg by 12 in. in height. The gold standard was "significant lower extremity PAD" as defined by the presence of monophasic Doppler signals. This group found that the presence of 1 or both criteria has an 86% sensitivity in identifying PAD and absence of both had a specificity of 92% (36). Another group of investigators examining 40 patients and 40 random volunteers found that all patients without PAD had normal toe oximetry readings but had only a 28% sensitivity in detecting moderate PAD (ABI 0.5 to 0.9) and 77% sensitivity in detecting severe PAD (ABI <0.5) (26).

Indocyanine green (ICG) imaging allows for real-time visualization of relative skin perfusion. Ratios of skin perfusion in various regions of interest can be calculated after some reference region, an area thought to have normal or sufficient skin perfusion, is identified. These measures therefore represent a relative value. Because the validity of these relative values is critically dependent on the reference region having normal or sufficient blood flow, this assessment should probably be paired with a more conventional test that at least assesses global foot perfusion. Additional quantitative methods of using the absolute rate of ICG influx and efflux have been described (40) as a means to circumvent this limitation, but these have not yet been well validated.

The quantitative assessment of skin temperature as a sign of PAD probably also has limited utility, as skin temperature varies significantly with ambient temperatures (39). Absolute temperatures by themselves probably have little role. Patients with PAD may display temperature decreases with exercise (24) and temperature increases following intervention (38) but mirror changes seen in ABIs, a much more standardized and well-accepted measurement.

Analysis of dorsal pedal venous blood gas (venous oximetry) has previously been described. Partial pressure of venous blood oxygen in patients included in this study increased after revascularization (15). No standardized values of venous oximetry for the foot or lower extremity have been evaluated, however, nor have levels or degrees of improvement that suggest an "adequate" revascularization. The clinical utility of venous oximetry in the diagnosis or quantification of lower extremity PAD is therefore limited at this time.

QUALITATIVE ASSESSMENT

Plethysmography (pulse volume recordings) provides a graphical representation of total blood flow at various levels of the limb. Similar to the measurement of ankle pressures or other segmental pressures, plethysmography is obtained by placing an appropriately sized cuff at the level of interest in the limb. Instead of measuring the pressure at which a systolic waveform returns after temporary occlusion, plethysmography graphs the rate and volume of displacement of air in the cuff throughout the cardiac cycle. Plethysmography recordings at various levels are frequently obtained in noninvasive vascular labs and reported along with their corresponding pressure measurements.

Plethysmography is considered a secondary measurement of arterial perfusion because its interpretation is ultimately quantitative. In general, normal waveforms have a sharp (brief) systolic upstroke and feature the dicrotic notch (representing reversal of flow during early diastole; Fig. 3.6A). Mildly impaired waveforms do not have a dicrotic notch but have an obvious systolic upstroke and a downward slope that is either convex or neutral (Fig. 3.6B). Moderately impaired plethysmography waveforms have a detectable systolic upstroke that is somewhat more rounded (longer duration) and a diastolic component that is concave (Fig. 3.6C). Severely impaired waveforms show little or no obvious systolic upstroke.

Although an assessment with handheld (continuous-wave) Doppler for the global assessment of blood flow has important limits mentioned earlier, handheld Doppler can be used for a qualitative assessment of the patency of the deep plantar arch or other collaterals in the foot when a foot operation may disrupt collaterals. Such situations may include a proximal transmetatarsal or Lisfranc amputation that will disrupt the deep plantar arch. Attinger et al. (3,5) have shown more details on how a handheld Doppler may be used to assess the patency of the pedal arch, and Roukis (36) has demonstrated details on how a handheld Doppler assessment may be used in preoperative planning prior to creation of local soft tissue flaps in the foot.

CROSS-SECTIONAL IMAGING

In general, noninvasive anatomic imaging should not be used as first-line testing in diabetic patients with foot ulcers. Although imaging can identify the presence of PAD, it cannot quantify the hemodynamic effects. As such, the clinical impact of atherosclerotic lesions is often unclear and may predispose to either under treatment or over treatment. There are roles for noninvasive anatomic imaging—at least after the presence of significant PAD has been noted from noninvasive arterial tests. In health care environments with suboptimal access to

angiographic suites for angiography and possible endovascular intervention, anatomic imaging may help elucidate the level(s) of atherosclerotic disease that will require intervention. Having this information may help in planning the optimal route of arterial access (e.g., retrograde via contralateral femoral versus antegrade via ipsilateral femoral). It may also help in planning efficient use of the angiography suite, as patients whose noninvasive anatomic imaging suggests surgical bypass may be the only feasible option can be scheduled for only as much time as is needed for a diagnostic angiogram, whereas those who seem to have endovascular options may need more time.

There are many limitations in the use of noninvasive anatomic imaging, especially in the setting of a diabetic foot ulcer. Computed tomography angiography (CTA; CT imaging with arterial-phase contrast) involves exposure to radiation and typically requires large doses (>100 mL) of iodinated contrast agents to image from the distal aorta to the feet. The spatial resolution of CTA and the presence of calcification of the media may impair the ability to accurately evaluate the patency of tibial and pedal arteries. Magnetic resonance angiography (MRA) uses a gadolinium, a noniodinated contrast agent that is safe to use in patients with an estimated glomerular filtration rate greater than 30 mL/min. MRA tends to overestimate the degree of stenosis. MRA cannot visualize areas with previously

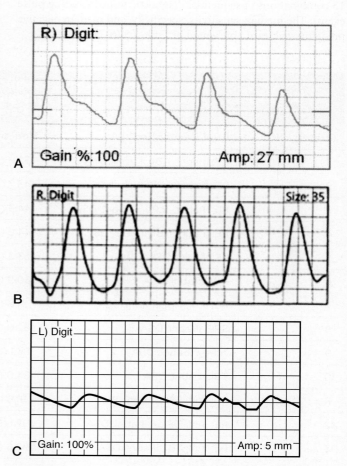

FIGURE 3.6 Plethysmography: normal **(A)**, mildly impaired **(B)**, and moderately impaired **(C)**.

placed stents and thus cannot be used to identify occlusions or stenosis within segments previously treated by stents.

WHEN TO ORDER NONINVASIVE STUDIES

Angiography is still considered the gold standard for the identification of significant PAD. Not all patients with diabetic foot ulcers should be subjected to angiography, however, because of its associated costs and invasive nature, a screening test is therefore helpful in this situation. In general, ideal screening tests are widely available and are low cost. Although angiography is the confirmatory test having 100% specificity, it is more important that a screening test used to determine the need for angiography have high *sensitivity*—that is, can rule out significant PAD with high levels of accuracy.

Our group has utilized probabilistic decision analysis models to estimate the composite (overall) sensitivity and specificity of various combinations of tests used to identify PAD among patients with diabetes mellitus. Diagnostic accuracy of individual tests, including pulse exam, were pooled from previously published studies (Table 3.2). These results were then included into a probabilistic Markov model to obtain estimates of various diagnostic strategies (i.e., the overall diagnostic accuracy of 13 combinations of sequential diagnostic tests, including pulse exam). The median sensitivity, specificity, and median negative predictive values are presented in Table 3.3 (6).

The results of this analysis suggested that employing certain strategies may increase the identification of PAD among those with foot ulcers, perhaps while also decreasing unnecessary costs:

1. Toe pressures and SPPs are preferable to ankle pressures/ABIs.
2. The sensitivity of SPPs, TBIs, and $TcPo_2$ measurement are similar, but specificities differ. Therefore, SPPs may be the single best noninvasive testing modality. TBIs/toe pressures should be used when SPP measurement is not available. $TcPo_2$ measurement can be used when SPP and TBI measurement is not available.
3. Performing noninvasive testing on all patients and using this to determine the need for angiography (regardless of the results of pulse exam; strategies 8 to 10) yields good levels of sensitivity (Table 3.3).
4. Excellent levels of sensitivity in the detection of PAD are obtained when noninvasive testing is used to corroborate the absence of PAD in patients with palpable pulses and when an angiography is performed in patients without palpable pulses (i.e., without using noninvasive testing to confirm PAD; strategies 11 to 13) (Table 3.3).

It may also be appropriate to perform noninvasive arterial testing after revascularization. Performing such testing early after revascularization may help ensure the procedure has augmented arterial perfusion that will be sufficient for wound healing. Testing may be helpful in patients with a remote history of revascularization and recent development of a foot ulcer to determine the current patency of the revascularization procedure.

TABLE 3.3	Cumulative Sensitivity, Specificity, and Negative Predictive Value of Various Combinatorial Testing Strategies, Ordered by Increasing Sensitivity, in the Base Case Scenario (Population Peripheral Arterial Disease Prevalence of 9.8%)			
Strategy No.	Brief Description	Median Sensitivity	Median Specificity	Median NPV
1	PE: if abnl, ABI; if abnl, DSA	32.6 (31.6–33.6)	97.4 (97.2–97.6)	69.9 (66.5–73.5)
2	PE: if abnl, SPP; if abnl, DSA	43.7 (42.4–45.1)	96.5 (96.0–96.8)	74.0 (70.0–76.6)
3	PE; if abnl, $TcPo_2$; if abnl, DSA	44.3 (43.0–45.7)	93.5 (93.2–93.9)	73.6 (70.0–76.2)
4	PE: if abnl, TBI; if abnl, DSA	44.8 (43.7–46.2)	96.1 (95.8–96.4)	74.3 (70.5–76.9)
5	PE: if abnl, DSA	53.3 (52.1–54.6)	82.6 (82.2–83.1)	74.7 (70.8–77.2)
6	ABI: if abnl, DSA	60.9 (59.9–62.1)	89.1 (88.6–90.0)	79.1 (75.7–81.2)
7	PE: if nl, ABI, if abnl, DSA	81.8 (81.1–82.5)	73.6 (73.0–74.2)	87.0 (84.7–88.6)
8	SPP: if abnl, DSA	82.0 (80.0–83.6)	89.1 (88.6–89.6)	89.1 (87.0–90.7)
9	$TcPo_2$: if abnl, DSA	83.1 (81.8–84.4)	62.8 (61.3–64.5)	86.1 (83.3–87.6)
10	TBI: if abnl, DSA	84.0 (83.0–85.2)	77.8 (76.1–79.4)	88.9 (86.9–90.3)
11	PE: if nl, SPP, if abnl, DSA	91.6 (90.7–92.4)	65.7 (63.7–67.2)	92.8 (91.2–93.9)
12	PE: if nl, $TcPo_2$, if abnl, DSA	92.1 (91.4–92.8)	51.9 (50.6–53.4)	91.7 (89.8–92.6)
13	PE: if nl, TBI, if abnl, DSA	92.6 (92.1–93.1)	64.2 (62.8–65.7)	93.4 (92.1–94.3)

Values in parentheses represent the 25%–75% interquartile range of values.
ABI, ankle-brachial index; abnl, abnormal; DSA, digital subtraction angiography; nl, normal; NPV, negative predictive value; PE, pulse exam; SPP, skin perfusion pressure; TBI, toe-brachial index; $TcPo_2$, transcutaneous oxygen pressure.

CLINICAL CASE SCENARIOS

Four cases are presented to further demonstrate some of the principles described earlier. All cases had some form of anatomic imaging available for correlation. Three of the 4 cases had either more than 1 noninvasive testing modality done at the

initial assessment or repeat assessment after revascularization. This frequency of testing is not always necessary and should not be interpreted as typical or recommended; rather, these cases are somewhat exceptional but are presented because comparing the results of the various noninvasive testing modalities helps demonstrate their respective strengths and weaknesses.

CASE STUDY 1

A 64-year-old man with diabetes mellitus (hemoglobin A_{1c} 5.7%) presented with gangrene of the tip of the left first toe and forefoot cellulitis. Transmetatarsal plethysmography suggested severe impairment (Fig. 3.7A,B). He underwent an initial open amputation of the first toe through the metatarsophalangeal joint to treat the infection, followed

by a bypass from the distal thigh portion of the superficial femoral artery to the tibioperoneal trunk using ipsilateral nonreversed great saphenous vein and subsequent amputation of the distal metatarsal with primary wound closure (Fig. 3.7C,D). The wound healed completely without recurrence of infection.

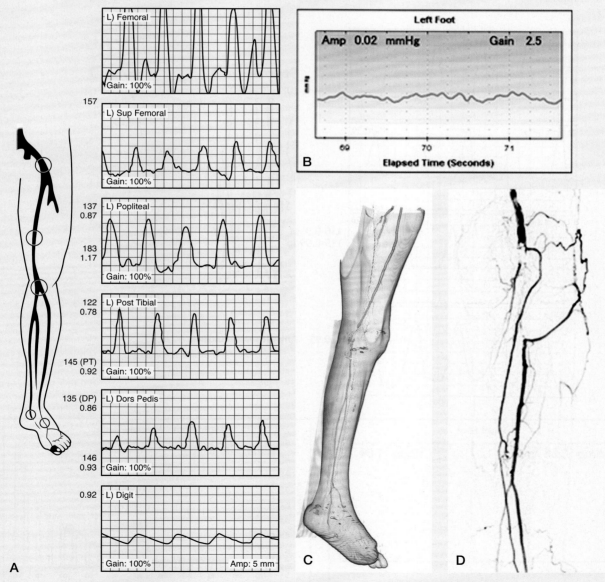

FIGURE 3.7 Demonstration of an arterial bypass from the distal thigh portion of the superficial femoral artery to the tibioperoneal trunk using an ipsilateral nonreversed great saphenous vein. **A.** Segmental pressures and plethysmography of the left leg; **(B)** transmetatarsal plethysmography of the left foot; **(C)** occlusion of the left popliteal artery as seen on 3-dimensional reconstruction of a computed tomography angiography; and **(D)** digital subtraction angiography.

CASE STUDY   2

A 65-year-old man with diabetes mellitus (hemoglobin A_{1c} 6.0%) and stage 3A chronic kidney disease (serum creatinine 1.8 mg/dL, estimated glomerular filtration rate of 46 mL/min) presented with a right second toe ulcer. He had a history of transtibial amputation of the left leg and partial right hallux amputation. The right femoral and popliteal pulses were palpable; pedal pulses were not palpable. Toe pressures could not be obtained because of swelling of the second toe and previous partial amputation of the hallux. The ABI was 0.99, and right fifth toe plethysmography suggested only mild impairment (Fig. 3.8A–C). Transmetatarsal plethysmography also showed mild impairment, but skin perfusion pressure (SPP) obtained along the medial aspect of the plantar forefoot (under the head of the second metatarsal) yielded a pressure of 38 mmHg. Because of somewhat discrepant results and the patient's previous history of contralateral leg amputation (i.e., at high risk for a significant change in functional status if amputation of the ipsilateral limb were to occur), angiography was performed. This demonstrated inline blood flow from the distal aorta to the right foot via patent tibial and pedal vessels that were without hemodynamically significant lesions (Fig. 3.8D; angled views at the level of the knee demonstrated a patent popliteal artery—not seen in the anteroposterior projection shown here because of a metallic knee prosthesis). The patient underwent second ray (toe and metatarsal) resection. The surgical site healed completely without the need for arterial intervention.

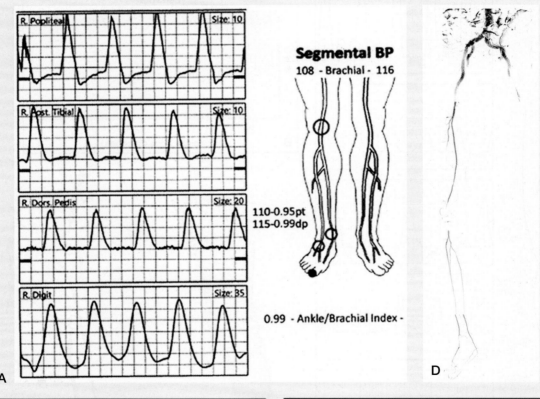

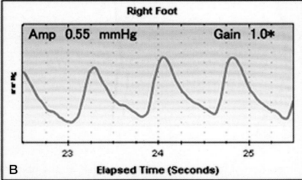

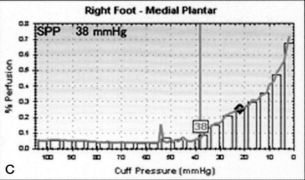

FIGURE 3.8 Demonstration of an angiography and noninvasive studies without the need of arterial intervention.

CASE STUDY 3

A 72-year-old man with diabetes mellitus (hemoglobin A_{1c} 7.6%) and peripheral neuropathy presented with a longstanding first toe ulcer and radiographic changes suggested of osteomyelitis in the first distal phalanx. Noninvasive vascular testing showed an ankle pressure of 43 mmHg and a second toe pressure of 16 mmHg. Plethysmography at the level of the ankle suggested severe impairment (Fig. 3.9A). Angiography showed occlusion of the superficial femoral artery from its origin through the level of the adductor hiatus, occlusion of the mid and distal anterior tibial artery and dorsalis pedis artery, and severe stenosis in the proximal posterior tibial artery (Fig. 3.9B). A bypass from the common femoral to the midcalf posterior tibial artery was performed; because of a history of saphenectomy for previous coronary artery bypass grafting, this was done using a prosthetic vascular graft conduit and a distal vein patch constructed from the upper arm basilic vein. Repeat noninvasive testing following bypass demonstrated significant increases in ankle and toe pressures (122 and 49 mmHg, respectively; Fig. 3.9C). A skin perfusion pressure (SPP) of 57 mmHg also suggested adequate arterial perfusion (Fig. 3.9D). Transmetatarsal plethysmography suggested only mild impairment (Fig. 3.9E). Partial hallux amputation with primary wound closure was performed. Complete wound healing was seen. Computed tomography angiography done to evaluate for seroma demonstrated a widely patent bypass graft (Fig. 3.9F).

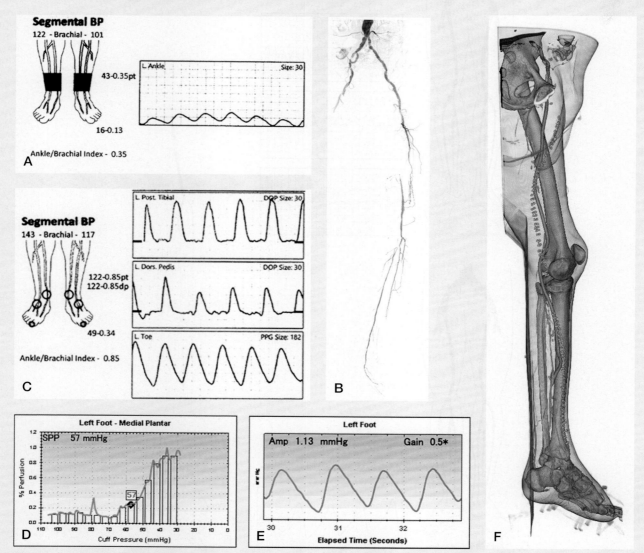

FIGURE 3.9 Demonstration of an arterial bypass from the common femoral to the midcalf posterior tibial artery by using a prosthetic vascular graft conduit and a distal vein patch constructed from the upper arm basilic vein. **A.** Ankle-level plethysmography prior at presentation; **(B)** composite of digital subtraction angiography demonstrating superficial femoral artery occlusion and occlusion of the peroneal and anterior tibial vessels; **(C)** ankle pressures and plethysmography following revascularization; **(D)** skin perfusion pressures following revascularization; **(E)** transmetatarsal plethysmography following revascularization; **(F)** three-dimensional reconstruction of a computed tomography angiography showing a patent femorotibial bypass graft.

An 85-year-old man with diabetes mellitus (hemoglobin A_{1c} of 6.8%) presented with a nonhealing wound and persistent cellulitis over the site of a fifth toe amputation performed 1 month prior at another hospital. First toe pressure was 25 mmHg, and ankle plethysmography showed severe impairment (Fig. 3.10A). Angiography showed inline flow from the aorta through the popliteal artery without hemodynamically significant lesions. Occlusions of all 3 tibial vessels were seen at the level of the mid to distal ankle with reconstitution of the dorsalis pedis artery, the pedal arch, and the lateral plantar artery (Fig. 3.10B). An attempt at angioplasty of the distal anterior tibial artery was unsuccessful. A bypass from the popliteal artery to the dorsalis pedis artery using nonreversed ipsilateral saphenous vein was performed. Repeat first toe pressure following bypass was 93 mmHg, and digit plethysmography was normal or mildly impaired (Fig. 3.10C). Ostectomy of the fifth metatarsal head with primary wound closure was performed. The wound healed completely and cellulitis resolved.

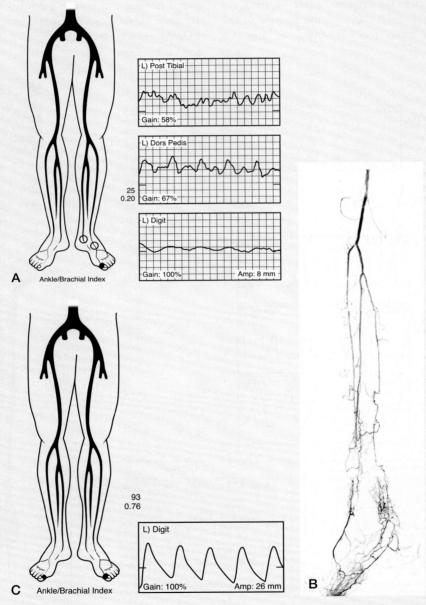

FIGURE 3.10 Demonstration of an arterial bypass from the popliteal artery to the dorsalis pedis artery using a nonreversed ipsilateral saphenous vein. **A.** Ankle and digit plethysmography showing severe impairments in arterial perfusion; **(B)** composite of digital subtraction angiography demonstrating occlusion of all tibial vessels at the ankle and reconstitution of the dorsalis pedis artery; **(C)** normalized toe pressures and digit plethysmography following revascularization.

Conclusion

Noninvasive vascular testing can be very helpful in assuring that arterial blood flow to the foot is adequate for wound healing. Nonetheless, these are only numeric representations of a complex physiologic process, and limitations are inherent to these testing modalities. Clinicians should have a high index of suspicion in identifying PAD. Palpable pedal pulses should be corroborated with noninvasive testing before significant PAD is ruled out. SPPs and toe pressures are probably the best noninvasive modalities for evaluating arterial perfusion in patients with diabetic foot ulcers. Anatomic imaging does not provide physiologic information and should therefore generally be reserved for preoperative planning.

References

1. Aragón-Sánchez J, Lázaro-Martínez JL. Factors associated with calcification in the pedal arteries in patients with diabetes and neuropathy admitted for foot disease and its clinical significance. Int J Low Extrem Wounds 2013;12:252–255.

2. Aro H, Eerola E, Aho AJ, et al. Tissue oxygen tension in externally stabilized tibial fractures in rabbits during normal healing and infection. J Surg Res 1984;37:202–207.

3. Attinger C, Cooper P, Blume P, et al. The safest surgical incisions and amputations applying the angiosome principles and using the Doppler to assess the arterial-arterial connections of the foot and ankle. Foot Ankle Clin 2001;6:745–799.

4. Attinger CE, Evans KK, Bulan E, et al. Angiosomes of the foot and ankle and clinical implications for limb salvage: reconstruction, incisions, and revascularization. Plast Reconstr Surg 2006;117(7 suppl):261–293.

5. Attinger CE, Meyr AJ, Fitzgerald S, et al. Preoperative Doppler assessment for transmetatarsal amputation. J Foot Ankle Surg 2010;49:101–105.

6. Barshes NR, Flores E, Belkin M, et al. The accuracy and cost-effectiveness of strategies used to identify peripheral artery disease among patients with diabetic foot ulcers. J Vasc Surg 2016;64:1682–1690.

7. Bianchi C, Montalvo V, Ou HW, et al. Pharmacologic risk factor treatment of peripheral arterial disease is lacking and requires vascular surgeon participation. Ann Vasc Surg 2007;21:163–166.

8. Blumenthal HT. More on microvascular disease of the foot in diabetes. N Engl J Med 1985;313:696–697.

9. Boyko EJ, Ahroni JH, Davignon D, et al. Diagnostic utility of the history and physical examination for peripheral vascular disease among patients with diabetes mellitus. J Clin Epidemiol 1997;50:659–668.

10. Boyko EJ, Ahroni JH, Stensel V, et al. A prospective study of risk factors for diabetic foot ulcer. The Seattle Diabetic Foot Study. Diabetes Care 1999;22:1036–1042.

11. Cormack GC, Lamberty BGH. The arterial anatomy of skin flaps. London, United Kingdom: Churchill Livingstone, 1989.

12. Demling RH. Nutrition, anabolism, and the wound healing process: an overview. Eplasty 2009;9:e9.

13. Diehm N, Rohrer S, Baumgartner I, et al. Distribution pattern of infrageniculate arterial obstructions in patients with diabetes mellitus and renal insufficiency—implications for revascularization. Vasa 2008;37:265–273.

14. Durrand JW, Batterham AM, O'Neill BR, et al. Prevalence and implications of a difference in systolic blood pressure between one arm and the other in vascular surgical patients. Anaesthesia 2013;68:1247–1252.

15. Ener BK. Dorsal pedal venous oximetry as an outcome index of lower extremity revascularizations. Vasc Surg 2001;35:37–41.

16. Espinola-Klein C, Rupprecht HJ, Bickel C, et al. Different calculations of ankle-brachial index and their impact on cardiovascular risk prediction. Circulation 2008;118:961–967.

17. Faglia E, Clerici G, Caminiti M, et al. Predictive values of transcutaneous oxygen tension for above-the-ankle amputation in diabetic patients with critical limb ischemia. Eur J Vasc Endovasc Surg 2007;33:731–736.

18. Faglia E, Favales F, Quarantiello A, et al. Angiographic evaluation of peripheral arterial occlusive disease and its role as a prognostic determinant for major amputation in diabetic subjects with foot ulcers. Diabetes Care 1998;21:625–630.

19. Fiordaliso F, Clerici G, Maggioni S, et al. Prospective study on microangiopathy in type 2 diabetic foot ulcer. Diabetologia 2016;59:1542–1548.

20. Fishbein MC, Fishbein GA. Arteriosclerosis: facts and fancy. Cardiovasc Pathol 2015;24:335–342.

21. Gray GH, Grant AA, Kalbaugh CA, et al. The impact of isolated tibial disease on outcomes in the critical limb ischemic population. Ann Vasc Surg 2010;24:349–359.

22. Hart CR, Layec G, Trinity JD, et al. Evidence of preserved oxidative capacity and oxygen delivery in the plantar flexor muscles with age. J Gerontol A Biol Sci Med Sci 2015;70:1067–1076.

23. Heinonen I, Saltin B, Kemppainen J, et al. Skeletal muscle blood flow and oxygen uptake at rest and during exercise in humans: a pet study with nitric oxide and cyclooxygenase inhibition. Am J Physiol Heart Circ Physiol 2011;300:H1510–1517.

24. Huang CL, Wu YW, Hwang CL, et al. The application of infrared thermography in evaluation of patients at high risk for lower extremity peripheral arterial disease. J Vasc Surg 2011;54:1074–1080.

25. Jaszczak P. Skin oxygen tension, skin oxygen consumption, and skin blood flow measured by a tc-pO2 electrode. Acta Physiol Scand Suppl 1991;603:53–57.

26. Jawahar D, Rachamalla HR, Rafalowski A, et al. Pulse oximetry in the evaluation of peripheral vascular disease. Angiology 1997;48:721–724.

27. Khan NA, Rahim SA, Anand SS, et al. Does the clinical examination predict lower extremity peripheral arterial disease? JAMA 2006;295:536–546.

28. Lo T, Sample R, Moore P, et al. Prediction of wound healing outcome using skin perfusion pressure and transcutaneous oximetry: a single-center experience in 100 patients. Wounds 2009;21:310–316.

29. LoGerfo FW, Coffman JD. Current concepts. Vascular and microvascular disease of the foot in diabetes. Implications for foot care. N Engl J Med 1984;311:1615–1619.

30. Marston WA, Davies SW, Armstrong B, et al. Natural history of limbs with arterial insufficiency and chronic ulceration treated without revascularization. J Vasc Surg 2006;44:108–114.

31. Mills JL Sr, Conte MS, Armstrong DG, et al. The Society for Vascular Surgery Lower Extremity Threatened Limb Classification

System: risk stratification based on wound, ischemia, and foot infection (WIfI). J Vasc Surg 2014;59:220–234.e1.

32. Norgren L, Hiatt WR, Dormandy JA, et al. Inter-society consensus for the management of peripheral arterial disease (TASC II). J Vasc Surg 2007;45S:S5–67.

33. Parameswaran GI, Brand K, Dolan J. Pulse oximetry as a potential screening tool for lower extremity arterial disease in asymptomatic patients with diabetes mellitus. Arch Intern Med 2005;165:442–446.

34. Pomposelli FB, Kansal N, Hamdan AD, et al. A decade of experience with dorsalis pedis artery bypass: analysis of outcome in more than 1000 cases. J Vasc Surg 2003;37:307–315.

35. Raffetto JD, Chen MN, LaMorte WW, et al. Factors that predict site of outflow target artery anastomosis in infrainguinal revascularization. J Vasc Surg 2002;35:1093–1099.

36. Roukis TS. The Doppler probe for planning septofasciocutaneous advancement flaps on the plantar aspect of the foot: anatomical study and clinical applications. J Foot Ankle Surg 2000;39:270–290.

37. Rueda CA, Nehler MR, Perry DJ, et al. Patterns of artery disease in 450 patients undergoing revascularization for critical limb ischemia: implications for clinical trial design. J Vasc Surg 2008;47:995–999.

38. Staffa E, Bernard V, Kubicek L, et al. Infrared thermography as option for evaluating the treatment effect of percutaneous transluminal angioplasty by patients with peripheral arterial disease. Vascular 2017;25:42–49.

39. Stoner HB, Barker P, Riding GS, et al. Relationships between skin temperature and perfusion in the arm and leg. Clin Physiol 1991;11(1):27–40.

40. Terasaki H, Inoue Y, Sugano N, et al. A quantitative method for evaluating local perfusion using indocyanine green fluorescence imaging. Ann Vasc Surg 2013;27:1154–1161.

41. Tsai FW, Tulsyan N, Jones DN, et al. Skin perfusion pressure of the foot is a good substitute for toe pressure in the assessment of limb ischemia. J Vasc Surg 2000;32:32–36.

42. Vierron E, Halimi JM, Giraudeau B. Ankle-brachial index and peripheral arterial disease. N Engl J Med 2010;362:471.

43. Weinberg I, Gona P, O'Donnell CJ, et al. The systolic blood pressure difference between arms and cardiovascular disease in the Framingham Heart Study. Am J Med 2014;127:209–215.

44. Yang C, Weng H, Chen L, et al. Transcutaneous oxygen pressure measurement in diabetic foot ulcers: mean values and cut-point for wound healing. J Wound Ostomy Continence Nurs 2013;40:585–589.

45. Zheng J, Hasting MK, Zhang X, et al. A pilot study of regional perfusion and oxygenation in calf muscles of individuals with diabetes with a noninvasive measure. J Vasc Surg 2014;59:419–426.

CHAPTER 4

Diabetic Lower Extremity Angioplasty and Bypass Reconstruction

Neal R. Barshes

INTRODUCTION

Peripheral arterial disease (PAD) is present in approximately 10% to 15% of people with diabetes mellitus and as many as 40% of those presenting with diabetic foot ulcers (DFUs) (12). Given this high prevalence, all clinicians managing patients with DFUs should have at least some rudimentary understanding of how PAD is managed among patients with a DFU. This chapter will review a variety of revascularization techniques and outcomes in patients with diabetes mellitus.

PERIOPERATIVE RISK AND PATIENT SELECTION FOR DIABETIC ARTERIAL SURGERY

Estimating the potential impact of diabetic lower extremity revascularization, it is best performed by the experienced clinician taking many different factors into consideration, including medical comorbidities, baseline functional status, social support, and the patient's preferences for various health outcomes. Perhaps the single most important consideration for revascularization is the baseline functional status of the patient. Patients with essentially no meaningful function in their lower extremity—not used for ambulation, transferring from bed or wheelchair and/or standing due to a previous cerebrovascular accident, spinal cord injury, or other severe deconditioning—would not benefit from lower extremity preservation. On the other end of the spectrum, diabetic patients with excellent functional status can undergo surgical reconstruction.

Many patients with DFUs and PAD have poor to average functional status prior to revascularization. The presence of several systemic comorbidities is the rule rather than the exception. Many clinicians view poor functional status and systemic comorbidities as posing risk to the performance of a leg bypass operation, thinking that because a leg amputation operation is briefer, the risk will be less. Mortality within 30 days after randomization in Bypass versus Angioplasty in Severe Ischemia of the Leg (BASIL) trial was no different for those who underwent angioplasty-first strategy and those that

underwent leg bypass surgery (2). Another study compared outcomes of infrainguinal bypass and above-ankle amputation among patients considered high risk for perioperative mortality per RAND (research and development) criteria using data from the American College of Surgeons National Surgical Quality Improvement Program. Propensity analysis was used to perform 1:1 matching of 792 patients who had undergone leg amputation and 781 patients who had undergone infrainguinal bypass. After matching, no significant differences existed in age, comorbidity presence/severity, functional status, or anesthetic technique (general versus regional) used for the operation. After matching, 30-day survival was 93.5% in those undergoing bypass and 90.0% in those undergoing leg amputation ($P = .01$) (10).

BENEFITS OF AND ALTERNATIVES TO DIABETIC LOWER EXTREMITY REVASCULARIZATION

Overall, revascularization and lower extremity preservation is quite effective at maintaining ambulatory function in the overwhelming majority of patients (1). Functional outcomes following revascularization are somewhat mitigated in elderly patients or those with poor baseline functional status, and those with little or no baseline function in the affected lower extremity should not be expected to improve following revascularization (Fig. 4.1). Patients with excellent baseline functional status (i.e., younger patients with diabetic foot complications or younger patients undergoing leg amputation following major trauma) also have excellent functional outcomes following primary leg amputation, whereas those with little or no baseline function are very unlikely to maintain or regain ambulatory function following major amputation. Patients with some poor (marginal) functional status are much less likely to maintain ambulatory ability following leg amputation compared to those with undergoing revascularization and lower extremity preservation.

A formal cost-effectiveness analysis based on these observations support the idea that marginal patients (i.e., elderly patients, those with advanced systemic comorbidities, or those

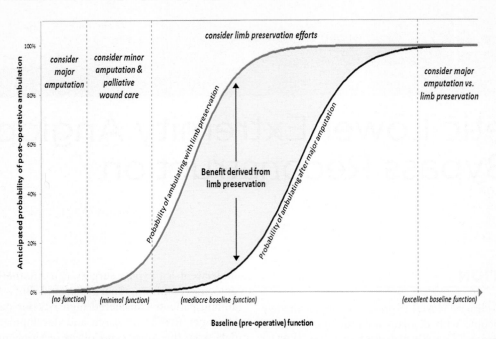

FIGURE 4.1 Functional outcomes following revascularization and lower extremity preservation *(top curve)* versus primary leg amputation *(bottom curve)*. The gap between the curves at any given point along the horizontal axis represents the potential benefit to lower extremity preservation in any given patient based on baseline functional status.

with poor levels of baseline function) may have the potential to benefit even *more* from revascularization and lower extremity preservation than patients that are younger, healthier, or have excellent baseline functional status (9). These potential benefits would not be apparent to those comparing outcomes among different populations of patients in absolute terms but only when comparing outcomes of one treatment for a specific group relative to outcomes of another treatment for that group. Together with the relatively higher morbidity and mortality associated with leg amputation in high-risk patients, these findings support a liberal approach to revascularization in circumstances when some degree of uncertainty about the benefit of revascularization exists.

Leg amputation for primary treatment of diabetic foot complications should be reserved to some rare situations. These might include clinical case scenarios where the patient has extremely limited lower extremity function or overall functional status (e.g., cerebrovascular accident with major residual deficit, history of spinal cord injury, bedbound due to medical illness, significant flexion contracture of the hip or knee), situations where the patient has a very low likelihood of surviving more than 2 years (e.g., pancreatic adenocarcinoma, glioblastoma of the brain, or metastases of certain tumors), or situations where the soft tissue and/or bony destruction of the foot is too advanced to allow for reconstruction attempts that will provide meaningful function in the lower extremity (e.g., extensive necrotizing soft tissue infection throughout the plantar aspect of the midfoot and hindfoot).

Our group has pursued a strategy of "palliative wound care" in selected patients with significant PAD, very advanced systemic comorbidities, and low functional level (8). This strategy consists of minor amputations or incision and drainage to remove obviously necrotic areas and treat infection with subsequent wound care. The wound care is very deliberately described as "palliative" to avoid the expectation that the wound will heal. Our published series compared 11 patients who received a strategy of palliative wound care to an age-matched group of 12 control patients who underwent primary leg amputations. The median age of these patients was 80 years old, and approximately half had stage 3 or higher chronic kidney disease (estimated glomerular filtration rate less than 60 mL/min). Half of the patients had some degree of heart failure, and approximately one quarter had a left ventricular ejection fraction of less than 30%. All of the patients had moderate or severe foot infections. All of the patients who lived independently in the community and were at least somewhat capable of using the affected lower extremity for transfers or ambulation remained so after a strategy of palliative wound care. In contrast, 75% of the group who underwent primary leg amputation experienced a change in ambulatory status, and half were no longer able to live independently. The lower extremity preservation rate at 2 years for those who received a strategy of palliative wound care was 66%, and no episodes of ascending lower extremity infection or systemic sepsis were seen. Based on this experience, we suggest a strategy of minor amputations and palliative wound care as an alternative to primary leg amputation for patients with foot infections, severe PAD, and advanced systemic comorbidities who live independently in the community and have some (albeit low) function in the affected lower extremity.

GENERAL CONCEPTS IN REVASCULARIZATION FOR PATIENTS WITH DIABETIC FOOT ULCERS

Endovascular Treatment

Endovascular intervention is becoming a more frequently used method of revascularization in patients with diabetic foot complications. In various health care settings, these interventions can be effectively and safely performed by surgeons, interventional radiologists, interventional cardiologists, or other physicians with the proper procedural training and experience. The procedures can also be performed in a variety of clinical settings, ranging from fluoroscopy-equipped operating rooms in hospital to procedural suites in outpatient facilities.

After infiltration with local anesthesia, access to the arterial system is first established using a needle and wire and then followed by placement of a sheath (cannula with a side port for aspiration and flushing). This access is very commonly established in the common femoral artery contralateral to the affected lower extremity, with the wire/catheter/sheath access being directed in a retrograde direction toward the aortic bifurcation, then through the iliac system on the affected side in an antegrade direction. The benefit of this access is that it not only allows for visualization of the entirety of the arterial system of the affected lower extremity but also establishes access for endovascular treatment of virtually all areas (all except the proximal common iliac artery of the affected side). Once an atherosclerotic lesion is visualized, a variety of wires and catheters are used to cross past the diseased area and to gain intraluminal access to a patent and relatively unaffected artery distal to this lesion. Wires and catheters are selected based on various qualities that may make them advantageous for crossing lesions in various areas, including length, diameter, shape, rigidity, and material coating the surface of the wire or catheter (Fig. 4.2).

Other locations of arterial access are frequently used. Accessing the ipsilateral common femoral artery or proximal superficial femoral artery in an antegrade direction allows for visualization of almost all of the infrainguinal circulation on the affected side. The shorter distance between this ipsilateral site of access may somewhat increase the chances of successfully treating more distal (especially infrapopliteal) lesions. Other sites of arterial access are also used, including access via pedal or tibial vessels on the affected lower extremity to allow infrainguinal lesions to be treated in a retrograde direction.

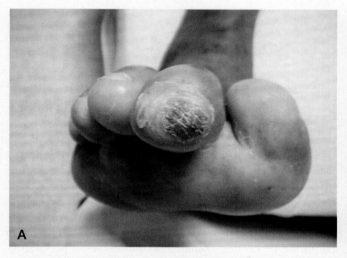

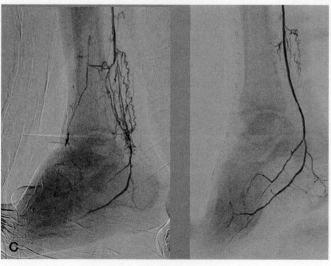

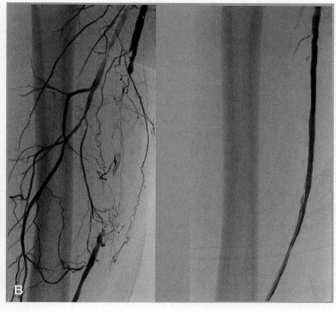

FIGURE 4.2 A 57-year-old male with diabetes mellitus (hemoglobin A_{1c} of 10.9%) presented with a 6-month history of severe pain and nonhealing ulcer at the tip of his right second toe **(A)**. The patient had previously undergone right partial hallux amputation. He had no history of coronary artery or cerebrovascular disease. A transmetatarsal pulse volume recording (plethysmography) suggested moderately impaired arterial perfusion to the right foot. An angiogram was performed via percutaneous retrograde access of the contralateral left common femoral artery that demonstrated occlusion of a long segment of the midthigh superficial femoral artery **(B)** *(left side)* and the distal posterior tibial artery **(C,D)** *(left side)*. *(continued)*

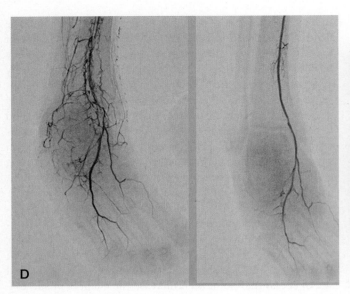

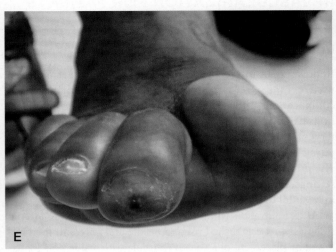

FIGURE 4.2 *(Continued)* No significant lesions were seen in the popliteal artery. The peroneal and anterior tibial arteries were occluded in the calf; no dorsalis pedis artery reconstitution was seen in the foot. The superficial femoral artery lesion was crossed with a wire, allowing for angioplasty and placement of a drug-eluting nitinol stent **(B)** *(right side)*. The distal posterior tibial artery lesion could not be successfully crossed through this approach. Clopidogrel was initiated. One week after the initial procedure, the patient underwent an additional endovascular intervention. Percutaneous access of the proximal portion of the ipsilateral right superficial femoral artery was performed, and an attempt at crossing the distal posterior tibial artery lesion was successful through this approach **(C,D)** *(right side)*. Because of significant residual stenosis after angioplasty, 2 drug-eluting stents were placed in the distal posterior tibial artery. Excellent filling of the lateral plantar artery and some segment of the medial plantar artery was seen. Both procedures were performed on an outpatient basis and were tolerated well. No complications were seen. The patient's pain resolved. Healing of the ulcer was seen within 1 month of the second procedure **(E)**.

Balloon angioplasty is often used as the primary means of treating an area of stenosis (narrowing) or occlusion (blockage) after a wire is adequately positioned across the atherosclerotic lesion. Inflation of the balloon over a wire effectively increases the luminal diameter not by decreasing the thickness of atherosclerotic plaques but rather by a controlled tear of fibers in the media layer of the wall of the artery, thereby increasing the total diameter of the vessel in that location, including the luminal diameter.

Based on the characteristics of the atherosclerotic lesion and the degree of response to balloon angioplasty, stents may also be used. Stents are composed of material that exerts a continuous outward (radial) force on the walls of the vessel, thereby attempting to increase or maintain luminal diameter. Balloon angioplasty and the use of stents are relatively conventional and accepted components of endovascular therapy for infrainguinal disease. Other modalities exist, but their relative benefits are not yet well established. Perhaps the most commonly used of these modalities is atherectomy. Atherectomy devices use laser or mechanical action to debulk the thickness of atherosclerotic lesions.

The inpatient hospital perioperative mortality of infrainguinal endovascular therapy is low (2.9%) and did not differ significantly from the inpatient hospital perioperative mortality of surgical bypass in the 1 existing randomized trial that compared the 2 modalities (2). Morbidity directly related to the procedure should be similarly low.

Access-related complications such as hematoma and vessel injury requiring surgical repair should occur in <5% of cases. Use of ultrasound to guide access increases the likelihood of successful access and significantly decreases the rate of access complications (16). Contrast-induced nephropathy may occur due to the use of iodinated contrast agents, especially considering the high prevalence of chronic kidney disease among patients with diabetic foot complications. This risk can be mitigated through the periprocedural administration of intravenous fluids and free radical scavengers such as *N*-acetylcysteine and vitamin C. The use of iodinated agents can be minimized or avoided by using carbon dioxide, gadolinium, or other non-nephrotoxic contrast agents for some or all of the procedure. Distal embolization, vessel perforation, or other complications occurring at the site of intervention have been reported but are rare. These procedures may be performed on an outpatient basis if not combined with inpatient treatment of diabetic foot infection or other medical issues.

Virtually all patients with PAD should receive aspirin therapy unless contraindications are present. Patients who have received stents may be prescribed clopidogrel, especially if drug-eluting stents were placed. Duplex ultrasound surveillance is not routinely performed following endovascular interventions but may be reasonable.

Surgical Bypass Treatment

Because of the infrainguinal and infrapopliteal lesions typical of PAD among patients with diabetes mellitus, surgical revascularization consists predominately of infrainguinal bypass procedures. Rather than directly addressing segments with occlusions or high-grade stenosis, leg bypass procedures establish a new high-caliber route of arterial blood flow past these areas. As described in Chapter 3, the large caliber and more direct route of a bypass graft relative to collateral vessels are some of the features that ensure that a bypass will effectively increase blood flow to the foot.

Nomenclature used to describe the surgical bypass operations specify the site of origination (the "inflow" site) and the site of termination (the "outflow" site, also referred to as the "distal target"). Femoropopliteal bypasses, originating from the common femoral or proximal superficial femoral artery and terminating in the popliteal artery, and femorotibial bypasses, terminating at a tibial vessel, are the most common types of leg bypass procedures performed in the setting of DFUs (Fig. 4.3). Femoropedal or popliteopedal bypasses, originating at the femoral or popliteal artery, respectively, and terminating in a pedal artery such as the dorsalis pedis artery or the lateral plantar artery, are also frequently performed.

As described earlier, a good distal target is necessary for a leg bypass to be effective in improving blood flow to the foot and for long-term patency of the bypass. An adequate distal target is defined as a large-caliber artery that is in continuity with the pedal vessels in the foot without hemodynamically significant lesions along its course. A femoropopliteal bypass, for example, would not be helpful or durable in a patient with

some segment of patent popliteal artery but occlusion of all three tibial vessels in the distal calf. Although some authors (13,18) have reported good outcomes with bypasses to isolated popliteal segments (i.e., popliteal arteries that are not continuous with tibial and pedal vessels), such bypasses are not conventional or widely performed.

The use of autologous, good-caliber single-segment great saphenous vein as the bypass conduit is preferred for all infrainguinal bypasses, regardless of their level or distal target. This preference is based on two features: First, the great saphenous vein is associated with higher long-term patency than prosthetic conduits at all levels; and second, whereas occlusion of a vein graft is often a clinically silent event, occlusion of a prosthetic conduit is much more often associated with lower extremity-threatening acute ischemia (17). Contralateral great saphenous vein is a good option in situations where the ipsilateral great saphenous vein is small in caliber or is absent because of previous use elsewhere or because of ablation or stripping as treatment for varicosities.

Prosthetic conduit—mainly expanded polytetrafluoroethylene (ePTFE), often with a covalently bonded heparin coating—or alternative autologous veins—including spliced segments of great saphenous veins, arm veins (forearm and/or upper arm segments of cephalic and/or basilic veins), and

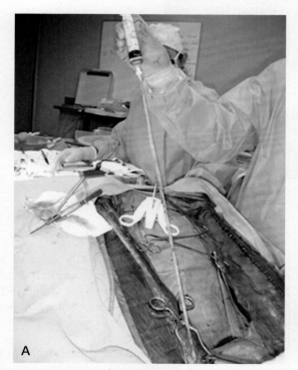
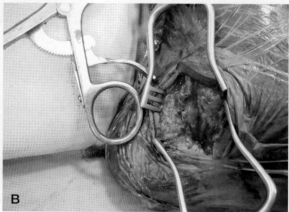

FIGURE 4.3 A 67-year-old male with diabetes mellitus (hemoglobin A_{1c} 8.7%) presented with a gangrenous left foot first toe, forefoot fluctuance, and surrounding cellulitis. The patient had a history of cigarette smoking (50 pack-year total) and history of prior coronary artery bypass grafting. Femoral pulses were palpable, but no palpable pedal pulses were appreciated. A guillotine amputation of the first toe was performed through the metatarsophalangeal joint for control of infection. An angiogram was also performed; this demonstrated occlusion of the popliteal artery and all 3 tibial vessels in the calf. Reconstitution of the distal posterior tibial artery at the ankle was seen. Ultrasound confirmed the absence of his left and right great saphenous veins (from previous coronary artery bypass surgery) but demonstrated good caliber left and right small saphenous veins. A leg bypass operation was performed. The bilateral small saphenous veins were harvested from the posterior calves with the patient in prone position **(A)**. The patient was then moved to supine position for a bypass from the midthigh superficial femoral artery to the posterior tibial artery **(B)** using the spliced small saphenous vein segments. *(continued)*

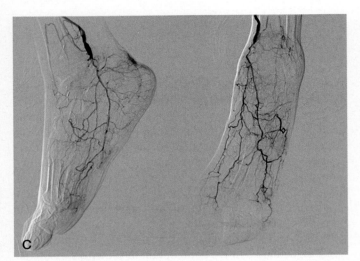

FIGURE 4.3 *(Continued)* Completion angiogram demonstrated good filling of the lateral and medial plantar arteries **(C)**. Wound débridement, resection of the distal first metatarsal, and primary wound closure was performed 4 days after the bypass operation **(D)** *(top left and right)*. Some initial wound dehiscence was noted **(D)** *(bottom left)*, but complete wound healing occurred within 3 months of the operation **(D)** *(bottom right)*. The patient's initial hospital stay was 10 days; the subsequent foot operation was performed on an outpatient basis. No complications were noted.

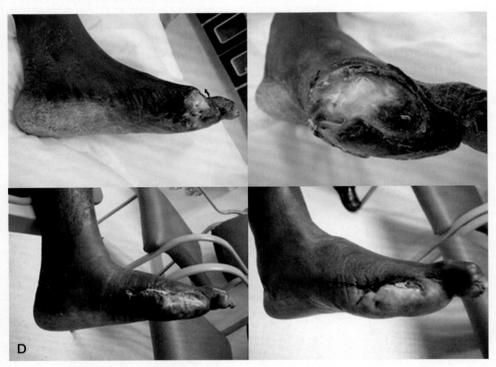

the small saphenous vein from the posterior calf—are good alternatives when no adequate caliber single-segment great saphenous vein is available. Compared to prosthetic conduits, alternative autologous veins have slightly higher patency and limb preservation rates but come at the cost of longer operative times and the need to perform adjuvant endovascular or surgical procedures to maintain patency. Small-caliber saphenous veins and allogenic (cadaveric) veins and arteries do not appear to be cost-effective options but may have some limited roles in very specific situations (11,19).

The average length of stay following infrainguinal bypasses is 5 to 7 days. The perioperative (30-day) mortality of patients undergoing in the infrainguinal bypass with saphenous vein in the Project of Ex Vivo Vein Graft Engineering via Transfection (PREVENT) III trial was 2.7% (15), and mortality among patients randomized to a surgical revascularization strategy in

the BASIL trial did not differ significantly compared to those randomized to an endovascular intervention strategy (2). Major morbidity occurred in 17% of the overall PREVENT III trial cohort, with the most common being graft occlusion, myocardial infarction, and major wound complications (approximately 5% incidence for each).

As mentioned earlier, virtually all patients with PAD should be receiving aspirin therapy unless contraindications are present. Aspirin therapy need not be discontinued prior to a leg bypass operation. There is some evidence to suggest that anticoagulation with warfarin may be helpful in optimizing patency in selected subgroups of patients undergoing bypass using autologous vein such as those with spliced vein conduits, those with suboptimal outflow vessels, and those with known hypercoagulable disorders (23). Follow-up after leg bypass using autologous vein often also includes surveillance duplex ultrasound to identify developing areas of stenosis due to neo-intimal hyperplasia that might threaten patency. These ultrasounds are typically performed at 6-month intervals during the first 2 years following bypass and yearly thereafter.

Other surgical procedures are occasionally needed in the setting of DFUs. A common femoral endarterectomy with profundoplasty and patch angioplasty addresses bulky plaques in the common femoral and proximal deep femoral arteries prior to closure with additional materials used to enlarge the caliber of the vessel. Several surgical options also exist to address hemodynamically significant aortoiliac disease when endovascular intervention is not possible. These procedures include aortobifemoral bypasses, femorofemoral bypasses, and axillobifemoral bypasses.

Comparisons of Surgical Bypass and Endovascular Treatments

To date, the BASIL trial (2) remains the only randomized study comparing endovascular intervention with surgical bypass for patients with infrainguinal PAD. Enrollment began in August 1999 and ended in June 2004. Criteria for inclusion were (a) severe limb ischemia, defined as ischemic rest pain or tissue loss (ulcer and/or gangrene) that was attributed to chronic ischemia at present for at least 2 weeks, and (b) an angiographic pattern of disease that could be treated equally well by infrainguinal bypass or balloon angioplasty. Approximately 70% of patients that were eligible based on these inclusion criteria were enrolled. Those patients meeting inclusion criteria and proving written informed consent were then allocated to surgical bypass versus endovascular in a 1:1 fashion in a randomization pattern stratified based on presentation (rest pain versus tissue loss) and ankle pressure (above/equal versus below 50 mmHg). The primary endpoint was major (above-ankle) amputation-free and overall survival after a minimum of 3 years follow-up. The trial was designed to have 90% power to detect a 15% difference in amputation-free survival. Secondary outcome measures included early (30-day) morbidity and mortality, reinterventions, health-related quality of life, and use of hospital resources.

In total, 224 patients were assigned to an angioplasty-first strategy, and 228 patients were assigned to a surgery-first strategy. Of those assigned to the surgery-first group, 85% underwent bypass surgery, whereas 96% of those randomized to the angioplasty-first strategy underwent an initial endovascular intervention. The mean amputation-free survival of the 2 groups did not differ significantly: 3.84 years for the surgery group and 3.62 years for the angioplasty group.

The results of the BASIL trial have been criticized as having low relevance to contemporary practice based on several features (14). The patient population consisted of those with "severe limb ischemia, defined as those with rest pain or tissue loss (ulcer or gangrene) of presumed arterial etiology for more than 2 weeks" (2). In contrast, PREVENT III and many observational studies have focused on the more restricted subgroup of "critical" limb ischemia, defined as those with ischemic rest pain alone and ankle or toe pressures less than 50 and 30 mmHg, respectively, or those with nonhealing ulcers or gangrene and ankle or toe pressures less than 70 and 50 mmHg, respectively (15). About

TABLE 4.1		
Comparison of Study Populations in the BASIL and PREVENT III Trials		
	BASIL (N = 452)	PREVENT III (N = 1,404)
Diabetes mellitus	190 (42.0%)	900 (64.1%)
Foot ulcer or gangrene	336 (74.3%)	1,046 (74.5%)
Current or former cigarette smoking	363 (80.3%)	1,033 (73.6%)
Tibial or pedal target for bypass	55 of 179 (30.7%)	914 (65.1%)
Vein conduit	136 of 179 (76.0%)	1,404 (100%)

BASIL, Bypass versus Angioplasty in Severe Ischemia of the Leg; PREVENT, Project of Ex Vivo Vein Graft Engineering via Transfection.

one quarter of patients in the BASIL trial did not meet criteria for critical limb ischemia (24).

Compared to the PREVENT III, the BASIL trial study sample had fewer bypasses to tibial or pedal targets (65.1% versus 30.7%, respectively) (Table 4.1) and somewhat fewer bypasses using vein conduit (100% versus 76.0%, respectively). Isolated infrapopliteal targets comprised only 7% of the endovascular interventions. Only 58% took antiplatelet medications, and 34% took statins in the BASIL study sample. The overwhelming majority of endovascular interventions consisted of balloon angioplasty alone; stents were used in only 3% of the group randomized to the endovascular cohort and 2% of the total cohort. The use of duplex ultrasound surveillance for bypass grafts was not standardized. Based on the BASIL trial, investigators in the United Kingdom are also now enrolling patients into the BASIL 2 trial. Similar to original BASIL trial, BASIL 2 is a randomized comparison of endovascular-first and vein bypass-first revascularization strategies but allows for stent placement (21).

The randomized, multicenter, controlled trial to compare Best Endovascular versus best Surgical Therapy in patients with Critical Limb Ischemia (BEST-CLI) trial (20) hopes to address some of the perceived limitations in the BASIL trial. Currently in the enrollment phase, the BEST-CLI trial is randomizing patients with significant PAD (so-called critical limb ischemia) and ischemic rest pain, nonhealing foot wounds, or gangrene to endovascular or surgical revascularization. Site study investigators must agree that a trial subject must have feasible endovascular and surgical treatment options prior to randomization. Randomization is stratified based on the presence of ischemic rest pain alone versus nonhealing foot wounds or gangrene as well as based on the presence or absence of adequate single-segment great saphenous vein.

Several good-quality meta-analyses provide composite estimates of outcomes for various surgical and endovascular revascularization options. Perhaps the most thorough of these studies are the meta-analyses that provide pooled analyses of outcomes following infrapopliteal bypass using alternative (i.e., nonsaphenous) autologous vein (4), infrapopliteal bypass using prosthetic conduit (3), infrapopliteal bypass using allogeneic vein (5), and infrapopliteal angioplasty (22).

Cost and Cost-effectiveness Considerations

Our group has performed a series of formal cost-effectiveness analyses using probabilistic Markov models to simulate events following various revascularization strategies. The rate of clinical events and the estimates of health utilities in the model were based on an extensive review of the best quality evidence available on the topic (6). Cost estimates were obtained from literature and from a single-center study of costs obtained using activity-based costing methodology (7). These analyses suggested that bypass using single-segment saphenous vein may be the most cost-effective revascularization strategy, but endovascular intervention may be reasonable for smaller foot wounds (7). These studies may be relevant to clinical settings with limited health care resources. The cost drivers identified in these studies may also be of interest to those looking for opportunities to contain costs and improve the value of revascularization strategies performed in the setting of nonhealing foot wounds.

Conclusion

Endovascular intervention and surgical bypass are both effective methods of improving arterial blood flow to the foot in patients with DFUs or areas of gangrene. Adequate distal targets are necessary for either form of revascularization to be effective. Revascularization should be considered in diabetic patients with some degree of lower extremity function (i.e., use in ambulation, transfers). Infrainguinal bypass is associated with a lower perioperative mortality than major (above-ankle) amputation in high-risk patients, so the presence of systemic comorbidities should generally not be interpreted as a contraindication to lower extremity surgical bypass procedures.

References

1. Abou-Zamzam AM Jr, Lee RW, Moneta GL, et al. Functional outcome after infrainguinal bypass for limb salvage. J Vasc Surg 1997;25:287–295.

2. Adam DJ, Beard JD, Cleveland T, et al. Bypass versus angioplasty in severe ischaemia of the leg (BASIL): multicentre, randomised controlled trial. Lancet 2005;366:1925–1934.

3. Albers M, Battistella VM, Romiti M, et al. Meta-analysis of polytetrafluoroethylene bypass grafts to infrapopliteal arteries. J Vasc Surg 2003;37:1263–1269.

4. Albers M, Romiti M, Brochado-Neto FC, et al. Meta-analysis of alternate autologous vein bypass grafts to infrapopliteal arteries. J Vasc Surg 2005;42:449–455.

5. Albers M, Romiti M, Pereira CA, et al. Meta-analysis of allograft bypass grafting to infrapopliteal arteries. Eur J Vasc Endovasc Surg 2004;28:462–472.

6. Barshes NR, Belkin M. A framework for the evaluation of "value" and cost-effectiveness in the management of critical limb ischemia. J Am Coll Surg 2011;213:552–566.

7. Barshes NR, Chambers JD, Cohen J, et al. Cost-effectiveness in the contemporary management of critical limb ischemia with tissue loss. J Vasc Surg 2012;56:1015.e1–1024.e1.

8. Barshes NR, Gold B, Garcia A, et al. Minor amputation and palliative wound care as a strategy to avoid major amputation in patients with foot infections and severe peripheral arterial disease. Int J Low Extrem Wounds 2014;13:211–219.

9. Barshes NR, Kougias P, Ozaki CK, et al. Cost-effectiveness of revascularization for limb preservation in patients with marginal functional status. Ann Vasc Surg 2014;28:10–17.

10. Barshes NR, Menard MT, Nguyen LL, et al. Infrainguinal bypass is associated with lower perioperative mortality than major amputation in high-risk surgical candidates. J Vasc Surg 2011;53:1251–1259.

11. Barshes NR, Ozaki CK, Kougias P, et al. A cost-effectiveness analysis of infrainguinal bypass in the absence of great saphenous vein conduit. J Vasc Surg 2013;57:1466–1470.

12. Boyko EJ, Ahroni JH, Stensel V, et al. A prospective study of risk factors for diabetic foot ulcer. The Seattle Diabetic Foot Study. Diabetes Care 1999;22:1036–1042.

13. Brewster DC, Charlesworth PM, Monahan JE, et al. Isolated popliteal segment v tibial bypass. Comparison of hemodynamic and clinical results. Arch Surg 1984;119:775–779.

14. Conte MS. Bypass versus angioplasty in severe ischaemia of the leg (BASIL) and the (hoped for) dawn of evidence-based treatment for advanced limb ischemia. J Vasc Surg 2010;51(5 suppl):69S–75S.

15. Conte MS, Bandyk DF, Clowes AW, et al. Results of PREVENT III: a multicenter, randomized trial of edifoligide for the prevention of vein graft failure in lower extremity bypass surgery. J Vasc Surg 2006;43:742–751.

16. Gedikoglu M, Oguzkurt L, Gur S, et al. Comparison of ultrasound guidance with the traditional palpation and fluoroscopy method for the common femoral artery puncture. Catheter Cardiovasc Interv 2013;82:1187–1192.

17. Jackson MR, Belott TP, Dickason T, et al. The consequences of a failed femoropopliteal bypass grafting: comparison of saphenous vein and PTFE grafts. J Vasc Surg 2000;32:498–505.

18. Kaufman JL, Whittemore AD, Couch NP, et al. The fate of bypass grafts to an isolated popliteal artery segment. Surgery 1982;92:1027–1031.

19. McPhee JT, Barshes NR, Ozaki CK, et al. Optimal conduit choice in the absence of single-segment great saphenous vein for below-knee popliteal bypass. J Vasc Surg 2012;55:1008–1014.

20. Menard MT, Farber A. The BEST-CLI trial: a multidisciplinary effort to assess whether surgical or endovascular therapy is better for patients with critical limb ischemia. Semin Vasc Surg 2014;27:82–84.

21. Popplewell MA, Davies H, Jarrett H, et al. Bypass versus angioplasty in severe ischaemia of the leg - 2 (BASIL-2) trial: study protocol for a randomised controlled trial. Trials 2016;17:11.

22. Romiti M, Albers M, Brochado-Neto FC, et al. Meta-analysis of infrapopliteal angioplasty for chronic critical limb ischemia. J Vasc Surg 2008;47:975–981.

23. Sarac TP, Huber TS, Back MR, et al. Warfarin improves the outcome of infrainguinal vein bypass grafting at high risk for failure. J Vasc Surg 1998;28:446–457.

24. Second European consensus document on chronic critical leg ischemia. Circulation 1991;84(4 suppl):IV1–IV26.

CHAPTER 5

Elective Surgical Reconstruction for the Diabetic Foot

Barry I. Rosenblum • John M. Giurini • Drew H. Taft

INTRODUCTION

Surgery on the diabetic foot has historically consisted of operating only in the presence of acute infection or when performing an amputation. Several misconceptions have perpetuated this, including the risk of infection or amputation if diabetic foot surgery was to fail, or the risk of performing an elective procedure in a diabetic patient that may not heal (30).

As our understanding of diabetes mellitus has improved, the medical community has realized that recurrent diabetic foot ulcerations treated with protracted conservative care instead of definitive surgery may be at higher risk for infections, hospitalizations, patient deconditioning, and amputations. Physicians and surgeons are beginning to recognize the importance of elective diabetic foot surgery in helping patients to stay active and ulcer-free (5,14,26,32,36).

Classification of Diabetic Foot Surgery

Corey (17) subdivided elective procedures into prophylactic, reconstructive, and traumatic. Later, Armstrong and Frykberg (3) classified diabetic foot procedures as being ablative, curative, or prophylactic/reconstructive (Table 5.1). More recently, Armstrong et al. (4) developed a classification system that was validated in 2006 and was based on the presence or absence of 3 characteristics: (a) sensory neuropathy, (b) open wound, and (c) acute or limb-threatening infection. According to this classification system, the vascular status of the lower extremity must be adequate for healing prior to surgery unless it is considered emergent in which case alternative measures should be used in the interim (4). This system is divided into 4 classes:

Class I (Elective): procedures for painful deformities in diabetic patients without neuropathy or open wounds

Class II (Prophylactic): procedures for prevention of ulceration in diabetic patients with neuropathy but no open wounds

Class III (Curative): procedures to help heal open ulcerations in diabetic patients with peripheral neuropathy

Class IV (Emergent): procedures performed in the setting of acute infection

Goals of Elective Surgery in the Diabetic Foot

The primary goals of elective foot surgery in the diabetic patient with peripheral neuropathy are to prevent foot ulceration, infection, and amputation by creating 1 or a combination of the following:

1. Stability
2. Realignment
3. Plantigrade foot amenable to bracing or shoe accommodation
4. Reduction of pressure points or "surgical off-loading"

This concept often requires correcting the underlying structural osseous deformities and/or tendon imbalances, which lead to skin breakdown. The goal of this surgical intervention is to eliminate increased areas of pressure and thereby reduce callus formation and subsequent diabetic foot ulcer development. If open wounds are already present, surgery may be necessary to excise wounds and address the underlying deformity. Elective diabetic foot surgery may also be utilized in the setting of previous amputations or Charcot neuroarthropathy (CN) where the residual deformities and tendon imbalances have created high-risk areas for ulcerations (4).

History and Physical Examination

Timing of surgical intervention is patient-specific, although the medical status and underlying pathology are clearly very important factors when considering surgery. When dealing with elective, prophylactic, and/or reconstructive surgeries, a multidisciplinary team approach for the medical and surgical management of the diabetic patient is the key for success. Further evaluation by the patient's primary care physician, cardiologist, nephrologist, nutritionist, or another specialist may be necessary prior to surgical intervention. Sadoskas et al. (52) found that perioperative hyperglycemia >200 mg/dL was associated with increased rates of surgical site infection after foot and ankle surgery. In addition, although glycemic control may influence postoperative complication rates in elective foot and ankle surgery, it has also been shown that medical

TABLE 5.1	
Classification of Diabetic Foot Surgery	
Class	**Examples**
Ablative	Amputations, surgical débridements, incision and drainage
Curative	Partial or complete removal of a bone such as a metatarsal head, sesamoid, accessory bone, exostosis, or calcanectomy
Prophylactic/ Reconstructive	Realignment osteotomies or tendon balancing procedures, arthrodesis, Charcot neuroarthropathy reconstruction

comorbid conditions and the presence of peripheral neuropathy also play a significant role (20,65).

Diabetic Foot Assessment and Surgical Timing

When considering elective or prophylactic foot surgery, every diabetic patient should be evaluated completely. Assessment of the entire patient, including his or her current medical status and social environment, must be fully understood and taken into consideration. Finally, evaluation of the lower extremity must confirm the absence of infection and ischemia.

Conservative measures such as ulcer débridement, lower extremity off-loading, and appropriate wound care should be attempted first. The percentage of wound healing achieved over time can serve as a general guide to help physicians decide when an alternative approach is necessary. If there has been less than 50% reduction in the size of an ulcer after 4 weeks of standard care, more aggressive therapies including surgical intervention should be entertained (56). However, this approach does not apply to every diabetic patient, whereas treatment and decision making must be adaptive, attentive, and flexible. Diabetic foot and/or ankle deformities that are unstable or severely malaligned may warrant more aggressive measures on initial presentation.

Prior to elective diabetic foot and/or ankle surgical procedures, acute infection should be controlled. When incision and drainage or surgical débridement procedures are contemplated, they should be planned with the final functional outcome in mind. However, a chronic wound without evidence of active infection may be present in the setting of an elective procedure, especially if the procedure will eliminate or aid in closure of the wound.

Evaluation of the patient's vascular status must also be carefully and thoroughly executed. Risk factors and history of peripheral arterial disease may give clues to vascular insufficiency. The absence of a palpable pedal pulse is not normal and warrants further investigation. Noninvasive vascular studies are often a good start and may include ankle-brachial indices, Doppler waveforms, pulse volume recordings, segmental

pressures, and transcutaneous tissue oxygen tension. Relying completely on ankle-brachial indices is not recommended because they may be falsely elevated due to noncompressible vessels. Segmental pressures can be obtained as distal as the toes if surgery involves the forefoot. If there are any concerns with the vascular testing results, diabetic patients should be referred for arteriography and vascular consultation. Surgery should be postponed in diabetic patients with questionable or poor vascular perfusion until adequately revascularized (33,40,49,66).

ELECTIVE SURGICAL PROCEDURES FOR THE DIABETIC FOOT

Forefoot

Lesser Toes

Toe deformities, in the presence of diabetic peripheral neuropathy, can lead to ulceration that may rapidly extend to the underlying phalanges. When conservative management fails, simple surgical procedures can be very effective at reducing the risk of future ulceration or infection.

Location of the ulceration may vary by the toe deformity type. Ulcerations can occur at the distal tip, at the apex of a flexed joint dorsally, or on the sides of adjacent toes (Fig. 5.1). An essential characteristic in choosing the appropriate procedure is the degree of toe rigidity, as determined by the Kelikian push-up test. Other factors also play a role in the surgical decision-making process including the location of the preulceration or ulcer, etiology, biomechanics, and degree of deformity. Special care should be taken to preserve the second toe when feasible. Absence of the second toe frequently contributes to the formation or progression of a hallux abductovalgus (HAV) deformity, which may then ulcerate.

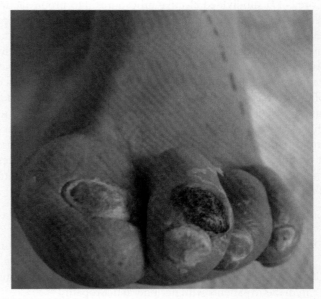

FIGURE 5.1 Infected ischemic ulcer occurring at the apex of a flexed second toe.

This elevated risk lowers the threshold for corrective procedures of the second toe relative to the other toes.

Flexible or reducible toe deformities tend to be supported by soft tissue contractures. These may be corrected by a number of procedures including, but not limited, to tenotomies, capsulotomies, tendon transfers, or lengthenings. Distal tuft toe ulcers frequently respond well to simple flexor tenotomies via stab incisions that may be performed in the clinical setting (59). This procedure is performed with the toe held in a slightly extended position to create tension on the flexor tendon. Using a no. 61 surgical blade, a small stab incision is made within the plantar skin crease beneath the proximal interphalangeal joint (PIPJ) or distal interphalangeal joint (DIPJ), corresponding to the level of deformity. Slight side to side motion is made to release the flexor tendon with care not to extend too far medially or laterally to compromise the neurovascular structures. Once the flexor tendon is transected, the surgeon should immediately see reduction of the deformity. Care should be taken not to drive the no. 61 surgical blade too deep to compromise the capsular structures as this could destabilize the joint.

A rigid toe deformity is indicative of severe soft tissue contractures as well as joint adaptation. These contractures are best managed with joint destructive procedures such as standard arthroplasty or arthrodesis at the site of maximal deformity. In most instances of a rigid hammertoe, a standard arthroplasty with resection of the underlying joint may suffice. If osteomyelitis is present, this procedure may help confirm the diagnosis and be therapeutic, may reduce the need for prolonged parenteral antibiotics, and may avoid amputation. Armstrong et al. (5) looked at the lesser toe arthroplasty in diabetic and nondiabetic patients and found that although diabetic patients with peripheral neuropathy were more likely to develop an infection postoperatively than diabetic patients with peripheral neuropathy with no history of ulceration and nondiabetic patients, the long-term outcome of a 96.3% success rate (remaining ulcer-free) at the previous site of ulceration was uniformly good. A distal Symes toe amputation should also be considered for rigid toe deformities. This procedure allows bone biopsy diagnosis and removal of a nonhealing ulcer, confirms clear margins regarding the osteomyelitis, and addresses the underlying toe deformity to minimize the chances of repeat ulceration (9).

If there are open ulcers or calluses present at the time of the procedure, they can either be allowed to heal by secondary intention or excised. If the ulcer or callus is located over the dorsal aspect of the PIPJ, it can often be easily excised by incorporating this into the incision planning. Converging semielliptical incisions are very effective in this clinical case scenario. Distal tuft toe ulcers may also be excised and primarily closed via a separate procedure or allowed to heal by secondary intention as the deforming forces have now alleviated pressure from this area.

Weight bearing in a postoperative shoe is generally allowed following toe surgery. The postoperative shoe prevents bending forces from exerting flexion of the toes. Cork or other padding may be built into the surgical shoe to allow the toes to float freely in space but is generally not necessary. Stabilization of toes may be maintained via Kirschner wires (K-wires) or dressings throughout the postoperative period. K-wires are often employed to help maintain correction postoperatively but are deferred if there are open toe ulcers at the time of surgery. If utilized, K-wires typically remain in place for at least 3 weeks following surgery. Betadine splints are frequently used in lieu of K-wires if open ulcerations are present and serve 2 important roles: (a) Betadine splints are effective for preventing infection in the setting of open ulcerations and (b) when Betadine splints are dried, the Betadine forms a stabilizing toe splint.

Hallux and First Metatarsophalangeal Joint

Dysfunction, faulty biomechanics, or absence of the hallux may predispose the patient to an altered gait pattern and pressure distribution. Most commonly, pronation increases during midstance and propulsion creates increased forces and pressures through the hallux. A number of structural deformities such as pes planovalgus, hallux rigidus, HAV, hallux malleus, pes cavus, and rigid plantarflexed first ray (hallux and metatarsal) increase the risk of hallux and first metatarsophalangeal joint (MTPJ) ulceration (Fig. 5.2). Preservation of the first ray is critical, and it is imperative to prevent ulceration with subsequent infection and amputation of this site.

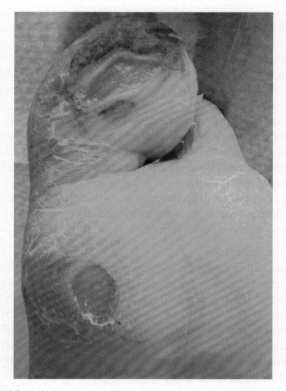

FIGURE 5.2 Structural deformities such as hallux abductovalgus, pes planovalgus, hallux malleus, hallux rigidus, and an elongated, plantarflexed first ray can predispose diabetic neuropathic patients to the development of hallux and/or first metatarsal ulcers.

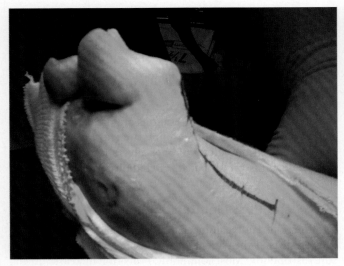

FIGURE 5.3 A hallux malleus deformity causing a dorsal hallux interphalangeal joint and plantar metatarsophalangeal joint ulcers requiring a Jones tenosuspension and hallux interphalangeal joint arthrodesis.

TABLE 5.2

Elective Surgical Options for Diabetic First Ray Pathology

Curative	Prophylactic/ Reconstructive
Exostectomy	Phalangeal osteotomies
Accessory bone excision	First metatarsal osteotomies
Condylectomy	Hallux interphalangeal joint arthrodesis
Sesamoidectomy or sesamoidal planing	First metatarsophalangeal joint arthrodesis
Hallux interphalangeal joint arthroplasty	First metatarsophalangeal joint release[a]
First metatarsophalangeal joint arthroplasty (Keller arthroplasty)	Tendon procedures[b]
First metatarsophalangeal joint cheilectomy	Tenotomies
First metatarsal head resection	Tendon transfers

[a]Including capsulotomies and capsulorrhaphies.
[b]Examples include Jones tenosuspension and peroneus longus lengthening for sub-first metatarsal head ulcers.

Ulceration of the hallux is most frequently seen at the plantar medial aspect because it is the widest part of the soft tissue envelope. It is further subjected to increased friction, especially in the presence of HAV, hallux limitus, or pes planovalgus deformities. Other sites such as the medial and plantar first MTPJ are prone to ulceration as well. Hallux malleus deformities can cause calluses or ulcerations around the distal tuft, dorsal interphalangeal joint (IPJ), or plantar MTPJ from retrograde pressures (Fig. 5.3). If joint contracture is absent, plantar IPJ ulceration in this area may be from an exostosis or accessory bone (25).

Surgical options for hallux or first MTPJ deformities and ulcerations may be thought of as either curative or prophylactic/reconstructive-type procedures. When partial or complete resection of bone is performed, it is classified as curative. However, when realignment is achieved, either through soft tissue or osseous procedures, it is considered as reconstructive. Some of the more common procedures on the first ray are shown in Table 5.2.

SESAMOIDECTOMY

As the hallux dorsiflexes, the sesamoid bones move distally and become more prominent. This may result in ulceration plantar to these bones. Chronic wounds in this location may benefit from removal of the associated sesamoid(s). Owing to its size and greater association with musculoskeletal deformity, the tibial sesamoid is more commonly associated with ulceration than its lateral counterpart. The advantages of this procedure include the ability to place incisions on non–weight-bearing surfaces, no hardware required, and no osteotomy to heal.

Incision placement primarily depends on whether an ulceration is present and its size and depth. A direct plantar approach is typically only advocated in the setting of an open ulceration, and absent infection will allow for ulcer excision and primary closure. If the fibular and/or tibial sesamoid(s) is to be removed, then incisions can be placed on non–weight-bearing surfaces medially. If an isolated fibular sesamoidectomy is planned without deep ulceration, then a dorsal approach through the first interspace may be considered but may be more difficult in the rectus first MTPJ.

Typically, a longitudinal incision is made along the plantar-medial junction of the first MTPJ. The nearby neurovascular elements are retracted inferiorly followed by incision of the joint capsule at this location. Soft tissue attachments are carefully released about the plantar surface to facilitate resection. Smaller surgical blades, such as a no. 64 Beaver blade, may aid in releasing the sesamoidal attachments in more confined areas. Removal of both sesamoids can be facilitated through this medial approach, but care must be taken to preserve the flexor tendons.

Because this surgical procedure does not require bone healing or fixation, the postoperative course is largely dictated by incision placement. Incisions placed in non–weight-bearing areas such as the plantar-medial or dorsal approaches permit immediate partial weight bearing in a postoperative shoe. However, complete non–weight-bearing of at least 3 to 4 weeks is required for plantar incisions. Plantar ulcers allowed to heal via secondary intention can be off-weighted with padding, felted foam dressings, traditional casting, posterior splint or total contact casting.

Whether 1 or both sesamoids are removed, the biomechanics of the first ray can become altered. Removal of a tibial sesamoid may worsen an HAV deformity, and fibular sesamoidectomy may cause a hallux varus deformity. Complete removal of both sesamoids, especially in pes cavus deformities, may be considered, but an adjunctive hallux IPJ arthrodesis should be performed concomitantly, along with transfer of the extensor hallucis longus tendon to the first metatarsal neck to avoid subsequent hallux malleus deformity. Failure to do this may increase the risk of transfer lesions plantar to the lesser metatarsals.

Giurini et al. (24) examined the sesamoidectomy procedure in 26 feet of 24 diabetic neuropathic patients, with 13 being tibial sesamoidectomies and 13 being total sesamoidectomies. With a mean follow-up of 33 months, a 16% reulceration rate was noted after a mean 22 months postoperatively. None of the study participants developed HAV; however, 8% did develop a hallux hammertoe (24).

HALLUX INTERPHALANGEAL JOINT ARTHROPLASTY

Plantar and dorsal hallux IPJ ulcerations in the presence of a normal first MTPJ may benefit from a hallux IPJ arthroplasty. Plantar hallux IPJ ulcerations from enlarged condyles or accessory bones often do well with this procedure because the bony prominence can be removed through the arthroplasty site. More common causes of plantar ulceration include IPJ hyperextension from hallux limitus/rigidus or pronation causing a plantar medial pinch callus or ulceration (19). Arthroplasty of the hallux IPJ, indicated in a foot without a significant biomechanical abnormality at the first MTPJ such as hallux valgus or hallux limitus/rigidus, may also be used when osteomyelitis is present at the hallux IPJ (11,38,47). Diabetic patients with a structural deformity at the first MTPJ may be best served with the Keller arthroplasty procedure, which will be described in the following section.

The hallux IPJ arthroplasty is typically approached via either a dorsal longitudinal or serpentine incision to allow for joint preparation. The extensor hallucis longus is either retracted laterally or tenotomized to gain access to the joint and repaired at the conclusion of the procedure. The head of the proximal phalanx is resected with the osteotomy perpendicular to the longitudinal axis of the phalanx. Stabilization following arthroplasty is discretionary and may require no more than splinting. The use of a single K-wire has also been described (38).

Arthroplasty of the hallux permits partial weight bearing in a postoperative shoe. A recurrent theme throughout these procedures that involve surgical off-loading is that weight bearing is protected until the index ulcer has healed. Following hallux IPJ arthroplasty, hallux shortening is an expected postoperative finding but is rarely problematic. Inadequate bone resection may allow ulcer recurrence. If hallux malleus develops as a complication from this procedure, transfer lesions or ulcerations may develop beneath the base of the proximal phalanx or first metatarsal head, necessitating arthrodesis of this joint. A study by Rosenblum et al. (47) examined outcomes of this procedure in 39 patients. Ninety-one percent of

patients healed without reulceration with a mean follow-up of 23.6 months (47). Other studies have shown success with this procedure as well (11,38).

FIRST METATARSOPHALANGEAL JOINT ARTHROPLASTY (KELLER ARTHROPLASTY)

If structural deformity of the first MTPJ exists, a Keller arthroplasty procedure, which resects a portion of the proximal phalanx base, may be appropriate. This procedure is primarily indicated when structural deformities, such as HAV or hallux rigidus, cause ulcerations of the first ray. Other general indications of the Keller arthroplasty include advanced degenerative changes of the first MTPJ, elderly patients with deformity, and an elongated hallux (6,8,25,60).

The surgical incision placement includes a linear or curvilinear incision medial to the extensor hallucis longus that allows for excellent visualization of the first MTPJ. A medially based U-capsulotomy provides good joint exposure and can be interposed within the first MTPJ joint at the conclusion of the surgical procedure. The proximal one-third of the proximal phalanx is resected. Depending on the primary deformity, additional bone cuts such as cheilectomies or medial eminence resections of the first metatarsal are performed. It is important to tether the flexor hallucis longus tendon to prevent a floating hallux or poor hallux purchase. This can be achieved either by suture routed through drill holes or attached to phalangeal soft tissue anchors. Finally, the U-capsulotomy is wrapped around the first metatarsal head and sutured into the soft tissues laterally. K-wires, Betadine splints, or taping techniques may be utilized to maintain the corrected position and is based on surgeon's preference, the presence of ulceration, and whether soft tissue anchors were utilized.

Because this procedure does not require bone healing and the incision is placed on non–weight-bearing areas, partial weight bearing in a postoperative shoe is permitted. Elevation and compression of the lower extremity will help minimize swelling. Sutures generally remain in place for 3 to 4 weeks. The patient may then transition to an athletic shoe based on symptoms and surgeon's preference.

Like the hallux IPJ arthroplasty, shortening of the hallux is expected and usually is asymptomatic. Other potential complications include reulceration, lesser metatarsalgia, poor hallux purchase, deformity recurrence, and flail toe. Many modifications of the Keller arthroplasty have been suggested to prevent these potential complications. One of the most important modifications is tethering or attaching the flexor hallucis longus tendon to the remaining proximal phalanx to improve toe purchase and digital stabilization.

Armstrong and colleagues (6) compared this technique to conservative care in 41 diabetic neuropathic patients. The surgical group healed in 24.2 (±9.9) days and reulcerated in 4.8% of subjects. This compared well to the 67.1 (±17.1) days and 35% reulceration rate of the conservative care group (6). Although there is the possibility of transfer ulcerations, the overall success rate has been shown to be significant, with resolution of the index ulcer as quickly as 3.1 weeks (8,60).

First Metatarsal Head Resection

Another option for an ulceration plantar or medial to the first metatarsal head is complete resection of the metatarsal head. This procedure is typically reserved for patients with existing ulcers that communicate with the first MTPJ or bone. Ulcer excision with metatarsal head resection is frequently performed concomitantly (18,25,34). This is appropriate in the absence of infection, and if the surrounding soft tissue envelop is amenable to a tension-free closure. If there are preulcerative lesions or superficial ulcerations, procedures which do not disrupt the metatarsal parabola are recommended over the metatarsal head resection.

The surgical incisional approach depends on the presence and depth of ulceration. If the patient has no open ulceration or a superficial plantar ulcer, either a standard dorsal or medial incision centered over the first MTPJ is performed (34). However, if there is a dorsal, medial, or deep plantar ulcer, an incision which encompasses the ulcer is preferred (18). This allows for direct exploration and débridement of soft tissue, excision of the ulcer, and primary closure. Because the metatarsal head is to be resected, there is less concern for contamination from the open wound. A biplanar osseous cut resects more bone plantarly and medially to avoid future prominences. K-wires, Steinmann pins, Betadine splints, or taping techniques may be utilized based on the individual situation and surgeon's preference (34). Adjunctive use of antibiotic-impregnated polymethylmethacrylate cemented beads and/or spacers and the use of an external fixator have been described with reasonably good results (18). Care must be taken with respect to the length of the remaining first metatarsal in order to minimize the risk of reulceration (42).

Curative type procedures, such as first metatarsal head resections, do not require healing of the bone, and hardware is not needed in most situations. Because of this, the postoperative course is primarily dependent on the location of the surgical incision. If plantar incisions were required, complete non–weight-bearing for at least 3 to 4 weeks is needed to allow coaptation. However, more commonly, dorsal and medial incisions will allow partial weight bearing in a postoperative shoe. Off-weighting with padding, felted foam dressings, or casting is recommended if plantar ulcers were allowed to heal by secondary intention (Fig. 5.4).

Potential complications following first metatarsal head resections include, but are not limited to, flail toe, hallux malleus, and decreased propulsion. One of the more difficult complications to manage is transfer ulcerations. Patients often require accommodative padding and custom-made extra-depth shoes with close postoperative monitoring. These transfer ulcerations can develop quickly, and if managed inappropriately, lead to infection and osteomyelitis. Future procedures may be necessary if padding cannot prevent these ulcerations from occurring.

Alternate Surgical Procedures Related to the First Ray

Osteotomies of the proximal phalanx and first metatarsal should be considered for preulcerative regions of the first metatarsal head and for ulcerations that do not extend to

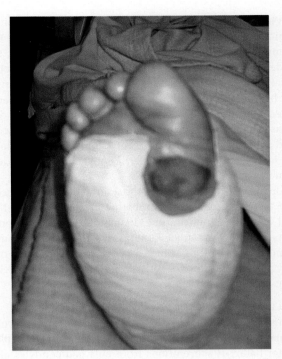

FIGURE 5.4 If ulcers are allowed to heal by secondary intention following surgical intervention, plantar ulcers must be off-weighted. A felted foam dressing or equivalent is recommended in this clinical case scenario.

the bone or joint, whereas arthrodesis of the first MTPJ may be performed as an effective and beneficial procedure with the understanding that those diabetic patients with peripheral neuropathy may be at increased risk for mild and moderate complications (1). Indications, surgical technique, postoperative management, and potential complications and outcomes for these osteotomies do not differ from patients without diabetic neuropathy. The various type of osteotomies described is quite expansive, and the osteotomy selected should address the underlying deformity.

Lesser Metatarsals

Diabetic neuropathy has been linked to intrinsic muscle wasting that leads to a cascade of biomechanical imbalances. Toe and MTPJ stabilization is largely mediated by these muscles. Failure of this balance promotes toe deformity such as hammertoes and clawtoes. As the toes dorsiflex, the fat pad migrates distally. Simultaneously, the dorsiflexed toes exert a retrograde buckling force onto the metatarsal heads further exaggerating plantar metatarsal head prominences (Fig. 5.5). Other causes of increased plantar pressures include plantarflexed or elongated metatarsals because they bear more pressure for a longer period during the gait cycle (25). Pressure is dependent on the force placed on the surface area of a structure such as a prominent lesser metatarsal head, and a biomechanical approach is a key element to the treatment of these problems. Failure to appreciate this concept will decrease the likelihood of success.

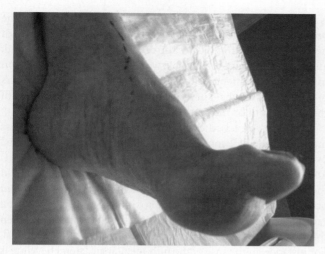

FIGURE 5.5 The development of toe contractures from intrinsic muscle wasting may lead to prominent plantar metatarsal heads from retrograde forces.

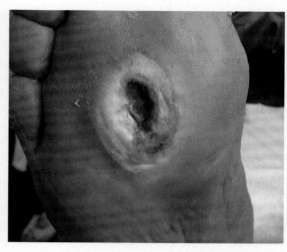

FIGURE 5.6 Example of a lesser metatarsal head plantar ulcer in a diabetic patient with peripheral neuropathy.

Ulcerations plantar to the lesser metatarsal head are among the most common problems encountered in diabetic patients with peripheral neuropathy (Fig. 5.6). Plain lower extremity radiographs can be used to rule out other clinically significant abnormalities such as osteomyelitis, stress fractures, and signs consistent with CN, but other more basic characteristics should be noted as well. Weight bearing lower extremity radiographs should be utilized to assess transverse, frontal, and sagittal plane alignment. Lesion markers are helpful in finding areas of plantar prominence. Special attention to the metatarsal parabola can identify elongated structures, whereas a lateral or axial projection may reveal a plantarflexed structure.

LESSER METATARSAL OSTEOTOMY

Metatarsal osteotomies should be considered for preulcerative regions of the metatarsal head and for ulcerations that do not extend to the bone or joint. If persistent serous drainage is present, this may indicate synovial fluid from joint involvement, and alternative procedures are recommended. As the options for different lesser metatarsal osteotomies are expansive, procedures will be limited to a select few that have been used specifically in the treatment of diabetic foot ulcers. Metatarsal osteotomies are selected based on the underlying deformity and the appearance of the plantar ulceration. In most cases, shortening osteotomies are preferred; however, elevating osteotomies may be performed as well. Most shortening metatarsal osteotomies are now based on the distal oblique method as described by Weil (63). For the insensate foot with either preulcerative or ulcerative lesions, this procedure achieves shortening of the metatarsal with reduction in plantar pressures. Modifications of the Weil lesser metatarsal osteotomy have also been described to correct transverse and frontal plane deformities as well as plantarflexed metatarsal heads (63).

Lesser metatarsal osteotomies are approached through a dorsal incision because these are considered "clean" procedures and utilize internal fixation. The dorsal incision avoids weight bearing surfaces and, more importantly, avoids contamination of the surgical site from the open ulceration. The Weil osteotomy involves an osteotomy starting 3 mm below the dorsal articular cartilage edge of the metatarsal head, directed plantarly and proximally. The osteotomy is oblique to the metatarsal shaft and kept parallel to the weight bearing surface in order to avoid plantarflexion. The capital fragment is then allowed to retract proximally a few millimeters. The metatarsal parabola is assessed, and the plantar aspect of the metatarsal head is palpated to feel for prominences while the foot is loaded. The osteotomy is typically fixated with a single screw. The procedure may also be performed without fixation, sometimes referred to as a "floating" Weil osteotomy. In the presence of osteopenic bone or history of infection, one may want to avoid internal fixation utilization. This is an inherently stable osteotomy as long as care is made to avoid excessive soft tissue dissection especially around the collateral ligaments of the associated MTPJ.

The Weil osteotomy of the second metatarsal head has been shown to decrease plantar pressures by 36% and 65% in stance phase and heel rise, respectively (35). A study by Vandeputte et al. (62) found that the Weil osteotomy resulted in a mean 52% reduction of plantar pressure from a preoperative pedobarographic examination. At a mean follow-up of 30 months, only 11% of the feet had developed a transfer lesion. Seventy-four percent of the patients were lesion-free, whereas only 5% had no visible improvement of their callus (62). Beyond the complications already mentioned, a floating toe believed to be secondary to the altered MTPJ axis has been reported in as many as 20% of these cases (55). Special attention is required to balance the soft tissue structures, with tendon transfers, lengthening, and tenotomies performed when necessary to minimize complications.

A more minimally invasive shortening metatarsal osteotomy has also been described. Tamir et al. (58) performed a perpendicular or short oblique osteotomy at the neck or diaphysis of the metatarsal with a Shannon burr through a 3-mm incision. The osteotomy results in a dorsally displaced metatarsal head. These patients had existing plantar head ulcerations of which 17/20 was healed at 6 weeks (58).

Shortening metatarsal osteotomies, such as the Weil osteotomy, allow partial weight bearing in a postoperative shoe due to its intrinsic stability. If ulcerations are present, off-loading techniques may be utilized in the postoperative period to off-weight the healing plantar wound. As with any surgery, edema control with lower extremity compressive dressings and elevation help minimize wound healing complications. Physical therapy or taping of the toes is sometimes necessary to improve toe purchase.

LESSER METATARSAL HEAD RESECTION

Lesser metatarsal head resections are considered when ulcers plantar to the metatarsal heads extend down to the bone or joint level or are infected (Fig. 5.7). In this clinical case scenario, a lesser metatarsal head resection or complete joint resection is performed. This procedure may be performed as both a therapeutic intervention, that is, to remove the underlying area of increased pressure, but also may be considered both diagnostic as well as therapeutic when dealing with the possibility of infected bone.

For solitary metatarsal head resections, 2 main surgical approaches are recommended. A dorsal curvilinear incision centered over the metatarsal allows for a "clean" approach but relies on the ulcer healing by secondary intention. This approach is typically reserved for diabetic patients unable to remain non–weight-bearing and healing of the index ulceration proceeds via secondary intention. The preferred surgical approach, however, is a plantar incision which incorporates ulcer excision, removal of the associated metatarsal head, and primary closure without skin tension (Fig. 5.8). This procedure

is particularly recommended if any concern exists about the presence of infection. This approach also allows for excision of necrotic, nonhealing tissues, direct inspection of the wound, and faster and more predictable wound healing. One exception may be the fifth metatarsal head ulcer, where it is the surgeon's preference as to what surgical approach is taken, regardless of the ulcer depth or the presence of osteomyelitis.

The ulcer is excised down to bone level via a full-thickness incision, made of 2 converging semielliptical incisions, centered over the ulceration with a length-to-width ratio of at least 3:1. The osteotomy itself should be made proximal enough within the metatarsal neck to remove any potentially infected bone and oriented dorsal-distal to plantar-proximal in order to prevent a prominent plantar edge. Slight modifications must be made when this procedure is performed on either the first or fifth metatarsal. For instance, in the case of the fifth metatarsal, lateral beveling is recommended to prevent a prominence in this location.

The base of the associated proximal phalanx at the lesser MTPJ should also always be inspected. This bone may be involved, especially if osteomyelitis is present in the metatarsal head region. If concern exists, the base of the proximal phalanx should also be removed. Other structures, such as the plantar plate and flexor tendons, should be resected if infection is present. All bone and soft tissues are sent to pathology and microbiology with separate clean margins if osteomyelitis is suspected to help determine antibiotic therapy and duration. Prior to wound closure, the area is inspected for any remaining bone spicules and aggressively irrigated. If a tourniquet was utilized, it should be deflated to ensure that resections were

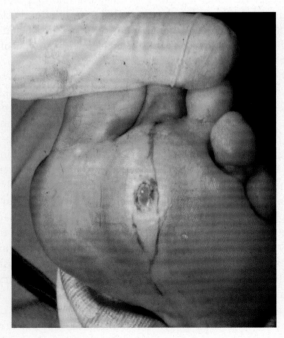

FIGURE 5.7 Lesser metatarsal ulcer with synovial-type exudate indicates deeper involvement warranting alternative procedures such as metatarsal head resections.

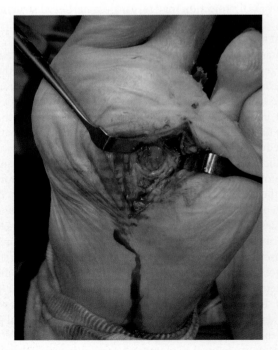

FIGURE 5.8 The direct plantar approach for metatarsal head resections allows ulcer excision, good visualization, surgical débridement, and primary closure of the wound all through 1 incision.

adequately performed to healthy bleeding bone and that there was adequate hemostasis (25).

The closure of these plantar wounds requires a simple technique. Full-thickness wide retention sutures are evenly interspaced with 2-0 or 0 nonabsorbable monofilament material, starting centrally. These large wide retention sutures allow the surgeon to avoid using deep-buried knots, which can serve as a nidus for infection. Smaller 3-0 monofilament suture is then placed in between these deeper retention sutures providing eversion of the skin edges. There is the potential for a significant dead space created from this procedure, and closed-suction surgical drains may be used to prevent hematoma. During the postoperative period, patients should be kept non–weight-bearing until the plantar skin incision has healed. Usually, sutures are removed after 3 to 4 weeks with partial weight bearing initiated by the fourth week. If a dorsal incision is utilized, weight bearing is dictated by the healing of the plantar ulcer.

Transfer lesions or ulcerations are the most commonly reported complications associated with lesser metatarsal head resections. Accommodative padding and orthotic devices are recommended with close follow-up postoperatively to assess plantar pressure distribution. Other complications include wound dehiscence, infection, flail or shortened toe, stress fractures, or development of CN. Wieman et al. (64) performed solitary and multiple metatarsal head resections in 101 patients with a mean follow-up of 35 months. They reported a 94% salvage rate but noted that ulcer recurrence was a problem in 8% and new ulcer formation was a problem in 52%. Part of the study design was such that all wounds were expected to heal by secondary intention; therefore, none of the ulcers in this study were excised (64). An earlier study by Patel and Wieman (44) reported the change in peak plantar pressure following metatarsal head resection. They noted a 70% reduction after a first metatarsal head resection, whereas resections of either the second or third metatarsals resulted in a 39% reduction. A 45% reduction was achieved by resection of either the fourth or fifth metatarsal heads (44). Faglia et al. (22) found that bone resection for osteomyelitis of the metatarsal and/or phalanx with preservation of the toe and soft tissue envelope did not result in any risk of major dehiscence or ulcer recurrence compared with ray or toe amputation.

Panmetatarsal Head Resection

Given the fact that isolated metatarsal resections may be associated with transfer ulcers, and that as a result, many patients may require repeat trips to the operating room as new ulcers form, it may be advisable to consider a panmetatarsal head resection in the presence of transfer ulcers or in feet that may be biomechanically predisposed to the development of increased pressure and therefore neuropathic and/or recurrent ulcers. Generally, once 2 or more metatarsal heads are resected, the authors advocate a panmetatarsal head resection, especially if it involves any of the 3 central metatarsals. It is in the best interest of the patient because we have found that this minimizes multiple surgical procedures and potential deconditioning of the patient. Before this procedure was popularized, transmetatarsal amputation was frequently performed for multiple

recurrent ulcerations. The panmetatarsal head resection is recommended over the transmetatarsal amputation because it maintains the metatarsal parabola and foot length. This permits easier fit in custom-made shoes and a more normal gait pattern. In addition, the panmetatarsal head resection may be psychologically more appealing to the patient, especially one who has undergone revascularization (48).

Many surgical approaches have been discussed and recommended for this procedure. These include dorsal, plantar, and combined incisions; the success of each is dictated by the desired exposure, but all are essentially equivalent. Utilizing the dorsal approach, 4 longitudinal incisions are placed in the following locations: (a) midline or medial over the first metatarsal, (b) midline over the second interspace, (c) midline over the fourth metatarsal, and (d) midline to slightly lateral over the fifth metatarsal. Each of these incisions allows for adequate exposure and minimizes excessive soft tissue retraction while preserving the vascularity of the dorsal skin.

If the plantar approach is preferred, then a transverse incision is made at the level of the toe sulcus. The exposure is not as extensive as the dorsal approach; however, careful planning allows for ulcer excision through the use of a transverse ellipse incision and without multiple incisions (Fig. 5.9). A combination of both dorsal and plantar incisions may also be employed. Plantar incisions are utilized to excise ulcers with resection of the metatarsal heads through this incision, as previously described, whereas dorsal incisions are strategically placed to remove the remaining "noncontaminated" metatarsal heads. Lastly, a creative approach to skin closure may be utilized including the possibility of a plantar rotation flap (12).

Resection of the metatarsal heads has been described in the individual metatarsal resection discussion. Bone cuts should be oriented dorsal-distal to plantar-proximal in order to prevent a plantar edge. Both the first and fifth metatarsals should

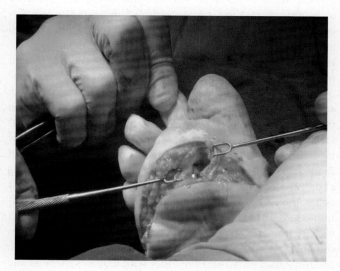

FIGURE 5.9 A transverse plantar incision can be used to excise plantar ulcers. Additional access may be obtained through dorsal incisions to remove metatarsal heads without associated ulcerations.

be beveled medially and laterally, respectively, to avoid prominences. Following metatarsal head resection, temporary toe stabilization with K-wires is recommended in the absence of deep ulcerations or osteomyelitis and is typically utilized for toes undergoing a dorsal approach.

Maintenance of the metatarsal parabola is imperative to the success of this procedure. A smooth parabola avoids creating new pressure points, and no metatarsal should be significantly longer than the adjacent one. In general, the second metatarsal is the longest. The first and third metatarsals are equal lengths and should be just slightly shorter than the second metatarsal. This is followed by the fourth and finally the fifth metatarsal being the shortest. Although the above metatarsal parabola is desired, it is not always possible due to prior surgical débridements, metatarsal, or ray resections. In these circumstances, the "desired metatarsal parabola" is created with the remaining metatarsals with padding and accommodation customized postoperatively.

Postoperative care typically should include non–weight-bearing until the plantar incision is healed. If open ulcerations were present with concern for osteomyelitis, bed rest, lower extremity elevation, compression dressings, and antibiotics are administered until the wounds are dry. Sutures typically remain for 3 to 4 weeks, and a traditional cast, posterior splint, or total contact cast may be utilized to off-load the lower extremity in the immediate postoperative period. Once incisions have healed, protected weight bearing in a postoperative shoe is initiated. Patients are gradually progressed to full weight bearing in an athletic shoe or accommodative footwear with padding, depending on the particular clinical case scenario. If another procedure such as posterior muscle group lengthening or tendon transfer has been performed, then immobilization may be dependent on that particular operation (31).

Several studies have examined outcomes following this procedure in the diabetic population with peripheral neuropathy. Giurini et al. (23) reported the outcomes of this technique in 34 procedures after a mean of 20.9 months. Sixty-one percent of the procedures included primary ulcer excision with no complications in healing. Of the remaining patients, delayed healing occurred in 1 patient, whereas another patient had recurrence of the original ulcer. None of the patients required any type of amputation by the end of the study period, and the overall salvage rate was 97%. A common complication of this procedure is new bone growth at the osteotomy metatarsal sites; in this series, 29% developed this resulting in new ulcerations. A single revisional exostectomy was required, but in most cases, conservative care was adequate (23). Armstrong et al. (2) also confirmed these results in a 2012 study. In this paper, the authors noted that patients in the surgery group exhibited faster healing and a lower reulceration rate. Petrov et al. (45), however, performed a retrospective review of 2 groups of patients undergoing panmetatarsal head resection: 1 with rheumatoid arthritis and the other with diabetes mellitus and peripheral neuropathy, examining 15 patients in the former group and 12 in the latter. The incidence of reulceration was 28% and 25%, respectively (45).

ALTERNATE SURGICAL PROCEDURES RELATED TO THE LESSER METATARSALS

Isolated or multiple metatarsal condylectomies may also be indicated in the presence of a plantar metatarsal ulceration. Prominent metatarsal condyles may be resected with either a direct approach through the plantar ulceration or through a dorsal approach in the absence of an infection or ulceration. The direct plantar approach for a metatarsal condylectomy and full-thickness excision of the concomitant ulceration is highly recommended for chronic nonhealing wounds. In addition, isolated or multiple lesser MTPJ arthrodesis procedures may be indicated in certain clinical case scenarios understanding the potential of complications in diabetic patients with peripheral neuropathy.

Midfoot/Hindfoot

When existing diabetic midfoot ulcers have failed conservative measures, they usually do not heal or become reulcerated unless the overall structure is assessed. If vascular perfusion is adequate and the soft tissues and bone are free of infection, then the primary problem is typically peripheral neuropathy combined with structural deformity.

CN is the most common structural cause of midfoot complications in diabetic patients with peripheral neuropathy. Collapse of the foot arch architecture creates increased plantar foot pressures and ulcerations from the CN rocker bottom deformity. Ulcerations can be found in any region, depending on the underlying osseous malalignment. The most frequent midfoot ulcer locations are plantar medial from either the first metatarsal-medial cuneiform joint or navicular-medial cuneiform joint (Fig. 5.10), followed by plantar lateral ulcers from cuboid dislocations or the styloid process of the fifth metatarsal. The least common ulcers are located more plantar central from collapse of the central tarsal-metatarsal region.

It is important to realize that a strict algorithm does not and should not exist for treatment of these diabetic foot complications. Instead, a more flexible approach is required, keeping in mind the goals of surgery: stability, realignment, a plantigrade foot amenable to bracing or accommodation, and reduction of pressure points. This task can be performed with or without ulcer excision combined with exostectomies, realignment osteotomies with arthrodeses, or a combination of these procedures depending on the clinical case scenario. Every diabetic CN deformity is different, and basic principles help guide the surgeon on the best procedure for each patient. Regardless of the procedure performed, an adjunctive tendo-Achilles lengthening (TAL) or gastrocnemius recession is usually indicated for many diabetic patients with peripheral neuropathy. Lengthening the Achilles tendon decreases the amount of propulsive forces transmitted to the forefoot and midfoot. Ulcer excision with primary closure is also preferred in cases without infection and may require additional skin grafting or flaps in a staged reconstruction.

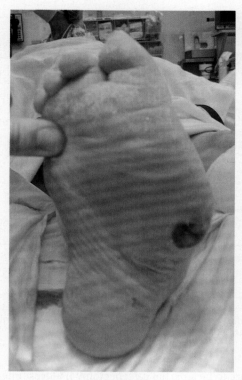

FIGURE 5.10 Collapse of the medial arch from Charcot neuro-arthropathy creates increased plantar pressures often resulting in ulcerations.

Exostectomy

The exostectomy procedure is a very simple technique to address osseous prominences within the diabetic foot where off-loading and conservative measures have failed. This surgical procedure can be very effective when used in the right circumstances. Diabetic patients with peripheral neuropathy and midfoot collapse will often have osseous prominences causing increased plantar pressures resulting in callus formation and ulceration. If the deformity is rigid and stable, an exostectomy may be the best choice. Exostectomies may also be considered in the very elderly and minimally ambulatory patient when the primary goal is to close a wound in an expedited manner in order to prevent infection. If osteomyelitis is present, an exostectomy can be curative as well as corrective. However, if any motion or joint instability exists or if the osseous resection has the potential to cause instability because of the size or location, then this isolated exostectomy procedure should be avoided. In this clinical setting, a more formal deformity correction including an arthrodesis should be considered.

Surgical incision placement for midfoot exostectomy is influenced by primarily the depth but also the size, location, and quality of the overlying soft tissues and ulcer. These 4 factors help determine whether to approach the exostectomy directly or indirectly. For indirect approaches, a separate skin incision is made away from the ulcer site, whereas direct approaches involve excising the ulcer and approaching the exostosis directly through this site.

Indirect surgical approaches are typically utilized when the midfoot exostosis is located on the plantar medial or plantar lateral aspects of the foot. Incisions can be placed on the side of the foot, avoiding the non–weight-bearing surface. These surgical approaches are reserved for more superficial ulcers that do not communicate with the bone. The overlying soft tissues should also be free of infected or nonviable tissues and bursa formation. Deeper ulcers or ulcers that can be excised with primary wound closure as previously discussed are more amenable to a direct surgical approach. If there is active infection or a history of osteomyelitis, the bone and ulcer can be directly excised. Underlying bursa tissue, even with overlying superficial granular tissue, should steer the surgeon into opting for a direct approach for concomitant bursa excision.

A variety of surgical techniques are available and dictated by the exposure and shape of the underlying midfoot osseous prominence. Osseous planing via saw is efficient, but the saw blade's excursion often limits its use. Thermal necrosis is not a concern because the goal is to prevent regrowth of the bone. However, the plantar location of these wounds often makes it very difficult to utilize power instrumentation and instead a combination of standard and curved osteotomes might be useful when osseous surfaces curve abruptly. The rongeur is appropriate for resection of small osseous prominences and shaping of residual bone. The goal of these procedures is to create a flat osseous surface without leaving a new osseous ridge or step-off. Following osseous resection, a bone rasp should smooth the surfaces as needed. The surgical site should be irrigated, and closure may include ulcer excision, and a local flap if deemed necessary.

Surgical drains are used if concern exists for hematoma formation, especially after resection of cancellous bone. Adequate compression over the incision, lower extremity elevation, and immobilization of the foot are critical. If surgical incisions are on weight bearing surfaces of the foot, non–weight-bearing is recommended for at least 3 to 4 weeks; however, typically, patients require an average of 6 to 8 weeks without placing weight on the foot.

In 1997, Rosenblum et al. (48) studied the outcomes following lateral column exostectomies of 32 feet in 31 patients who underwent an exostectomy alone ($n = 7$), with primary closure ($n = 17$), or a rotational flap ($n = 8$). They concluded that 25% of these patients required additional resection or flap coverage with an overall success rate of 89% (48). Catanzariti et al. (15) performed 27 procedures: 18 were for the treatment of medial column ulcerations, whereas the remaining 9 were lateral column wounds. They reported a 74% healing rate. However, 85% of those patients who did not heal, initially had a lateral column ulceration. Fifty-five percent of the patients with lateral column ulcers initially required some revisional surgery to facilitate healing. They reported a statistically significant difference in the rate of complication based on ulcer location. They concluded that the lateral column is less predictable and often requires an adjunctive soft tissue procedure to be successful (15). Pinzur et al. (46) used exostectomy in 8 patients and found that 100% were ambulatory in accommodative footwear after 3.6 years (46). Brodsky and Rouse (13) found that 11 of 12 patients remained healed after a mean follow-up of 25 months.

In the hindfoot, calcaneal ulcerations are a frequently encountered clinical entity, often the result of prolonged static bed rest. These ulcers are typically located along the posterior calcaneal surface; however, plantar calcaneal ulcers occur too. Nonhealing calcaneal wounds should be evaluated for chronic infection or osteomyelitis. Most importantly, the vascular status must be carefully assessed in this clinical setting. Depending on the size of the involved calcaneal ulceration, a simple exostectomy may be adequate; however, for more extensive involvement, some type of calcanectomy may be required (Fig. 5.11). Calcanectomies are only recommended for well-perfused lower extremities when ulceration with osteomyelitis exists or if the patient is minimally to nonambulatory and primary wound closure is desired. The goals of a calcanectomy are to remove infected bone and create redundancy for primary wound closure, which should help facilitate wound healing to avoid more proximal lower extremity amputations.

There are 3 types of calcanectomy, the most extreme being the total calcanectomy. Indications for a total calcanectomy are limited and often result in destabilization of the subtalar and even ankle joint. More commonly, the partial and subtotal calcanectomies are used to achieve the goals previously mentioned. The exact definition of each procedure has not been previously described and is generally related to the amount of bone resected. At our institution, we consider the

Class	Definition
Total calcanectomy	Complete removal of the calcaneus
Subtotal calcanectomy	Partial resection of the calcaneus including removal of the calcaneal tuberosity with detachment of the Achilles tendon
Partial calcanectomy	At least one-third of the calcaneus resected but Achilles tendon still intact. This may include plantar fascia detachment.
Calcaneal débridement	Removal of less than one-third of the calcaneus with an intact Achilles tendon

TABLE 5.3

Calcanectomy Classification

Adapted from Cook J, Cook E, Landsman AS, et al. A retrospective assessment of partial calcanectomies and factors influencing postoperative course. J Foot Ankle Surg 2007;46:248–255.

procedure to be a partial calcanectomy if at least one-third of the calcaneus is resected. However, if the resection requires removal of the calcaneal tuberosity and therefore Achilles tendon detachment, it is classified as subtotal calcanectomy (Table 5.3).

The surgical approach to calcanectomies includes a longitudinal elliptical incision encompassing the ulceration made on the posterior surface of the calcaneus. Additionally, alternative incisions have been described, each dealing with a different type of calcaneal ulcer, but all leading to closure of these difficult wounds after calcanectomy has been performed (10). After isolation of the calcaneus, an oblique osteotomy, large enough to include all infected bone, is oriented dorsal-proximal to plantar-distal (Fig. 5.12). This may be performed with a power saw starting laterally but should be finished off with an osteotome

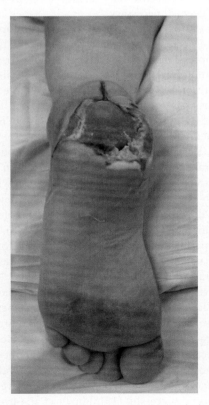

FIGURE 5.11 Example of a large posterior heel ulcer requiring subtotal calcanectomy.

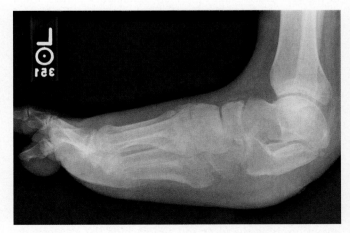

FIGURE 5.12 Plain radiograph of a subtotal calcanectomy without any bony prominences.

or laminar spreader to avoid damaging the medial neurovascular structures. The planter osseous edges are then rounded off with a rongeur and smoothed with a bone rasp.

If possible, the wound is closed using nonabsorbable suture over a closed suction surgical drain. If infection or significant loss of soft tissue was present, the wound may be left open to heal by secondary intention. Once infection has been eradicated, open wounds should be closed in an expedited manner, and adjunctive measures are indicated in these clinical case scenarios. Whether negative pressure wound therapy, advanced wound care products, or skin grafts or flaps are utilized, the goal is to prevent further patient deconditioning and reinfection from open ulcerations. If the procedure is a subtotal calcanectomy, the Achilles tendon is typically not reattached but allowed to fibrose to surrounding tissues. Reattachment would require an advancement of the Achilles tendon and an anchoring device which could serve as a nidus for infection. In these cases, long-term lower extremity bracing is necessary and/or definitive treatment with an ankle arthrodesis might be performed if feasible.

Postoperative care consists of prolonged non–weight-bearing and immobilization until the soft tissues heal. Patient counseling regarding a realistic postoperative course must be discussed. Wound healing complications are frequent and especially when surgical sites cannot be primarily closed. Certain factors can predictably lengthen the recovery period including concomitant osteomyelitis, patients with poor albumin levels, those infected with methicillin-resistant *Staphylococcus aureus*, and those with peripheral arterial disease. Long-term postoperative care requires the use of an accommodative shoe or ankle-foot orthosis (16).

Cook et al. (16) reported the results of 51 calcanectomies (39 partial, 12 subtotal) with a mean follow-up of 33 months. Overall, lower extremity salvage was achieved at 1 and 4 years in 89% and 80%, respectively. There was a 69% healing rate with 65% of the patients being ambulatory by the conclusion of the study. Thirty-five percent of patients required some form of revision, most frequently skin grafting or local flap to achieve wound closure (16).

Arthrodesis

Double (talonavicular and subtalar) or triple (talonavicular, subtalar, and calcaneocuboid) joint arthrodesis can be a powerful procedure, achieving all goals of midfoot/hindfoot surgery in the diabetic patient with peripheral neuropathy: stability, realignment of the hindfoot to the leg and midfoot, and prevention of infection from skin breakdown secondary to underlying deformity. These types of procedures are usually performed in combination with a TAL or gastrocnemius recession for many diabetic patients with peripheral neuropathy. Lengthening the Achilles tendon first often helps mobilize the calcaneus in order to aid in deformity correction as well as decrease the amount of propulsive forces transmitted to the forefoot following arthrodesis of these joints (Fig. 5.13). In addition, a modified triple arthrodesis is sometimes necessary in diabetic neuropathic patients, especially in the clinical setting

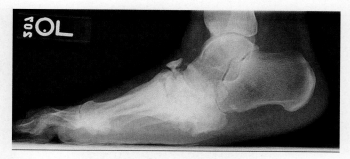

FIGURE 5.13 Example of a Charcot neuroarthropathy with equinus deformity creating increased forefoot and midfoot pressures.

of CN. By extending the arthrodesis procedures to additional adjacent joints, internal fixation purchase and stability improve because the fixation construct is bypassing the underlying pathologic bone (Fig. 5.14).

Following the TAL or gastrocnemius recession, the triple arthrodesis classically begins with a lateral incision which starts just inferior to the lateral malleolus and ends at the base of the fourth and fifth metatarsals. Excellent exposure of the calcaneocuboid and subtalar joints can be obtained through this approach. The lateral aspect of the talonavicular joint may also be visualized, but a second medial incision is often required to gain full access to this joint, especially with an abducted foot. Exposure is obtained in layered dissection, reflecting the extensor digitorum brevis superiorly and the peroneal tendons inferiorly at the lateral aspect of the foot. Sometimes, it is necessary to transect the calcaneofibular ligament to gain access to the subtalar joint, and should therefore be repaired at the conclusion of the case, to avoid future lateral ankle instability. The medial incision begins just anterior to the medial malleolus and curves over the talonavicular joint, ending at the inferior aspect of the naviculocuneiform joint. This incision can be extended distally if additional medial column joints require formal arthrodesis. Complete visualization of the talonavicular joint as well as the dorsal aspect of the talar neck can be achieved through this medial incision (27).

With the calcaneocuboid, subtalar, and talonavicular joints exposed, the surgeon may use their method of choice to remove the cartilaginous joint surfaces. If wedges of bone are removed to correct osseous malalignment, a power saw instrumentation or osteotome may be used, but care must be taken to avoid thermal necrosis. Wedging osseous procedures can be very effective in correcting all planes of deformities. Alternatively, if osseous shortening is not necessary, a curettage technique may be employed. This will preserve osseous contours and prevent loss of foot height that may sometimes cause shoe irritation from the malleoli postoperatively. Regardless of the surgical technique, all cartilage is denuded and the osseous surfaces are fenestrated with a K-wire or shingled with a small osteotome to promote subchondral bleeding.

Malalignments can also be corrected with interpositional bone allografts. An interpositional bone allograft placed within

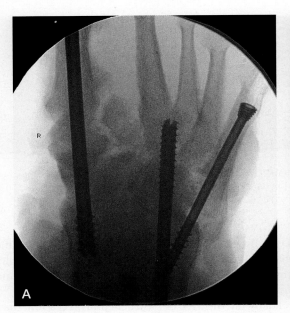
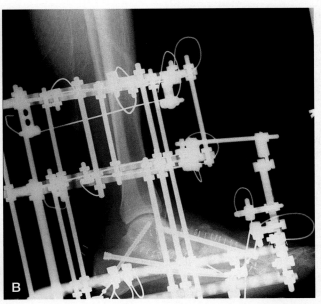

FIGURE 5.14 When dealing with Charcot neuroarthropathy of the midfoot, additional joints both distal and proximal to the pathologic bone should be included into the surgical planning along with larger fixation for long-term success and stability. **A.** Example of a combination of multiple joints intramedullary screw fixation. **B.** This fixation was further secured with a static circular external fixation device. (Courtesy of Barry Rosenblum, DPM, and Philip Basile, DPM.)

the subtalar joint can help correct varus or valgus deformities. Allograft is also frequently interposed between the calcaneus and cuboid to lengthen the lateral column in severely abducted feet. Sliding of the tarsal bones can also be used to alter arch height but can be difficult to perform if the deformity is very rigid.

Whether osseous wedging, sliding, interpositional bone grafting, or preservation of bone contours is employed, the ultimate goal is to achieve anatomic alignment, thus preventing skin breakdown and future ulcerations. First, alignment of the hindfoot to the leg should be assessed. The calcaneus is best evaluated from a posterior orientation and should be rectus to slightly everted position in relation to the leg. In the sagittal plane, the calcaneal inclination angle should be 15 to 20 degrees, and the lateral process of the talus should bisect the longitudinal axis of the tibia. Finally, the foot should be placed in 10 to 15 degrees of abduction in the transverse plane. With the hindfoot now aligned to the leg, the forefoot–hindfoot relationship should be assessed. The subtalar joint is placed in 5 to 10 degrees of valgus position, with the talocalcaneal angle 15 to 35 degrees. The longitudinal bisection of the talus should be as close to collinear as possible to the first metatarsal on the sagittal plane views.

Once proper alignment of the double or triple arthrodesis has been achieved, a number of different fixation modalities have been effective. Traditionally, the subtalar joint is fixed first, however, in severe deformity correction; the fixation order may need to be altered. Particularly in the setting of CN, our institution advocates fixation across the joint with the primary deformity first. Because a collapsed medial arch is often the most severe aspect of these deformities, fixation

of the medial column is often addressed initially. Achieving collinearity of the talus and first metatarsal is stressed and sometimes requires a more extended arthrodesis of the medial column. Furthermore, like in midfoot arthrodesis procedures, it is our institution's experience that it is necessary to use additional and larger fixation than what is traditionally used in nonneuropathic patients. Whether screws, staples, plates, wires, pins, intramedullary nail(s), or external fixation is used, it is important to have compression, strength, and stability across the arthrodesis sites. Wound healing problems in this patient population are essentially expected but with proper débridement and wound care is seldom an issue. Other complications include, but are not limited to, postoperative infection, edema, nonunions, delayed unions, malunions, and hardware complications.

If necessary, surgical drains are used to prevent hematoma formation, and the incisions are closed in a layered fashion. The foot is dressed with a dry sterile dressing and a compressive posterior splint is applied to the leg. The patient is kept non–weight-bearing with elevation, and once the surgical drain is removed and swelling is controlled, a below-the-knee fiberglass cast is applied. It is important to cast only after swelling has significantly decreased because severe wound problems can occur from cast irritations in diabetic neuropathic patients. If concern exists, a bivalve cast may be applied until the patient is ready to be placed in an enclosed lower extremity fiberglass cast. Sutures may need to remain in for 3 to 4 weeks, and the patient is kept immobilized and non–weight-bearing until plain radiographs demonstrate evidence of consolidation. Typically, the patients are progressed to partial weight bearing at 6 to 8 weeks with full weight bearing in a below-the-knee walking boot or cast at 10 to 12 weeks. Physical therapy is frequently needed during the postoperative period due to activity adjustments and deconditioning.

Realignment Osteotomies

Realignment calcaneal osteotomies are an effective and powerful way to realign the hindfoot to the leg. These procedures may be isolated in certain clinical case scenarios but usually are combined or incorporated into an arthrodesis procedure, depending on the underlying deformity (67). Two procedures that are commonly used in diabetic neuropathic patients are the Evans lateral column lengthening and posterior calcaneal displacement osteotomy (PCDO).

The Evans lateral column lengthening can achieve triplanar correction when there is primarily forefoot abduction combined with some valgus deformity and sagittal collapse. Although, the lateral column lengthening is traditionally recommended for flexible deformities, it can be built into double or triple arthrodesis procedures as well by lengthening through the calcaneocuboid arthrodesis. The lateral column lengthening swings the forefoot out of abduction and concomitantly tightens the peroneus longus. This technique indirectly increases the foot arch height by plantarflexing the first ray while supination of the subtalar joint is also achieved. A concomitant medial column arthrodesis or plantarflexory osteotomy may be necessary to achieve balance and avoid new areas of preulcerative lesions in diabetic neuropathic patients (61).

When dealing with primarily frontal plane valgus deformities, a PCDO may be beneficial. Like the Evans calcaneal osteotomy, the PCDO is also typically recommended for flexible deformities without arthritic hindfoot changes. However, this osteotomy may be used in conjunction with subtalar, double, or triple arthrodesis. In fact, this is preferred over trying to obtain frontal plane correction through the subtalar joint arthrodesis site with bone resection and/or bone allograft wedges. Correcting frontal plane deformities through the subtalar joint arthrodesis site can be very difficult and technically demanding due to its shape. Instead, a PCDO may be performed in addition to the planned subtalar joint arthrodesis with 1 or 2 large screws capturing both the osteotomy and subtalar joint arthrodesis sites. It is also recommended to bevel and smooth the prominent cortical shelf after medial translation of the calcaneus. Any remaining osseous prominence can lead to future ulceration in diabetic neuropathic patients.

Hindfoot/Ankle

More extensive arthrodesis procedures such as ankle, tibiotalocalcaneal, tibiocalcaneal with talectomy, or pantalar arthrodesis may be necessary when malalignment or significant instability of the hindfoot/ankle joints exists to the point that there are preulcerative regions or ulcerations with bracing. Multiple studies have evidenced that CN deformity of the ankle, which accounts for 5% of the patterns, can have the most devastating results (43,53,54). The goals of surgery

and indications are similar to those in the midfoot/hindfoot arthrodesis procedures. However, it cannot be emphasized enough that positioning of the joints is critical and malalignment can cause problems that are worse than the original deformity. The location of the primary deformity must be determined and more proximal malalignments should be addressed first. More detailed description of the CN hindfoot/ankle procedures is defined in great depth in later chapters of this textbook.

Fixation devices for the types of arthrodesis procedures may include internal fixation such as screws, plates, intramedullary nailing, Steinmann pins, external fixation, or a combination of internal and external fixation constructs. Staged reconstruction is advisable in the presence of an ankle infection or osteomyelitis with or without the utilization of antibiotic-impregnated polymethylmethacrylate cemented beads and/or spacers. The use of autogenous or allogenic bone grafts may also be applied at the time of definitive reconstructive procedure. If an external fixation was utilized, patients should be placed in either a protective lower extremity cast or below-the-knee brace following the external fixation removal until a custom locked articulating ankle foot orthosis is constructed.

Mendicino et al. (41) illustrated the increased risk of diabetic patients to develop major complications in intramedullary nailing procedures. Stuart and Morrey (57) experienced a complication rate of 78% if CN was present. This includes, but is not limited to, nonunions, delayed unions, malunions, infections, wound healing and hardware complications, pin track infections, tibia fractures, postoperative edema, and a number of serious medical complications including the increased risk of deep venous thrombosis and pulmonary embolism.

Posterior Muscle Group Lengthening

In many of these diabetic patients, there coexists an equinus deformity, and consideration should be given to the performance of a lengthening of the posterior muscle groups. The 2 primary methods to accomplish this are by TAL or performing a gastrocnemius recession. Regardless of the procedure performed, an adjunctive TAL or gastrocnemius recession may be indicated for many diabetic neuropathic patients. Lengthening the posterior muscle group by either method decreases the propulsive force transmitted to the forefoot and midfoot and reduces plantar foot pressures. Increased plantar foot pressures in diabetic patients are thought to be caused by a number of reasons, including structural deformities and limited joint mobility (37). Glycation of the Achilles tendon, thus causing inelasticity, stiffening, and shortening of this tendon, may further contribute to this problem (28).

There are many ways to lengthen the Achilles tendon, but one of the simplest and quickest techniques is the percutaneous triple-hemi incisional approach (Fig. 5.15). The medial one-half of the Achilles tendon is transected via a stab incision approximately 1 cm from the superior aspect of the calcaneus. A second stab incision, 3 cm superior to this incision, transects the lateral half of the Achilles tendon. Finally, a third medial stab incision is made 3 cm superior

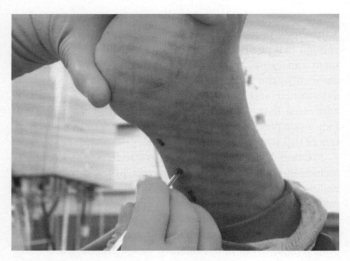

FIGURE 5.15 An adjunctive tendo-Achilles lengthening may be performed with the patient in a supine position. A minimally invasive approach with 3 small stab incisions can effectively and efficiently lengthen the Achilles tendon.

to the second incision. The foot is then dorsiflexed under controlled pressure until the desired amount of dorsiflexion is achieved. Patients are immobilized with the foot 90 degrees to slightly dorsiflexed and kept non–weight-bearing for a period of 3 to 4 weeks. However, weight bearing status is often dictated by concomitant procedures.

Minimal complications are associated with this TAL procedure. The most devastating is overlengthening or tendon rupture causing the development of a calcaneal ulceration from a calcaneal gait. The incidence of calcaneal ulceration following TAL is unknown but is anecdotally reported to range anywhere from 2% to 10%. Of greater concern is the recurrence of equinus and only transient relief of increased forefoot plantar pressures following this procedure. TAL may also decrease propulsion and reduce plantarflexory power. This is not considered a complication but a desired effect in this diabetic population with peripheral neuropathy in order to reduce the risk for plantar pressures and ulcerations.

In a study by Armstrong et al. (7), mean plantar forefoot pressures decreased from $86 \pm 9.4 \, \text{N/cm}^2$ to $63 \pm 13.2 \, \text{N/cm}^2$ ($p <.001$) following TALs. Other studies have found similar results with subsequent healing of forefoot ulcerations and prevention of recurrence of plantar foot ulcerations (21,39). Certainly, the benefits of TAL outweigh the potential risks and are highly recommended to reduce plantar foot pressures in many clinical case scenarios.

Gastrocnemius recession may be considered over a TAL in that it offers a more controlled lengthening. It spares the soleus muscle, maintains plantarflexory strength, and potentially spares an already likely diseased tendon. If performed endoscopically, the amount of tissue exposure is significantly reduced. The question of vascularity around the Achilles tendon is also eliminated with a gastrocnemius recession (29). DiDomenico et al. (19) showed an average increase of

18 degrees of ankle dorsiflexion from 31 endoscopic gastrocnemius recessions in 28 patients.

For an open technique of gastrocnemius recession, the patient is positioned supine and with the lower extremity slightly externally rotated. A 3 to 4 cm incision is made 1 to 2 cm medial to the midline of the leg and 1 to 2 cm distal to the inferior margin of the gastrocnemius muscle belly. Blunt dissection is performed through the subcutaneous layer until the deep fascia is identified. Care is taken to avoid the lesser saphenous vein and nerve. The deep fascia is then incised in line with the skin incision and retracted medially and laterally with the subcutaneous tissues exposing the underlying gastrocnemius aponeurosis. The medial and lateral borders of the aponeurosis should be identified at this time. With the knee in an extended position and the foot slightly dorsiflexed at the ankle, a surgical blade or scissor is used to transect the aponeurosis usually from medial to lateral. The plantaris tendon is usually appreciated medially which is also transected. Layered closure is performed starting with the deep fascia.

For the endoscopic gastrocnemius recession technique, a single portal is generally used. A 1 cm incision is made about 1 to 2 cm inferior to the medial belly of the gastrocnemius and 1 cm posterior to the medial border of the aponeurosis. Blunt dissection is made down through the subcutaneous tissues until the deep fascia is identified. A small incision is made through the deep fascia which is then elevated and retracted exposing the underlying aponeurosis. A fascial elevator is then passed deep to the deep fascia along the aponeurosis to the lateral side making way for insertion of the obturator and cannula. The obturator is removed, and a 4 mm, 30 degree endoscope is inserted with the camera facing anterior to identify the aponeurosis and also to ensure any neurovascular structures are not injured. A knife blade is then mounted on the endoscope and advanced from medial to lateral. As the blade and scope are being removed, one should see the underlying soleus muscle. Patients may be full weight bearing in a tall pneumatic walking boot for 2 to 4 weeks, assuming no other restrictions for concomitant procedures are encountered.

Overall, there is a low associated morbidity with both open and endoscopic gastrocnemius recession procedures. Roukis and Schweinberger (50) reported complications on 23 uniportal endoscopic gastrocnemius recessions with 3 conversions to open, 3 delayed healing of incisions and no neurovascular injuries. Rush et al. (51) reported complications for 126 patients who underwent open gastrocnemius recessions with and without other procedures with a 6% complication rate: 6 (4%) had scar problems, 2 (1.33%) had wound dehiscence, 2 (1.33%) had infection, 3 (2%) had nerve problems, and 1 (0.67%) developed complex regional pain syndrome.

In conclusion, this chapter highlights the important role of elective diabetic foot surgery and emphasizes the multidisciplinary team approach for the diabetic patient's overall successful outcome.

References

1. Anderson JJ, Hansen M, Rowe GP, et al. Complication rates in diabetics with first metatarsophalangeal joint arthrodesis. Diabet Foot Ankle 2014;5.

2. Armstrong DG, Fiorito JL, Leykum BJ, et al. Clinical efficacy of the pan metatarsal head resection as a curative procedure in patients with diabetes mellitus and neuropathic forefoot wounds. Foot Ankle Spec 2012;5:235–240.

3. Armstrong DG, Frykberg RG. Classifying diabetic foot surgery: toward a rational definition. Diabet Med 2003;20:329–331.

4. Armstrong DG, Lavery LA, Frykberg RG, et al. Validation of a diabetic foot surgery classification. Int Wound J 2006;3:240–246.

5. Armstrong DG, Lavery LA, Stern S, et al. Is prophylactic diabetic foot surgery dangerous? J Foot Ankle Surg 1996;35:585–589.

6. Armstrong DG, Lavery LA, Vazquez JR, et al. Clinical efficacy of the first metatarsophalangeal joint arthroplasty as a curative procedure for hallux interphalangeal joint wounds in patients with diabetes. Diabetes Care 2003;26:3284–3287.

7. Armstrong DG, Stacpoole-Shea S, Nguyen H, et al. Lengthening of the Achilles tendon in diabetic patients who are at high risk for ulceration of the foot. J Bone Joint Surg Am 1999;81:535–538.

8. Berner A, Sage R, Niemela J. Keller procedure for the treatment of resistant plantar ulceration of the hallux. J Foot Ankle Surg 2005;44:133–136.

9. Boffeli TJ, Abben KW, Hyllengren SB. In-office distal Symes lesser toe amputation: a safe, reliable, and cost-effective treatment of diabetes-related tip of toe ulcers complicated by osteomyelitis. J Foot Ankle Surg 2014;53:720–726.

10. Boffeli TJ, Collier RC. Near total calcanectomy with rotational flap closure of large decubitus heel ulcerations complicated by calcaneal osteomyelitis. J Foot Ankle Surg 2013;52:107–112.

11. Boffeli TJ, Hyllengren SB. Unilobed rotational flap for plantar hallux interphalangeal joint ulceration complicated by osteomyelitis. J Foot Ankle Surg 2015;54:1166–1171.

12. Boffeli TJ, Reinking R. Plantar rotation flap technique for pan-metatarsal head resection and transmetatarsal amputation: a revision approach for second metatarsal head transfer ulcers in patients with previous partial first ray amputation. J Foot Ankle Surg 2014;53:96–100.

13. Brodsky JW, Rouse AM. Exostectomy for symptomatic bony prominences in diabetic Charcot feet. Clin Orthop Relat Res 1993;296:21–26.

14. Catanzariti AR, Blitch EL, Karlock LG. Elective foot and ankle surgery in the diabetic patient. J Foot Ankle Surg 1995;34:23–41.

15. Catanzariti AR, Mendicino R, Haverstock B. Ostectomy for diabetic neuroarthropathy involving the midfoot. J Foot Ankle Surg 2000;39:291–300.

16. Cook J, Cook E, Landsman AS, et al. A retrospective assessment of partial calcanectomies and factors influencing postoperative course. J Foot Ankle Surg 2007;46:248–255.

17. Corey S. Elective surgery in the diabetic patient. In: McGlamry ED, ed. Reconstructive surgery of the foot and leg, update. Tucker, GA: Podiatry Institute Inc, 1989;159–167.

18. Dalla Paola L, Carone A, Morisi C, et al. Conservative surgical treatment of infected ulceration of the first metatarsophalangeal joint with osteomyelitis in diabetic patients. J Foot Ankle Surg 2015;54:536–540.

19. DiDomenico LA, Adams HB, Garchar D. Endoscopic gastrocnemius recession for the treatment of gastrocnemius equinus. J Am Podiatr Med Assoc 2005;95:410–413.

20. Domek N, Dux K, Pinzur M, et al. Association between hemoglobin A1c and surgical morbidity in elective foot and ankle surgery. J Foot Ankle Surg 2016;55:939–943.

21. Duckworth T, Boulton AJ, Betts RP, et al. Plantar pressure measurements and the prevention of ulceration in the diabetic foot. J Bone Joint Surg Br 1985;67:79–85.

22. Faglia E, Clerici G, Caminiti M, et al. Feasibility and effectiveness of internal pedal amputations of phalanx or metatarsal head in diabetic patients with forefoot osteomyelitis. J Foot Ankle Surg 2012;51:593–598.

23. Giurini JM, Basile P, Chrzan JS, et al. Panmetatarsal head resection. A viable alternative to the transmetatarsal amputation. J Am Podiatr Med Assoc 1993;83:101–107.

24. Giurini JM, Chrzan JS, Gibbons GW, et al. Sesamoidectomy for the treatment of chronic neuropathic ulcerations. J Am Podiatr Med Assoc 1991;81:167–173.

25. Giurini JM, Rosenblum BI. Surgical treatment of the diabetic foot. In: McGlamry ED, ed. McGlamry's comprehensive textbook of foot and ankle surgery. Philadelphia: Lippincott Williams & Wilkins, 2001:1595–1616.

26. Giurini JM, Rosenblum BI. The role of foot surgery in patients with diabetes. Clin Podiatr Med Surg 1995;12:119–127.

27. Goecker RM, Ruch JA. Rearfoot arthrodesis. Part 1. Triple arthrodesis In: McGlamry ED, ed. McGlamry's comprehensive textbook of foot and ankle surgery. Philadelphia: Lippincott Williams & Wilkins, 2001:1167–1192.

28. Grant WP, Sullivan R, Sonenshine DE, et al. Electron microscopic investigation of the effects of diabetes mellitus on the Achilles tendon. J Foot Ankle Surg 1997;36:272–278.

29. Greenhagen RM, Johnson AR, Bevilacqua NJ. Gastrocnemius recession or tendo-Achilles lengthening for equinus deformity in the diabetic foot? Clin Podiatr Med Surg 2012;29:413–424.

30. Gudas CJ. Prophylactic surgery in the diabetic foot. Clin Podiatr Med Surg 1987;4:445–458.

31. Hamilton GA, Ford LA, Perez H, et al. Salvage of the neuropathic foot by using bone resection and tendon balancing: a retrospective review of 10 patients. J Foot Ankle Surg 2005;44:37–43.

32. Henke PK, Blackburn SA, Wainess RW, et al. Osteomyelitis of the foot and toe in adults is a surgical disease: conservative management worsens lower extremity salvage. Ann Surg 2005;241:885–894.

33. Hingorani A, LaMuraglia GM, Henke P, et al. The management of diabetic foot: a clinical practice guideline by the Society for Vascular Surgery in collaboration with the American Podiatric Medical Association and the Society for Vascular Medicine. J Vasc Surg 2016;63(2 suppl):3–21.

34. Johnson J, Anderson SA. One stage resection and pin stabilization of first metatarsophalangeal joint for chronic plantar ulcer with osteomyelitis. Foot Ankle Int 2010;31:973–979.

35. Khalafi A, Landsman AS, Lautenschlager EP, et al. Plantar forefoot pressure changes after second metatarsal neck osteotomy. Foot Ankle Int 2005;26:550–555.

36. Kravitz SR, McGuire JB, Sharma S. The treatment of diabetic foot ulcers: reviewing the literature and a surgical algorithm. Adv Skin Wound Care 2007;20:227–237.

37. Lavery LA, Armstrong DG, Boulton AJ, et al. Ankle equinus deformity and its relationship to high plantar pressure in a large population with diabetes mellitus. J Am Podiatr Med Assoc 2002;92:479–482.

38. Lew E, Nicolosi N, McKee P. Evaluation of hallux interphalangeal joint arthroplasty compared with nonoperative treatment of recalcitrant hallux ulceration. J Foot Ankle Surg 2015;54: 541–548.

39. Lin SS, Lee TH, Wapner KL. Plantar forefoot ulceration with equinus deformity of the ankle in diabetic patients: the effect of tendo-Achilles lengthening and total contact casting. Orthopedics 1996;19:465–475.

40. Markakis K, Bowling FL, Boulton AJ. The diabetic foot in 2015: an overview. Diabetes Metab Res Rev 2016;32(suppl 1):169–178.

41. Mendicino RW, Catanzariti AR, Saltrick KR, et al. Tibiotalocalcaneal arthrodesis with retrograde intramedullary nailing. J Foot Ankle Surg 2004;43:82–86.

42. Molines-Barroso RJ, Lázaro-Martínez JL, Aragón-Sánchez J, et al. The influence of the length of the first metatarsal on the risk of reulceration in the feet of patients with diabetes. Int J Low Extrem Wounds 2014;13:27–32.

43. Myerson MS, Edwards WH. Management of neuropathic fractures in the foot and ankle. J Am Acad Orthop Surg 1999;7:8–18.

44. Patel VG, Wieman TJ. Effect of metatarsal head resection for diabetic foot ulcers on the dynamic plantar pressure distribution. Am J Surg 1994;167:297–301.

45. Petrov O, Pfeifer M, Flood M, et al. Recurrent plantar ulceration following pan metatarsal head resection. J Foot Ankle Surg 1996;35:573–602.

46. Pinzur MS, Sage R, Stuck R, et al. A treatment algorithm for neuropathic (Charcot) midfoot deformity. Foot Ankle 1993;14:189–197.

47. Rosenblum BI, Giurini JM, Chrzan JS, et al. Preventing loss of the great toe with the hallux interphalangeal joint arthroplasty. J Foot Ankle Surg 1994;33:557–560.

48. Rosenblum BI, Giurini JM, Miller LB, et al. Neuropathic ulcerations plantar to the lateral column in patients with Charcot foot deformity: a flexible approach to limb salvage. J Foot Ankle Surg 1997;36:360–363.

49. Rosenblum BI, Pomposelli FB Jr, Giurini JM, et al. Maximizing foot salvage by a combined approach to foot ischemia and neuropathic ulceration in patients with diabetes. A 5-year experience. Diabetes Care 1994;17:983–987.

50. Roukis TS, Schweinberger MH. Complications associated with uni-portal endoscopic gastrocnemius recession in a diabetic patient population: an observational case series. J Foot Ankle Surg 2010;49:68–70.

51. Rush SM, Ford LA, Hamilton GA. Morbidity associated with high gastrocnemius recession: retrospective review of 126 cases. J Foot Ankle Surg 2006;45:156–160.

52. Sadoskas D, Suder NC, Wukich DK. Perioperative glycemic control and the effect on surgical site infections in diabetic patients undergoing foot and ankle surgery. Foot Ankle Spec 2016;9: 24–30.

53. Schon LC, Cohen I, Horton GA. Treatment of the diabetic neuropathic flatfoot. Tech Orthop 2000;15(3):277–289.

54. Schon LC, Easley ME, Weinfeld SB. Charcot neuroarthropathy of the foot and ankle. Clin Orthop Relat Res 1998;349:116–131.

55. Sharma DK, Roy N, Shenolikar A. Weil osteotomy of lesser metatarsals for metatarsalgia: a clinical and radiological follow-up. The Foot 2005;15:202–205.

56. Sheehan P, Jones P, Giurini JM, et al. Percent change in wound area of diabetic foot ulcers over a 4-week period is a robust predictor of complete healing in a 12-week prospective trial. Plast Reconstr Surg 2006;117(7 suppl):239–244.

57. Stuart MJ, Morrey BF. Arthrodesis of the diabetic neuropathic ankle joint. Clin Orthop Relat Res 1990;253:209–211.

58. Tamir E, Finestone AS, Avisar E, et al. Mini-invasive floating metatarsal osteotomy for resistant or recurrent neuropathic plantar metatarsal head ulcers. J Orthop Surg Res 2016;11:78.

59. Tamir E, McLaren AM, Gadgil A, et al. Outpatient percutaneous flexor tenotomies for management of diabetic claw toe deformities with ulcers: a preliminary report. Can J Surg 2008;51: 41–44.

60. Tamir E, Tamir J, Beer Y, et al. Resection arthroplasty for resistant ulcers underlying the hallux in insensate diabetics. Foot Ankle Int 2015;36:969–975.

61. Tien TR, Parks BG, Guyton GP. Plantar pressures in the forefoot after lateral column lengthening: a cadaver study comparing the Evans osteotomy and calcaneocuboid fusion. Foot Ankle Int 2005;26:520–525.

62. Vandeputte G, Dereymaeker G, Steenwerckx A, et al. The Weil osteotomy of the lesser metatarsals. Foot Ankle Int 2000;21: 370–374.

63. Weil LS Sr. Weil head-neck oblique osteotomy: technique and fixation. Paper presented at: Techniques of Osteotomies of the Forefoot. October 20–22, 1994; Bordeaux, France.

64. Wieman TJ, Mercke YK, Cerrito PB, et al. Resection of the metatarsal head for diabetic foot ulcers. Am J Surg 1998;176: 436–441.

65. Wukich DK, Crim BE, Frykberg RG, et al. Neuropathy and poorly controlled diabetes increase the rate of surgical site infection after foot and ankle surgery. J Bone Joint Surg Am 2014;96A: 832–839.

66. Wukich DK, Shen W, Raspovic KM, et al. Noninvasive arterial testing in patients with diabetes: a guide for foot and ankle surgeons. Foot Ankle Int 2015;36:1391–1399.

67. Zwipp H, Rammelt S. Subtalar arthrodesis with calcaneal osteotomy [in German]. Orthopade 2006;35:400–404.

CHAPTER 6

Lower Extremity Nerve Decompression in Patients with Diabetic Peripheral Neuropathy

Wenchuan Zhang

INTRODUCTION

Diabetic peripheral neuropathy (DPN) is one of the common complications of diabetes mellitus with the occurrence rate of up to 60%. DPN is mainly characterized by the sensory, motor, and autonomic nerve dysfunction of bilateral lower extremities. Sensory dysfunction includes typical behavior such as "socks-type" sensory abnormalities, absence of light touch, temperature sense, proprioception, and pain perception. The motor dysfunction is manifested in intrinsic muscle atrophy, whereas the autonomic nerve dysfunction is characterized by the absence of skin temperature, microcirculation, and normal perspiration (26).

In the past, neurology specialists used to treat DPN with nerve nutrition, microcirculation improvement, and pain management. When diabetic patients present with foot ulcers (Fig. 6.1), surgeons are faced with a great challenge for salvaging the diabetic lower extremity (13,30). In 1992, Dellon (9), a professor of neurosurgery at Johns Hopkins University, applied the lower limb peripheral nerve microscopic decompression treatment for DPN for the first time with significant results in the diabetic population. Most experts around the world have confirmed that the lower limb peripheral nerve microscopic decompression treatment can change the natural course of a patient with DPN (11,12,14,27,29,34).

CLINICAL ASSESSMENT

The Toronto Clinical Scoring System (TCSS) is more widely applied in the clinical assessment treatment. The TCSS includes the neurologic symptoms, neural reflexes, and sensory function tests. Neurologic signs include lower limb pain, numbness, tingling, weakness, ataxia, and upper extremity symptoms; the nerve reflexes include the knee jerk and ankle reflex; and the sensory function test includes pain, temperature sense, light touch, vibration sense, and position sense (Table 6.1). The TCSS can relatively accurately reflect the severity of patients with DPN; however, it is subjective, and it is difficult to become objective (3,15).

The nerve electrophysiology examination is an important examination method to diagnose the peripheral nerve entrapment by recording the electrical activity in the associated nerve and muscle as it reflects the nerve and muscle function to determine the neural function. Nerve conduction velocity (NCV), incubation, and amplitude are commonly used indicators of the electrophysiologic examination, which can reflect the transmission function of the peripheral electroneurographic signal. This test can be objective, quantitative, and reliable as well as the "gold standard" in the diagnosis of peripheral neuropathy. The revised DPN simple diagnosis standard of Japan in 2002 and Chinese Medical Doctor Association in 2009 pointed out that if 2 or more nerves suffer abnormality in the NCV, incubation, and amplitude, this can be identified as DPN (4,17,18,20). Xinhua Hospital, affiliated to Shanghai Jiao Tong University School of Medicine, followed up to 560 patients with DPN from 2007 to 2012 and found that the NCV of patients with DPN is significantly lower than normal (Table 6.2).

Quantitative sensory testing (QST) is a technological tool that can quantitatively judge the sense function and evaluate the nerve sensory function through the measurement of skin temperature and vibration sense (Fig. 6.2). QST usually adopts the bound and level methods. The stimulus intensity in the bound method increases or decreases gradually, and when the patients feel the change of stimulus intensity, the examiner should stop immediately and record the stimulus intensity as the threshold value. Following this test, the stimulus intensity should be reset in the level method and measuring of the threshold value is performed by adjusting the stimulus intensity. Although the level method can more accurately determine the threshold value, it also needs testing more times than the bound method, and patients may therefore distract their attention and produce an erroneous measurement. The bound method is more often used in the clinical treatment and settings (16,18,28). Xinhua Hospital, affiliated to Shanghai Jiao Tong University School of Medicine, followed up to 560 patients with DPN from 2007 to

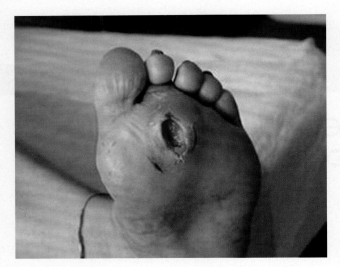

FIGURE 6.1 Left foot ulcer in a patient with diabetic peripheral neuropathy.

2012 and found that patients with DPN suffer abnormal sensation threshold, thermal sensation threshold, and vibration sensation threshold, verifying that the QST can be used for preoperative screening (Table 6.3).

The nerve electrophysiology examination and quantitative sensory examination can only obtain the change of neural function in patients with DPN, but the high-frequency nerve ultrasound can get the condition of nerve morphosis (Fig. 6.3). The high-frequency nerve ultrasound is noninvasive, convenient, and objective, and it has been increasingly used in the preoperative diagnosis of peripheral nerve disease because it provides the basis for the choice of operation. In addition, the high-frequency nerve ultrasound is also applied in the postoperative follow-up to assess the nerve edema of patients that have undergone peripheral nerve surgery (2,32,33,35). Xinhua Hospital, affiliated to Shanghai Jiao Tong University School of Medicine, followed up to 560 patients with DPN from 2007 to 2012 and found that the nerve transverse diameter, anteroposterior diameter, and the cross-sectional area of patients with preoperative DPN are greater than the normal but improved in their postoperative follow-up visits.

The use of the plantar pressure measuring instrument is to measure the mechanics, geometry, and time parameters of plantar pressure in the static and dynamic process of the human body as well as to obtain the plantar pressure distribution status and characteristics (Fig. 6.4). By analyzing the parameters and distribution characteristics of plantar pressure, the etiologic factors of increased plantar pressure can be determined and thus provide the corresponding preventive measures in time. The plantar pressure detection has important significance for assessing foot ulcer risk in patients with DPN and preventing amputation (31).

Surgical Indications and Contraindications

Indications

All of the abnormal neurologic signs must be caused by diabetes mellitus including DPN. The common symptoms of DPN include, but are not limited, to pain, numbness, dysesthesia, absence of ankle reflex, with temperature and vibration sense abnormalities. In addition, the tibial nerve at the medial malleolus area is producing a positive Tinel sign and, by taping the tibial nerve at the medial malleolus, is causing pain and numbness in the innervation area. Other surgical indications include a 2-point discrimination loss more than 9 mm, an abnormal NCV through electrophysiologic examination, and a fasting blood glucose controlled below 8 mmol/L 2 weeks before the surgery.

Contraindications

Contraindications to surgical decompression of patients with DPN include, but are not limited to, a history of cervical and lumbar vertebrae diseases, nervous system lesion caused by other systemic diseases (familial, nutritional, alcoholic, uremic), and lower extremity peripheral arterial disease. Finally, uncontrolled blood glucose levels are expected to affect the postoperative wound and nerve repair (1,7–10,21).

Preoperative Assessment

Conventional surgical preparation before lumbar or general anesthesia includes medical optimization, psychological

TABLE 6.1			Toronto Clinical Scoring System						
Symptom			**Reflex**				**Sensory test**		
Lower Extremity	N	Y	Knee	(+)	(±)	(−)		(+)	(−)
Pain	0	1	L	0	1	2	Pain	0	1
Numbness	0	1	R	0	1	2	Temperature	0	1
Tingling	0	1	Ankle				Touch	0	1
Weakness	0	1	L	0	1	2	Vibration	0	1
Ataxia	0	1	R	0	1	2	Position	0	1
Upper Extremity	0	1							

TABLE 6.2

Nerve Conduction Velocities of Patients with Diabetic Peripheral Neuropathy

Nerves	Control NCV (m/s)	Preoperative NCV (m/s)	Abnormal Ratio n (%)
Posterior tibial nerve	43.8 ± 3.9	28.2 ± 7.2	843 (75.3%)
Common peroneal nerve	46.6 ± 4.1	33.3 ± 5.3	768 (68.6%)
Superficial peroneal nerve	47.4 ± 3.9	35.2 ± 8.1	865 (77.2%)
Sural nerve	50.1 ± 4.9	40.3 ± 16.6	879 (78.3%)

NCV, nerve conduction velocities.

TABLE 6.3

Quantitative Sensory Testing Used for Preoperative Screening

QST	Control	DPN
Cold perception threshold (°C)	28.8 ± 2.5	21.1 ± 0.6
Warm sensation threshold (°C)	40.1 ± 1.3	46.3 ± 2.3
Vibratory perception threshold (μm)	3.0 ± 2.8	9.8 ± 8.2

DPN, diabetic peripheral neuropathy; QST, quantitative sensory testing.

teaching, preoperative fasting, and normalization of blood glucose levels before surgery. Intraoperative patient positioning is supine for the release of the tibial and deep peroneal nerves and bending the knee for the release of the common peroneal nerve. The incisional designs include a 3-cm-long incision below the fibular head, oblique 3-cm-long incision between the first and second metatarsals dorsally, and a 7-cm-long incision in the posterior medial malleolus (Figs. 6.5 to 6.7).

Operating Technique

All surgical procedures are performed with the use of a microscope under continuous epidural anesthesia or general anesthesia. The common peroneal nerve trunk is exposed and decompressed after the fascia above the common peroneal nerve and the peroneus longus muscle is excised. For releasing the deep peroneal nerve, superficial and deep fascia layers are resected to expose the tendon of the extensor hallucis brevis muscle. The tendon is then excised to decompress the deep peroneal nerve. For the tibial nerve decompression, after the flexor retinaculum is identified and excised behind the medial malleolus, the posterior tibial artery and veins and the tibial nerve are then identified and decompressed. An epineurium

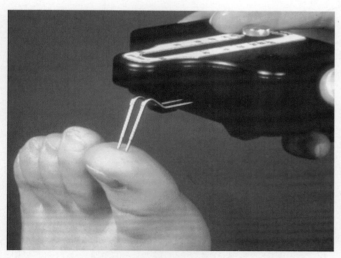

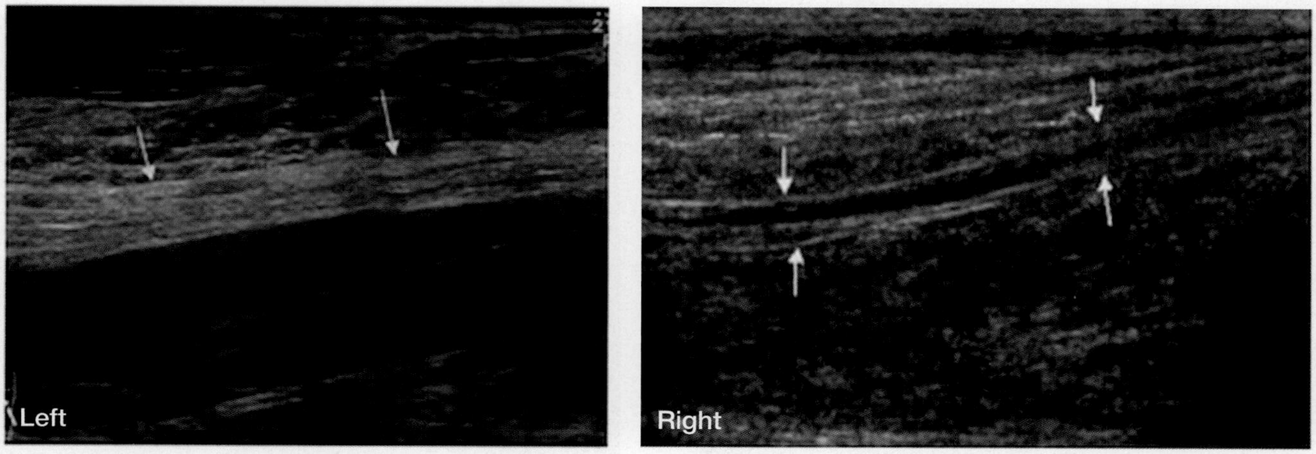

FIGURE 6.2 Quantitative sensory testing on the plantar aspect of the left hallux.

FIGURE 6.3 The *left* image shows the appearance of a normal nerve (*yellow arrows*) in ultrasonography, whereas the *right* ultrasonographic image shows the appearance of an edematous nerve (*white arrows*) in a patient with diabetic peripheral neuropathy.

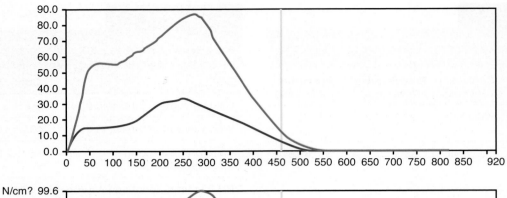

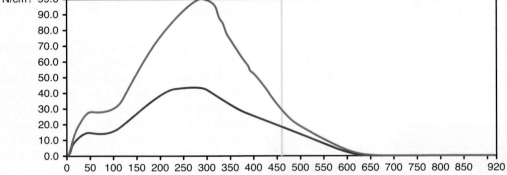

FIGURE 6.4 Plantar pressure increases in patients with diabetic peripheral neuropathy.

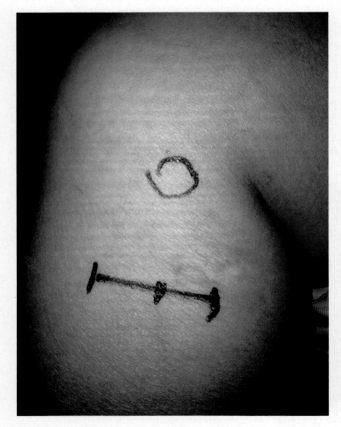

FIGURE 6.5 Incision for common peroneal nerve decompression.

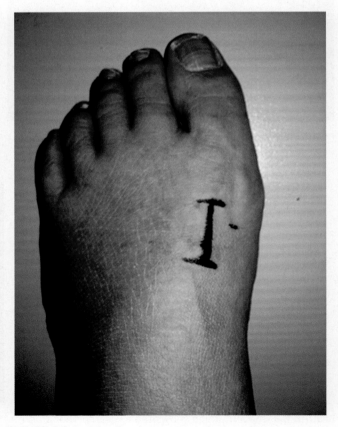

FIGURE 6.6 Incision for deep peroneal nerve decompression.

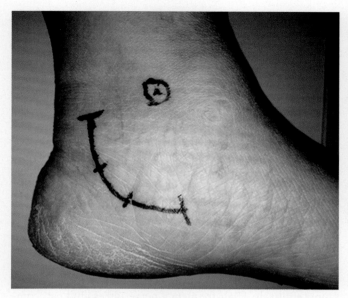

FIGURE 6.7 Incision for tibial nerve decompression.

decompression is also performed if there are signs of epineurial thickening (Figs. 6.8 to 6.10).

Postoperative Complications and Treatments

Nerve injuries can be divided into permanent and transient nerve damage characterized by the sensory dysfunction of the dominance area, numbness, and muscle weakness. For example, the tibial nerve injury can cause foot hypoesthesia and numbness, whereas the common peroneal nerve injury can cause loss of sensation and movement of the foot and/or leg. The permanent nerve damage is caused by intraoperative contusion, thermosetting conduction, and sharpness damage, and if happened, it is more difficult to be improved. Routine peripheral nerve surgery is conducted under the utilization of a microscope with intraoperative electrophysiologic monitoring for limbs while surgical experience is paramount for the patient's overall successful outcome. The transient nerve

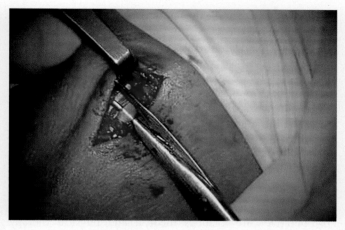

FIGURE 6.9 Decompression of deep peroneal nerve.

damage is mainly caused by intraoperative excessive force and can be alleviated with postoperative medications. The intraoperative pulling angle should be controlled according to the principles of atraumatic technique and correcting it in a timely manner when the electrophysiologic monitoring finds excessive pulling.

Microscopic lower limb peripheral nerve decompression causes minimal blood loss, but due to the anatomic close proximity of the artery, vein, and nerve at the time of surgical decompression, injuries to the vascular bundle may cause a serious incidence and especially to the posterior tibial artery within the tarsal tunnel. If happened, in order to prevent nerve damage caused by thermal condensation, the bleeding can be stopped through compression and hemostatic materials.

Postoperative nerve edema is a common finding, but if there is adequate nerve decompression, it will not generally cause any symptoms in the patients. Individual patients with peripheral edema or patients with obvious nerve edema before the operation will probably have aggravated symptoms within 2 weeks after the operation; however, with the recession of edema, the aforementioned symptoms are gradually eased.

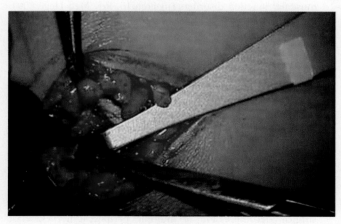

FIGURE 6.8 Decompression of common peroneal nerve.

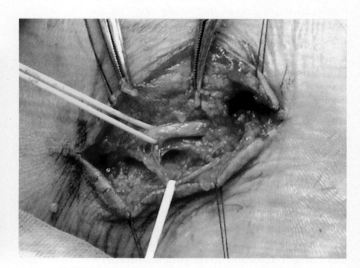

FIGURE 6.10 Decompression of the tibial nerve.

Fully releasing the nerve during the operation can prevent or reduce the nerve edema.

Postoperative wound infections can be associated in patients with peripheral arterial disease and uncontrolled blood glucose levels that might lead to nonhealing wounds and eventual amputation. Preventive measures to minimize postoperative wound complications may include, but are not limited to, intraoperative aseptic technique, mattress-suturing wound closure techniques, local wound care of the incisional sites, and minimal weight bearing status until postoperative wounds have healed completely.

Postoperative Care and Follow-up

Postoperative care includes medical and physical therapy modalities. Currently, the most common medicines for DPN include vitamins, calcium antagonists, vasodilator substance, nerve growth factor, ganglioside treatment, and aldose reductase inhibitors. Vitamin B_{12} improves glucose metabolism and enhances nerve energy supply mainly in the form of a coenzyme; calcium antagonists improve the nerve ischemic hypoxia and protect the nerve by increasing nerve blood flow; vasodilator substances lower the peripheral resistance and strengthen the nerve blood oxygen by blocking α-adrenergic receptors; nerve growth factors and gangliosides can promote nerve repair; and aldose reductase inhibitors reduce the deposit of sorbitol and fructose in peripheral nerve tissue by inhibiting the activity of aldose reductase.

Physical therapy modalities include the electromagnetic wave therapy, aquatic therapy, electrical stimulation therapy, and many others. Through the stimulation of electromagnetic waves, the electromagnetic wave therapy expands the local small blood vessels and thus promotes the blood circulation of nervous tissue, improving the nerve anaerobic condition while accelerating the metabolism of tissue. The aquatic therapy uses the buoyancy of water to relieve muscle tension and speed up the circulation of blood and lymphatic return, whereas the electrical stimulation therapy improves blood circulation and strengthens the nutrition of the nerve while promoting the bioelectricity of nerves, improving nerve excitability, and restoring nerve function (5,22,24,25,27).

Maintaining normal blood glucose levels includes diet control, medical therapy, and exercise therapy. Diet control is the foundation of normalizing blood glucose levels in patients with diabetes mellitus. Reasonably calculating the proportion of carbohydrate, fat, and protein intake is the main way of diet control. Specific methods mainly include choosing the diet rich in cellulose and protein and low fat, choosing the food easier to be digested, and eating in small proportions but frequently and in a set quantity and time. Drug therapy is the main way to control blood glucose levels in the normal range through a variety of hypoglycemic agents or insulin. Hypoglycemic agents mainly include the sulfonylureas, biguanides, glycosidase inhibitors, thiazolidinediones, and non-sulfonylureas insulin promoters, which is necessary to select one or more types and adjust them in time according to the patients' needs. Exercise therapy can improve blood glucose level control as well as improve the body's sensitivity to insulin. It is advisable to choose aerobic exercises and adjust the appropriate exercise intensity according to the patient's demands with diabetes mellitus.

The postoperative follow-up items for patients with DPN mainly include the following (4,6,18,19,23): (a) neural electrophysiologic examination—as the "gold standard" of peripheral nerve disease diagnosis, needs the perfect electrophysiologic technique and supporting professionals but may cause a certain degree of pain, and therefore, it cannot be conducted many times and is more suitable for the long-term follow-up; (b) quantitative sensory examination—compared to the neural electrophysiologic examination, it can directly reflect the change of nerve sensory function more sensitively, simpler, and accepted by patients more easily. However, the test result is closely related to the patients' cooperation directly and is vulnerable to testing environment, people's attention, and instrumentation; (c) high-frequency nerve ultrasound—by showing nerve edema, it can present the neural morphologic changes more intuitively. High-frequency nerve ultrasound can compensate for the nerve electrophysiologic and quantitative sensory examinations and assess the nerve edema in the postoperative period by directly displaying the nerve morphosis of patients with DPN; and lastly, (d) foot-scan—plantar foot pressure increase is the independent risk factor for development of foot ulcers in patients with DPN that may lead to a lower extremity amputation. Plantar pressure examination can detect the plantar foot pressure abnormality in the early stages and thus prevent the risk of ulceration and/or amputation.

References

1. Aszmann O, Tassler PL, Dellon AL. Changing the natural history of diabetic neuropathy: incidence of ulcer/amputation in the contralateral limb of patients with a unilateral nerve decompression procedure. Ann Plast Surg 2004;53:517–522.

2. Baker N. An alternative to a 10-g monofilament or tuning fork? Two new, simple, easy-to-use screening tests for determining foot ulcer risk in people with diabetes. Diabet Med 2012;29:1477–1479.

3. Bril V, Perkins BA. Validation of the Toronto Clinical Scoring System for diabetic polyneuropathy. Diabetes Care 2002;25:2048–2052.

4. Chauplannaz G, Vial C. Electrodiagnostic assessment of neuromuscular junction disorders [in French]. Rev Med Liege 2004;59(suppl 1):184–189.

5. Chong MS, Hester J. Diabetic painful neuropathy: current and future treatment options. Drugs 2007;67:569–585.

6. Chong PS, Cros DP. Technology literature review: quantitative sensory testing. Muscle Nerve 2004;29:734–747.

7. Dellon AL. Neurosurgical prevention of ulceration and amputation by decompression of lower extremity peripheral nerves in diabetic neuropathy: update 2006. Acta Neurochir Suppl 2007;100:149–151.

8. Dellon AL. Preventing foot ulceration and amputation by decompressing peripheral nerves in patients with diabetic neuropathy. Ostomy Wound Manage 2002;48:36–45.

9. Dellon AL. Treatment of symptomatic diabetic neuropathy by surgical decompression of multiple peripheral nerves. Plast Reconstr Surg 1992;89:689–697.

10. Dellon AL, Aszmann OA, Tassler P. Outcome of surgical decompression of nerves in diabetic on incidence of ulceration and amputation. J Reconstr Microsurg 2003;19:350–355.

11. Dellon AL, Mackinnon SE. Chronic nerve compression model for the double crush hypothesis. Ann Plast Surg 1991;26:259–264.

12. Dellon AL, Muse VL, Nickerson DS, et al. Prevention of ulceration, amputation, and reduction of hospitalization: outcomes of a prospective multicenter trial of tibial neurolysis in patients with diabetic neuropathy. J Reconstr Microsurg 2012;28:241–246.

13. Driver VR, Fabbi M, Lavery LA, et al. The cost of diabetic foot: the economic case for the limb salvage team. J Am Podiatr Med Assoc 2010;100:335–341.

14. Dyck PJ, Giannini C. Pathologic alterations in the diabetic neuropathies of humans: a review. J Neuropathol Exp Neurol 1996;55:1181–1193.

15. Guyatt GH, Townsend M, Berman LB, et al. A comparison of Likert and visual analogue scales for measuring change in function. J Chronic Dis 1987;40:1129–1133.

16. Kamei N, Yamane K, Nakanishi S, et al. Effectiveness of Semmes-Weinstein monofilament examination for diabetic peripheral neuropathy screening. J Diabetes Complications 2005;19:47–53.

17. Kincaid JC, Price KL, Jimenez MC, et al. Correlation of vibratory quantitative sensory testing and nerve conduction studies in patients with diabetes. Muscle Nerve 2007;36:821–827.

18. Onde ME, Ozge A, Senol MG, et al. The sensitivity of clinical diagnostic methods in the diagnosis of diabetic neuropathy. J Int Med Res 2008;36:63–70.

19. Ørstavik K, Norheim L, Jørum E. Pain and small-fiber neuropathy in patients with hypothyroidism. Neurology 2006;67:786–791.

20. Perkins BA, Olaleye D, Zinman B, et al. Simple screening tests for peripheral neuropathy in the diabetes clinic. Diabetes Care 2001;24:250–256.

21. Rader AJ. Surgical decompression in lower-extremity diabetic peripheral neuropathy. J Am Podiatr Med Assoc 2005;95:446–450.

22. Reiber GE. The epidemiology of diabetic foot problems. Diabet Med 1996;13(suppl 1):6–11.

23. Rutkove SB, Veves A, Mitsa T, et al. Impaired distal thermoregulation in diabetes and diabetic polyneuropathy. Diabetes Care 2009;32:671–676.

24. Sangiorgio L, Iemmolo R, Le Moli R, et al. Diabetic neuropathy: prevalence, concordance between clinical and electrophysiological testing and impact of risk factors. Panminerva Med 1997;39:1–5.

25. Siemionow M, Zielinski M, Sari A. Comparison of clinical evaluation and neurosensory testing in the early diagnosis of superimposed entrapment neuropathy in diabetic patients. Ann Plast Surg 2006;57:41–49.

26. Singh N, Armstrong DG, Lipsky BA. Preventing foot ulcers in patients with diabetes. JAMA 2005;293:217–228.

27. Sinnreich M, Taylor BV, Dyck PJ. Diabetic neuropathies. Classification, clinical features, and pathophysiological basis. Neurologist 2005;11:63–79.

28. Sorensen L, Molyneaux L, Yue DK. The level of small nerve fiber dysfunction does not predict pain in diabetic neuropathy: a study using quantitative sensory testing. Clin J Pain 2006;22:261–265.

29. Upton AR, McComas AJ. The double crush in nerve entrapment syndromes. Lancet 1973;2:359–362.

30. Valensi P, Le Devehat C, Richard JL, et al. A multicenter, double-blind, safety study of QR-333 for the treatment of symptomatic diabetic peripheral neuropathy. A preliminary report. J Diabetes Complications 2005;19:247–253.

31. Viswanathan V, Snehalatha C, Sivagami M, et al. Association of limited joint mobility and high plantar pressure in diabetic foot ulceration in Asian Indians. Diabetes Res Clin Pract 2003;60:57–61.

32. Volpe A, Rossato G, Bottanelli M, et al. Ultrasound evaluation of ulnar neuropathy at the elbow: correlation with electrophysiological studies. Rheumatology (Oxford) 2009;48:1098–1101.

33. Wiesler ER, Chloros GD, Cartwright MS, et al. Ultrasound in the diagnosis of ulnar neuropathy at the cubital tunnel. J Hand Surg Am 2006;31:1088–1093.

34. Wood WA, Wood MA. Decompression of peripheral nerves for diabetic neuropathy in the lower extremity. J Foot Ankle Surg 2003;42:268–275.

35. Yoon JS, Walker FO, Cartwright MS. Ultrasonographic swelling ratio in the diagnosis of ulnar neuropathy at the elbow. Muscle Nerve 2008;38:1231–1235.

CHAPTER 7

Stepwise Surgical Approach to Diabetic Foot Infections and Osteomyelitis

Javier Aragón-Sánchez

INTRODUCTION

Diabetic foot infections (DFIs) are a worrying complication of diabetes mellitus. This clinical manifestation requires a comprehensive medical and surgical team approach and surgery may be necessary in the treatment of many types of DFIs (49,52,91). The initial patient evaluation, type of infection (6), and its severity are some of the key points in order to decide the best treatment options for the diabetic patient. The ultimate goal is to save the life of the diabetic patient achieving limb salvage if possible. In addition to antibiotic therapy, initially empiric and further treatment based on soft tissue and/or bone cultures and biopsies, many types of DFIs will require some type of surgical intervention, ranging from minor surgical débridement to major surgical resection, amputation, or revascularization (92). This is especially true in cases of deep DFIs because they rarely respond to antimicrobial therapy alone and generally require surgical procedures to drain purulence, débride necrotic tissue, and minimize the risk for further infection spreading (30,49). Delay in the implementation of appropriate surgery may be responsible for the high percentage of amputations because it allows the infection to proliferate and further devitalize the surrounding soft tissues and/or bone (47,114,119). This clinical case scenario is especially true in cases of DFIs associated with peripheral arterial disease.

Osteomyelitis is one of the most frequent DFIs, accounting for 10% to 15% of mild infections and almost 50% of severe infections (90). The treatment of diabetic foot osteomyelitis continues to spur debate, and currently, optimal treatment is yet to be defined (65,66,91,112). The major continuing controversy on the management of diabetic foot osteomyelitis is based on the relative roles of surgery and antibiotic treatment (66). A recent study supports the treatment of diabetic foot osteomyelitis exclusively with antibiotics (79), but surgery still has an important role in treating such patients. The combination of antibiotics with surgical resection of the infected bone may cure most cases of diabetic foot osteomyelitis (59,64,123).

The surgeon who treats patients with diabetes mellitus and DFIs should have a thorough knowledge of the foot and ankle anatomy and should be able to identify the ways in which DFIs spread throughout the foot (6,13). Many diabetic patients must undergo more than one surgical procedure in order to save the infected diabetic foot (12), and revision surgeries should be based on the same anatomic principles.

CLINICAL PRESENTATION OF DIABETIC FOOT INFECTIONS AND OSTEOMYELITIS

Noninfectious causes of inflammation, such as acute diabetic Charcot neuroarthropathy changes, superimposed gouty arthritis, inappropriate footwear, and excessive weight bearing on a foot osseous prominence, can cause localized changes mimicking an infection (69). DFIs can be classified into 2 main groups: soft tissue and bone infections (Table 7.1). Soft tissue infections are then classified as cellulitis, abscess, tenosynovitis, and necrotizing soft tissue infections (NSTIs) (necrotizing cellulitis, necrotizing fasciitis, necrotizing tenosynovitis, and myonecrosis) (4,16). Cellulitis is a diffuse inflammation of the skin and subcutaneous tissue. Abscess is a purulent collection in the soft tissues, either beneath the epidermis, in the subcutaneous tissue, or beneath the fascia layers. Subepidermal abscess and paronychia should be considered as a mild infection. Abscesses can be confined to the subcutaneous tissues. In such cases, the infection is not deep but if it is not adequately treated may become complicated. A deep abscess is located below the fascia level. NSTIs are associated with extensive tissue destruction. The typical signs of NSTIs are a foul smell, extensive cellulitis, skin necrosis, bluish patches, and hemorrhagic bullae. Necrotizing cellulitis is diagnosed when the necrotizing changes only involve the skin and subcutaneous tissue. Necrotizing fasciitis is diagnosed when there is involvement of the fascia, necrotizing tenosynovitis when there is involvement of the tendons and their associated sheaths, and

TABLE 7.1

Clinical-Pathologic Classification of Diabetic Foot Infections

Soft Tissue Infections	• Cellulitis
	• Abscess
	  • Superficial
	    ○ Subepidermal abscess
	    ○ Subcutaneous abscess
	  • Deep tissue abscess
	• Tenosynovitis
	• Necrotizing soft tissue infections
	  • Necrotizing cellulitis
	  • Necrotizing fasciitis
	  • Necrotizing tenosynovitis
	  • Myonecrosis

Joint Infections	• Septic arthritis
Bone Infections	• Osteitis • Osteomyelitis

myonecrosis when the necrotizing process involves the muscle. Deep NSTIs are dangerous and life-threatening infections that spread throughout and necrotizing the fascial planes. In one series involving 223 patients with DFIs, necrotizing tenosynovitis/fasciitis affected 20% of the patients (44). In another study of 145 patients with NSTIs, 109 patients (75.2%) had necrotizing cellulitis, 25 (17.2%) had necrotizing fasciitis, and 11 (7.6%) were consisted with myonecrosis (16). Osteomyelitis associated with NSTIs was diagnosed in 55 patients (38%); however, osteomyelitis was not associated with limb loss and mortality.

The pathophysiology of diabetic foot osteomyelitis is different from other types of osteomyelitis. Hematogenous osteomyelitis is rare in adults and most frequently involves vertebral bodies (87). Diabetic foot osteomyelitis is almost always associated with an ulceration due to peripheral neuropathy, peripheral arterial disease, or both, and/or penetrating injury inoculating bacteria from the skin into the bone. This entails that soft tissues, periosteum, cortical bone, and bone marrow are sequentially involved by the infection before it reaches the bone. The first osseous layer affected by the infection is the periosteum (periostitis). Subsequently, the cortical bone may be affected (osteitis), and then if the infection progresses into the medullar bone, the infection is defined as osteomyelitis. In a cohort study of 1,666 diabetic patients, osteomyelitis was diagnosed in 20% of the patients who developed a foot infection. The risk factors for developing osteomyelitis were the following: wounds that extended to a bone or joint (relative risk = 23.1), previous history of a wound prior to enrolment (relative risk = 2.2), and recurrent or multiple wounds during the study period (relative risk = 1.9) (78). The clinical presentation of osteomyelitis may vary considerably and become complicated when it is associated with a soft tissue infection (4). A classification

system has been proposed based on the presence of ischemia and soft tissue infection (5), and the outcomes of the surgical treatment were related to the presence of both complications.

Initial Evaluation of a Patient with a Diabetic Foot Infection

Systemic manifestations such as fevers and chills, general malaise, nausea, and vomiting may suggest a more serious infection, but ≥50% of patients with a limb-threatening infection do not manifest systemic signs or symptoms (90). Physical examination of the DFI must include seeking out the point of entry of the infection and evaluating the appearance of the entire foot and lower extremity. The point of entry of the infection is frequently an ulcer but may be another type of a wound, for example a nail puncture. The location of the ulcer, whether it is plantar, dorsal, medial, lateral, or interdigital must be defined. Suppuration through the ulcer while palpating at a location distant from the ulcer is consistent with spreading of the infection while the clinician takes into account the pathway of the involved tendons. Infection always spreads from a high pressure to a lower pressure area meaning that when the infection is initially located in the plantar aspect of the foot and no off-loading has been implemented, the infection can spread to the dorsal aspect of the foot. Pressure develops while walking over the inflamed foot and thus spreading the infection to the dorsal aspect of the foot. In addition, it is uncommon that infections arising on the dorsal aspect of the foot to spread to the plantar area because the dorsum of the foot does not sustain a high pressure. In cases of diabetic neuropathic plantar ulcers beneath the metatarsal heads complicated by osteomyelitis, the joint capsule ruptures and purulence may drain to the dorsum of the foot. The evaluation of the depth of the DFI is important because this has been a significant factor in the outcome for the treatment of diabetic foot ulcers (18). However, it has been reported that nearly 90% of the diabetic foot wounds in one series were not evaluated for involvement of underlying structures (43). The depth of a diabetic foot ulcer can be sometimes difficult to determine due to the presence of an overlying hyperkeratosis or necrosis. Therefore, diabetic foot ulcers with associated hyperkeratosis and necrosis should be débrided as soon as possible (3) to facilitate determination of the ulcer depth. The Halsted-Mosquito forceps is a very useful tool for detecting fistulous tracks, cavities, and pathways of infection spreading throughout the foot. A fistulous track from a plantar ulcer to the dorsum of the diabetic foot can be seen in Figure 7.1.

Osteomyelitis is almost always present if the bone can be visualized underneath the associated diabetic foot ulcer. In one study, the bone was exposed in 31% of cases of diabetic foot osteomyelitis (4). The probe-to-bone (PTB) test (15,58,77,110) is a potentially useful tool for diagnosing osteomyelitis underlying a diabetic foot ulcer. When first described 15 years ago, this test showed a positive predictive value of 0.89 in detecting bone involvement in patients

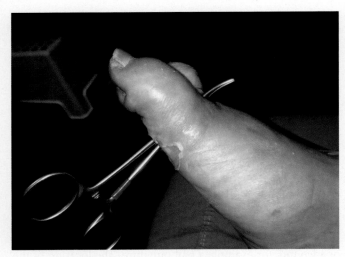

FIGURE 7.1 A fistulous track from a diabetic plantar ulcer to the dorsum of the right foot.

with limb-threatening infections (58). The positive predictive value of PTB in 2 subsequent studies (77,110), however, was considerably lower (0.50 and 0.62). One recent study performed in an outpatient clinical setting using histopathologic analysis as the standard criterion has reported a predictive value of 0.95 (96). PTB had a sensitivity of 0.95, a specificity of 0.93, positive predictive value of 0.97, and a negative predictive value of 0.83 in another study (33). The PTB test was originally described using a sterile, blunt, 14-cm, 5-Fr, stainless-steel eye probe (58), but a Halsted-

Mosquito forceps can also be used (2,15). The surgical instrument is gently introduced through the wound, and the PTB is considered "positive" if bone (a hard or gritty surface) is touched.

Classifying the Severity of Diabetic Foot Infections

DFIs have been classified into 3 types: non–limb-threatening, limb-threatening, and life-threatening (71). This well-accepted scheme is simplistic, but it provides the essentials in determining the severity of DFIs and subsequent treatments (52). Recently, the Infectious Diseases Society of America (IDSA) proposed a newer classification. DFIs are classified according to their severity as mild, moderate, and severe (90), and this classification had been validated (76). The International Working Group on Diabetic Foot (IWGDF) has proposed the perfusion, extent, depth, infection, and sensation (PEDIS) scheme for classifying diabetic foot ulcers and DFI is divided into 4 types. Classification of the severity of DFIs according to IDSA and the international consensus is shown in Table 7.2 (90). These 2 classifications are similar and very useful for the clinicians in order to decide the need for hospitalization and the route of administration of antibiotics but do not clearly indicate the need for surgical treatment. Mild and severe infections are clearly outlined but defining infections as "moderate" poses a great difficulty because this term covers a broad spectrum of wounds, some of which can be quite complicated and even limb-threatening (90). Furthermore, this type of DFIs may get worse in a short period of time and become severe.

TABLE 7.2	Classification of Diabetic Foot Infections According to Their Severity		
		IDSA	PEDIS Grade (IWGDF)
Wound without purulence or any manifestations of inflammation		Uninfected	1
Two or more manifestations of inflammation (purulence or erythema, pain, tenderness, warmth, or induration); any cellulitis or erythema extends ≤2 cm around ulcer, and infection is limited to skin or superficial subcutaneous tissues; no local complications or systemic illness		Mild	2
Infection in a patient who is systemically well and metabolically stable but has ≥1 of the following: cellulitis extending ≥2 cm; lymphangitis; spread beneath fascia; deep tissue abscess; gangrene; muscle, tendon, joint, or bone involvement		Moderate	3
Any foot infection in the presence of a systemic inflammatory response manifested by at least 2 of the following characteristics: • Temperature >38°C or <36°C • Pulse >90 bpm • Respiratory rate >20/min • pCO_2 <32 mmHg • Leukocytes >12,000 or <4,000/mm^3 • 10% of immature (band) forms		Severe	4

IDSA, Infectious Diseases Society of America; IWGDF, International Working Group on Diabetic Foot; pCO_2, partial pressure of carbon dioxide; PEDIS, perfusion, extent, depth, infection, and sensation.

Need for Hospitalization

The IWGDF recommends patient hospitalization in cases of severe DFIs, metabolic or hemodynamic instability, in cases in which intravenous antibiotic therapy is needed, when diagnostic tests and imaging are needed and not available as outpatient, when critical limb ischemia is present, and when surgical procedures are required. Hospital admission is also necessary in cases of unsuccessful treatment as an outpatient, when the patient is unable or unwilling to comply with outpatient-based treatment, when there is a need for more complex dressing changes than patient/caregivers can provide, or when a careful, continuous observation is needed (88).

Medical Imaging Studies for Diabetic Foot Infections and Osteomyelitis

The basic imaging study for treating patients with DFIs is a plain pedal radiograph (x-ray) in 3 standard views. This should be part of the initial consultation whenever a foot infection is suspected in a diabetic patient. Three important signs should be looked for in a plain pedal radiograph: presence of a foreign body, free gas in the soft tissues, and bone destruction. The presence of soft tissue gas in an x-ray alerts the clinician to the presence of a severe, limb-threatening infection, which should be treated immediately with surgical intervention (42). An x-ray showing free gas in the plantar space and osteomyelitis is shown in Figure 7.2. Appropriate aggressive surgical débridement of the pedal compartments is necessary in order to avoid adverse conditions for the growth of anaerobic bacteria (93).

In cases of diabetic foot osteomyelitis, x-rays show cortical disruption, periosteal elevation, a sequestrum and/or involucrum, or gross destruction of the bone. However, these radiologic changes do not appear until 10 to 14 days after the onset of the bone infection (42,90). The reported sensitivity of plain radiography in the diagnosis of osteomyelitis is usually low, especially in the early stages of infection (28,41). This may be attributed to several factors, including how positive signs are defined, the timing of the x-rays in relation to the duration of the diabetic foot ulcer, the radiographic technique used, and the skill of the radiologist reading the plain films (41). The radiologic diagnosis of bone infection in diabetic patients is difficult due to complications of Charcot neuroarthropathy, previous bone and/or soft tissue infections, previous bone trauma, and bone deformities (1,115). In cases where no positive findings are found, follow-up plain radiography is usually performed 2 to 6 weeks later, although there is no universal agreement for the best interval of follow-up radiographic imaging. If the diagnosis of diabetic foot osteomyelitis still remains in doubt, further investigations may be needed (125).

Magnetic resonance imaging (MRI) has been suggested as the most useful imaging study to evaluate both soft tissue and bone-related infections, especially in the early stages (42,70,87). Meta-analyses have found that the sensitivity of an MRI for diabetic foot osteomyelitis is about 90% and the specificity about 85%, diagnostic odds ratio (OR) of 24, and likelihood rations estimated at positive of 3.8 and negative of 0.14 (70). Abscesses associated with osteomyelitis (81), necrosis (83), and tendon involvement (82) are also identified effectively using an MRI. In some diabetic foot cases, MRI can play a role in surgical planning (122), but no studies have proved its usefulness. MRI has also been used for guiding the duration of antibiotics in cases of forefoot osteomyelitis in diabetic patients (118), but the cost-effectiveness of this approach should be evaluated taking into account that the PTB test was used as a sign suggestive of bone infection and to indicate the need of MRI (118). Despite the generalized opinion that MRI may help surgeons to plan the surgical procedure, the exact role of advanced imaging studies in order to determine the level of resection and thus minimizing the infection recurrence has still not been clarified with only a few studies reported on this topic. One study reported that 13 out of 21 diabetic feet were operated on the level of amputation/resection that was limited to the specific region of infection demonstrated at MRI (97). There were no recurrences at the surgical margins during 9 months of follow-up. However, in this study, no information about the type of surgical resection, that is, whether the wound was closed or open in order to heal by secondary intention, was provided (97). Furthermore, the authors recognized that the extent of infection could have been overestimated with the MRI and no histologic correlation with regard to the extent of involvement was found. Additionally, a preoperative MRI in cases of diabetic foot osteomyelitis with associated ischemia may be less effective for distinguishing osteomyelitis from bone marrow edema than in cases of neuropathic ulcers (53). Recently, a group of authors suggested a surgical strategy for diabetic foot osteomyelitis based on MRI findings. They recommended that the appropriate surgical margin performing amputations should be set in the area of bone marrow edema based on MRI examination after

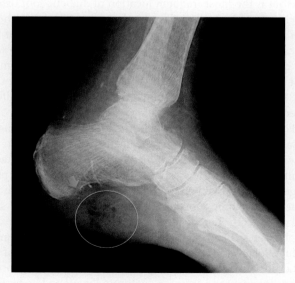

FIGURE 7.2 A lateral view of a plain pedal x-ray showing free gas in the plantar space *(encircled in yellow)* with calcaneal osteomyelitis *(blue arrow)*.

revascularization if needed (54). However, in this study, it is very difficult to extract definitive conclusions in a very short retrospective period.

Nuclear medical imaging used in the diabetic foot pathology includes 3-phase technetium bone scan, gallium scan, and indium-labeled leukocyte scan. Of the 3 nuclear imaging studies, the indium scan is the most sensitive and specific for diagnosing diabetic foot osteomyelitis (42). Newer hybrid imaging techniques (single-photon emission computed tomography/computed tomography [SPECT/CT], positron emission tomography/computed tomography [PET/CT], and PET/ MRI) seem to be very useful in the diagnosis of diabetic foot osteomyelitis, but more research is needed (57). When MRI is not available or contraindicated, white blood cell–labeled nuclear medical imaging, SPECT/CT, or 18F-fluorodeoxyglucose (18F-FDG) PET scans should be considered (88).

Empiric Antibiotic Treatment for Diabetic Foot Infections

Antibiotics must be initiated at the moment in which infection is diagnosed. Selection of an initial antibiotic regimen is usually empiric covering the most common infecting organisms but can be modified according to the DFI severity and available clinical or microbiologic information (88). Several conditions should be taken into account when selecting empiric antibiotics. In cases in which maceration of the ulcer exists and/or there is a warm climate, the presence of *Pseudomonas* species should be considered. Anaerobes must be covered by antibiotics in cases of ischemia, necrosis, or gas-forming DFIs. The physician needs to consider adding an agent active against methicillin-resistant *Staphylococcus aureus* (MRSA) if there is a substantial risk of infection with this organism (e.g., high local prevalence of MRSA, a patient with a recent stay in a health care institution, recent antibiotic therapy, or known MRSA colonization) (88). Empiric antibiotic treatment of moderate/ severe DFIs based on several preoperative conditions and according to the recommendations of the IWGDF 2015 is shown in Table 7.3. Soft tissue and/or bone specimens with bone biopsy to be analyzed in a microbiology/histopathology laboratory must be taken during surgery.

Anatomic Surgical Principles for Diabetic Foot Infections

The foot is divided into rigid compartments. When an infection penetrates into a compartment, there is an increase of the compartmental pressure. When compartmental pressure exceeds the capillary pressure, necrosis occurs. Bacterial growth, toxins, and leukocyte response may also produce necrosis. The pressure in the foot compartments in a patient with diabetic neuropathy may also be increased due to edema caused by the sorbitol pathway and disturbances in the capillary permeability (106).

The anatomic floor of the foot compartments is the plantar aponeurosis, which is attached to the calcaneus and spreads distally to the toes. The plantar aponeurosis is the outermost fascia,

and it is the anatomic layer located beneath the subcutaneous tissue. The medial and central foot compartments are separated by the medial intermuscular septum, which extends from the medial calcaneal tuberosity to the first metatarsal head. The central and lateral compartments are separated by the lateral intermuscular septum, which extends from the calcaneus to the fifth metatarsal head. The medial compartment contains the flexor hallucis brevis muscle, abductor hallucis muscle, and flexor hallucis longus tendon. The central compartment contains the flexor digitorum brevis muscle, lumbrical muscles, flexor digitorum longus tendons, and quadratus plantae muscle. It has been argued that the central compartment has 2 subcompartments, superficial and deep or "calcaneal" section (94), although this subdivision was not recognized by other authors (60). The lateral compartment contains the flexor digiti minimi brevis muscle and abductor digiti minimi muscle. The interosseous compartment is located between the metatarsal bones and contains the interossei muscles. Figure 7.3 shows a cross-section of the compartments of the foot.

The fascial planes do not contain the infection in the forefoot as has been reported in 1 study using MRI (80). The dorsal foot compartment (23,24) is also very important in some types of DFIs. The dorsal aspect of the foot has a thin layer of subcutaneous tissue, and the tendons contained in this space can be easily exposed in the presence of an infection. The tendons of the great toe are the extensor hallucis longus and extensor hallucis brevis. From the second through the fifth toes, the tendons are the extensor digitorum longus and extensor digitorum brevis.

In cases of a bone infection, the first layer affected by the infection is the periosteum. Subsequently, the cortical bone may be affected, and if the infection progresses into the medullar bone, osteomyelitis is strictly defined and established. This sequence is very important because the soft tissues around the bone may be affected by the infection. The forefoot is the most frequent location of diabetic foot osteomyelitis (4,118). A surgical series demonstrated that diabetic foot osteomyelitis was located at the forefoot in 90% of the cases, midfoot in 5%, and hindfoot in the remaining 5% of the cases (4). Other reports have had higher figures of midfoot and hindfoot osteomyelitis with 1 study describing that 21.8% of their patients presented with midfoot and hindfoot osteomyelitis (71).

Forefoot osteomyelitis involves the toe phalanges and metatarsal heads. When analyzing the anatomy of the forefoot, the only location in which there is neither joint nor tendon attachments is the tip of the toes, which is the tip of the distal phalanges. Ulcers located on the tip of the toe can easily reach the bone because only subcutaneous tissue lies between the skin and periosteum. Tendon attachments are on the base of the distal phalanges. The flexor hallucis longus (plantar) and extensor hallucis longus (dorsal) tendons are attached to the base of the distal phalanx of the hallux (great toe). The flexor digitorum longus (plantar) and extensor digitorum longus and brevis tendons (dorsal) are attached to the base of the distal phalanges of the lesser toes. Osteomyelitis may spread proximally through

TABLE 7.3	Empiric Antibiotic Treatment of Moderate/Severe Diabetic Foot Infections Based on Several Preoperative Conditions and According to the Recommendations of the International Working Group on Diabetic Foot 2015
No complicating clinical features	• Amoxicillin/clavulanate • Ampicillin/sulbactam • Second-/third-generation cephalosporin
Recent antibiotics	• Ticarcillin/clavulanate • Piperacillin/tazobactam • Third-generation cephalosporin • Ertapenem
Macerated ulcer Warm climate	• Ticarcillin/clavulanate • Piperacillin/tazobactam • Semisynthetic penicillinase-resistant penicillin + ceftazidime • Semisynthetic penicillinase-resistant penicillin + antipseudomonal fluoroquinolone • Imipenem, meropenem, doripenem
Ischemic limb Necrosis Gas-forming infections	• Amoxicillin/clavulanate • Ampicillin/sulbactam • Ticarcillin/clavulanate • Piperacillin/tazobactam • Ertapenem, imipenem, meropenem, doripenem • Second-/third-generation cephalosporin + clindamycin or metronidazole
Risk factors for methicillin-resistant *Staphylococcus aureus* (MRSA)	• Consider addition/or substituting with • Glycopeptides • Linezolid • Daptomycin • Fusidic acid • Trimethoprim/sulfamethoxazole • Doxycycline • Fluoroquinolone • ±Rifampin
Risk factors for resistant gram-negative rods	• Carbapenems • Fluoroquinolone • Aminoglycoside • Colistin

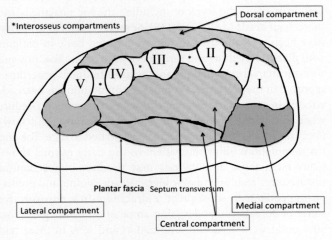

FIGURE 7.3 A cross-section of the compartments of the foot.

these tendons. Ulcers located in the interphalangeal joints on the dorsum of the toes may easily involve the joint. This is frequently found in cases of toe deformities, such as claw toes or hammertoes, subjected to trauma with the shoes.

Another common location in which the ulcers can easily reach the joint and the bone is the space located between the lesser toes. These interdigital ulcers appear on the lateral side of the lesser toes due to high pressure from the adjacent phalangeal condyle as a result of wearing tight shoes. Lateral hallux deformities such as bunions are high-risk locations for osteomyelitis. Plantar ulcers with osteomyelitis may become especially difficult to treat because before reaching the bone, the infection may involve the tendons inside the compartments and can spread both proximally and distally from the point of entry. Osteomyelitis of the first ray (great toe and first metatarsal) may spread through the medial compartment;

osteomyelitis of the second to fourth rays may spread through the central compartment, whereas those of the fifth ray can spread through the lateral compartment (6).

Timing for Surgical Interventions in Patients with Diabetic Foot Infections

The timing for performing surgery in DFIs is not well defined, but it has been reported that prompt surgical treatment including extensive use of revascularization may reduce the need for above-the-ankle amputations (33,56,114,116). Delay in diabetic patient referrals to a specialized department has been reported on the Eurodiale study. Causes for delays in diabetic patient referrals usually include the local health care organization, availability of resources, personal beliefs of the health care professionals, and training of primary care teams. On average, more than 1 in 4 individuals was treated for >3 months before a referral was made to a diabetic foot clinic (103). Delay in patient referral is considered a risk factor for amputation (67), and this is especially true in cases of DFIs and peripheral arterial disease.

Diabetic foot surgery has been categorized into 4 classes (17). Nonvascular surgical interventions due to acutely DFIs are classified as class III or curative (procedures performed to assist in healing open wound) and as class IV or emergency (procedures performed to limit progression of acute infection) (17). They include incision and drainage, surgical débridement, bone resections, and minor or major amputations. Currently, no classification system exists in order to determine either the point at which surgery becomes absolutely necessary or when surgery is likely to produce a better outcome than further prolonged treatment with antibiotics.

Conversely, there is agreement that when the DFI is potentially life-threatening, immediate surgery should be indicated (52). Delay in the implementation of appropriate diabetic foot surgery may be responsible for the high percentage of lower extremity amputations. Guidelines for treating diabetic foot osteomyelitis suggest urgent surgery for necrotizing fasciitis, deep soft tissue abscesses, or gangrene accompanying osteomyelitis. Nonurgent surgery may be necessary if there is a significant compromise of the soft tissue envelope (26). When diabetic foot osteomyelitis is not linked to such complicating factors, some researchers advocate antibiotic treatment, whereas others recommend surgical débridement or combined approaches. The IDSA guidelines state that there are 4 clinical case scenarios in which nonsurgical management of osteomyelitis might be considered (89): (a) There is no acceptable surgical target (i.e., radical cure of the infection would cause unacceptable loss of function); (b) the patient has ischemia caused by nonreconstructable vascular disease but wishes to avoid amputation; (c) infection is confined to the forefoot, and there is minimal soft tissue loss; and (d) the patient and health care professionals agree that surgical management carries excessive risk or is otherwise not appropriate or desirable.

Based on the clinical presentation of diabetic foot osteomyelitis, surgery is required when the bone is protruding through the ulcer, when there is extensive bone destruction seen on x-ray or progressive bone destruction on sequential x-ray while undergoing antibiotic treatment, or when the soft tissue envelope is compromised and there is gangrene or spreading of the soft tissue infection (7). When some of these factors are present, this indicates that the clinical case scenario is advanced and the only possible curative option is amputation. Indeed, bone exposed through the diabetic foot ulcer and soft tissue infections associated with osteomyelitis are risk factors for amputation that have been encountered previously (4,10).

The optimum timing for vascular surgery in diabetic patients with ischemia and foot osteomyelitis has not yet been identified. In cases of severe DFIs, it is important to proceed with surgical débridement as soon as possible with the intention of performing revascularization after adequate surgical débridement. For a diabetic patient with a severely infected dysvascular foot, it is preferable to perform revascularization within 1 to 2 days of the initial surgical débridement (127). When the patient is metabolically stable and osteomyelitis is not accompanied by necrotizing changes, deep abscesses, or systemic response to infection, it is preferable to start antibiotic treatment and perform revascularization as soon as possible.

Increased distal blood flow to the lower extremity can be attained to promote wound healing after a surgical procedure on the infected bone. A health care team in Rome monitored transcutaneous oxygen tension (TcPo$_2$) after percutaneous transluminal angioplasty (PTA) in diabetic patients with ischemic foot ulcers (74). They found that in the group of patients with successful revascularization, the percentage of patients with a TcPo$_2$ greater than or equal to 30 mmHg was 38.5% 1 week after PTA, although this increased to 75% after 3 weeks. They concluded that when it is possible to delay surgery, the best time to perform a more aggressive débridement or minor amputations is 3 to 4 weeks after successful revascularization (31). Conversely, there is a lack of evidence related to the optimum time for performing bone surgery in a diabetic patient after a lower extremity revascularization.

Surgery of Diabetic Forefoot Osteomyelitis

The most frequent location of osteomyelitis in the feet of diabetic patients is the forefoot including the toe phalanges and metatarsal heads (4,19,55,86,118). Several types of amputation have been typically used to remove infected bone in patients with diabetes mellitus and forefoot osteomyelitis. Toe, ray, and transmetatarsal amputations are the most frequent procedures reported in the literature. Prompt toe amputation has been advocated in cases of toe osteomyelitis as a cost-saving procedure when compared to long-term antibiotic therapy (72); however, this has not been prospectively validated to date. Toe and ray amputations allow the patient to use fairly normal shoes. Conversely, these amputations may produce biomechanical disturbances resulting in new high-pressure points and predisposing patients to subsequent reulceration. In a retrospective study of 90 patients undergoing amputation of the great toe, 60% underwent a second amputation and 17% of these had a below-the-knee amputation (98). In addition, various reulcerations and reamputations could probably be reduced with a specialized multidisciplinary postoperative treatment based on custom-made shoes and diabetic foot care (38).

In cases of toe phalangeal involvement, the toe can be amputated through the phalanx, interphalangeal joint, metatarsophalangeal joint, or the metatarsal bone. The decision of closing the wound primarily will depend on whether there is no infected bone and/or soft tissue in the surgical wound. It was reported that 10.3% (10/97) of dehiscence of surgical wounds occurred when treating diabetic foot osteomyelitis using at least 4 weeks of antibiotic therapy and local dressing before performing the amputation (47). In a series of 185 patients, minor amputations consisted of 70 partial or total amputations of toes and 9 open transmetatarsal amputations combined with healing by secondary intention (4). Healing was achieved in 120 days (range 21 to 365) in the cases of open minor amputations. Open transmetatarsal amputations with subsequent closure techniques may be useful in cases of advanced forefoot DFIs.

Surgical treatment of diabetic foot osteomyelitis without amputation is an alternate option to remove infected bone while conserving the soft tissue envelope and maintaining the external appearance of the foot. The term "internal pedal amputation" has been used by some authors (45,74) even though the term "conservative surgery" could be more appropriate for defining this type of diabetic foot surgery without amputation. Conservative surgical treatment was initially defined as a limited resection of the infected part of the phalanx or the metatarsal bone under the wound, without any other resection associated with the excision of the ulcer site (62). Other authors later defined this type of surgery as any procedure in which only the infected bone and nonviable soft tissue are removed but no amputation of any part of the foot is undertaken (4). Surgery without amputation may be a positive outcome for a patient with diabetes mellitus because it is aesthetically acceptable (47), although the impact of this type of surgery on the quality of life has not been addressed. In theory, a conservative surgical approach also changes the foot biomechanics, even though the risk of reulceration may be lower than amputation, where more bone segments are removed.

Removing the distal phalanx can be successfully carried out to treat osteomyelitis of the distal phalanx of any toe. Percutaneous tenotomy can be performed in an outpatient clinic in cases of claw toe deformities with distal phalangeal osteomyelitis (113). In this study (113), the authors did not report on whether infected bone on the tip of the toes was removed in addition to tenotomy or was treated exclusively with antibiotics. In cases of involvement of the interphalangeal joint, a resection arthroplasty can be carried out (4,13,73,95). Other authors have reported using a modified arthroplasty to treat osteomyelitis of the proximal and distal interphalangeal joint and the tip of the second, third, fourth, and fifth toes. In one such study, no great toe osteomyelitis was included in a group of 52 patients (57 feet and 72 toes). The bone was removed through a dorsal wound, the wound was irrigated, and a Kirschner wire 1.2 mm in diameter was inserted (85). Healing was achieved in 25.6 ± 6.2 days (73). Another common location of osteomyelitis in the foot of diabetic patients is the lesser metatarsal heads. Metatarsal head resection is a very useful procedure employed by different study groups in cases with

or without osteomyelitis (4,19,47,51,124). Dorsal or plantar approach can be used to remove the infected metatarsal head.

The location of diabetic forefoot osteomyelitis that is the most difficult to treat is the first metatarsophalangeal joint, which is the largest joint and the most complex. Osteomyelitis involving the hallux is a serious condition because it has an important role in the biomechanics of the foot (84), and its amputation is associated with significant biomechanical disturbances. Furthermore, osteomyelitis of the hallux and first metatarsophalangeal joint can be associated with longer healing times (32). One-stage resection and pin stabilization was reported in a retrospective series consisting of 15 patients (18 feet) with an average follow-up of 48.8 months (68). Only 1 patient required a transmetatarsal amputation after the procedure for worsening infection and wound complications. Another option is to use external fixation after removing the infected bone (108). The authors (108) used staged surgical procedures consisting of ulcer excision, removal of all necrotic soft tissue and bone, followed by pulse lavage irrigation, culturing, and polymethylmethacrylate antibiotic cement application. The staged procedure included a mini-external fixator that was placed in 4 out of 6 cases. When the infection was eradicated, the authors subsequently used allogenic bone graft, iliac crest bone graft, or arthroplasty without bone grafting with the external fixator. None of the surviving patients developed a recurrent ulceration or required amputation after 14 months of follow-up (108). Another study reported a cohort including 28 patients with osteomyelitis of the first ray treated by a technique requiring a one-stage surgical approach (37). After surgical débridement with removal of the infected bone, the authors inserted an antibiotic-loaded bone cement and stabilized the treated area with an external fixator. Four patients developed a relapse of the ulceration after the procedure. During the follow-up period, no ulceration recurrences, transfer ulcerations, shoe gear problems, or gait abnormalities were detected in the other 24 patients (37).

Using an antibiotic-impregnated cement spacer to fill the cavity resulting from the removal of the infected bone is another option. The authors (95) describing this therapy treated 7 out of 20 patients who presented with osteomyelitis of the first metatarsophalangeal joint. Bone débridement and antibiotic-impregnated cement spacer were used in every patient, and Kirschner wire was used in 3 patients. Five patients required further surgeries including cement removal and first metatarsophalangeal joint arthrodesis (95). The outcomes in this subgroup of patients were good and 1 of these patients required a below-the-knee amputation due to complications arising from a new ulcer under the fifth metatarsal head.

A usual case where conservative surgery was performed is shown in the following clinical case study. A 52-year-old male had a diabetic foot ulcer on the plantar aspect of his left foot for 3 months. The ulcer was located under the second metatarsal head and was initiated after walking during holidays. He had been treated as an outpatient in another hospital department using several types of dressings and periods of oral antibiotic therapy. Two months after developing the plantar ulceration, the patient presented with severe edema of the left foot and fever (38.5°C) requiring admission to the hospital. MRI was performed with only soft tissue infection involvement. No signs of osteomyelitis were found in the MRI. Cultures of suppuration were taken, and *Streptococcus* species and MRSA were isolated. Treatment with linezolid and clindamycin was implemented. Systemic and inflammatory signs of the foot were improved, and the patient was discharged from the hospital 10 days after being admitted. Outpatient wound care for the left foot was provided and the plantar ulcer healed, but 3 days after healing, suppuration on the dorsum of the left foot was evident.

New hospital admission was required while another health care provider recommended a transmetatarsal amputation to the left foot. The patient sought consultation in our department to avoid amputation. At physical examination, the left foot was edematous, a fistula on the dorsum of the foot was evident (Fig. 7.4), and the dorsal tendons were visible at the bottom of the fistula. There was also associated erythema on the dorsum of the foot, the second toe was swollen, and the plantar ulcer was healed (Fig. 7.5). In our department, we performed instrumental exploration of the fistula, and a track along the tendons (proximally and distally) was detected (Fig. 7.6). Lower extremity distal pulses were palpable to the left foot.

The patient had hypertension and a 2-year history of diabetes mellitus controlled with oral hypoglycemic agents. During his hospital admission, the laboratory test results were as follows: glucose, 125 mg/dL; blood urea nitrogen, 48 mg/dL; creatinine, 1 mg/dL; sodium, 143 mEq/L; hemoglobin, 12.9 g/dL; white blood cell count, 6,600 cells/µL; platelet

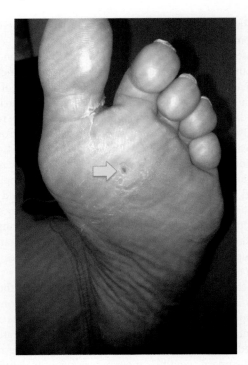

FIGURE 7.5 Clinical picture of the healed ulceration at the plantar aspect of the left foot *(yellow arrow)*.

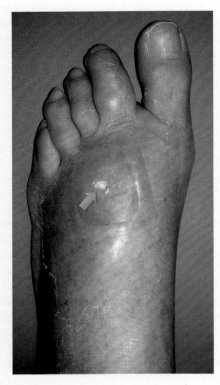

FIGURE 7.4 Clinical picture of the fistula on the dorsum of the left foot *(blue arrow)* with visualization of the extensor tendon at the bottom of the fistula.

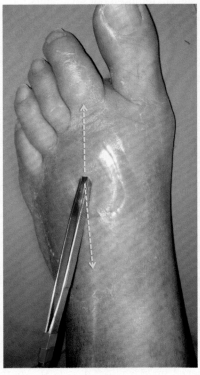

FIGURE 7.6 Instrumental exploration of the dorsal left foot fistula with a track along the extensor tendons (proximally and distally).

count, 202,000 cells/μL; and an erythrocyte sedimentation rate, 60 mm/h. An x-ray of the left foot was taken (Fig. 7.7), revealing dislocation of the second metatarsophalangeal joint and cortical disruption of the second metatarsal head. Minor cortical disruption could also be seen at the base of the proximal phalanx of the second toe (see Fig. 7.7). Osteomyelitis with fistulization to the dorsum of the foot with tenosynovitis and proximal spreading was diagnosed, and surgical treatment was offered to the patient.

Our department's surgical approach is based on the following several steps (9):

1. Early conservative surgery (attempt to minimize resection): Surgical treatment of diabetic foot osteomyelitis without amputation is an alternate option for the removal of infected bone while conserving the soft tissue envelope and maintaining the external appearance of the foot.
2. Total or partial removal of the infected bone and soft tissues: The surgical procedure is planned based on plain pedal x-rays, but the final procedure is carried out according to intraoperative findings.

3. Intraoperative bone biopsy for microbiology and pathology: Surgical margins are not specifically studied.
4. The wound is left open to heal by secondary intention; this permits drainage of any residual infection, especially when infected bone has not been completely resected.
5. Efficient local wound care and off-loading
6. Postoperative systemic antibiotic treatment based on intraoperative bone cultures
7. Assume that the infection is resolved when the surgical wound is epithelized for 6 months.
8. Customized insoles and shoes to reduce further transfer lesions in the foot

The first step during this patient's surgery was to explore the distal and proximal track from the fistulous wound (Fig. 7.8). After exploring the track, a dorsal incision was made covering the entire fistulous track (Fig. 7.9). Extensor tendon involvement was evident, and the tendon involved by the infection (Fig. 7.10) was resected (Fig. 7.11). The periosteum was enlarged and was dissected before approaching the second metatarsal bone (Fig. 7.12). Osteotomy was performed in an apparent healthy zone using a power saw (Fig. 7.13), and the second metatarsal head was removed (Fig. 7.14). The resected second metatarsal head and tendon were sent to the pathology department with a portion of the bone to the microbiology department. The base of the proximal phalanx of the second toe was also removed, and the resected space was irrigated with super-oxidized water (Fig. 7.15). Packing with calcium alginate was placed in the residual space of the resected second metatarsophalangeal joint (Fig. 7.16).

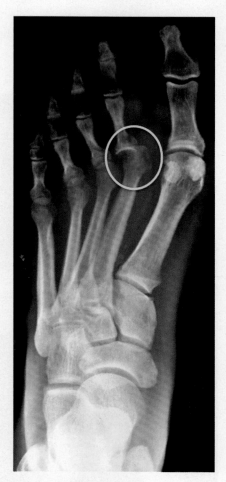

FIGURE 7.7 A plain pedal x-ray of the left foot revealed dislocation of the second metatarsophalangeal joint and cortical disruption of the second metatarsal head. Minor cortical disruption could also be seen at the base of the proximal phalanx of the second toe (*encircled in yellow*).

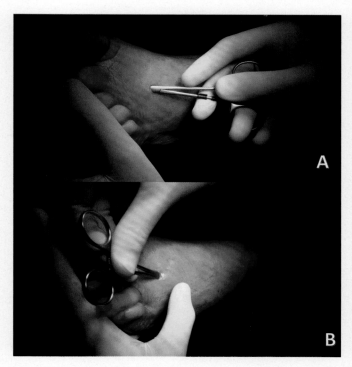

FIGURE 7.8 Intraoperative pictures showing exploration of the distal **(A)** and proximal **(B)** track from the dorsal fistulous wound.

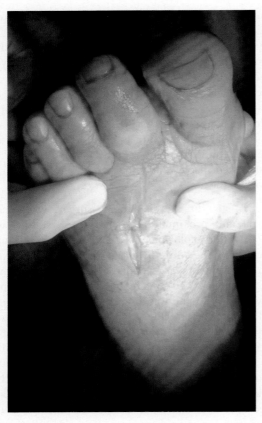

FIGURE 7.9 Intraoperative picture showing the dorsal incision covering the entire fistulous track.

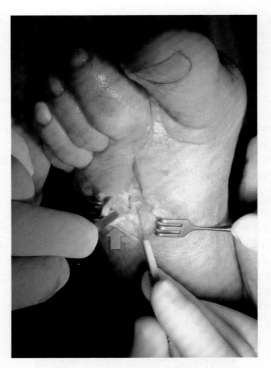

FIGURE 7.10 Intraoperative picture showing the extensor tendon involvement with infection *(blue arrow)*.

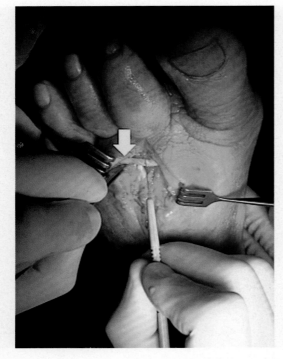

FIGURE 7.11 Intraoperative picture showing the resection of the infected extensor tendon *(yellow arrow)*.

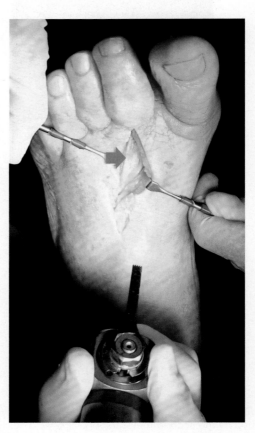

FIGURE 7.12 Intraoperative picture showing the enlarged periosteum which was dissected before approaching the second metatarsal bone *(red arrow)*.

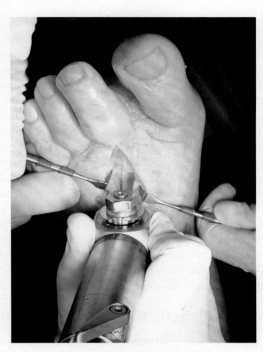

FIGURE 7.13 Intraoperative picture showing the second metatarsal osteotomy which was performed in an apparent healthy zone using a power saw.

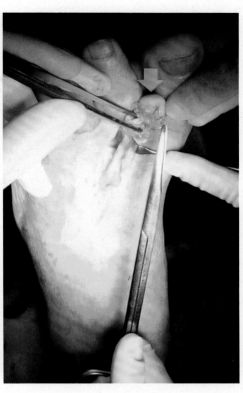

FIGURE 7.14 Intraoperative picture showing the resection of the second metatarsal head *(blue arrow)*.

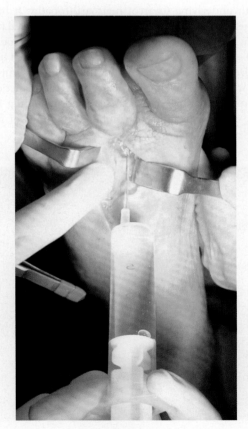

FIGURE 7.15 The base of the proximal phalanx of the second toe was also removed. This intraoperative picture is showing irrigation of the resected second metatarsophalangeal joint with super-oxidized water.

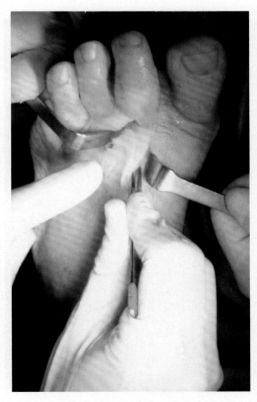

FIGURE 7.16 Intraoperative picture showing packing with calcium alginate in the residual space of the resected second metatarsophalangeal joint.

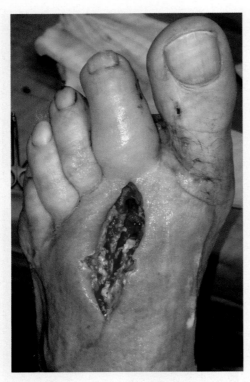

FIGURE 7.17 Initial postoperative picture 2 days after the surgical procedure. The associated left foot edema had been improved, and the wound bed was clean without necrosis.

Empiric intravenous levofloxacin was administered before surgery. Final microbiology cultures revealed no growth in the bone cultures, and the intravenous levofloxacin was changed to oral administration after 7 days. Final pathology reports revealed a polymorphonuclear neutrophil infiltrate over a background of chronic inflammatory cells involving the periosteum and cortical bone, extending to the medullar bone. These findings were compatible with acute exacerbation of chronic osteomyelitis. Necrotizing changes were also found on the extensor tendon.

The first postoperative wound assessment was carried out 48 hours after surgery. The associated foot edema had been improved, and the wound bed was clean without necrosis (Fig. 7.17). Negative pressure wound therapy (NPWT) was then applied (Fig. 7.18). Four days after applying the NPWT, the wound had a satisfactory healing course and the foot edema was totally resolved (Fig. 7.19). The wound finally healed 60 days after the original surgery (Fig. 7.20), whereas the oral levofloxacin was administered for a total of 37 days.

Surgery of Diabetic Midfoot Osteomyelitis

Large series including patients with diabetes mellitus and midfoot osteomyelitis has not been reported in the medical literature. Most studies including these patients are case reports making it difficult to extract definitive conclusions. Cases involving midfoot osteomyelitis are frequently associated with underlying Charcot neuroarthropathy. It has been recommended that repeated bone resections followed by using antibiotic cement spacer or beads in such cases may be beneficial (96). As a consequence of bone resection, the foot becomes destabilized and lower extremity immobilization is implicated. Several ways of stabilizing and correcting the diabetic Charcot neuroarthropathy have been reported, including internal fixation, external fixation, or combined methods of fixation.

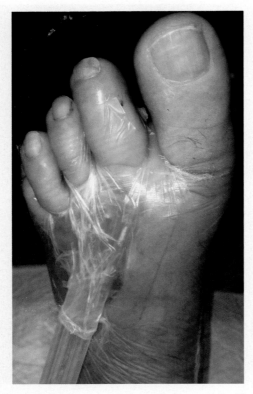

FIGURE 7.18 Postoperative picture showing application of the negative pressure wound therapy at the first postoperative wound dressing change.

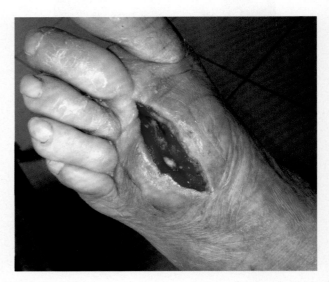

FIGURE 7.19 Postoperative picture 4 days after application of the negative pressure wound therapy. The surgical wound had a satisfactory healing course and the foot edema was totally resolved.

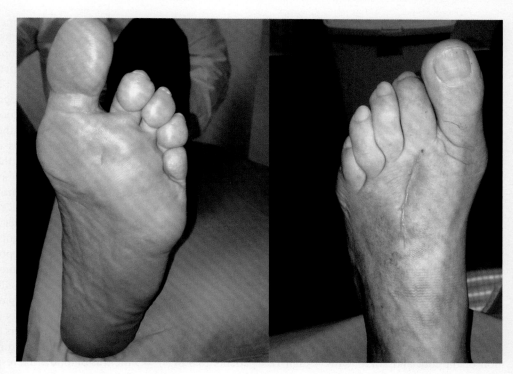

FIGURE 7.20 Postoperative clinical pictures of the left foot showing complete healing of the wound 60 days after the original surgery.

Internal fixation is contraindicated in an area of previous osteomyelitis (29). Circular external fixation based on Ilizarov principles provides stabilization following correction of deformities (102). Complex procedures of plastic surgery closure can be used together with external fixation to achieve diabetic limb salvage (29,104). A group of authors reported 2 cases of extensive midfoot osteomyelitis and unstable foot successfully treated by a different approach. Most of the part of the infected bone was surgically removed, and a windowed total contact casting was used to stabilize extensive bone destruction and achieve a stable foot following surgery (11).

Surgery of the Diabetic Hindfoot and Ankle Osteomyelitis

Saving the diabetic foot in cases of calcaneus ulcers and osteomyelitis is a challenge because failure frequently leads to a major amputation. Subtotal and total calcanectomy has been suggested as an option to achieve limb salvage in patients, including those with diabetes mellitus (21,27,50,85,101,105). A systematic review of partial or total calcanectomy as an alternative to below-the-knee amputation was recently reported (107). The combined data represented 100 patients who had undergone 76 partial and 28 total calcanectomies, giving a total of 104 calcanectomies. Forty-nine out of 76 partial calcanectomies (64.4%) did not have complications. Total calcanectomy was carried out without complications in 14 out of 28 cases (50%). Minor complications were skin breakdown, subcutaneous abscess, papilloma, postoperative hematoma, and delayed healing. Regarding major complications, the rate was 36.1% after total calcanectomy and 15.8% after

a partial calcanectomy. Seven cases of partial calcanectomy (9.2%) and 4 cases of total calcanectomy (14.3%) subsequently required a major amputation (14.3%). Patients with diabetes mellitus had a fivefold greater risk of undergoing a major amputation (107). Another study also reported that patients with diabetes mellitus and those with peripheral arterial disease are at high risk of failure after undergoing partial calcanectomy (105). Seventy-five percent of patients maintained their preoperative ambulatory status postoperatively following either partial or total calcanectomy (107).

In another study, a group of authors reported a series that was not included in the aforementioned review, which consisted of 24 patients who had undergone a partial calcanectomy (120). Using a midline incision, they removed the necrotic soft tissue and calcaneal bone. Resection of the insertion of the Achilles tendon was sometimes required when it was involved in the infection. If primary closure was possible, closure was achieved in a single layer with 2-0 nylon. If not possible, the wound was left open and repeated surgical débridement with secondary closure was planned. Only 1 out of 24 patients underwent a below-the-knee amputation. In addition, only in 1 out of the 8 patients with diabetes mellitus the infection was not controlled and required further resection. Four patients with diabetes mellitus required secondary suturing. The mean hospital stay in patients with diabetes mellitus was 56.7 days and healing was achieved in 118 days. There was no major difference in the failure rate between patients with and without diabetes mellitus. All patients were able to walk with or without external support (120).

When the surgical wound is healed, the diabetic patient will need regular foot care, customized insoles, and adequate footwear to minimize the risk of reulceration. Orthotic devices, custom-made shoes, ankle-foot orthosis, and Charcot restraint orthotic walkers were used to assist the patients to maintain their ambulatory status after total or partial calcanectomy (107).

Charcot neuroarthropathy of the ankle is a severe complication that becomes limb-threatening when it is complicated by osteomyelitis. A group of authors reported a prospective cohort of 45 patients with Charcot neuroarthropathy foot and ankle osteomyelitis (36). The location of the ulcer complicated by osteomyelitis was plantar at the hindfoot in 13 cases, 18 in the medial malleolus, and 13 in the lateral malleolus. The authors used extensive débridement of the infected bone, and the foot was subsequently stabilized with external fixation. The authors reported the key elements of their successful experience including complete surgical débridement of the infected tissue, application of the external fixator with pins and wires not interfering with the infection site, use of only tensioned thin wires on the foot, 6 to 8 weeks of parenteral antibiotics in the postoperative period, and use of NPWT for the postoperative treatment of open wounds. Fifteen patients had critical limb ischemia and underwent 12 percutaneous transluminal angioplasties and 3 bypasses before the surgical reconstruction of the foot and ankle. Only 4 high-risk patients (8.8%) required a major amputation (36).

Outcomes of Surgical Treatment for Diabetic Foot Infections

Amputation rates may depend on the particular surgical approach (22), but the experience and skills of the surgeon should also be taken into consideration (119). A group of authors included in their series 114 diabetic patients who underwent emergency surgery for indications of infection, gangrene, or infected neurotrophic ulcers (116). Surgery was always performed within 48 hours of admission in the operating room under regional (never local) anesthesia, and 47% of those patients underwent 2 or more surgical procedures. The authors stated that early aggressive incision and drainage, surgical débridement, and local foot amputations combined with use of revascularization resulted in cumulative diabetic limb salvage of 74% at 5 years (64). This aggressive method of treatment in this series was safe because only 1 patient died due to myocardial infarction. A group of authors (44) published a series involving 223 patients treated for DFIs. They reported that 43% of their patients healed after an amputation (major or minor) and the total rate of major amputations was 10.7% (44). Another group reported the outcomes of diabetic patients with presumed adequate circulatory status undergoing toe amputations. Complete healing was achieved in only 34%, infection persisted in 36% of the operated limbs (99), whereas 24% of their patients underwent a major amputation (99). A higher amputation rate was found in 1 study in which life-threatening infections were excluded, where 33% of their patients underwent amputations although the level where these were performed was not stated (22). Despite peripheral arterial disease being the cause of most of their wounds, an arterial bypass was performed on only 1 of the 26 patients who underwent amputation (3.8%) and on only 2 of the 52 patients who did not undergo amputation (22). In the multivariate analysis, the presence of peripheral arterial disease increased the risk of amputation by 12.5 times (22). These results highlight the importance of appropriate vascular treatment in the treatment of the diabetic foot.

Another group of authors reported that when aggressive revascularization was carried out, deep foot infections in ischemic patients had the same prognosis as in nonischemic patients (47). Early surgical débridement of deep foot abscesses and revascularization were the keys to achieving good results (47). Only 4.7% in a group of 106 patients with deep foot infections underwent major amputation, whereas revascularization was performed in 60.3% of the patients (47). Other authors have also reported high short-term limb salvage rate with aggressive treatment of invasive foot infection during a period of less than 48 hours from admission followed by autogenous arterial bypass (33). Another group of authors using extensive angioplasty in patients with critical limb ischemia and severe foot ulcers reported 15.7% of major amputations and 60.8% of wound healing after 4.9 ± 0.9 and 9.4 ± 0.5 months of follow-up, respectively (117).

These aforementioned studies remark the fact that careful vascular status determination must be made before performing a diabetic foot amputation. It has been shown that the combination of peripheral arterial disease and infection has a major impact on healing rates. Ischemia has long been recognized as a factor contributing to prolonged hospitalization, spread of infection, and avoidable amputation in diabetic patients with foot ulcers. The possibility of the presence of ischemia should always be completely ruled out in diabetic patients with infected foot ulcers. In cases where pedal pulses are absent, a vascular surgeon should be consulted. Minor amputations in a foot without adequate foot perfusion may be complicated by nonhealing wounds, spread of infection, and necrosis, with major amputation subsequently being required. Failure of treatment was linked to values of ankle systolic blood pressure <50 mmHg, toe systolic blood pressure <30 mmHg, ankle-brachial index <0.5, and transcutaneous oxygen pressure (TcPo$_2$) <20 mmHg in a prospective series of DFIs, including 58% of osteomyelitis (40). Other authors also reported peripheral arterial disease as a risk factor for failure of conservative surgery and amputation (4,5,8). Hartemann-Heurtier et al. (61) showed that an increase in the time to heal correlated with the existence of peripheral arterial disease and end-stage renal disease treated with hemodialysis. In this study, the outcomes of 6 patients with osteomyelitis and ischemia were not reported because these patients were included in the group of 30 patients with severe peripheral arterial disease. In this ischemic group, 24 patients had undergone bypass vascular surgery with a limb salvage rate of 97.5% with this aggressive approach (61). Henke et al. (63) demonstrated that peripheral arterial disease was associated with a lower rate of wound healing and limb salvage. In their sample, bypass arterial surgery was linked to wound healing and limb salvage.

Aggressive surgical débridement accompanied by early revascularization can achieve a high rate of limb salvage (61,63). The decision to intervene with an open bypass arterial surgery rather than endovascular revascularization depends primarily with the pattern of arterial occlusion along with the experience of the surgical team and is best made in a multidisciplinary approach of surgeons and interventionists.

NSTIs in the feet of patients with diabetes mellitus are critical infections. In 1 series of diabetic patients with necrotizing fasciitis of the leg, all 16 patients underwent major amputation (39). Other authors have reported 64.28% of below-the-knee amputations (100). The major amputation rate in another series of 145 patients was 18.6%. These authors classified the infections according to the depth of the necrotizing infection. In the necrotizing cellulitis group (N = 109), 8 (7.3%) major amputations were performed. In the necrotizing fasciitis group (N = 25), 13 (52%) major amputations were undertaken. In the myonecrosis group (N = 11), 6 (54.5%) major amputations were performed. Predictive variables related to limb loss were fasciitis (OR = 20, 95% confidence interval [CI] [3.2 to 122.1]) and myonecrosis (OR = 53.2, 95% CI [5.1 to 552.4]).

In an analysis of randomized controlled trials of antibiotic treatment, MRSA isolation was described as a significant factor associated with the failure of treatment in patients with DFIs (121). However, little evidence exists about the impact of surgical treatment on these worrying infections. In one study, MRSA was isolated in 35 cases (36.8% of *Staphylococcus aureus* isolated and 18% of the total bacteria isolated) and was the only pathogen on 22 occasions. MRSA osteomyelitis was associated with a higher body temperature, raised white blood cell counts, fetid smell, and cutaneous necrosis than the methicillin-sensitive *Staphylococcus aureus*. Moreover, MRSA osteomyelitis was not associated with a worse prognosis in this study (14). Another group of authors found that MRSA osteomyelitis was associated with poorer prognosis (34).

The location of diabetic foot osteomyelitis is related to the outcome of treatment. Karchmer and Gibbons (71) reported the outcomes of surgical treatment of diabetic foot osteomyelitis in 110 patients, with diagnosis proven by biopsy in 96% of the cases. In this group, 88% of minor and 12% of major amputations were performed in 86 cases of forefoot osteomyelitis (71). Another study reported that 48.5% of 167 patients with forefoot osteomyelitis underwent conservative surgery without amputation, 45.5% underwent minor amputations, and 6% had major amputations (4). Faglia et al. (46) stated that toe or ray amputation was performed in 198 out of 234 patients with forefoot osteomyelitis (84.6%), whereas the rest of the patients underwent 25 transmetatarsal and 1 Lisfranc amputations.

Midfoot and hindfoot osteomyelitis were associated with worse prognosis than forefoot osteomyelitis (4,7,71). Conservative management based only on antibiotics prior to admission worsened the lower extremity salvage rate in adults with osteomyelitis of the foot and toe in a group that was not exclusively diabetic (63). The authors reported on a sample of 237 patients who were treated for osteomyelitis over a period of 7 years. In this data set, the patients were treated using 1 of 2 methods

of treatment: medical or surgical. Of the 237 patients, 13 were excluded because they could not be followed postoperatively and another 14 were excluded who had undergone an immediate major amputation. Thus, the sample contained 210 patients of whom 80% were diabetic. Fifty-two percent of the patients had previously been given antibiotics, 19% intravenous, and 33% oral with a mean treatment time of 5 ± 2 months. On admission, 95 patients were treated surgically and 115 were given only antibiotics. In the surgical group, 77% underwent conservative surgery and 23% a minor amputation. Subsequently, 18% of the patients in this group underwent a major amputation, so the rate of limb salvage was 82% after 31 months of follow-up. In the 115 patients receiving medical treatment, the limb salvage rate was 81%. Thus, there was no statistically significant difference between the 2 groups. The initial débridement and bypass arterial surgery were associated with wound healing. Previous antibiotic treatment was associated with limb amputation in the logistic regression model (*P* = .009). The authors suggested that this finding may be related to the development of antibiotic-resistant organisms and the delayed removal of an infected bone nidus that allows advanced contiguous spread of osteomyelitis. The overall rate of major amputations in the 224 patients was 23.6% (63).

Osteomyelitis of the toes is usually treated by amputation of the affected toe (35). Another different approach (61,62) is to perform conservative surgery in cases of diabetic foot osteomyelitis (4,7). The outcome of conservative surgery treating diabetic foot osteomyelitis is not well defined. One report investigated a group of 185 patients, including those with severe soft tissue infections accompanying osteomyelitis. After excluding the patients for whom conservative surgery was found to be not feasible on admission, 111 patients underwent conservative surgery as the first choice. Of those, only 20 (18%) required subsequent amputations, with 13 minor (11.7%) and 7 major amputations (6.3%). Conservative surgery was successful in 82% of the cases (4).

The same working group (4) reported a new cohort of 81 patients with the same characteristics (10). Forty-eight patients (59.3%) had conservative surgery, 32 (39.5%) had minor amputations, and 1 (1.2%) had major amputation (19). The factors associated with amputation in the logistic regression model were previous ulceration (*P* = .03, OR 0.23, 95% CI [0.06 to 0.9]), soft tissue infection accompanying osteomyelitis (*P* = .02, OR 4.9, 95% CI [1.2 to 20]), capillary glucose monitoring in quartiles 2 to 4 (*P* = .04, OR 5.9, 95% CI [1.6 to 24.7]), peripheral arterial disease (*P* < .01, OR 6.2, 95% CI [1.6 to 24.7]), and skin necrosis (*P* < .01, OR 12.2, 95% CI [2.9 to 50.9]). The authors also found that the bone changes seen in pedal x-rays with associated osteomyelitis did not have any prognostic value when surgical treatment was undertaken. The outcomes were more related to soft tissue involvement than the bone destruction seen in pedal x-rays (10). The presence of limb ischemia and soft tissue infections associated to osteomyelitis are associated with a worse prognosis and amputation in cases of diabetic foot osteomyelitis (4,5). Patients with diabetic foot osteomyelitis and deep soft tissue infections have worse prognosis than those with isolated bone infections (44). Other authors have also concurred on this where patients with diabetic foot osteomyelitis have better prognosis than those with deep soft tissue abscesses (46). Deep soft tissue abscesses had a higher rate of major amputations and a much more proximal level of minor amputations. However, the authors also mentioned the possibility that some patients with soft tissue abscesses also had infection in the bone, but this overlap was not considered because the clinical pattern of the abscess was prevalent (46).

These aforementioned outcomes highlight the need for defining the type of osteomyelitis present in order to compare different series. An attempt to characterize the grading of the severity of osteomyelitis was made recently. Osteomyelitis was classified as follows: osteomyelitis without ischemia and without soft tissue involvement (class 1), osteomyelitis with ischemia without soft tissue involvement (class 2), osteomyelitis with soft tissue involvement (class 3), and osteomyelitis with ischemia and soft tissue involvement (class 4). No amputation was required in a subgroup of 25 out of 81 patients without ischemia and soft tissue infections. The characterization of osteomyelitis into 4 classes showed a statistically significant trend toward increased severity and increased amputation rate and mortality (5).

When lower extremity ischemia is not present, the outcomes reported in the literature are optimal. A group of authors (62) retrospectively compared the results of the treatment of osteomyelitis without ischemia over 2 different periods. Thirty-two patients belonged to a past group (1986 to 1993) of patients treated with antibiotic therapy, off-loading, and local wound care. The second group consisted of 32 patients who underwent conservative surgery followed by the same regimen of care (September 1993 to March 1995). Healing rates were 57% for the former group and 78% for the latter ($P < .008$), and there was also a significant difference in healing time: 462 ± 98 days and 181 ± 30 days ($P < .008$), respectively. In the group who underwent conservative surgery, only 2 patients (6.25%) required a minor amputation. In the antibiotic group, failure of the medical management resulted in 40% of patients undergoing amputations: 9 toes, 3 transmetatarsal, and 2 below-the-knee. These authors concluded that in the case of diabetic foot osteomyelitis, conservative surgery reduced the healing time, duration of antibiotic therapy, and the number of secondary surgical procedures. Healing was achieved in 181 ± 30 days (62).

Other authors reported that open wounds healed by secondary intention over a median period of 90 days. The median wound healing times in patients with successful conservative surgery was 80 days (12 to 365) compared to 120 days (21 to 365 days) for those who had minor amputations ($P = .003$). Median wound healing times were longer in cases where there was associated soft tissue infection ($P = .0005$) and limb ischemia ($P = .001$) (4). Another investigation assessed 157 patients with complicated diabetic foot ulcers and 51 patients of whom had osteomyelitis. Forty-five patients had osteomyelitis without foot ischemia, and 41 of these (91%) underwent

surgical treatment with 28 having conservative surgery (68%) and 13 having minor amputations (32%) (61).

Little information is currently available on osteomyelitis remission in the feet of diabetic patients, although its potential to recur is widely accepted (25). Rates of recurrence of diabetic foot osteomyelitis have been reported as 12.1% (75), 30% (109) and 31% (55) after antibiotic treatment, and 60.7% after surgery (55). There are 2 possible explanations for why the ulcer and/or surgical wound may be complicated by osteomyelitis after initial surgery. First, infection may have remained in the operated bone and "persistent infection" would need to be diagnosed. Impaired immune and inflammatory responses, bacterial factors such as biofilms and persistent phenotypes (25), or insufficient surgery (7,75) may be some of the causes for recurrent diabetic foot osteomyelitis. Second, in cases where the infected bone is totally resected, nonhealing wounds may act as a point of entry for reinfection. One study reported that healing was complete in only 57% of 168 patients with limb salvage (63). Eighty-two percent of those whose wounds did not heal had persistent complications as a result of osteomyelitis. Persistent osteomyelitis or insufficient surgery should always be suspected when the wound does not heal. One study dealt specifically with the issue of diabetic foot osteomyelitis recurrence after surgery. Recurrence of osteomyelitis was defined as the appearance of bone infections at the same or adjacent site after healing of both the ulcer and the surgical wound. In cases of recurrence, the ray, bone, and/or joint affected was the same as that operated on in the initial surgery. Reulceration was defined as any ulcer, regardless of depth, appearing during follow-up at the same or other sites including the contralateral foot. A new episode of osteomyelitis was defined in cases where the new ulcer was complicated by bone infection, but this was not considered as a recurrence (19). Osteomyelitis was located on the forefoot in 74 patients (91.3%), midfoot in 4 patients (4.9%), and hindfoot in 3 patients (3.7%). Forty-eight patients (59.3%) underwent conservative surgery, 32 (39.5%) had minor amputations, including 9 open transmetatarsal amputations, and there was 1 (1.2%) major amputation. Recurrence was diagnosed in 3 out of 65 patients (4.6%), 51, 71, and 105 days after healing. No recurrences were observed after this period. Twenty-four out of 65 patients developed reulceration (36.9%) at a new site after a median period of 46.5 weeks. Reulceration was associated with plantar location of the ulcer during the first episode ($P = .02$, hazard ratio [HR] 2.4, 95% CI [1.1 to 5.1]) and Charcot neuroarthropathy ($P = .002$, HR 4.3, 95% CI [1.6 to 10.9]). A new episode of osteomyelitis was diagnosed in 11 patients (17%). There was no doubt about the new site of infection in all the cases, and limb salvage was achieved in each case (19).

Recent studies have highlighted the fact that patients with bone margins affected by infection after undergoing amputation for osteomyelitis have poor prognosis. Wide excision of necrotic and infected bone with 5 mm or greater of clearance has been shown to reduce the risk for recurrence in cases of chronic osteomyelitis (111), but in this study, only 7 out of 50 patients (14%) had chronic osteomyelitis which had spread from an overlying ulcer. However, it is difficult to extract any conclusion from this study for the treatment of bone infection in the feet of patients with diabetes mellitus. A group of researchers reported a retrospective series of 111 patients, evaluating the impact of residual osteomyelitis on surgical margins after surgical resection of infected bone (75). Forty-seven patients underwent digital amputation, 21 partial ray amputations, 38 ray resections, and 5 other procedures. Of the 111 patients included in the study, 39 (35.14%) had pathologic confirmed margins positive for residual osteomyelitis. Patients with positive margins presented significantly higher rates of proximal amputations as well as skin and soft tissue infections. The authors concluded that residual osteomyelitis at the pathologic margin was associated with a higher rate of treatment failure, despite the longer duration of antibiotic therapy (75). Another retrospective observational study involving 27 patients with diabetes mellitus showed that the overall rate of residual osteomyelitis was 40.7% (11/27). Nine out of 11 patients (81.8%) with positive margins had poor outcomes, including 3 reamputations, 3 wound dehiscences, 1 reulceration, 1 death, and 1 chronic wound that required skin grafting (20).

In conclusion, it has been reported that the level of surgical experience may play a role in the outcomes after amputations due to DFIs (126). Taylor et al (116) have also had similar findings regarding surgery in the diabetic foot. The outcomes of performing diabetic foot surgery without surgical experience and appropriate training may be unsuccessful for the patient because inadequate surgical débridement and medical optimization rarely achieves healing in the diabetic patient with multiple medical comorbidities. Patient referral and consultation to a medical center with experience in managing diabetic foot problems and with the input of a multidisciplinary health care team may be the best way to achieve diabetic limb salvage. Specialized teams in the management of acute diabetic foot problems may result in a reduction of diabetic lower extremity amputations (48,61).

References

1. Alazraki N, Dalinka MK, Berquist TH, et al. Imaging diagnosis of osteomyelitis in patients with diabetes mellitus. American College of Radiology. ACR Appropriateness Criteria. Radiology 2000;215(suppl):303–310.

2. Álvaro-Afonso FJ, Lázaro-Martínez JL, Aragón-Sánchez J, et al. Inter-observer reproducibility of diagnosis of diabetic foot osteomyelitis based on a combination of probe-to-bone test and simple radiography. Diabetes Res Clin Pract 2014;105:e3–e5.

3. Apelqvist J, Bakker K, van Houtum WH, et al. Practical guidelines on the management and prevention of the diabetic foot: based upon the International Consensus on the Diabetic Foot (2007) prepared by the International Working Group on the Diabetic Foot. Diabetes Metab Res Rev 2008;24(suppl 1):181–187.

4. Aragón-Sánchez FJ, Cabrera-Galván JJ, Quintana-Marrero Y, et al. Outcomes of surgical treatment of diabetic foot osteomyelitis: a series of 185 patients with histopathological confirmation of bone involvement. Diabetologia 2008;51:1962–1970.

5. Aragón-Sánchez J. Clinical-pathological characterization of diabetic foot infections: grading the severity of osteomyelitis. Int J Low Extrem Wounds 2012;11:107–112.

6. Aragón-Sánchez J. Seminar review: a review of the basis of surgical treatment of diabetic foot infections. Int J Low Extrem Wounds 2011;10:33–65.

7. Aragón-Sánchez J. Treatment of diabetic foot osteomyelitis: a surgical critique. Int J Low Extrem Wounds 2010;9:37–59.

8. Aragón-Sánchez J, Lázaro-Martínez JL. Impact of perioperative glycaemia and glycated haemoglobin on the outcomes of the surgical treatment of diabetic foot osteomyelitis. Diabetes Res Clin Pract 2011;94:e83–e85.

9. Aragón-Sánchez J, Lázaro-Martínez JL, Alvaro-Afonso FJ, et al. Conservative surgery of diabetic forefoot osteomyelitis: how can I operate on this patient without amputation? Int J Low Extrem Wounds 2015;14:108–131.

10. Aragón-Sánchez J, Lázaro-Martínez JL, Campillo-Vilorio N, et al. Controversies regarding radiological changes and variables predicting amputation in a surgical series of diabetic foot osteomyelitis. Foot Ankle Surg 2012;18:233–236.

11. Aragón-Sánchez J, Lázaro-Martínez JL, Cecilia-Matilla A, et al. Limb salvage for spreading midfoot osteomyelitis following diabetic foot surgery. J Tissue Viability 2012; 21:64–70.

12. Aragón-Sánchez J, Lázaro-Martínez JL, Hernández-Herrero C, et al. Does osteomyelitis in the feet of patients with diabetes really recur after surgical treatment? Natural history of a surgical series. Diabet Med 2012;29:813–818.

13. Aragón-Sánchez J, Lázaro-Martínez JL, Hernández-Herrero C, et al. Surgical treatment of limb- and life-threatening infections in the feet of patients with diabetes and at least one palpable pedal pulse: successes and lessons learnt. Int J Low Extrem Wounds 2011;10:207–213.

14. Aragón-Sánchez J, Lázaro-Martínez JL, Quintana-Marrero Y, et al. Are diabetic foot ulcers complicated by MRSA osteomyelitis associated with worse prognosis? Outcomes of a surgical series. Diabet Med 2009;26:552–555.

15. Aragón-Sánchez J, Lipsky BA, Lázaro-Martínez JL. Diagnosing diabetic foot osteomyelitis: is the combination of probe-to-bone test and plain radiography sufficient for high-risk inpatients? Diabet Med 2011;28:191–194.

16. Aragón-Sánchez J, Quintana-Marrero Y, Lázaro-Martínez JL, et al. Necrotizing soft-tissue infections in the feet of patients with diabetes: outcome of surgical treatment and factors associated with limb loss and mortality. Int J Low Extrem Wounds 2009;8:141–146.

17. Armstrong DG, Frykberg RG. Classifying diabetic foot surgery: toward a rational definition. Diabet Med 2003;20:329–331.

18. Armstrong DG, Lavery LA, Harkless LB. Validation of a diabetic wound classification system. The contribution of depth, infection, and ischemia to risk of amputation. Diabetes Care 1998;21:855–859.

19. Armstrong DG, Rosales MA, Gashi A. Efficacy of fifth metatarsal head resection for treatment of chronic diabetic foot ulceration. J Am Podiatr Med Assoc 2005;95:353–356.

20. Atway S, Nerone VS, Springer KD, et al. Rate of residual osteomyelitis after partial foot amputation in diabetic patients: a standardized method for evaluating bone margins with intraoperative culture. J Foot Ankle Surg 2012;51;749–752.

21. Baravarian B, Menendez MM, Weinheimer DJ, et al. Subtotal calcanectomy for the treatment of large heel ulceration and calcaneal osteomyelitis in the diabetic patient. J Foot Ankle Surg 1999;38:194–202.

22. Barberán J, Granizo JJ, Aguilar L, et al. Predictive model of short-term amputation during hospitalization of patients due to acute diabetic foot infections. Enferm Infecc Microbiol Clin 2010;28:680–684.

23. Bartolomei FJ. Compartment syndrome of the dorsal aspect of the foot. J Am Podiatr Med Assoc 1991;81:556–559.

24. Bartolomei FJ, Colley JO III. Compartment syndrome. A dorsal pedal presentation. J Am Podiatr Med Assoc 1989;79:139–141.

25. Berendt AR, Peters EJ, Bakker K, et al. Diabetic foot osteomyelitis: a progress report on diagnosis and a systematic review of treatment. Diabetes Metab Res Rev 2008;24(suppl 1):S145–S161.

26. Berendt AR, Peters EJ, Bakker K, et al. Specific guidelines for treatment of diabetic foot osteomyelitis. Diabetes Metab Res Rev 2008;24(suppl 1):S190–S191.

27. Bollinger M, Thordarson DB. Partial calcanectomy: an alternative to below knee amputation. Foot Ankle Int 2002;23:927–932.

28. Butalia S, Palda VA, Sargeant RJ, et al. Does this patient with diabetes have osteomyelitis of the lower extremity? JAMA 2008;299:806–813.

29. Capobianco CM, Stapleton JJ, Zgonis T. Surgical management of diabetic foot and ankle infections. Foot Ankle Spec 2010;3:223–230.

30. Caputo GM, Cavanagh PR, Ulbrecht JS, et al. Assessment and management of foot disease in patients with diabetes. N Engl J Med 1994;331:854–860.

31. Caselli A, Latini V, Lapenna A, et al. Transcutaneous oxygen tension monitoring after successful revascularization in diabetic patients with ischaemic foot ulcers. Diabet Med 2005;22:460–465.

32. Cecilia-Matilla A, Lázaro-Martínez JL, Aragón-Sánchez J, et al. Influence of the location of nonischemic diabetic forefoot osteomyelitis on time to healing after undergoing surgery. Int J Low Extrem Wounds 2013;12:184–188.

33. Chang BB, Darling RC III, Paty PS, et al. Expeditious management of ischemic invasive foot infections. Cardiovasc Surg 1996;4:792–795.

34. Couret G, Desbiez F, Thieblot P, et al. Emergence of monomicrobial methicillin-resistant *Staphylococcus aureus* infections in diabetic foot osteomyelitis (retrospective study of 48 cases) [in French]. Presse Med 2007;36:851–858.

35. Cuttica DJ, Philbin TM. Surgery for diabetic foot infections. Foot Ankle Clin 2010;15:465–476.

36. Dalla Paola L, Brocco E, Ceccacci T, et al. Limb salvage in Charcot foot and ankle osteomyelitis: combined use single stage/double stage of arthrodesis and external fixation. Foot Ankle Int 2009;30:1065–1070.

37. Dalla Paola L, Carone A, Morisi C, et al. Conservative surgical treatment of infected ulceration of the first metatarsophalangeal joint with osteomyelitis in diabetic patients. J Foot Ankle Surg 2015;54:536–540.

38. Dalla Paola L, Faglia E, Caminiti M, et al. Ulcer recurrence following first ray amputation in diabetic patients: a cohort prospective study. Diabetes Care 2003;26:1874–1878.

39. Demirağ B, Tirelioğlu AO, Sarisözen B, et al. Necrotizing fasciitis in the lower extremity secondary to diabetic wounds [in Turkish]. Acta Orthop Traumatol Turc 2004;38:195–199.

40. Diamantopoulos EJ, Haritos D, Yfandi G, et al. Management and outcome of severe diabetic foot infections. Exp Clin Endocrinol Diabetes 1998;106:346–352.

41. Dinh MT, Abad CL, Safdar N. Diagnostic accuracy of the physical examination and imaging tests for osteomyelitis underlying diabetic foot ulcers: meta-analysis. Clin Infect Dis 2008;47:519–527.

42. Dinh T, Snyder G, Veves A. Current techniques to detect foot infection in the diabetic patient. Int J Low Extrem Wounds 2010;9:24–30.

43. Edelson GW, Armstrong DG, Lavery LA, et al. The acutely infected diabetic foot is not adequately evaluated in an inpatient setting. J Am Podiatr Med Assoc 1997;87:260–265.

44. Eneroth M, Larsson J, Apelqvist J. Deep foot infections in patients with diabetes and foot ulcer: an entity with different characteristics, treatments, and prognosis. J Diabetes Complications 1999;13:254–263.

45. Faglia E, Clerici G, Caminiti M, et al. Feasibility and effectiveness of internal pedal amputation of phalanx or metatarsal head in diabetic patients with forefoot osteomyelitis. J Foot Ankle Surg 2012;51:593–598.

46. Faglia E, Clerici G, Caminiti M, et al. Prognostic difference between soft tissue abscess and osteomyelitis of the foot in patients with diabetes: data from a consecutive series of 452 hospitalized patients. J Foot Ankle Surg 2012;51:34–38.

47. Faglia E, Clerici G, Caminiti M, et al. The role of early surgical debridement and revascularization in patients with diabetes and deep foot space abscess: retrospective review of 106 patients with diabetes. J Foot Ankle Surg 2006;45:220–226.

48. Faglia E, Favales F, Aldeghi A, et al. Change in major amputation rate in a center dedicated to diabetic foot care during the 1980s: prognostic determinants for major amputation. J Diabetes Complications 1998;12:96–102.

49. Fisher TK, Scimeca CL, Bharara M, et al. A step-wise approach for surgical management of diabetic foot infections. J Vasc Surg 2010;52(3 suppl):72S–75S.

50. Fleischli JG, Laughlin TJ. Subtotal calcanectomy for the treatment of large heel ulceration and calcaneal osteomyelitis in the diabetic patient. J Foot Ankle Surg 1999;38:373–374.

51. Freeman GJ, Mackie KM, Sare J, et al. A novel approach to the management of the diabetic foot: metatarsal excision in the treatment of osteomyelitis. Eur J Vasc Endovasc Surg 2007;33:217–219.

52. Frykberg RG, Wittmayer B, Zgonis T. Surgical management of diabetic foot infections and osteomyelitis. Clin Podiatr Med Surg 2007;24:469–482.

53. Fujii M, Armsrong DG, Terashi H. Efficacy of magnetic resonance imaging in diagnosing diabetic foot osteomyelitis in the presence of ischemia. J Foot Ankle Surg 2013;52:717–723.

54. Fujii M, Terashi H, Yokono K. Surgical treatment strategy for diabetic forefoot osteomyelitis. Wound Repair Regen 2016;24:447–453.

55. Game FL, Jeffcoate WJ. Primarily non-surgical management of osteomyelitis of the foot in diabetes. Diabetologia 2008;51:962–967.

56. Gibbons GW. The diabetic foot: amputations and drainage of infection. J Vasc Surg 1987;5:791–793.

57. Glaudemans AW, Uçkay I, Lipsky BA. Challenges in diagnosing infection in the diabetic foot. Diabet Med 2015;32:748–759.

58. Grayson ML, Gibbons GW, Balogh K, et al. Probing to bone in infected pedal ulcers. A clinical sign of underlying osteomyelitis in diabetic patients. JAMA 1995;273:721–723.

59. Grayson ML, Gibbons GW, Habershaw GM, et al. Use of ampicillin/sulbactam versus imipenem/cilastatin in the treatment of limb-threatening foot infections in diabetic patients. Clin Infect Dis 1994;18:683–693.

60. Guyton GP, Shearman CM, Saltzman CL. The compartments of the foot revisited. Rethinking the validity of cadaver infusion experiments. J Bone Joint Surg Br 2001;83:245–249.

61. Hartemann-Heurtier A, Ha Van G, Danan JP, et al. Outcome of severe diabetic foot ulcers after standardised management in a specialised unit. Diabetes Metab 2002;28:477–484.

62. Ha Van G, Siney H, Danan JP, et al. Treatment of osteomyelitis in the diabetic foot. Contribution of conservative surgery. Diabetes Care 1996;19:1257–1260.

63. Henke PK, Blackburn SA, Wainess RW, et al. Osteomyelitis of the foot and toe in adults is a surgical disease: conservative management worsens lower extremity salvage. Ann Surg 2005;241: 885–892.

64. Hill SL, Holtzman GI, Buse R. The effects of peripheral vascular disease with osteomyelitis in the diabetic foot. Am J Surg 1999;177:282–286.

65. Jeffcoate WJ, Lipsky BA. Controversies in diagnosing and managing osteomyelitis of the foot in diabetes. Clin Infect Dis 2004;39(suppl 2):S115–S122.

66. Jeffcoate WJ, Lipsky BA, Berendt AR, et al. Unresolved issues in the management of ulcers of the foot in diabetes. Diabet Med 2008;25:1380–1389.

67. Jeffcoate WJ, van Houtum WH. Amputation as a marker of the quality of foot care in diabetes. Diabetologia 2004;47: 2051–2058.

68. Johnson JE, Anderson SA. One stage resection and pin stabilization of first metatarsophalangeal joint for chronic plantar ulcer with osteomyelitis. Foot Ankle Int 2010;31:973–979.

69. Joseph WS, Tan JS. Infections in diabetic foot ulcerations. Curr Infect Dis Rep 2003;5:391–397.

70. Kapoor A, Page S, Lavalley M, et al. Magnetic resonance imaging for diagnosing foot osteomyelitis: a meta-analysis. Arch Intern Med 2007;167:125–132.

71. Karchmer AW, Gibbons GW. Foot infections in diabetes: evaluation and management. Curr Clin Top Infect Dis 1994;14:1–22.

72. Kerstein MD, Welter V, Gahtan V, et al. Toe amputation in the diabetic patient. Surgery 1997;122:546–547.

73. Kim JY, Kim TW, Park YE, et al. Modified resection arthroplasty for infected non-healing ulcers with toe deformity in diabetic patients. Foot Ankle Int 2008;29:493–497.

74. Koller A. Internal pedal amputations. Clin Podiatr Med Surg 2008;25:641–653.

75. Kowalski TJ, Matsuda M, Sorenson MD, et al. The effect of residual osteomyelitis at the resection margin in patients with surgically treated diabetic foot infection. J Foot Ankle Surg 2011;50:171–175.

76. Lavery LA, Armstrong DG, Murdoch DP, et al. Validation of the Infectious Diseases Society of America's diabetic foot infection classification system. Clin Infect Dis 2007;44:562–565.

77. Lavery LA, Armstrong DG, Peters EJ, et al. Probe-to-bone test for diagnosing diabetic foot osteomyelitis: reliable or relic? Diabetes Care 2007;30:270–274.

78. Lavery LA, Peters EJ, Armstrong DG, et al. Risk factors for developing osteomyelitis in patients with diabetic foot wounds. Diabetes Res Clin Pract 2009;83:347–352.

79. Lázaro-Martínez JL, Aragón-Sánchez J, García-Morales E. Antibiotics versus conservative surgery for treating diabetic foot osteomyelitis: a randomized comparative trial. Diabetes Care 2014;37:789–795.

80. Ledermann HP, Morrison WB, Schweitzer ME. Is soft-tissue inflammation in pedal infection contained by fascial planes? MR analysis of compartmental involvement in 115 feet. AJR Am J Roentgenol 2002;178:605–612.

81. Ledermann HP, Morrison WB, Schweitzer ME. Pedal abscesses in patients suspected of having pedal osteomyelitis: analysis with MR imaging. Radiology 2002;224:649–655.

82. Ledermann HP, Morrison WB, Schweitzer ME, et al. Tendon involvement in pedal infection: MR analysis of frequency, distribution, and spread of infection. AJR Am J Roentgenol 2002;179:939–947.

83. Ledermann HP, Schweitzer ME, Morrison WB. Nonenhancing tissue on MR imaging of pedal infection: characterization of necrotic tissue and associated limitations for diagnosis of osteomyelitis and abscess. AJR Am J Roentgenol 2002;178:215–222.

84. Lee DK, Mulder GD, Schwartz AK. Hallux, sesamoid, and first metatarsal injuries. Clin Podiatr Med Surg 2011;28:43–56.

85. Lehmann S, Murphy RD, Hodor L. Partial calcanectomy in the treatment of chronic heel ulceration. J Am Podiatr Med Assoc 2001;91:369–372.

86. Lesens O, Desbiez F, Vidal M, et al. Culture of per-wound bone specimens: a simplified approach for the medical management of diabetic foot osteomyelitis. Clin Microbiol Infect 2011;17:285–291.

87. Lew DP, Waldvogel FA. Osteomyelitis. Lancet 2004;364:369–379.

88. Lipsky BA, Aragón-Sánchez J, Diggle M, et al. IWGDF guidance on the diagnosis and management of foot infections in persons with diabetes. Diabetes Metab Res Rev 2016;32(suppl 1):45–74.

89. Lipsky BA, Berendt AR, Cornia PB, et al. 2012 Infectious Diseases Society of America clinical practice guideline for the diagnosis and treatment of diabetic foot infections. Clin Infect Dis 2012;54:e132–e173.

90. Lipsky BA, Berendt AR, Deery HG, et al. Diagnosis and treatment of diabetic foot infections. Clin Infect Dis 2004;39:885–910.

91. Lipsky BA, Berendt AR, Deery HG, et al. Diagnosis and treatment of diabetic foot infections. Plast Reconstr Surg 2006;117(7 suppl):212S–238S.

92. Lipsky BA, Peters EJ, Senneville E, et al. Expert opinion on the management of infections in the diabetic foot. Diabetes Metab Res Rev 2012;28(suppl 1):163–178.

93. Liu YM, Chi CY, Ho MW, et al. Microbiology and factors affecting mortality in necrotizing fasciitis. J Microbiol Immunol Infect 2005;38:430–435.

94. Manoli A II, Weber TG. Fasciotomy of the foot: an anatomical study with special reference to release of the calcaneal compartment. Foot Ankle 1990;10:267–275.

95. Melamed EA, Peled E. Antibiotic impregnated cement spacer for salvage of diabetic osteomyelitis. Foot Ankle Int 2012;33: 213–219.

96. Morales Lozano R, González Fernández ML, Martinez Hernández D, et al. Validating the probe-to-bone and other tests for diagnosing chronic osteomyelitis in the diabetic foot. Diabetes Care 2010;33:2140–2145.

97. Morrison WB, Schweitzer ME, Wapner KL, et al. Osteomyelitis in feet of diabetics: clinical accuracy, surgical utility, and cost-effectiveness of MR imaging. Radiology 1995;196:557–564.

98. Murdoch DP, Armstrong DG, Dacus JB, et al. The natural history of great toe amputations. J Foot Ankle Surg 1997;36:204–208.

99. Nehler MR, Whitehill TA, Bowers SP, et al. Intermediate-term outcome of primary digit amputations in patients with diabetes mellitus who have forefoot sepsis requiring hospitalization and presumed adequate circulatory status. J Vasc Surg 1999;30:509–517.

100. Ozalay M, Ozkoc G, Akpinar S, et al. Necrotizing soft-tissue infection of a limb: clinical presentation and factors related to mortality. Foot Ankle Int 2006;27:598–605.

101. Perez ML, Wagner SS, Yun J. Subtotal calcanectomy for chronic heel ulceration. J Foot Ankle Surg 1994;33:572–579.

102. Pinzur MS. Circular fixation for the nonplantigrade Charcot foot. Hosp Pract (1995) 2010;38:56–62.

103. Prompers L, Huijberts M, Apelqvist J, et al. Delivery of care to diabetic patients with foot ulcers in daily practice: results of the Eurodiale study, a prospective cohort study. Diabet Med 2008;25:700–707.

104. Ramanujam CL, Facaros Z, Zgonis T. Abductor hallucis muscle flap with circular external fixation for Charcot foot osteomyelitis: a case report. Diabet Foot Ankle 2011;2.

105. Randall DB, Phillips J, Ianiro G. Partial calcanectomy for the treatment of recalcitrant heel ulcerations. J Am Podiatr Med Assoc 2005;95:335–341.

106. Rauwerda JA. Foot debridement: anatomic knowledge is mandatory. Diabetes Metab Res Rev 2000;16(suppl 1):S23–S26.

107. Schade VL. Partial or total calcanectomy as an alternative to below-the-knee amputation for limb salvage: a systematic review. J Am Podiatr Med Assoc 2012;102:396–405.

108. Schweinberger MH, Roukis TS. Salvage of the first ray with external fixation in the high-risk patient. Foot Ankle Spec 2008;1:210–213.

109. Senneville E, Lombart A, Beltrand E, et al. Outcome of diabetic foot osteomyelitis treated nonsurgically: a retrospective cohort study. Diabetes Care 2008;31:637–642.

110. Shone A, Burnside J, Chipchase S, et al. Probing the validity of the probe-to-bone test in the diagnosis of osteomyelitis of the foot in diabetes. Diabetes Care 2006;29:945.

111. Simpson AH, Deakin M, Latham JM. Chronic osteomyelitis. The effect of the extent of surgical resection on infection-free survival. J Bone Joint Surg Br 2001;83:403–407.

112. Snyder RJ, Cohen MM, Sun C, et al. Osteomyelitis in the diabetic patient: diagnosis and treatment. Part 2: medical, surgical, and alternative treatments. Ostomy Wound Manage 2001;47:24–30.

113. Tamir E, McLaren AM, Gadgil A, et al. Outpatient percutaneous flexor tenotomies for management of diabetic claw toe deformities with ulcers: a preliminary report. Can J Surg 2008;51:41–44.

114. Tan JS, Friedman NM, Hazelton-Miller C, et al. Can aggressive treatment of diabetic foot infections reduce the need for above-ankle amputation? Clin Infect Dis 1996;23:286–291.

115. Tan PL, Teh J. MRI of the diabetic foot: differentiation of infection from neuropathic change. Br J Radiol 2007;80:939–948.

116. Taylor LM Jr, Porter JM. The clinical course of diabetics who require emergent foot surgery because of infection or ischemia. J Vasc Surg 1987;6:454–459.

117. Uccioli L, Gandini R, Giurato L, et al. Long-term outcomes of diabetic patients with critical limb ischemia followed in a tertiary referral diabetic foot clinic. Diabetes Care 2010;33:977–982.

118. Valabhji J, Oliver N, Samarasinghe D, et al. Conservative management of diabetic forefoot ulceration complicated by underlying osteomyelitis: the benefits of magnetic resonance imaging. Diabet Med 2009;26:1127–1134.

119. van Baal JG. Surgical treatment of the infected diabetic foot. Clin Infect Dis 2004;39(suppl 2):S123–S128.

120. Van Riet A, Harake R, Stuyck J. Partial calcanectomy: a procedure to cherish or to reject? Foot Ankle Surg 2012;18:25–29.

121. Vardakas KZ, Horianopoulou M, Falagas ME. Factors associated with treatment failure in patients with diabetic foot infections: an analysis of data from randomized controlled trials. Diabetes Res Clin Pract 2008;80:344–351.

122. Vartanians VM, Karchmer AW, Giurini JM, et al. Is there a role for imaging in the management of patients with diabetic foot? Skeletal Radiol 2009;38:633–636.

123. Venkatesan P, Lawn S, Macfarlane RM, et al. Conservative management of osteomyelitis in the feet of diabetic patients. Diabet Med 1997;14:487–490.

124. Wieman TJ, Mercke YK, Cerrito PB, et al. Resection of the metatarsal head for diabetic foot ulcers. Am J Surg 1998;176:436–441.

125. Williams DT, Hilton JR, Harding KG. Diagnosing foot infection in diabetes. Clin Infect Dis 2004;39(suppl 2):S83–S86.

126. Wong YS, Lee JC, Yu CS, et al. Results of minor foot amputations in diabetic mellitus. Singapore Med J 1996;37:604–606.

127. Zgonis T, Stapleton JJ, Rodriguez RH, et al. Plastic surgery reconstruction of the diabetic foot. AORN J 2008;87:951–966.

CHAPTER 8

Negative Pressure Wound Therapy Applications for the Diabetic Foot

Crystal L. Ramanujam • Thomas Zgonis

LITERATURE REVIEW AND CLINICAL OUTCOMES

Negative pressure wound therapy (NPWT) plays a vital role in today's adjunctive management of diabetic foot wounds. In 1993, Fleischmann et al. (10) first published the use of subatmospheric pressure applied to wounds in the context of open fractures. Their technique consisted of a suction system delivering 600 millimeter of mercury (mmHg) to a wound dressed with porous polyvinyl alcohol foam wrapped around suction drains that was sealed with a polyurethane drape, subsequently showing increased granulation tissue and no infections in 15 patients (10). The landmark work of Argenta and Morykwas (1) in 1997 demonstrated how NPWT could be useful for a variety of difficult soft tissue defects including acute, subacute, and chronic wounds. Their extensive clinical and laboratory work over a 9-year period using the vacuum-assisted wound closure device (VAC; KCI, San Antonio, TX) became the basis for some of NPWT's reported benefits including improved local blood flow, decreased edema, and reduction of bacterial load (1,24).

Some of the earliest traces of NPWT date back to 600 bc in Assyria and Babylon where wound drainage through suction was routinely performed. In 400 BC, the Greeks developed the cupping technique in which wounds were treated through a vacuum using heated copper bowls (17). In its simplest form, NPWT involves a closed environment in which a dressing is secured to a wound through which negative pressure is applied and fluids are drained into a collection container. Since its inception, a number of advancements have been made for the application of NPWT including but not limited to types of foam dressings, adherent materials for fixation to the wound, tubing modifications, and smaller, more portable units for delivery of negative pressure. The concept of creating a negative pressure environment at the wound site appears simple; however, explanation of the true mechanism(s) of action for the benefits of NPWT is still a work in progress. Existing data supports that the benefits of NPWT are multifactorial and may be related to the following areas: improved perfusion, increased granulation tissue, decreased bacterial count, and reduction of edema involved in wound healing (Table 8.1).

Morykwas and colleagues (24) utilized laser Doppler probes in their initial laboratory work with a swine model, demonstrating increased blood flow at the subcutaneous tissue adjacent to wounds treated with subatmospheric pressure. An experimental study by Chen et al. (6) using microcirculation microscope and image pattern analysis in a rat model also demonstrated NPWT promoted capillary blood flow velocity, stimulated endothelial proliferation, and angiogenesis. Zöch (37) measured an increased in blood flow through indocyanine-green (IC-view) perfusography in diabetic foot wounds treated with NPWT. However, an experimental study of NPWT in healthy volunteers by Kairinos et al. (13) has challenged the prior studies by showing a decrease in local perfusion with increased suction pressure.

Statistically significant increase in granulation tissue formation has been found in NPWT-treated wounds through numerous studies. For example, Morykwas et al. (24) measured this by wound volume in a swine model, whereas Fabian et al. (9) measured the increased granulation tissue using a lens micrometer in their rabbit model. Morykwas et al. (25) went on to analyze the effects of different levels of subatmospheric pressure on swine wounds, determining 125 mmHg as the ideal level for clinical use.

Several animal studies report reduction in bacterial bioburden with the use of NPWT, including Morykwas et al. (24) who demonstrated decreased bacterial counts by day 5 of NPWT in a swine model in a nonrandomized, controlled, prospective study. NPWT in humans shows conflicting results, particularly a study by Weed et al. (35) which demonstrated increased bacterial loads in quantitative cultures of 25 wounds undergoing NPWT; however, this increase did not seem to affect the overall wound healing. Furthermore, a randomized, controlled, and blinded clinical trial by Mouës et al. (26) including 29 patients treated with NPWT versus a saline gauze control group showed no difference in bacterial concentration between the 2 groups. Interestingly, the concentration of *Staphylococcus aureus* increased, whereas the concentration of gram-negative cocci decreased significantly in the NPWT group. Studies like these have sparked debate on whether other factors such as more frequent dressing changes

TABLE 8.1	Selected Evidence for Effects of Negative Pressure Wound Therapy		
Increase Local Blood Flow Wound Perfusion	**Increase Granulation Tissue**	**Decrease Tissue Bacterial Count**	**Decrease Edema**
• Morykwas et al. Ann Plast Surg 1997: animal study (24) • Chen et al. Asian J Surg 2005: animal study (6). • Zöch G. Zentralblatt Chir 2004: human study (37)	• Morykwas et al. Ann Plast Surg 1997: animal study (24) • Fabian et al. Am Surg 2000: animal study (9) • Morykwas et al. Ann Plast Surg 2001: animal study (25)	• Morykwas et al. Ann Plast Surg 1997: animal study (24)	• Lu et al. Chin J Clinic Rehab 2003: animal study (20) • Chen et al. Asian J Surg 2005: animal study (6) • Kamolz et al. Burns 2004: human study (14)

or topical antimicrobials applied simultaneously with NPWT would decrease bacterial counts and increase healing time.

Wounds with local inflammation and/or infection often produce high levels of exudates that effectively increase edema. NPWT is thought to facilitate edema control by removing excessive fluids, thereby improving local perfusion and decreasing accumulation of proteolytic enzymes that can be detrimental to normal cellular wound healing processes (20). Kamolz et al. (14) studied drained fluid in human burn wounds which demonstrated reduced edema; however, they could not conclude whether this phenomenon was directly related to the effects of NPWT or due to leakage of fluid from vessels within the wounds.

NPWT causes macrodeformation which leads to wound contraction and effectively reduces the surface area of the wound (12). Ongoing research is necessary to elucidate the true mechanism(s) behind NPWT's efficacy and further clarify the existing controversies in the treatment of diabetic foot wounds.

Although the current literature is replete with reports of NPWT for use in secondary healing of diabetic foot wounds, high-level evidence for this modality in the clinical setting is limited (Table 8.2). In a randomized control trial of NPWT versus saline gauze dressings for postoperative diabetic foot wounds, McCallon et al. (21) found the NPWT group to have faster healing times and greater reduction in wound surface area. Eginton et al. (8) published a small prospective randomized control trial for NPWT in diabetic foot wounds, showing NPWT caused decreased wound depth and volume in the early weeks of therapy more effectively than conventional moist gauze dressings. However, the results of these studies should be carefully considered because both studies contained very small sample sizes. Armstrong and Lavery (2) provided a large multicenter randomized control trial for diabetic wounds after partial foot amputation that demonstrated NPWT led to more healed patients, faster wound healing, faster formation of granulation tissue, and potentially fewer reamputations when compared to standard moist wound care.

TABLE 8.2	Published Clinical Trials for Negative Pressure Wound Therapy in Diabetic Foot Wounds				
Year	**Author**	**Location**	**Study Type**	**Wound Type**	**Sample Analyzed**
2000	McCallon et al. (21)	United States	RCT, single center	Postoperative diabetic foot wounds	10 patients
2003	Eginton et al. (8)	United States	RCT, single center	Diabetic foot wounds	6 patients
2005	Armstrong and Lavery (2)	United States	RCT, multicenter	Wounds after partial diabetic foot amputation	162 patients
2008	Blume et al. (5)	United States, Canada	RCT, multicenter	Diabetic foot ulcers	335 patients
2008	Mody et al. (22)	India	RCT, single center	Diabetic foot ulcers	15 patients
2010	Paola et al. (28)	Italy	RCT, single center	Diabetic open minor amputations	130 patients
2010	Novinscak et al. (27)	Croatia	RCT, single center	Complicated diabetic foot ulcers	19 patients
2011	Karatepe et al. (16)	Turkey	RCT, single center	Diabetic foot ulcers	67 patients

RCT, randomized controlled trial.

An even larger multicenter randomized control trial by Blume et al. (5) for diabetic foot ulcers found that NPWT achieved complete closure in more patients, fewer secondary amputations, and reduced home therapy days compared to advanced moist wound therapy. In both of these large clinical trials, the type and occurrence of adverse events such as infection were similar in both treatment groups. Mody et al. (22) provided data on NPWT compared to wet-to-dry gauze for wounds of different etiologies, including 15 diabetic foot ulcers. A randomized control trial by Paola et al. (28) comparing either surgical débridement with NPWT to surgical débridement with semi-occlusive silver dressing for treatment of infected open minor amputations found rapid granulation tissue formation, better and more rapid control of infections, and reduced time to complete wound closure in the NPWT group. A study by Novinscak et al. (27) also analyzed NPWT compared to standard moist gauze dressings in diabetic foot ulcers; however, little information was provided regarding the flow of patients through the study and certain outcomes were not accounted for. Karatepe et al. (16) demonstrated statistically significant reduction in healing time for diabetic foot ulcers treated with NPWT compared to standard wound care; furthermore, these authors reported improvement in quality of life measures for the NPWT group.

INDICATIONS

NPWT is indicated for diabetic foot wounds anywhere on the spectrum of acute to chronic, including but not limited to neuropathic ulcers, pressure ulcers, traumatic wounds, surgical wounds (Fig. 8.1), and postamputation wounds (Figs. 8.2

and 8.3). Surgical débridement of tissues in cases of diabetic foot infection, specifically abscess and osteomyelitis, can create wounds of varied size and depth. NPWT can be utilized for these soft tissue or osseous defects, especially in facilitating closure of large and irregular wounds. This modality is extremely helpful in wound bed preparation prior to autogenous or allogenic skin graft and flap application (Fig. 8.4). NPWT may be also useful in wounds with exposed bone, tendon, or hardware. In cases of exposed bone and tendon, NPWT promotes the formation of granulation tissue, which can either reduce the time to definitive wound closure or allow a more simple surgical option such as split-thickness skin grafting (STSG) rather than formal flap closure. In some cases of exposed hardware, NPWT may be able to induce enough health granulation tissue to allow for secondary wound closure or flap coverage. However, in the setting of large areas of exposed hardware or infection, hardware removal and other fixation techniques such as external fixation should be considered.

NPWT can be used over antibiotic-impregnated cement beads and/or spacers in diabetic foot wounds with bone loss. NPWT is also indicated for use over certain high-risk closed surgical incisions and can be used as a bolster dressing to secure flaps, STSGs, and/or bioengineered alternative tissues (Figs. 8.5 and 8.6). In addition, NPWT can be used to facilitate secondary wound healing after the modified Papineau technique, which involves open cancellous bone grafting in the treatment of septic bone defects. For infected tibial nonunions, Karargyris et al. (15) demonstrated that combination of the Papineau technique and Ilizarov bone transport with postoperative NPWT could successfully address the infections and bone defects along with achieving complete wound closure with minimal complications.

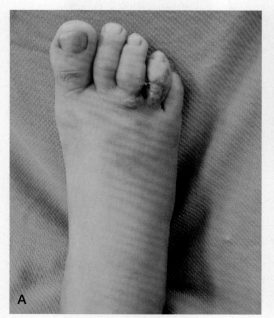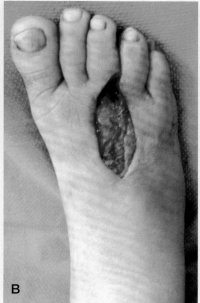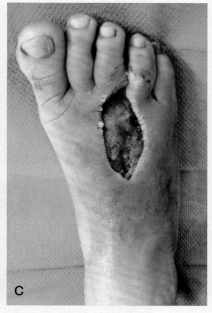

FIGURE 8.1 Preoperative clinical picture **(A)** showing a dorsal diabetic foot infection with extensive cellulitis and edema. Patient underwent an initial incision and drainage procedure with excisional débridement of all nonviable tissues **(B)** being followed by a revisional surgical débridement 2 days after the initial surgery **(C)**. *(continued)*

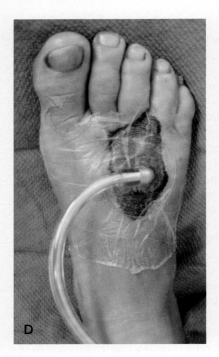

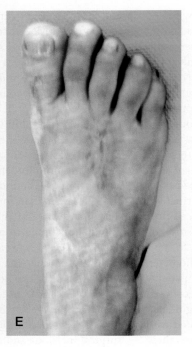

FIGURE 8.1 *(Continued)* At the second staged procedure, an intraoperative negative pressure wound therapy (NPWT) device was applied to the surgical wound bed **(D)**. The patient was followed closely in the outpatient and wound care specialty clinics with the NPWT being discontinued approximately 2 weeks postoperatively and followed by local wound care dressings. **E.** Final postoperative clinical outcome at 9 weeks.

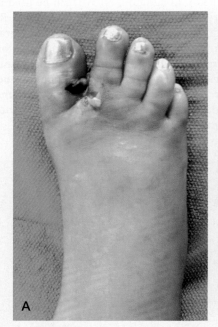

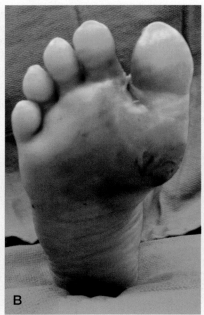

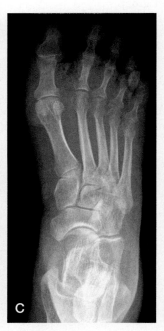

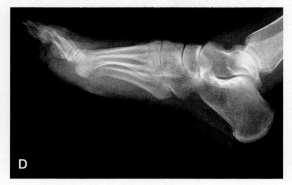

FIGURE 8.2 Preoperative clinical **(A,B)** and radiographic **(C,D)** pictures showing a severe diabetic foot infection with soft tissue gas of the entire forefoot. Patient underwent an initial open amputation of toes one through five at the metatarsophalangeal joint level **(E)** being followed by a partial resection of metatarsals one through five **(F)**, excision of sesamoids, and application of an intraoperative negative pressure wound therapy (NPWT) device 2 days after the initial surgery **(G)**. *(continued)*

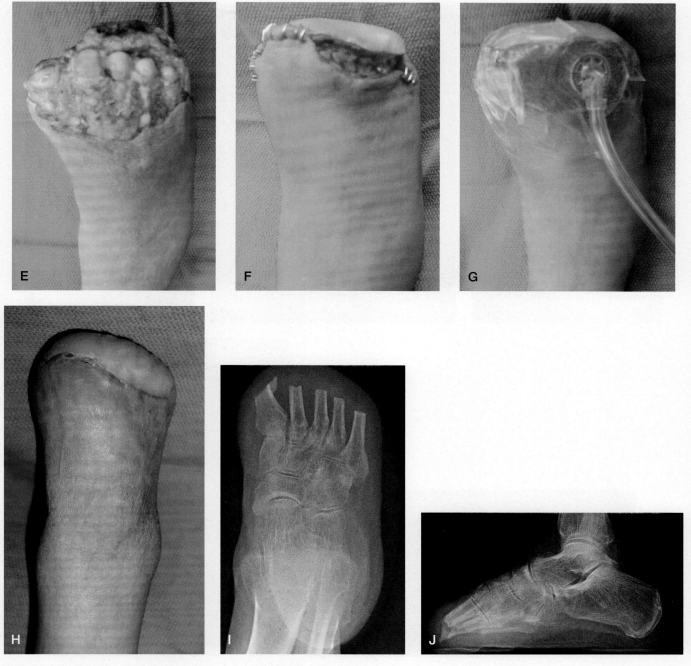

FIGURE 8.2 *(Continued)* The patient was followed closely in the outpatient and wound care specialty clinics with the NPWT being discontinued approximately 2 weeks postoperatively and followed by local wound care dressings. Final postoperative clinical **(H)** and radiographic **(I,J)** outcomes at approximately 19 weeks.

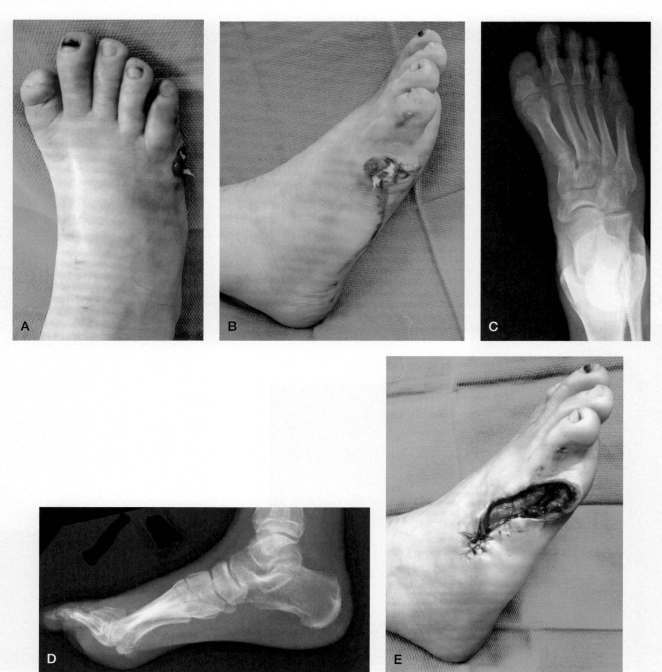

FIGURE 8.3 Preoperative clinical **(A,B)** and radiographic **(C,D)** pictures showing a diabetic foot infection with subcutaneous soft tissue gas and osteomyelitis of the fifth metatarsophalangeal joint. Patient underwent an initial open partial fifth ray (toe and metatarsal) amputation being followed by a revisional partial fifth ray amputation **(E)** and application of an intraoperative negative pressure wound therapy (NPWT) device 2 days after the initial surgery **(F)**. *(continued)*

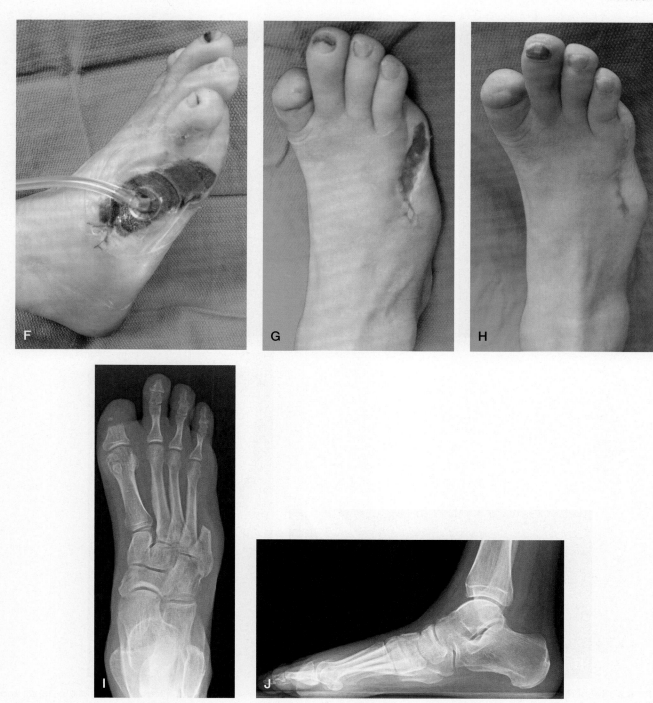

FIGURE 8.3 *(Continued)* The patient was followed closely in the outpatient and wound care specialty clinics with the NPWT being discontinued approximately 6 weeks postoperatively and followed by local wound care dressings **(G)**. Final postoperative clinical **(H)** and radiographic **(I,J)** outcomes at approximately 21 weeks.

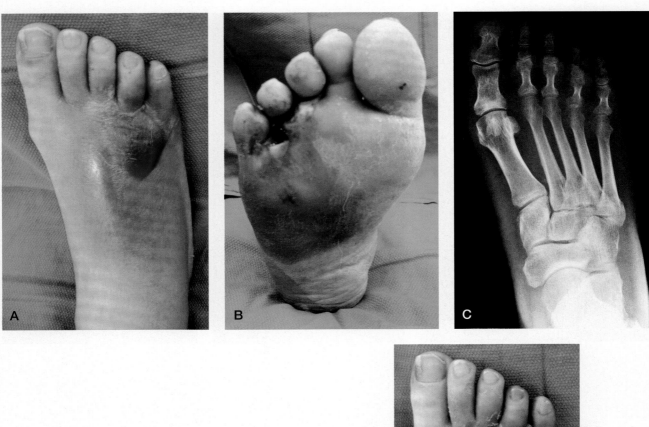

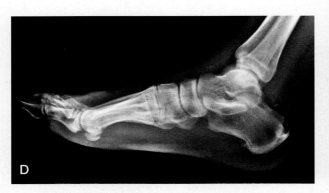

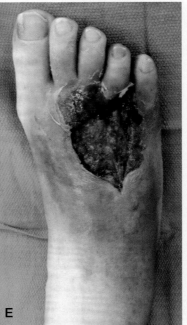

FIGURE 8.4 Preoperative clinical **(A,B)** and radiographic **(C,D)** pictures showing a severe diabetic foot infection at the dorsal and plantar aspect of the third and fourth interspaces with extensive cellulitis. Patient underwent an initial incision and drainage procedure with excisional débridement of all nonviable tissues **(E,F)** being followed by a partial fourth and fifth ray (toe and metatarsal) amputations **(G)** and application of an intraoperative negative pressure wound therapy (NPWT) device 2 days after the initial surgery **(H,I)**. *(continued)*

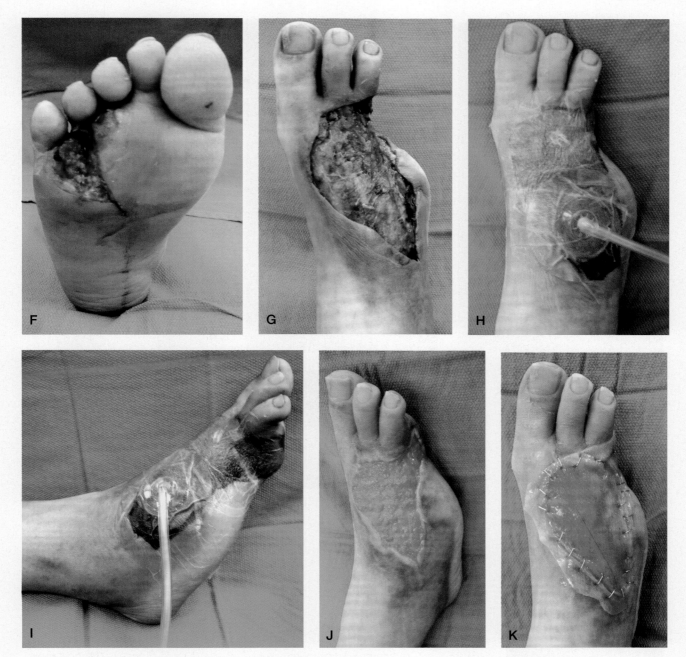

FIGURE 8.4 *(Continued)* The patient was followed closely in the outpatient and wound care specialty clinics with the NPWT being discontinued approximately 11 weeks postoperatively and followed by local wound care dressings. The patient underwent further hydrosurgical débridement of the wound and application of an acellular dermal replacement at 12 weeks postoperatively **(J,K)**. *(continued)*

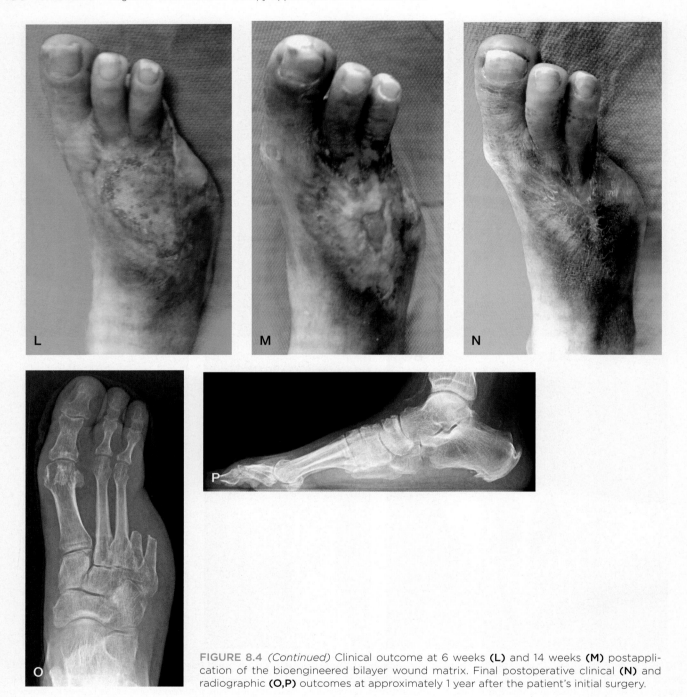

FIGURE 8.4 *(Continued)* Clinical outcome at 6 weeks **(L)** and 14 weeks **(M)** postapplication of the bioengineered bilayer wound matrix. Final postoperative clinical **(N)** and radiographic **(O,P)** outcomes at approximately 1 year after the patient's initial surgery.

Increased experience and advancements in NPWT over the years have expanded the application of this modality for the treatment of diabetic foot wounds. As NPWT has been shown to assist in creating more vascular and granular wound beds prior to definitive wound closure techniques, these same characteristics can augment incorporation of autogenous or allogenic skin grafts with simultaneous application. Additionally, NPWT can be used as an excellent bolster dressing for these grafts in the first 5 to 7 days (Fig. 8.7). The vacuum-sealed sponge conforms the graft to the wound bed and also reduces

movement at the graft–wound interface. Fluid collection is also controlled by NPWT, thereby reducing hematoma and seroma formation, in addition to preventing contamination. In 2002, Scherer et al. (31) demonstrated improved outcomes with NPWT securing skin grafts compared to traditional bolster dressings for wounds due to traumatic or thermal injury, noting better graft survival and reduction in the need for repeated skin grafting. In a 10-year retrospective review of foot and ankle reconstructive surgeries, Blume et al. (4) showed NPWT as an excellent alternative for securing autogenous

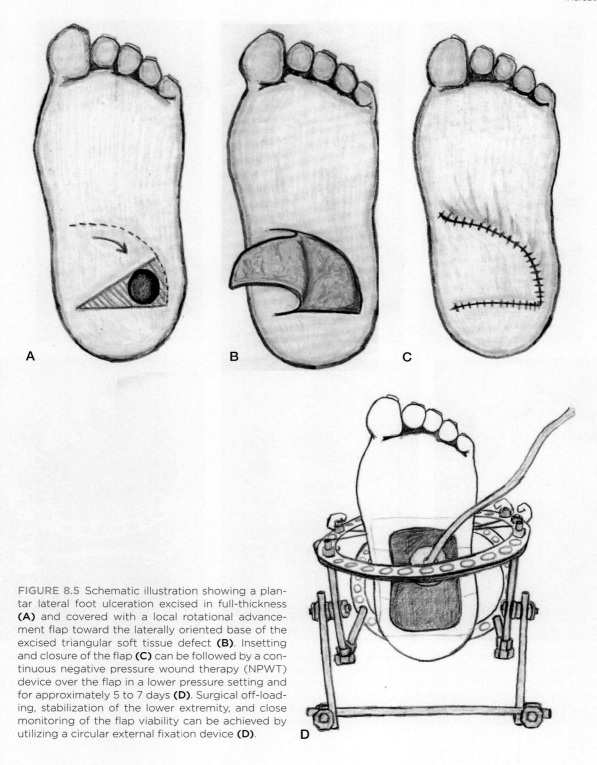

FIGURE 8.5 Schematic illustration showing a plantar lateral foot ulceration excised in full-thickness **(A)** and covered with a local rotational advancement flap toward the laterally oriented base of the excised triangular soft tissue defect **(B)**. Insetting and closure of the flap **(C)** can be followed by a continuous negative pressure wound therapy (NPWT) device over the flap in a lower pressure setting and for approximately 5 to 7 days **(D)**. Surgical off-loading, stabilization of the lower extremity, and close monitoring of the flap viability can be achieved by utilizing a circular external fixation device **(D)**.

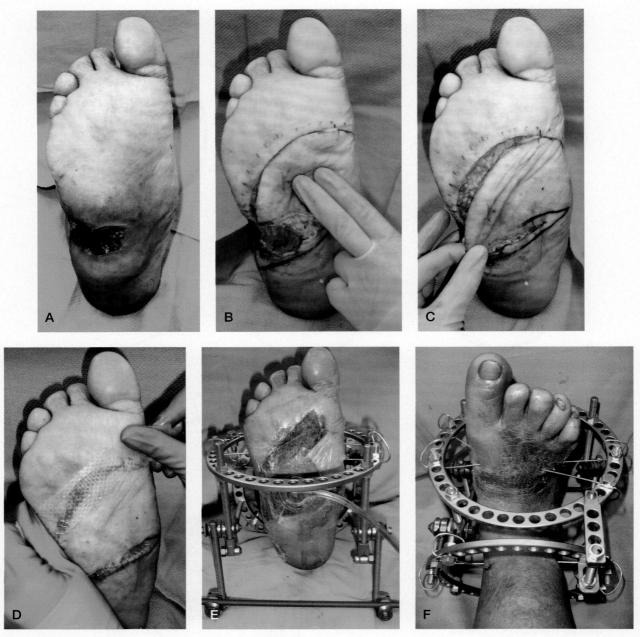

FIGURE 8.6 Preoperative clinical picture **(A)** showing a plantar centrolateral foot ulceration in a diabetic Charcot neuroarthropathy excised in triangular full-thickness fashion with the base of the triangle oriented laterally. A local rotational advancement flap based on the medial plantar artery **(B)** is raised and rotated toward the base of the excised triangular soft tissue recipient site **(C)**. The donor site distally can be covered by either an allogenic **(D)** or autogenous split-thickness skin graft. Continuous negative pressure wound therapy (NPWT) device over the flap and donor sites can be set in a lower pressure (mmHg) and for approximately 5 to 7 days. Circular external fixation can be utilized as a surgical off-loading device **(E,F)**.

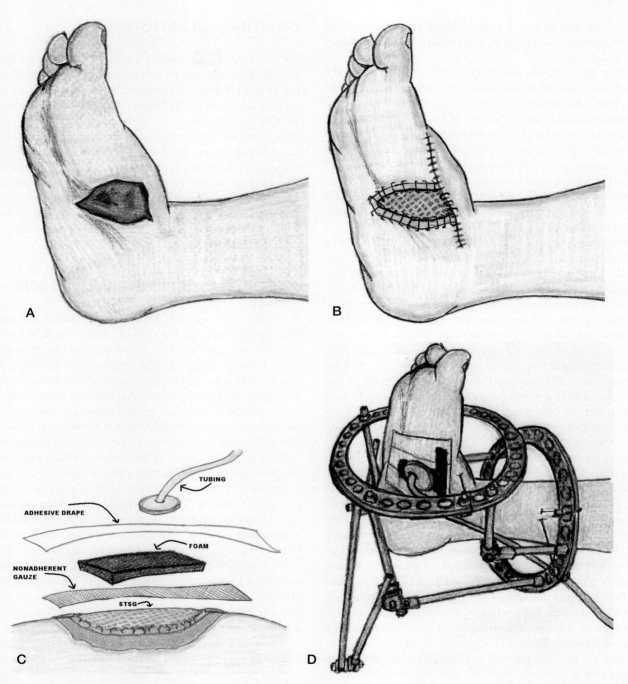

FIGURE 8.7 Schematic illustration showing a medial foot ulceration **(A)** excised in full-thickness and covered with an abductor hallucis muscle flap and split-thickness skin graft **(B)**. Illustration **(C)** shows the application of the negative pressure wound therapy (NPWT) device over the muscle flap and split-thickness skin graft being followed by a circular external fixation for surgical offloading, lower extremity stabilization, flap monitoring, and/or reconstruction **(D)**.

STSG compared to conventional dressings, with improved graft survival, reduced number of repeated STSG, and reduced graft complications.

When patients are medically compromised and/or the diabetic foot wound is not suitable for STSG or flap coverage, other bioengineered alternative tissues can be applied to expedite wound closure. Molnar et al. (23) applied NPWT directly over artificial skin substitutes in 8 patients for complex wounds, showing accelerated graft incorporation and low complication rates. Similarly, staged use of the aforementioned surgical techniques has been successfully performed to cover extensive wounds produced from diabetic foot infections (30). NPWT has also been reported safe in securing flaps for complex wound closure (18,34).

Using the same principles, another use of NPWT has been in closed surgical incisions to reduce rates of surgical site infections and dehiscence. The first published report of this technique was a randomized control study by Stannard et al. (33) for high-energy orthopedic trauma, procedures with inherent risks of drainage, infection, and wound dehiscence. Since that time, several publications attribute improved outcomes to reduced edema, reduced incision line tension, and providing an airtight seal with use of incisional NPWT. In 2016, an international multidisciplinary panel including surgical and infectious disease experts published a consensus document emphasizing the consideration of NPWT on closed incisions for management of high-risk patients and high-risk surgical procedures (36).

Many diabetic patients undergoing reconstruction for treatment of lower extremity traumatic injuries, deformity correction, and/or infection fall into these categories. A review by Ramanujam et al. (29) mentioned diabetic Charcot foot and ankle reconstructions including arthrodesis procedures provide an ideal clinical setting for use of incisional NPWT because these procedures may carry high-risk of surgical wound dehiscence and significant postoperative edema. Despite the rise in use of NPWT over closed incisions, grafts and flaps, and the current commercial availability of single-use NPWT devices, further clinical studies are still needed to determine its efficacy and optimal levels of pressure (mmHg) for application in the diabetic foot.

Based on the concept that regular cleansing of wounds reduces risk of contamination and infection, a recent development in conjunction with NPWT has been the instillation of sterile water, saline, antibiotics, or antiseptic solutions. In 2005, Bernstein and Tam (3) reported the successful use of NPWT combined with instillation of saline, polymyxin B, and bacitracin for the adjunctive treatment of 5 patients with postsurgical diabetic foot wounds. Dalla Paola (7) more recently published a case series in 2013 using NPWT with instillation of polyhexanide in 2 patients with diabetic foot ulcers. Future research with large studies on diabetic foot wounds is necessary to determine the efficacy of NPWT with instillation and to provide specific recommendations for specific solution types, duration of therapy, and pressure settings.

CONTRAINDICATIONS

NPWT is contraindicated for use in wounds with malignancy, critical ischemia, and/or untreated infection. NPWT should not be used directly over exposed nerve, blood vessel, or vascular anastomosis. NPWT may also be avoided in patients on continuous antiplatelet or anticoagulant therapy because the topical suction can further increase risk of bleeding. For the same reason, proper hemostasis at the surgical site should be achieved prior to any application of NPWT. This modality is also contraindicated in patients with allergies to any of the components used for NPWT such as the foam and adhesives materials. Furthermore, NPWT may not be used in patients who have a psychological aversion to the device or cannot endure the dressing changes.

PREOPERATIVE CONSIDERATIONS

It is vital that surgeons take into consideration not only the characteristics of the diabetic foot wound but also the medical status of the entire patient prior to the application of NPWT. Preoperative medical optimization through a multidisciplinary approach is recommended to achieve successful outcomes in the surgical management of diabetic foot and ankle wounds. Adequate perioperative glycemic control is important because hyperglycemia is known to interfere with fibroblast function, neovascularization, and inflammatory cells in all of the stages of the wound healing process (11). Because diabetes mellitus also affects the macro- and microcirculatory systems, potentially causing cardiovascular and peripheral arterial disease, a thorough vascular assessment should be undertaken, including clinical evaluation and noninvasive and invasive vascular studies when indicated. Any deficiencies should warrant a formal vascular surgery consultation to consider the likelihood of revascularization procedures prior to initiation of NPWT. Preoperative nutritional status and hydration of the patient should also be considered to improve immune function and increase tissue perfusion, respectively.

Chronic kidney disease is also a known risk factor for impaired wound healing in the diabetic foot and may also impact antibiotic therapy options (19). Patients with significant cardiac history such as occurrence of myocardial infarction or prior cardiac interventions often necessitate cardiology consultation prior to surgical wound management. Smoking cessation should be encouraged because nicotine is known to cause microvascular vasoconstriction (32). Current smoking or history of heavy smoking place patients at increased risk for fat necrosis, wound infection, and flap necrosis.

Persistent diabetic foot infections with large soft tissue and/or osseous defects may necessitate infectious disease consultation for further management of systemic or oral antibiotics. Multiple intraoperative soft tissue and bone cultures as well as bone biopsies are necessary in order to guide the duration and type of definitive antibiotic therapy. The recipient wound bed should be free of any infected or necrotic tissue before the application of an allogenic graft, STSG, and flap reconstruction.

DETAILED SURGICAL TECHNIQUE

In order to optimize diabetic foot and ankle wounds for NPWT application, thorough surgical débridement should be performed (Fig. 8.8). This surgical wound bed preparation should include removal of any infected and/or necrotic tissues

via sharp instrumentation and can be augmented by ultrasonic or hydrosurgical means for precise excision. Soft tissue and/or bone infection should also be addressed with systemic antibiotic therapy based on intraoperative culture results. Antibiotic-impregnated cement beads or spacers may be utilized for local delivery of specific antibiotics and can help stabilize surrounding structures in cases of significant bone and soft tissue loss. Multiple surgical débridements may be warranted in severe diabetic foot infections in order to produce an ideal wound for NPWT. Local hemostasis can be achieved with electrocautery and/or hemostatic agents such as topical thrombin. Efforts to

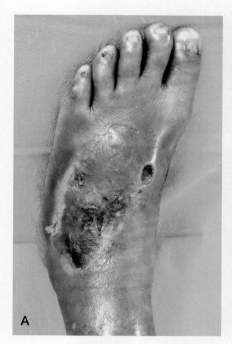
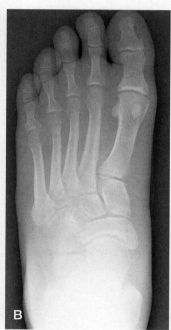
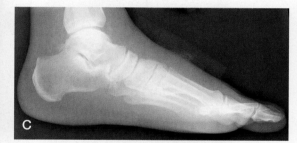
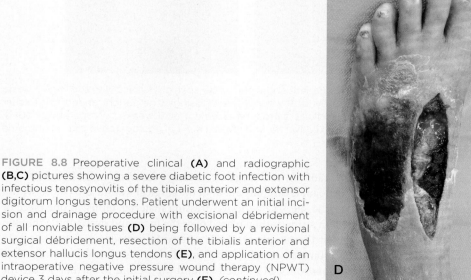
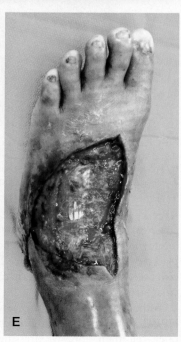

FIGURE 8.8 Preoperative clinical **(A)** and radiographic **(B,C)** pictures showing a severe diabetic foot infection with infectious tenosynovitis of the tibialis anterior and extensor digitorum longus tendons. Patient underwent an initial incision and drainage procedure with excisional débridement of all nonviable tissues **(D)** being followed by a revisional surgical débridement, resection of the tibialis anterior and extensor hallucis longus tendons **(E)**, and application of an intraoperative negative pressure wound therapy (NPWT) device 3 days after the initial surgery **(F)**. *(continued)*

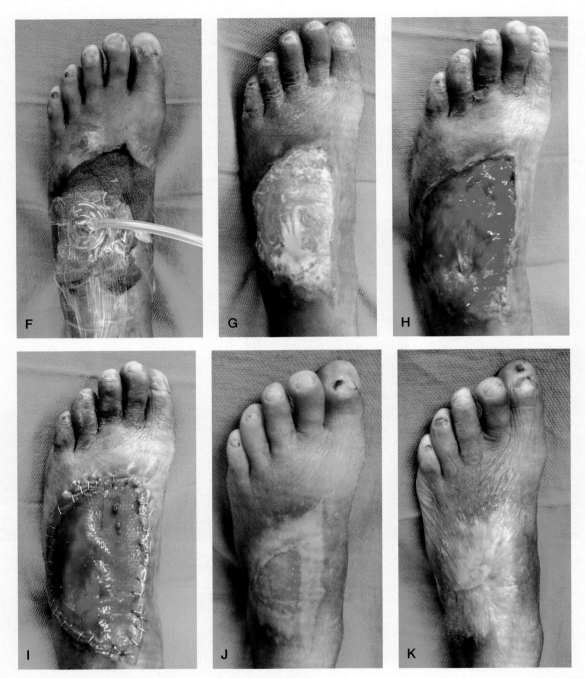

FIGURE 8.8 *(Continued)* The patient was followed closely in the outpatient and wound care specialty clinics with the NPWT being discontinued approximately 7 weeks postoperatively and followed by local wound care dressings. The patient underwent further hydrosurgical débridement of the wound and application of an acellular dermal replacement at 9 weeks postoperatively **(G–I)**. **J.** Clinical outcome at 14 weeks postapplication of the bioengineered bilayer wound matrix. **K.** Final postoperative clinical outcome at approximately 11 months.

cover exposed avascular structures such as tendons, bone, and joints should be made; however, non-adherent dressings can be placed over these areas prior to NPWT application if soft tissue coverage is lacking. NPWT is avoided over exposed neurovascular structures.

Although there are now several commercially available NPWT systems, all are composed of similar basic components: open-cell foam, adhesive dressing material, tubing, collection canister, and negative pressure delivery unit (Fig. 8.9). The foam is carefully cut to fit the surgical wound and placed within the site. The adhesive dressing material, either in one piece or in strips, is then placed over the foam and overlapping the skin at the periphery of the wound to provide an airtight seal. In some cases, adhesive products such as Mastisol or tincture of benzoin can be used around the wound to further secure the dressing material. Sometimes, it is also helpful to apply pieces

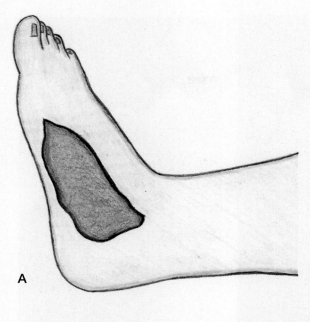

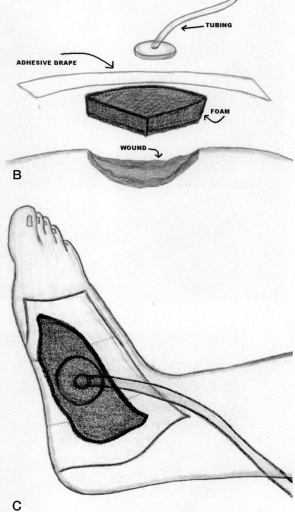

FIGURE 8.9 Schematic illustration of a medial foot ulceration with granulation tissue **(A)** being covered by a negative pressure wound therapy (NPWT) device **(B,C)**. The adhesive dressing material is placed over the selected foam and overlapping the skin at the periphery of the wound to provide an airtight seal. In some cases, adhesive products such as Mastisol or tincture of benzoin can be used around the wound to further secure the dressing material. The tube is then connected to a collection canister in the NPWT device and set in the desired pressure (mmHg).

of the adhesive dressing at the skin outlining the wound for further protection and promotion of a closed environment. Care should be taken when applying NPWT to wounds at interdigital locations so as not to place the adhesive dressing material in a fashion that may impair perfusion to the toes. A small slit in the adhesive material directly into the foam is then cut for placement of the tubing.

If there are multiple wounds necessitating NPWT or if the wound is located at a difficult location for direct placement of the tubing, bridging techniques can be utilized in which foam can be placed over the skin between 2 wounds and secured with adhesive material to join them (Fig. 8.10). Some of the NPWT devices also have available specialized connectors for multiple wounds. The opposite end of the tubing is then attached to the NPWT delivery unit which is powered on and set to the desired pressure setting. The initial pressure setting for NPWT used in diabetic wounds for secondary intention is typically continuous at 120 to 125 mmHg. Most NPWT devices have an indicator which can alert the surgeons of any leakage, and these areas can then be further secured with additional adhesive dressing.

The approach for NPWT over closed incisions (Fig. 8.11), grafts, and flaps in the diabetic foot is similar to that used in secondary intention, however, with the following exceptions: (a) A non-adherent dressing should be placed directly over the surgical incisional site prior to application of the foam, and (b) possible pressure settings can have a much larger range from 50 to 125 mmHg. Depending on the extent of the wound and any other concomitant procedures performed at the time of NPWT application, off-loading devices such as a posterior lower extremity splint or circular external fixation can also be applied at the time of surgery.

POSTOPERATIVE CARE AND COMPLICATIONS

When NPWT is used for secondary intention in diabetic foot wounds, dressings are usually changed every 2 days. For its use in high-risk closed surgical incisions, NPWT is a one-time application typically ranging from 5 to 7 days and usually set

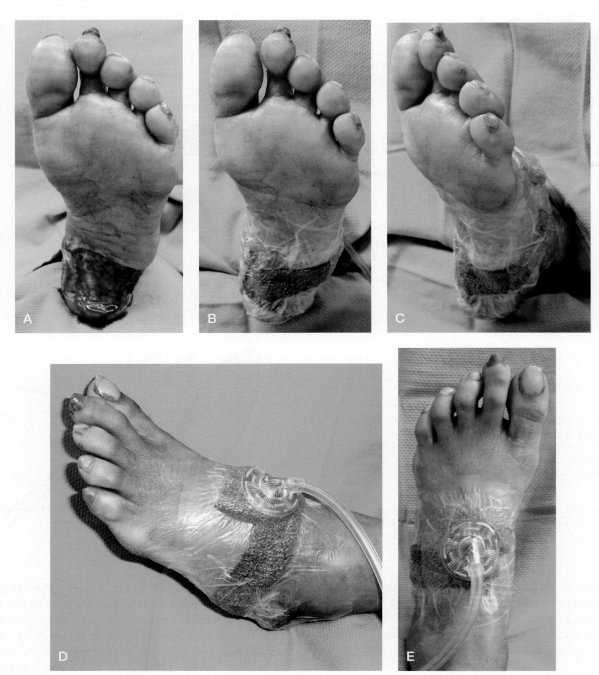

FIGURE 8.10 Intraoperative clinical picture **(A)** of a plantar foot wound with hydrosurgical débridement prepared for the application of a negative pressure wound therapy (NPWT) device **(B)**. Due to the anatomic location on the plantar aspect of the foot and difficult area for direct placement of the tubing, a bridging technique was utilized in which the foam over the wound was connected to a foam over the adhesive material starting laterally and ending on the dorsal aspect of the foot **(C-E)**.

in a lower pressure. Dressing changes should be performed by trained personnel in a clinical, wound care facility or home health care agency because most adverse effects reported in NPWT have been related to improper application and removal of the dressings. Bleeding can occur if the sponge is placed directly over exposed blood vessels. Infection can occur if pieces of the dressing are left behind with dressing changes. Regular

thorough evaluation of the surgical site can avoid vascular and infectious complications. For sensate patients, pressure settings can be reduced for better tolerance.

Methods for off-loading or immobilization of the affected lower extremity depends on the type(s) of surgical procedure performed. Patients undergoing major reconstructive surgery and NPWT may require close monitoring and can be

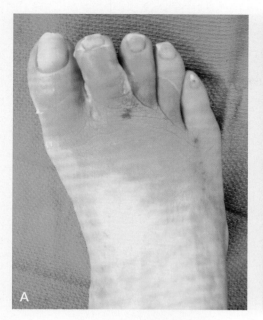

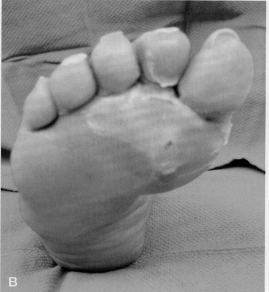

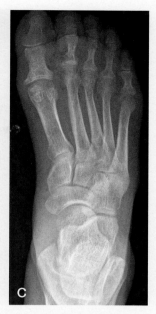

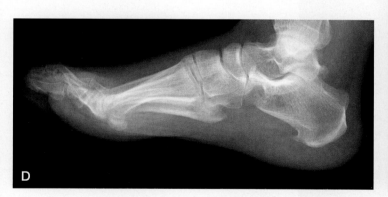

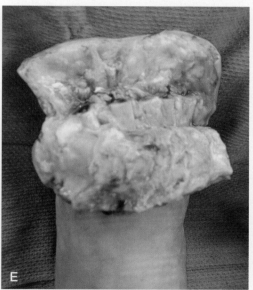

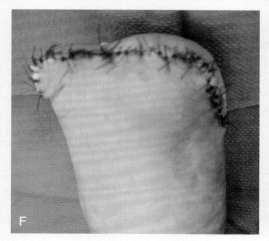

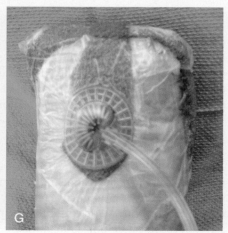

FIGURE 8.11 Preoperative clinical **(A,B)** and radiographic **(C,D)** pictures showing a severe diabetic foot infection with soft tissue gas of the entire forefoot. Patient underwent an initial transmetatarsal (toes and metatarsals one through five) amputation **(E)** being followed by a revisional amputation with delayed primary closure **(F)** and application of an incisional negative pressure wound therapy (NPWT) device **(G)**. Please note the bridging technique and application of tubing at the dorsal aspect of the foot **(G)**.*(continued)*

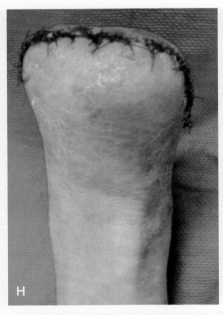
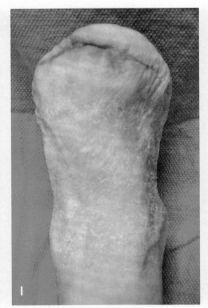
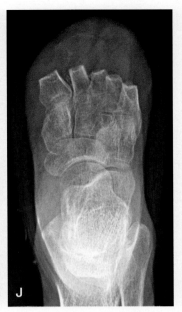

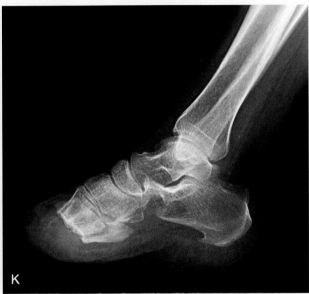

FIGURE 8.11 *(Continued)* The NPWT was left at a continuous setting and was removed postoperatively at 5 days. **H.** Clinical outcome at 6 weeks postapplication of the incisional NPWT device. Final postoperative clinical **(I)** and radiographic **(J,K)** outcomes at approximately 7 months after the patient's initial surgery.

considered for placement in assisted care facilities for proper rehabilitation. Patients and their families should be educated on the operational basics of the NPWT device including how to charge the battery, possible meanings of certain alarms, and personnel to contact in case of malfunction.

Conclusion

Although NPWT has entertained widespread use with several indications in the diabetic foot and ankle, surgeons should remember that this is an adjunctive modality and should be used in conjunction with sound surgical principles. Careful patient selection, medical optimization, adequate wound bed preparation with proper application, and postoperative care should minimize complications and improve patient outcomes.

References

1. Argenta LC, Morykwas MJ. Vacuum-assisted closure: a new method for wound control and treatment: clinical experience. Ann Plast Surg 1997;38:563–576.

2. Armstrong DG, Lavery LA. Negative pressure wound therapy after partial diabetic foot amputation: a multicentre, randomised controlled trial. Lancet 2005;366:1704–1710.

3. Bernstein BH, Tam H. Combination of subatmospheric pressure dressing and gravity feed antibiotic instillation in the treatment of post-surgical diabetic foot wounds: a case series. Wounds 2005;17:37–48.

4. Blume PA, Key JJ, Thakor P, et al. Retrospective evaluation of clinical outcomes in subjects with split-thickness skin graft: comparing V.A.C.® therapy and conventional therapy in foot and ankle reconstructive surgeries. Int Wound J 2010;7:480–487.

5. Blume PA, Walters J, Payne W, et al. Comparison of negative pressure wound therapy using vacuum-assisted closure with advanced moist wound therapy in the treatment of diabetic foot ulcers: a multicenter randomized controlled trial. Diabetes Care 2008;31:631–636.

6. Chen SZ, Li J, Li XY, et al. Effects of vacuum-assisted closure on wound microcirculation: an experimental study. Asian J Surg 2005;28:211–217.

7. Dalla Paola L. Diabetic foot wounds: the value of negative pressure wound therapy with instillation. Int Wound J 2013;10(suppl 1): 25–31.

8. Eginton MT, Brown KR, Seabrook GR, et al. A prospective randomized evaluation of negative-pressure wound dressings for diabetic foot wounds. Ann Vasc Surg 2003;17:645–649.

9. Fabian TS, Kaufman HJ, Lett ED, et al. The evaluation of subatmospheric pressure and hyperbaric oxygen in ischemic full-thickness wound healing. Am Surg 2000;66:1136–1143.

10. Fleischmann W, Strecker W, Bombelli M, et al. Vacuum sealing as a treatment of soft tissue damage in open fractures [in German]. Unfallchirurg 1993;96:488–492.

11. Greenhalgh DG. Wound healing and diabetes mellitus. Clin Plast Surg 2003;30:37–45.

12. Hasan MY, Teo R, Nather A. Negative-pressure wound therapy for management of diabetic foot wounds: a review of the mechanism of action, clinical applications, and recent developments. Diabet Foot Ankle 2015;6:27618.

13. Kairinos N, Voogd AM, Botha PH, et al. Negative-pressure wound therapy II: negative-pressure wound therapy and increased perfusion. Just an illusion? Plast Reconstr Surg 2009;123:601–612.

14. Kamolz LP, Andel H, Haslik W, et al. Use of subatmospheric pressure therapy to prevent burn wound progression in human: first experiences. Burns 2004;30:253–258.

15. Karargyris O, Polyzois VD, Karabinas P, et al. Papineau debridement, Ilizarov bone transport, and negative-pressure wound closure for septic bone defects of the tibia. Eur J Orthop Surg Traumatol 2014;24:1013–1017.

16. Karatepe O, Eken I, Acet E, et al. Vacuum assisted closure improves the quality of life in patients with diabetic foot. Acta Chir Belg 2011;111:298–302.

17. Kucharzewski M, Mieszczański P, Wilemska-Kucharzewska K, et al. The application of negative pressure wound therapy in the treatment of chronic venous leg ulceration: authors experience. Biomed Res Int 2014;2014:297230.

18. Lance S, Harrison L, Orbay H, et al. Assessing safety of negative-pressure wound therapy over pedicled muscle flaps: a retrospective review of gastrocnemius muscle flap. J Plast Reconstr Aesthet Surg 2016;69:519–523.

19. Lewis S, Raj D, Guzman NJ. Renal failure: implications of chronic kidney disease in the management of the diabetic foot. Semin Vasc Surg 2012;25:82–88.

20. Lu X, Chen S, Li X. The experimental study of the effects of vacuum-assisted closure on edema and vessel permeability of the wound. Chin J Clinic Rehab 2003;7:1244–1245.

21. McCallon SK, Knight CA, Valiulus JP, et al. Vacuum-assisted closure versus saline-moistened gauze in the healing of postoperative diabetic foot wounds. Ostomy Wound Manage 2000;46:28–32, 34.

22. Mody GN, Nirmal IA, Duraisamy S, et al. A blinded, prospective, randomized controlled trial of topical negative pressure wound closure in India. Ostomy Wound Manage 2008;54:36–46.

23. Molnar JA, DeFranzo AJ, Hadaegh A, et al. Acceleration of Integra incorporation in complex tissue defects with subatmospheric pressure. Plast Reconstr Surg 2004;113:1339–1346.

24. Morykwas MJ, Argenta LC, Shelton-Brown EI, et al. Vacuum-assisted closure: a new method for wound control and treatment: animal studies and basic foundation. Ann Plast Surg 1997;38: 553–562.

25. Morykwas MJ, Faler BJ, Pearce DJ, et al. Effects of varying levels of subatmospheric pressure on the rate of granulation tissue formation in experimental wounds in swine. Ann Plast Surg 2001;47:547–551.

26. Mouës CM, Vos MC, van den Bemd GJ, et al. Bacterial load in relation to vacuum-assisted closure wound therapy: a prospective randomized trial. Wound Repair Regen 2004;12:11–17.

27. Novinscak T, Zvorc M, Trojko S, et al. Usporedba troska i koristi (cost-benefit)triju nacina lijecenja dijabetickog vrijeda: suhim prevojem, vlaznim prevojem i negativnim tlakom. Acta Medica Croatica 2010;64(suppl 1):113–115.

28. Paola LD, Carone A, Ricci S, et al. Use of vacuum assisted closure therapy in the treatment of diabetic foot wounds. J Diabet Foot Complications 2010;2:3–44.

29. Ramanujam CL, Stapleton JJ, Zgonis T. Negative-pressure wound therapy in the management of diabetic Charcot foot and ankle wounds. Diabet Foot Ankle 2013;23:4.

30. Ramanujam CL, Zgonis T. Surgical soft tissue closure of severe diabetic foot infections: a combination of biologics, negative pressure wound therapy, and skin grafting. Clin Podiatr Med Surg 2012;29:143–146.

31. Scherer LA, Shiver S, Chang M, et al. The vacuum assisted closure device: a method of securing skin grafts and improving graft survival. Arch Surg 2002;137:930–934.

32. Siana JE, Rex S, Gottrup F. The effect of cigarette smoking on wound healing. Scand J Plast Reconstr Surg Hand Surg 1989;23:207–209.

33. Stannard JP, Robinson JT, Anderson ER, et al. Negative pressure wound therapy to treat hematomas and surgical incisions following high-energy trauma. J Trauma 2006;60:1301–1306.

34. Webster J, Scuffham P, Stankiewicz M, et al. Negative pressure wound therapy for skin grafts and surgical wounds healing by primary intention. Cochrane Database Syst Rev 2014;(10): CD009261.

35. Weed T, Ratliff C, Drake DB. Quantifying bacterial bioburden during negative pressure wound therapy: does the wound VAC enhance bacterial clearance? Ann Plast Surg 2004;52: 276–280.

36. Willy C, Agarwal A, Andersen CA, et al. Closed incision negative pressure therapy: international multidisciplinary consensus recommendations. Int Wound J 2017;14:385–398.

37. Zöch G. V.A.C.-therapy and laser-induced fluorescence of indocyanine-green (IC-view), an assessment of wound perfusion in diabetic foot syndrome [in German]. Zentralblatt Chir 2004;129(suppl 1):80–81.

CHAPTER 9

Surgical Débridement and Bioengineered Alternative Tissues for the Acute and Chronic Diabetic Foot Wounds

Caitlin S. Zarick • John S. Steinberg • Paul J. Kim

INTRODUCTION

Diabetic wound healing and limb salvage has gained attention over the last decade because of the potential for devastating end results and the increase in the number of people living with diabetes mellitus. It is estimated that by the year 2035, nearly 417 million people will be living with diabetes mellitus, increased from 382 million people in 2013 (26). Diabetic foot ulcers (DFUs) have become a significant public health concern and are estimated to occur in approximately 25% of people with diabetes mellitus and is the number one cause for hospitalization in these patients (40,63). Approximately one-quarter of all hospital days for diabetic patients are related to foot complications (36). The advancement of wound healing has focused on decreasing the time to wound closure, improving the cost-effectiveness of treatment options, and improving limb salvage rates.

Patients with diabetes mellitus have an impaired ability to heal wounds because of both intrinsic and extrinsic factors. High levels of glucose can stimulate production of inflammatory markers, inhibit collagen synthesis, decrease cellular proliferation, and inhibit differentiation of keratinocytes (24,64). Diabetic patients are also at higher risk for infection due to their impaired immune response system. Similarly, they often have compromised vasculature, neuropathy, and biomechanical abnormalities. The combination of these factors is what makes healing DFUs an ever-growing challenge.

The goal of treating any type of wound is to create an environment that is conducive to healing. The focus of this chapter will be on the role of surgical débridement and adjunctive wound therapy with application of cellular and tissue-based products (CTPs) for wounds. Normal wound healing should be assessed on a weekly basis with wound measurements. Normal healing is said to occur at a rate of 10% to 15% or more per week (29,55,56,61,67). If this rate is not seen or the

wound is stalled, one should consider adjunctive therapies such as CTPs. Prior to surgical débridement or adjunctive therapies, it is critical to ensure that the etiology of the wound has been properly diagnosed and treated, blood flow to the area is optimized, biomechanical abnormalities have been recognized with appropriate off-loading or correction performed, and any underlying medical or nutritional deficits have been addressed.

SURGICAL DÉBRIDEMENT

Surgical débridement has come to be known as a critical portion of wound care and wound bed preparation. Both acute and chronic wounds require efficient débridement to facilitate appropriate treatment and healing. The definition of débridement is "the removal of foreign material and devitalized tissue from or adjacent to a traumatic or infected lesion until surrounding healthy tissue is exposed" (12). The generally accepted principles of surgical débridement are as follows: early and frequent management, remove all necrotic tissue, inspect deep structures such as muscle and bone, preserve all viable skin and soft tissue, plan incisions and débridement for later reconstruction, and repeat as necessary (3,4,21). For acute wound débridement, the goal is to remove infected and necrotic tissue and get to healthy tissue. For chronic wounds, débridement converts these challenging wounds to acute wounds so that they can then progress through the normal stages of healing (60). One of the keys to débridement for surgeons is to be aggressive and to not let the residual soft tissue defect limit the amount of débridement performed.

Surgical débridement has long been considered an essential step in the management of DFUs but the evidence to support this argument is lacking. The beneficial effect of surgical débridement was first supported by a trial in 1996 by Steed et al. (65). The study was a randomized, prospective, double-blind trial comparing the use of recombinant human platelet-derived growth factor (rhPDGF) and placebo, both in combination with sharp débridement. They observed that a lower rate of healing was seen in centers that performed less frequent débridement (65). Another study in 1998 compared the effect of surgical and nonsurgical approaches to the healing of DFUs (51). Group A was treated with 1 initial clinic débridement, saline wet-to-dry dressings, and off-loading. Group B was treated with complete surgical excision of the ulceration with closure. Group A was found to have higher infection rates, lower healing rates, and increased healing time over 6 months compared to Group B. Group B was also noted to have lower recurrence rate (51). Several other studies exist that give marginal evidence toward the benefits of surgical débridement (8,11,51,52,57).

Emergent surgical débridement is needed when an acute infection is noted in the presence of a DFU. These acute wounds must be cleansed of contaminants and dead tissue as soon as possible. This is most appropriately carried out in the operating room to ensure adequate sterility, débridement, and lavage of the area. An incision and drainage of the area with or without complete excision of the ulceration is typically performed. Deep abscess and necrosis may be present and must be thoroughly explored during the acute surgical débridement. The goal of the initial surgical débridement is to remove all dead skin, subcutaneous tissue, muscle, fascia, and bone while ensuring preservation of all potential viable tissues. After adequate débridement, the wound is typically cleansed with pulse lavage and dressed appropriately. Repeat surgical débridements are typically performed every 24 to 72 hours as deemed necessary by the surgeon until only healthy, bleeding, viable tissue remains.

For chronic DFUs, débridement is usually initiated after addressing the underlying etiology or medical condition. Débridement of these wounds stimulates the conversion to an acute wound so they are no longer halted in the nonhealing state. Débridement also removes any surface contaminants or biofilm, which often impedes the healing process as well (33). The removal of bacteria allows local resources such as oxygen and nutrients to be available for healing instead of being consumed by the bacteria. Similar to acute surgical débridement, the goal is to achieve bleeding, normal-colored tissue that could progress through the normal wound healing stages or that could be amenable to grafting or advanced reconstructive closure techniques (3,4).

Techniques for Surgical Débridement

Many uncertainties exist regarding the evidence for the use and method of débridement for the treatment of DFUs. It is clear from multiple guidelines such as the American Diabetes Association, the American College of Foot and Ankle Surgeons, and Wound Healing Society that débridement should be included in protocols for the care of patients with DFUs (36). Most uncertainty pertains to the frequency, extent, and types of débridements performed. The operative

techniques are often guided by the practitioners' training, experience, and comfort level (8). Several techniques exist to carry out surgical débridement, and the instruments and techniques are important to successful débridement.

Depending on a surgeon's training, experience, and operating room setup, different surgical instruments will be available and used by the surgeon. A scalpel, forceps, scissors, and curettes are some of the basic instruments typically used to remove nonviable tissue from a wound base. For example, a no. 10 blade is useful for cutting thin layers of tissue until clean, healthy tissue remains. Sharp scissors and forceps are especially good for cutting eschar, desiccated tendons, and clean skin edges. Wound surfaces can be scraped with a large, sharp curette to facilitate removal of biofilm and superficial wound slough. This often stimulates wound bed bleeding. A variety of rongeurs can also be used to remove tissue in difficult-to-reach areas or deep spaces. They can also be used to resect pieces of bone or obtain tissue or bone biopsies. Elevators can be helpful for lifting tissue to expose areas of concern or to expose bone. A sagittal saw or osteotomes should also be available in order to resect bone when necessary. Pulse irrigation is then used to irrigate the surface of the wound from debris, tissue, and bacteria (5).

The VERSAJET (Smith & Nephew, Cambridge, England) is a hydrosurgical water knife (34). This instrument forces a narrow stream of water across a small opening at the tip of the instrument. The pressure from the water stream also creates a vacuum that sucks in the wound bed tissue and mills it. The VERSAJET is extremely useful for accurate control of débridement depth and minimizes accidental removal of healthy tissue. It is especially useful for preparation of wound beds for skin grafting or for larger wound surface areas (14,18,34,42,46). It helps to create a smooth wound bed with an even contour throughout.

Similarly, the use of methylene blue dye has been a very helpful tool to ensure adequate débridement is completed. The dye is applied with a cotton tip applicator to the entire surface of the wound and can also be injected into pockets or cavities. Débridement is then performed ensuring that all of the dye is removed from within the wound bed, which allows for complete removal of biofilm and surface contaminants (Fig. 9.1). The authors also employ a "two-table" surgical setup where a separate set of instruments, gloves, drapes, Bovie electrocautery, and suction are used after surgical débridement and lavage to avoid recontamination. It has been speculated that instruments used to débride the contaminated wounds harbor bacteria on their surfaces. The two-table surgical setup eliminates any potential for iatrogenic inoculation of the newly débrided wound.

Preparing the wound bed for healing is a vital part of wound care. Surgical débridement is the most accurate and effective method for preparing the wound bed as it allows for an appropriate setting to perform an extensive and thorough débridement as necessary. Adequate and successful débridement renders the wound bed with healthy, bleeding skin, subcutaneous tissue, fat, fascia, muscle, and bone. It is only after the wound is sufficiently prepared that one can consider adjunctive

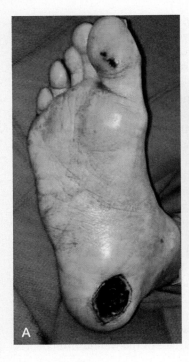
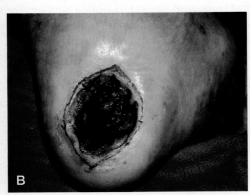
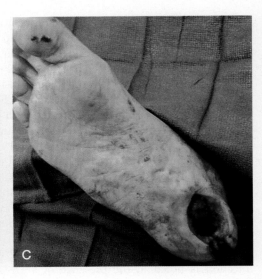

FIGURE 9.1 **A,B.** Application of methylene blue to wound bed of heel ulcer. **C.** Complete excision and débridement performed of the ulcer removing all methylene blue.

wound therapies such as application of CTPs. These therapies will only be successful if the wound is clean and healthy and in an environment conducive to anabolic metabolism.

Cellular and Tissue-Based Products for Diabetic Foot Wounds

One of the most rapidly growing and changing topics in wound care today is the use of CTPs in the form of grafting or topical application. Science has allowed the introduction of bioengineering and other graft harvesting as much research is focused on their use in temporary and permanent wound coverage and in augmentation of wound healing. There is also a new focus on stem cell–based wound care products that may be shaping the future of wound healing. All of these new products have a high potential for enhancing wound healing and facilitating skin regeneration. Advantages of these CTPs include decrease in bacterial counts while promoting a sterile wound environment. They can also help reduce pain associated with wounds, decrease scarring, and help restore function or motion. The ideal product would be cost-effective, have no antigenicity or toxicity, lack disease transmission, and be compatible with multiple tissue types (10,19).

Many of these products can be costly; thus, careful consideration must be taken in regard to the specific wound and timing prior to application. The use of these products is mostly reserved for recalcitrant wounds that have stalled in their normal healing rate. Some products are also used to help prepare the wound bed for later split-thickness skin grafting (STSG) or closure. A definitive treatment plan for closure and prevention of reulceration must be considered prior to application of CTPs due to their high cost. An autograft, such as a STSG,

is still an ideal closure method. However, autografts are not always the best or feasible option in the high-risk diabetic patients (Fig. 9.2).

Bioengineered alternative tissues can be categorized into 3 subsets, dermoinductive, dermoconductive, and dermogenic (Table 9.1). Kim and colleagues (32) in 2007 defined the terms *dermoinductive* and *dermoconductive* to help classify the many different available products and to help determine their appropriate use. Products are termed as dermoinductive if they have cells and other growth factors imbedded into the materials. Such cells may include fibroblasts or keratinocytes that are essential for skin development and wound healing (59). Dermoconductive refers to products that have no active cells within them and essentially serve as scaffolding for host cells to grow into (32,59). Each product has advantages and disadvantages.

Dermoinductive Products

Dermoinductive products include Apligraf (Organogenesis, Inc., Canton, MA), Dermagraft (Organogenesis, Inc., Canton, MA), TheraSkin (Soluble Systems, LLC, Newport News, VA), BIOBRANE (Smith & Nephew, Memphis, TN), and Epicel (Genzyme, Cambridge, MA). The 2 products with the most substantial clinical data and the most widely used of the dermoinductive agents are Apligraf and Dermagraft.

Apligraf was the first commercially available bioengineered biologic dressing for wound healing. It is a 2-layer product made from neonatal foreskin and bovine collagen (32,66,72). Cell proliferation and differentiation are stimulated within the wound by producing growth factors and proteins (16). The U.S. Food and Drug Administration has approved its use for DFUs (16,68).

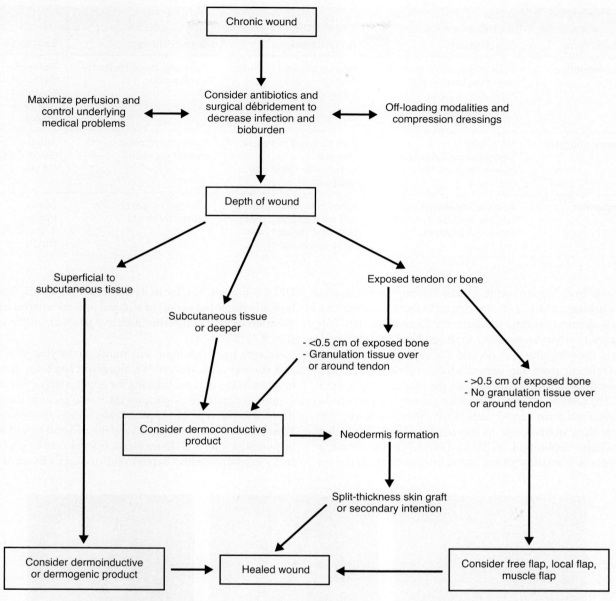

FIGURE 9.2 An algorithm for the use of bioengineered alternative tissues in diabetic foot wounds.

Three randomized controlled trials support the use of Apligraf for DFUs as a fast method of healing compared to standard wound care alone. Veves and colleagues (68) in 2001 performed a randomized, prospective controlled clinical trial at 24 centers in the United States looking at the use of Apligraf on DFUs compared to saline-moistened gauze. Two hundred and eight diabetic patients were included, and the results showed that the Apligraf group had 56% of patients healed at 12 weeks compared to 38%. They also found that it only took 65 days for the Apligraf group to heal compared to 90 days for the control group (68). The remaining 2 studies had similar results showing increased healing in the Apligraf group (13,58).

Dermagraft is made of human fibroblasts from neonatal foreskin, an extracellular matrix, and a bioabsorbable polyglactin mesh scaffold. Similar to Apligraf, epithelialization is stimulated by proteins and growth factors within the graft (17). One of the largest studies performed on Dermagraft looked at 314 diabetic patients with plantar ulcerations that had been nonhealing for 6 weeks. A randomized, prospective, multicenter trial was performed and found 30% of wounds treated with Dermagraft were closed at 12 weeks compared to 18.3% in the control group (38). Numerous studies exist analyzing the effectiveness of Dermagraft on DFUs (2,20,23,38,47,53).

Dermoconductive Products

Many dermoconductive products exist, but the most widely used and most abundant in the literature include Integra (Integra LifeSciences, Plainsboro, NJ), GRAFTJACKET (Wright Medical Technology, Arlington, TN), and OASIS (Smith & Nephew, Memphis, TN). These products merely provide a matrix for

TABLE 9.1	Summary of Bioengineered Alternative Tissue Products			
Product Type	**Description**	**Advantages**	**Disadvantages**	**Examples**
Dermoinductive	Cells and growth factors are imbedded in the products	Can be applied in clinic setting Easy application	Typically need multiple applications	Apligraf Dermagraft TheraSkin Biobrane Epicel
Dermoconductive	No active cells Serve as scaffolding or a matrix for host cells	Can be used in deeper wounds Often only need one application	Typically applied in the operating room	Integra GRAFTJACKET OASIS
Dermogenic	Releases or stimulates release of growth factors Stem cell products	Stem cells can differentiate into many different tissue types Easy application	Minimal research currently exists	Grafix EpiFix AmnioClear NEOX

which cells from the surrounding tissue can migrate across and create a neodermis (19,32,66). In contrast to the dermoinductive products, dermoconductive products contain no living cells (66).

Integra is a bilayer, acellular graft made of bovine type I collagen, chondroitin-6-sulfate, and a semipermeable silicone layer. Different from the dermoinductive products, Integra relies on the vascular ingrowth from the surrounding wound edges. The scaffolding effect allows for cells to migrate across the wound and form a neodermis (43,49,50,70,71). It was first used on burn wounds, but its use has now vastly expanded and includes application on DFUs (44,62,71). The research on Integra is extensive, but the literature specific to its use on DFUs is limited. Similar to its use in burn wounds, Integra is typically employed as part of a staged process where a later application of STSG or dermoinductive product will be applied (Fig. 9.3) (37,70,71).

Integra has been used on wounds of varying size, depth, and etiology with success. An algorithm has been developed to assist in the decision making for application of this dermoconductive graft. The algorithm takes into account the wound depth and the type of exposed tissue within the wound bed. Wounds must first be adequately débrided and free of biofilm or potential infection. Once clean, Integra may be applied directly to wounds with a depth to subcutaneous tissue or fascia.

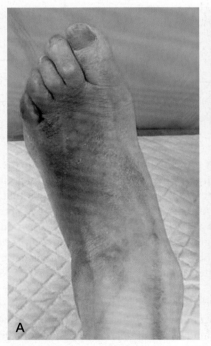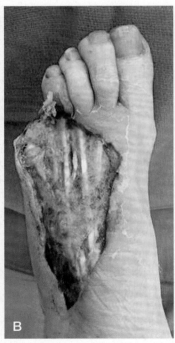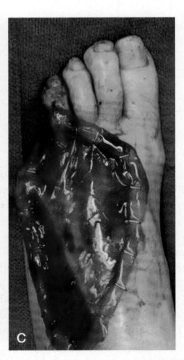

FIGURE 9.3 **A.** Left foot gas gangrene with ascending cellulitis. **B.** After initial incision and drainage and 2 surgical débridements, the patient was left with exposed tendons and fascia. **C.** Integra dermal regenerative matrix was applied to the wound bed to prepare the wound for later split-thickness skin grafting.

Deeper wounds that have exposed tendon or bone pose more of a challenge. It is recommended that for wounds with exposed tendon, there must be granulation tissue present. For larger wounds, the granulation should be present over the tendon, and for smaller wounds, it should be present around the tendon. The algorithm also recommends that application of Integra over bone may be utilized when there is 0.5 cm or less of exposed bone (31) (Fig. 9.4).

Another recent study performed at the authors' institution evaluated the use of Integra for diabetic limb salvage cases (27). One hundred five diabetic patients with 121 wounds that received Integra application for complex lower extremity wounds were retrospectively reviewed. For the entire population studied, the salvage rate was 77%. When categorized into low-risk versus high-risk wounds, the authors found an 83% salvage rate in the low-risk population compared to a 46% salvage rate in the high-risk group (27).

GRAFTJACKET is an acellular dermal matrix derived from human cadaveric dermis. During processing, all epidermal and cellular components are removed leaving only matrix and biochemical components (66). Several studies including 2 randomized controlled trials have shown the successful outcomes of GRAFTJACKET on DFUs (7,39,69).

Dermogenic Products

Many different aspects of medicine are now investigating the use of stem cell therapy for advancements in treatment options.

Wound care is one of those areas with the introduction of amniotic membrane products derived from placental tissue. The term *dermogenic* is used to describe a novel CTP category that can induce healing through direct application of growth factors or by eliciting growth factor release from the host tissue. Dermogenic products include those derived from placental tissue, amnion, chorion, and amniotic membranes. Several of these products include Grafix (Osiris Therapeutics, Inc., Columbia, MD), EpiFix (MiMedx Group, Inc., Marietta, GA), AmnioClear (Liventa Biosciences, Inc., Conshohocken, PA), and NEOX (Amniox Medical, Inc., Atlanta, GA). Stem cells are unique in that they can differentiate into different cell types while producing high quantities of growth factors and chemokines (6,9,22,25,41,54). During processing, several components of the placental membrane are preserved including vascular endothelial growth factor, platelet-derived growth factor, basic fibroblast growth factor, epidermal growth factor, transforming growth factor, and nerve growth factor (35,41,73). The goals of amniotic membrane products include decreasing wound closure time, enhancing healing potential, regeneration of skin, and decreasing wound contracture (9,25). Figure 9.5 demonstrates the use of Grafix to a chronic hallux ulceration.

The literature is still in the early phases with few substantial clinical trials available. One study looked at the use of Grafix on chronic DFUs compared to control treatment (35). They compared 50 diabetic patients who received Grafix in the weekly clinic setting compared to 47 who received stan-

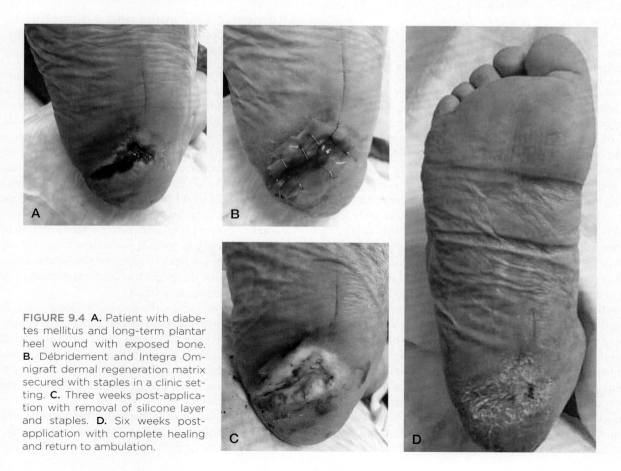

FIGURE 9.4 A. Patient with diabetes mellitus and long-term plantar heel wound with exposed bone. **B.** Débridement and Integra Omnigraft dermal regeneration matrix secured with staples in a clinic setting. **C.** Three weeks post-application with removal of silicone layer and staples. **D.** Six weeks post-application with complete healing and return to ambulation.

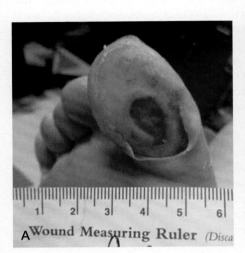
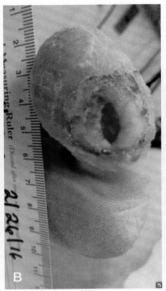
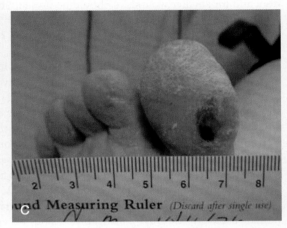

FIGURE 9.5 **A.** Right chronic hallux ulceration remained nonhealing with conservative care for 5 months. **B.** Weekly Grafix applications were started along with local débridements and appropriate off-loading. **C.** After 5 Grafix applications, the hallux ulcer healed.

dard of care wound treatments. Overall, the Grafix group had 62% of the wounds healed at an average of 42 days compared to 21% healed at 69.5 days in the standard of care group (35). Amniotic membrane products have shown early promise in advancing wound care and could prove beneficial in the years to come.

When, Where, and How to Apply Bioengineered Alternative Tissues

As mentioned previously, the decision to use a CTP is typically based on decrease percentage in wound size. There should be an observed 10% to 15% wound closure rate weekly (29,55,56,61,67). Typically, if this is not observed after 4 to 6 weeks of standard wound therapy, one should consider adjunctive therapies, including CTPs. Many CTPs are designed to be applied in the clinic setting, usually on a weekly basis. Examples of such products include Apligraf, Dermagraft, and Grafix. The authors have found greater success with these products when used on small ulcers with limited depth. By following standard guidelines, the wounds must be sharply débrided prior to application.

Other products, such as Integra, are meant to be applied in the operating room setting to maintain sterility. This is advantageous because wounds can be appropriately and thoroughly débrided prior to application of the graft. This will ensure removal of all nonviable tissue and elimination of infection or biofilm to increase the success of the graft. After adequate débridement, the product can be applied to the wound bed.

Some products will need fenestration with a no. 15 blade, whereas others come prefenestrated. This allows for drainage through the graft and reduction of a seroma or hematoma formation. Once the graft is in contact with the wound bed, it should be secured to the surrounding skin with Steri-Strips,

sutures, or staples. Typically, a nonadherent dressing is applied over the dorsal aspect of the graft and surrounding skin and dressing materials applied as deemed appropriate by the physician.

Alternative Therapies and Adjunctive Modalities for Soft Tissue Coverage of Diabetic Foot Wounds

It is important to remember that many CTPs can merely be applied in preparation for future STSG (Fig. 9.6). Autografts are typically more desirable, heal faster, and are less expensive than their bioengineered counterparts. They are ideal and facilitate faster wound closure in wounds with large surface areas. Typical STSG thickness can range from 0.012 to 0.018 in. based on reconstructive needs (Fig. 9.7). They should only be considered in granular, infection-free wound beds and in diabetic patients who have the capability to heal a donor site. For DFUs of increased size and depth with potentially exposed tendon or bone, other reconstructive options may be of more benefit. Such options include local flaps (Fig. 9.8) and free tissue transfers. Careful preoperative assessment and patient selection must be undertaken prior to performing these advanced wound closure methods.

As mentioned earlier, the successful closure of a diabetic foot wound is dependent on several factors. The simple act of applying a CTP does not always equal successful closure of a wound and does not necessarily prevent reulceration in the future. The fundamental principles of diabetic wound healing and limb salvage must first be addressed prior to attempting wound closure with CTPs.

One of the fundamental concepts that must be addressed is ensuring adequate blood flow to the lower extremity. Without sufficient arterial perfusion, diabetic wounds will not heal

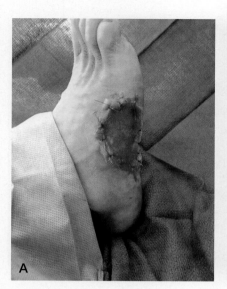
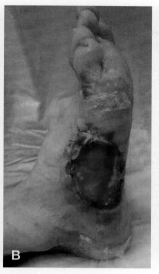
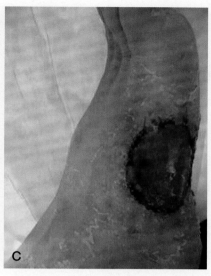

FIGURE 9.6 Complex wound reconstruction using Integra bilayer wound matrix. The bovine collagen product was applied to this deep wound after staged débridement of infected soft tissue and bone from the site **(A)**. After 14 days, the neodermis was formed under the Integra as illustrated by the red color adherent to the overlying graft **(B)**. The patient was then taken back to the operating room for application of a split-thickness skin graft to the site and rapid graft healing was observed **(C)**.

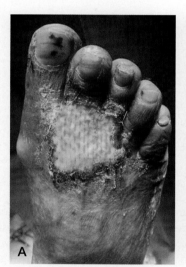
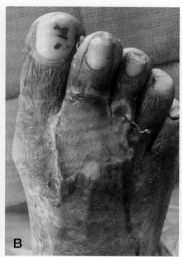
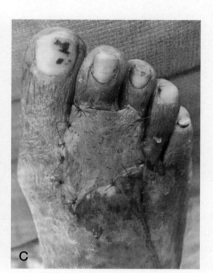

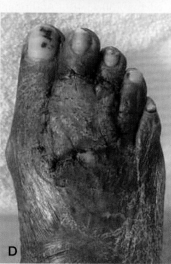

FIGURE 9.7 Patient with diabetes mellitus and dorsal forefoot wound. Local infected soft tissues and skin necrosis was débrided prior with application of porcine fenestrated xenograft **(A)**. The xenograft was left intact and then débrided from the wound base 5 days later to reveal granular wound base **(B)**. **C.** Split-thickness skin graft 0.012 in. was harvested from the thigh and secured to wound base. **D.** Two weeks post-application of the autogenous skin graft with complete wound healing.

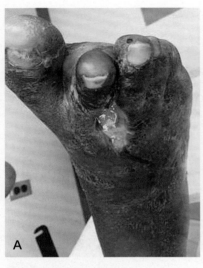
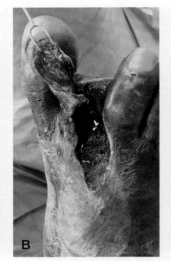
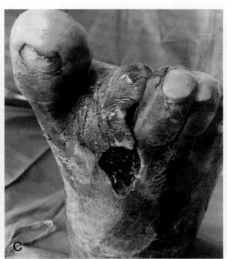
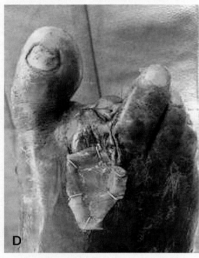

FIGURE 9.8 **A.** Patient with diabetes mellitus and second ray (metatarsal and toe) wound with infection requiring removal of the second meta-tarsal. **B.** Second toe fillet flap to preserve soft tissue as flap for partial closure of the surgical defect. **C.** Inset of second toe fillet flap. **D.** Final closure of the second toe fillet flap and residual proximal soft tissue defect covered with Integra bilayer wound matrix.

despite the modality used for closure. If necessary, a vascular consult should be obtained. Lower extremity biomechanical and structural deformities must also be addressed. This may be as simple as providing appropriate off-loading to the wound site through casting or splints. Surgical procedures may need to be performed including tendon balancing or lengthening, osseous reconstruction, or exostectomy. These considerations must also be addressed in order to prevent future complications. Other factors also play significance in wound healing including medical comorbidities and nutritional status. The patient must be medically and nutritionally optimized prior to, during, and after attempts at wound healing. All of these factors can often be overlooked but are crucial in the multifactorial approach to wound care.

Adjunctive therapies can also assist in the success of CTPs. These therapies include negative pressure wound therapy (NPWT) and hyperbaric oxygen therapy (HBOT). Oftentimes, they are used prior to the application of CTPs, but they can also be used in conjunction with certain grafts. NPWT is now very widely accepted for advanced wound care. It has a wide variety of uses, but importantly for DFUs, it is

useful for preparing the wound bed for delayed closure, skin grafting, or flap coverage. NPWT provides increased rate of granulation tissue, increase in vascularity to the wound bed, control of bacterial growth, less frequent dressing changes, and reduction in edema (30,45,48). Additionally, NPWT can be applied over a CTP or STSG to increase the take of the graft during the initial few days of healing and longer if needed. HBOT has been shown to have beneficial effects on diabetic wound healing. It may be specifically useful in patients with microvascular disease as long as any large vessel disease has been addressed. HBOT causes an increased level of oxygenation to the tissues and can have positive effects on wound healing. It should be used in combination with other modalities (1,15,28).

Conclusion

DFUs remain to be a complex and challenging entity of medicine. There is not 1 single way to heal a diabetic wound, and the physician must have a wide knowledge of available modalities to treat these difficult to heal DFUs. One must also be aware of the constant advances and new products that are available on the market in order to choose the best option for the patient. The use of these technologies should be based on evidence-based medicine with large randomized, prospective studies. CTPs will continue to be challenged as medicine continues to advance. Sound principles on fundamental wound care with adequate clinical or surgical débridement and the adjunctive use of CTPs when deemed necessary are paramount to the patient's successful outcome.

References

1. Abidia A, Laden G, Kuhan G, et al. The role of hyperbaric oxygen therapy in ischaemic diabetic lower extremity ulcers: a double-blind randomised-controlled trial. Eur J Vasc Endovasc Surg 2003;25:513–518.

2. Allenet B, Parée F, Lebrun T, et al. Cost-effectiveness modeling of Dermagraft for the treatment of diabetic foot ulcers in the French context. Diabetes Metab 2000;26:125–132.

3. Attinger CE, Bulan EJ. Débridement. The key initial step in wound healing. Foot Ankle Clin 2001;6:627–660.

4. Attinger CE, Bulan E, Blume PA. Surgical débridement. The key to successful wound healing and reconstruction. Clin Podiatr Med Surg 2000;17:599–630.

5. Attinger CE, Janis JE, Steinberg JS, et al. Clinical approach to wounds: débridement and wound bed preparation including the use of dressings and wound-healing adjuvants. Plast Reconstr Surg 2006;117:72–109.

6. Blumberg SN, Berger A, Hwang L, et al. The role of stem cells in diabetic foot ulcers. Diabetes Res Clin Pract 2012;96:1–9.

7. Brigido SA. The use of acellular dermal regenerative tissue matrix in the treatment of lower extremity wounds: a prospective 16-week pilot study. Int Wound J 2006;3:181–187.

8. Cardinal M, Eisenbud DE, Armstrong DG, et al. Serial surgical debridement: a retrospective study on clinical outcomes in chronic lower extremity wounds. Wound Repair Regen 2009;17:306–311.

9. Chen M, Przyborowski M, Berthiaume F. Stem cell for skin tissue engineering and wound healing. Crit Rev Biomed Eng 2009;37:399–421.

10. Cook EA, Cook JJ, Badri H, et al. Bioengineered alternative tissues. Clin Podiatr Med Surg 2014;31:89–101.

11. Cornell RS, Meyr AJ, Steinberg JS, et al. Débridement of the noninfected wound. J Vasc Surg 2010;52(3 suppl):31–36.

12. Dorland's illustrated medical dictionary, 27th ed. Philadelphia: Saunders, 1988.

13. Edmonds M. Apligraf in the treatment of neuropathic diabetic foot ulcers. Int J Low Extrem Wounds 2009;8:11–18.

14. Eneroth M, van Houtum WH. The value of debridement and vacuum-assisted closure (V.A.C.) therapy in diabetic foot ulcers. Diabetes Metab Res Rev 2008;24(suppl 1):76–80.

15. Faglia E, Favales F, Aldeghi A, et al. Adjunctive systemic hyperbaric oxygen therapy in treatment of severe prevalently ischemic diabetic foot ulcer. A randomized study. Diabetes Care 1996;19:1338–1343.

16. Falanga V, Isaacs C, Paquette D, et al. Wounding of bioengineered skin: cellular and molecular aspects after injury. J Invest Dermatol 2002;119:653–660.

17. Felder JM III, Goyal SS, Attinger CE. A systematic review of skin substitutes for foot ulcers. Plast Reconstr Surg 2012;130:145–164.

18. Fraccalvieri M, Serra R, Ruka R, et al. Surgical debridement with VERSAJET: an analysis of bacteria load of the wound bed pre- and post-treatment and skin graft taken. A preliminary pilot study. Int Wound J 2011;8:155–161.

19. Garwood CG, Steinberg JS, Kim PJ. Bioengineered alternative tissues in diabetic wound healing. Clin Podiatr Med Surg 2015;32:121–133.

20. Gentzkow GD, Iwasaki SD, Hershon KS, et al. Use of Dermagraft, a cultured human dermis, to treat diabetic foot ulcers. Diabetes Care 1996;19:350–354.

21. Granick M, Boykin J, Gamelli R, et al. Toward a common language: surgical wound bed preparation and debridement. Wound Repair Regen 2006;14(suppl 1):1–10.

22. Gu C, Huang S, Gao D, et al. Angiogenic effect of mesenchymal stem cells as a therapeutic target for enhancing diabetic wound healing. Int J Low Extrem Wounds 2014;13:88–93.

23. Hanft JR, Surprenant MS. Healing of chronic foot ulcers in diabetic patients treated with a human fibroblast-derived dermis. J Foot Ankle Surg 2002;41:291–299.

24. Hennessey PJ, Ford EG, Black CT, et al. Wound collagenase activity correlates directly with collagen glycosylation in diabetic rats. J Pediatr Surg 1990;25:75–78.

25. Huang L, Burd A. An update of stem cell applications in burns and wound care. Indian J Plast Surg 2012;45:229–236.

26. International Diabetes Federation. IDF diabetes atlas. 6th ed. Brussels, Belgium: International Diabetes Federation, 2013. Available at: http://www.idf.org/diabetesatlas.

27. Iorio ML, Goldstein J, Adams M, et al. Functional limb salvage in the diabetic patient: the use of a collagen bilayer matrix and risk factors for amputation. Plast Reconstr Surg 2011;127:260–267.

28. Kang TS, Gorti GK, Quan SY, et al. Effect of hyperbaric oxygen on growth factor profile of fibroblasts. Arch Facial Plast Surg 2004;6:31–35.

29. Kantor J, Margolis DJ. A multicentre study of percentage change in venous leg ulcer area as a prognostic index of healing at 24 weeks. Br J Dermatol 2000;142:960–964.

30. Kaplan M, Daly D, Stemkowski S. Early intervention of negative pressure wound therapy using vacuum-assisted closure in trauma patients: impact on hospital length of stay and cost. Adv Skin Wound Care 2009;22:128–132.

31. Kim PJ, Attinger CE, Steinberg JS, et al. Integra bilayer wound matrix application for complex lower extremity soft tissue reconstruction. Surg Technol Int 2014;24:65–73.

32. Kim PJ, Heilala M, Steinberg JS, et al. Bioengineered alternative tissues and hyperbaric oxygen in lower extremity wound healing. Clin Podiatr Med Surg 2007;24:529–546.

33. Kim PJ, Steinberg JS. Wound care: biofilm and its impact on the latest treatment modalities for ulcerations of the diabetic foot. Semin Vasc Surg 2012;25:70–74.

34. Klein MB, Hunter S, Heimbach D, et al. The Versajet trademark water dissector: a new tool for tangential excision. J Burn Care Rehabil 2005;26:483–487.

35. Lavery LA, Fulmer J, Shebetka KA, et al. The efficacy and safety of Grafix® for the treatment of chronic diabetic foot ulcers: results of a multi-centre, controlled, randomised, blinded, clinical trial. Int Wound J 2014;11:554–560.

36. Lebrun E, Tomic-Canic M, Kirsner RS. The role of surgical debridement in healing of diabetic foot ulcers. Wound Repair Regen 2010;18:433–438.

37. Lee LF, Porch JV, Spenler CW, et al. Integra in lower extremity reconstruction after burn injury. Plast Reconstr Surg 2008;121: 1256–1262.

38. Marston WA, Hanft J, Norwood P, et al. The efficacy and safety of Dermagraft in improving the healing of chronic diabetic foot ulcers: results from a prospective randomized trial. Diabetes Care 2003;26:1701–1705.

39. Martin BR, Sangalang M, Wu S, et al. Outcomes of allogenic acellular matrix therapy in treatment of diabetic foot wounds: an initial experience. Int Wound J 2005;2:161–165.

40. Martins-Mendes D, Monteiro-Soares M, Boyko EJ, et al. The independent contribution of diabetic foot ulcer on lower extremity amputation and mortality risk. J Diabetes Complications 2014;28:632–638.

41. Maxson S, Lopez EA, Yoo D, et al. Concise review: role of mesenchymal stem cells in wound repair. Stem Cells Transl Med 2012;1:142–149.

42. McCardle JE. Versajet hydroscalpel: treatment of diabetic foot ulcerations. Br J Nurs 2006;15:S12–S17.

43. Menn ZK, Lee E, Klebuc MJ. Acellular dermal matrix and negative pressure wound therapy: a tissue-engineered alternative to free tissue transfer in the compromised host. J Reconstr Microsurg 2012;28:139–144.

44. Molnar JA, DeFranzo AJ, Hadaegh A, et al. Acceleration of Integra incorporation in complex tissue defects with subatmospheric pressure. Plast Reconstr Surg 2004;113:1339–1346.

45. Morykwas MJ, Simpson J, Punger K, et al. Vacuum-assisted closure: state of basic research and physiologic foundation. Plast Reconstr Surg 2006;117(7 suppl):121S–126S.

46. Mosti G, Iabichella ML, Picerni P, et al. The debridement of hard to heal leg ulcers by means of a new device based on Fluidjet technology. Int Wound J 2005;2:307–314.

47. Naughton G, Mansbridge J, Gentzkow GD. A metabolically active human dermal replacement for the treatment of diabetic foot ulcers. Artif Organs 1997;21:1203–1210.

48. Niezgoda JA. The economic value of negative pressure wound therapy. Ostomy Wound Manage 2005;51(2A suppl):44–47.

49. Parrett BM, Matros E, Pribaz JJ, et al. Lower extremity trauma: trends in the management of soft tissue reconstruction of open tibia-fibula fractures. Plast Reconstr Surg 2006;117:1315–1322.

50. Parrett BM, Pomahac B, Demling RH, et al. Fourth degree burns to the lower extremity with exposed tendon and bone: a ten-year experience. J Burn Care Res 2006;1:34–39.

51. Piaggesi A, Schipani E, Campi F, et al. Conservative surgical approach versus non-surgical management of diabetic neuropathic foot ulcers: a randomized trial. Diabet Med 1998;15:412–417.

52. Piaggesi A, Viacava P, Rizzo L, et al. Semiquantitative analysis of the histopathological features of the neuropathic foot ulcer: effects of pressure relief. Diabetes Care 2003;26:3123–3128.

53. Pollak RA, Edington H, Jensen JL, et al. A human dermal replacement for treatment of diabetic foot ulcers. Wounds 1997;9:175–191.

54. Reyzelman A, Crews RT, Moore JC, et al. Clinical effectiveness of an acellular dermal regenerative tissue matrix compared to standard wound management in healing diabetic foot ulcers: a prospective, randomised, multicentre study. Int Wound J 2009;6:196–208.

55. Robson MC, Hill DP, Woodske ME, et al. Wound healing trajectories as predictors of effectiveness of therapeutic agents. Arch Surg 2000;135:773–777.

56. Robson MC, Steed DL, Franz MG. Wound healing: biologic features and approaches to maximize healing trajectories. Curr Probl Surg 2001;38:72–140.

57. Saap LJ, Falanga V. Debridement performance index and its correlation with complete closure of diabetic foot ulcers. Wound Repair Regen 2002;10:354–359.

58. Sams HH, Chen J, King LE. Graftskin treatment of difficult to heal diabetic foot ulcers: one center's experience. Dermatol Surg 2002;28:698–703.

59. Schilling JA. Wound healing. Surg Clin North Am 1976;56:859–874.

60. Schultz GS, Sibbald RG, Falanga V, et al. Wound bed preparation: a systematic approach to wound management. Wound Repair Regen 2003;11(suppl 1):1–28.

61. Sheehan P, Jones P, Caselli A, et al. Percent change in wound area of diabetic foot ulcers over a 4-week period is a robust predictor of complete healing in a 12-week prospective trial. Diabetes Care 2003;26:1879–1882.

62. Silverstein G. Dermal regeneration template in the surgical management of diabetic foot ulcers: a series of five cases. J Foot Ankle Surg 2006;45:28–33.

63. Singh N, Armstrong DG, Lipsky BA. Preventing foot ulcers in patients with diabetes. JAMA 2005;293:217–228.

64. Spravchikov N, Sizyakov G, Gartsbein M, et al. Glucose effects on skin keratinocytes: implications for diabetes skin complications. Diabetes 2001;50:1627–1635.

65. Steed DL, Donohoe D, Webster MW, et al. Effect of extensive debridement and treatment on the healing of diabetic foot ulcers. J Am Coll Surg 1996;183:61–64.

66. Steinberg JS, Werber B, Kim PJ. Bioengineered alternative tissues for the surgical management of diabetic foot ulceration. In: Zgonis T, ed. Surgical reconstruction of the diabetic foot and ankle. Philadelphia: Lippincott Williams & Wilkins, 2009: 100–118.

67. van Rijswijk L. Full-thickness leg ulcers: patient demographics and predictors of healing. Multi-center leg ulcer study. J Fam Pract 1993;36:625–632.

68. Veves A, Falanga V, Armstrong DG, et al. Graftskin, a human skin equivalent, is effective in the management of noninfected neuropathic diabetic foot ulcers: a prospective randomized multicenter clinical trial. Diabetes Care 2001;24:290–295.

69. Winters CL, Brigido SA, Liden BA, et al. A multicenter study involving the use of a human acellular dermal regenerative tissue matrix for the treatment of diabetic lower extremity wounds. Adv Skin Wound Care 2008;21:375–381.

70. Yannas IV, Burke JF. Design of an artificial skin. I. Basic design principles. J Biomed Mater Res 1980;14:65–81.

71. Yannas IV, Burke JF, Gordon PL, et al. Design of an artificial skin. II. Control of chemical composition. J Biomed Mater Res 1980;14:107–131.

72. Zaulyanov L, Kirsner RS. A review of a bi-layered living cell treatment (Apligraf) in the treatment of venous leg ulcers and diabetic foot ulcers. Clin Interv Aging 2007;2:93–98.

73. Zelen CM, Snyder RJ, Serena TE, et al. The use of human amnion/chorion membrane in the clinical setting for lower extremity repair: a review. Clin Podiatr Med Surg 2015;32:135–146.

CHAPTER 10

Autogenous Split-Thickness Skin Grafting for Diabetic Foot Wounds

David C. Hatch Jr • Vlad Sauciuc • Jennifer L. Pappalardo • David G. Armstrong

INTRODUCTION

The history of skin graft use can be traced as far back as 3000 years ago with the tilemaker caste of India using gluteal skin to reconstruct nose amputations (10,30). In the more modern era of the 19th century, Reverdin is credited for his use of skin transfer for the coverage of arm wounds and leg ulcerations (31). During that same century, Wolfe (39) and Krause (15) provided accounts of the use of full-thickness skin grafts (2). Thiersch is the literary originator of the use of split-thickness skin grafts (STSGs) that, although is under continual modernizing evolution, is so widely used today (36).

The use of STSG increased in popularity after the invention of a calibrated dermatome in 1939 (26), which allowed a surgeon with an increased ability to harvest a graft of a specified depth and size. Prior to dermatome use, a surgeon relied on obtaining a graft with a freehand technique using a grafting knife. This technique subsequently yielded irregular results in graft depth and thickness (13). The dermatome has since continued to be improved and remains the cornerstone for proper and accurate harvesting of an STSG. Skin grafting is now a medical mainstay in plastic and wound reconstructive strategies.

LITERATURE REVIEW

Considering the time-honored efficacy and utility of skin grafting, there is remarkably little published on the application of STSG for the treatment of diabetic foot ulcerations (DFUs). Historically, the use of STSG for coverage of DFUs had come with little recommendation, in particular on the plantar or weight bearing surface of the foot. This may be due to impressions that patients with diabetes mellitus, neuropathy, and plantar foot wounds experience higher rates of skin graft failure. The lack of evidence-based uniformity in postoperative management, incidence of complications, as well as generalized variance in the definition of "success" when it comes to STSG and DFUs likely propagates this notion.

There is, however, current literature in which several groups have reported success in healing diabetic wounds with STSG placement. Ramanujam et al. (30), in a review of 83 diabetic patients who underwent STSG placement for closure of diabetic foot wounds, found that 65% experienced initial skin graft take within 7 weeks postoperatively and progressed to wound closure uneventfully. Although all patients had a successful surgical outcome, being complete closure of the wound, 28% required some form of additional grafting procedure. This study noted an increase in skin graft failure incidence in smokers and patient level of amputation, when amputation was a factor (30).

A systematic review of the Cochrane Database by Santema et al. (34) revealed 17 studies in which 1655 randomized participants with a DFU received either a skin graft or tissue replacement versus standard wound care. The compiled data demonstrated an increase in healing rate with decreased rate of amputation with the use of grafts (34). McCartan and Dinh (20), in an effort to clarify risks unique to the diabetic population performed a meta-analysis of available publications on STSG placement for diabetic wounds. They concluded that STSG, when utilized as a method of primary healing of a DFU, demonstrated a 78% rate of success in reaching 90% closure (20).

Additional report by Mahmoud et al. (19), describing the use of STSG for DFU versus iodine-gauze therapy, found 86% of patients who received STSG healed at 8 weeks, compared to 46% in the iodine-gauze group. Further decreased hospital length of stay and overall decreased cost of care were also noted secondary to faster healing rates in the STSG group (19). In a retrospective examination of 107 patients with non-healing diabetic foot or leg ulcer who underwent STSG placement after débridement and infection control, Anderson et al. (2) calculated that the mean time to healing among all patients was 5.1 weeks with overall complication incidence of 2.8%.

Rose et al. (32), in a review of patients who underwent STSG placement by vascular and podiatric surgeons for chronic wounds of the lower extremity and foot, reported on a total of 94 patients, 66 patients with diabetes mellitus of which 13 were dialysis-dependent; the remaining 28 had other chronic complex nondiabetic wounds. During the 12-month follow-up after STSG placement, 65 (69.1%) experienced complete skin graft incorporation and healing, and 18 (19.1%) required revision, 5 (5.3%) of whom ultimately required major limb amputation. No statistically significant difference in healing of wounds with diabetes mellitus, compared to without, as well as in comparing plantar versus nonplantar skin graft application site was noted. However, patients with end-stage renal disease requiring dialysis experienced a threefold higher rate of STSG revision (46.2% versus 14.8%). It is critical to note from this study that the cumulative rate of wound healing as a function of time was unbiased concerning end-stage renal disease (32).

ANATOMIC CONSIDERATIONS

Human skin is composed of 2 distinct layers: epidermis and dermis. Each layer contains specialized cells or structures to facilitate protection, temperature control, sensation, perfusion, and moisture balance. The epidermis is the outermost layer and is mainly stratified squamous epithelium. The bulk of epithelium is formed by keratinocytes that provide sheets of keratinized cells to produce a water-tight barrier as well as exfoliation capability. Keratinocytes further comprise five distinct microscopic layers: the strata corneum, lucidum, granulosum, spinosum, and basale from superficial to deep, respectively. These layers are divided based on histologic findings of cellular differentiation from single layer columnar keratinocytes (basale) to flat, keratinized, specialized outermost (corneum) layer. The epidermis also contains melanocytes and Langerhans cells. Melanocytes are specialized pigment producing cells that facilitate filtering ultraviolet light, whereas Langerhans cells are a type of dendritic cells responsible for phagocytization of foreign substances in the epidermis. The thickness of the epidermis varies depending on anatomic location as well as an individual's age.

Just deep to the epidermis is the dermis. The dermal layer is composed mainly of connective and fibrous tissue but also contains specialized adnexa. Fibroblasts, the most abundant cells in the dermis, produce collagen and elastin that makes up the bulk of the dermal extracellular matrix. The dermis contains the most superficial blood vessels that provide vascular and nutritional support to the avascular epidermis as well as facilitate temperature regulation. Specialized structures include hair follicles, erector pili, apocrine glands, sebaceous glands, and sweat glands. Nerves in this layer include mechanoreceptors such as Meissner's corpuscles that relay tactile sensation and light touch and Pacinian corpuscles that transmit sensations of deep pressure and vibrations. Free nerve endings in the dermis are responsible for providing information concerning itching, pain, and temperature change.

The dermis is thicker than the epidermis, and the 2 are firmly connected by a basement membrane. The basement membrane is composed of 2 lamina formed by structural stabilizing molecules including integrins, dystroglycan, laminin, and type IV collagen. These structures provide cushioning, structural stability, and durability to both layers of the skin.

TYPES OF SKIN GRAFTING

Full-Thickness Skin Graft

As first described by Wolfe (39) and Krause (15), a full-thickness skin graft (FTSG) is sufficiently deep to include the epidermis and all of the dermis (39). Benefits of the FTSG include decreased graft contraction and often a result of more "normal" appearing tissue upon incorporation (33). The depth of a FTSG is 0.8 to 1.1 mm in most cases. The harvesting of a FTSG results in a full-thickness wound, which must be then closed surgically. This limits donor site availability that must be considered during the operative process, and the appropriate tissue advancement or closure method should be evaluated.

Due to the increased thickness of FTSGs, increased perfusion is required to ensure graft viability until incorporation. For this reason, recipient sites should be well prepared. Patients with questionable vascular status or decreased evidence of perfusion must be evaluated for possible vascular intervention prior to considering the application of an FTSG.

Pinch Graft

A "pinch" graft is the method of utilizing areas of redundant tissue or tissue with greater plasticity as donor tissue. Typical donor sites for pinch grafts include just distal and anterior to the lateral malleolus and posterior auricular soft tissue. This graft is by nature equivalent to FTSG as all subcutaneous fat and soft tissue must be removed leaving only dermis and epidermis. Pinch graft donor sites must be closed primarily after harvesting, which is a consideration during the graft harvesting procedure.

Split-Thickness Skin Graft

First described by Carls Thiersch in the 1800s, the STSG has increased in popularity and utility over the last 20 years (36). The STSG includes the entire epidermis and varying portions of the dermis. STSG depth is between 0.2 and 0.7 mm, with 0.2 to 0.3 mm, 0.4 to 0.5 mm, and 0.6 to 0.7 mm being thin, intermediate, or thick STSG, respectively.

Due to the thin nature and historically challenging task of maintaining skin graft regularity, the power dermatome has proven a revolutionary instrument in affording consistent and relatively easy harvesting of skin grafts of regular depth and shape. When harvesting a STSG, the power dermatome is adjusted to a surgeon selected depth (Fig. 10.1).

The STSG has been found to contract more than the FTSG, however, much less than after the complete reepithelialization of an open wound (33). Postoperative STSG tissue often remains thin and depending on depth is frequently devoid of tissue adnexa. Furthermore, the use of a STSG often results in visually unappealing tissue coverage. In contrast to these differences, the benefits of the use of STSG include

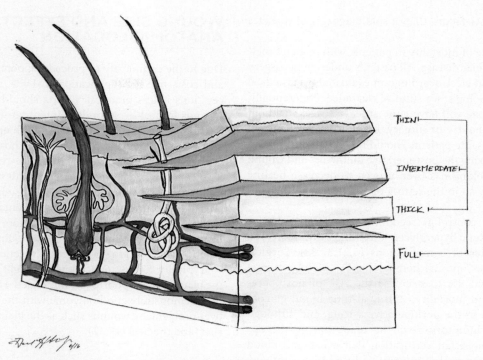

FIGURE 10.1 Split-thickness skin graft (STSG) depth is typically 0.2 to 0.3 mm, 0.4 to 0.5 mm, and 0.6 to 0.7 mm, being thin, intermediate, or thick STSG, respectively, with each layer containing the entire epidermis and varying portions of the underlying dermis.

the spontaneous healing of donor site, the availability of transferring hairless tissue, the potential to cover large soft tissue deficits with varying post-harvest graft manipulation techniques, and wider indication for application compared to other grafting modalities. All of these benefits are of critical importance during the soft tissue reconstruction of the diabetic foot.

SPLIT-THICKNESS SKIN GRAFT INDICATIONS

The use of STSG is indicated in the coverage of vascularized healthy tissue that present with evidence of persistently delayed epidermal migration or those that have completed the vertical phase of defect healing but require advanced therapy to complete horizontal healing. Although healthy recipient site perfusion must be optimized, STSGs require less vascular supply for survival due to the decreased thickness of the graft. It is for this reason that STSG can successfully be applied directly over periosteum, paratenon, as well as perichondrium. Generally, however, STSG application over these areas should be avoided due to higher incidence of graft failure.

The application of STSG is ideal over large areas of skin deficit due to easily being meshed to provide expansive coverage. This is particularly ideal where healing by secondary intention, the use of other soft tissue coverage techniques, or local tissue advancement flaps are insufficient in soft tissue coverage.

SPLIT-THICKNESS SKIN GRAFT CONTRAINDICATIONS

Although STSGs have greater likelihood of incorporation in areas of decreased blood supply compared to other grafts, the application in dysvascular areas should generally be avoided. These areas include large areas of exposed bone, tendon, and cartilage, which are insufficient in vascular supply to promote skin graft survival. In cases of small avascular coverage, a STSG may survive via blood supply from adequately vascularized nearby tissue; however, the patient should be aware of the associated risks of skin graft failure. The lack of subcutaneous tissue and thin nature of a STSG compared to normal skin predisposes it to breakdown from excess pressure. In most clinical indications, the routine application of a STSG to high-pressure areas, such as the plantar foot, comes with historically decreased recommendation.

PREOPERATIVE CONSIDERATIONS

The preoperative evaluation of a patient undergoing STSG for the treatment of DFU must include a thorough review of systems and physical examination. In a retrospective review of approximately 200 diabetic patients with foot wounds who underwent subsequent STSG placement, Ramanujam et al. (29) found that the comorbidities associated with diabetes mellitus, such as peripheral arterial disease, retinopathy, nephropathy, and cardiovascular disease, were a greater indication of STSG failure than a sole diagnosis of diabetes mellitus (29).

A leading cause of mortality in patients with diabetes mellitus is cardiovascular disease. All patients undergoing surgery must have a recent electrocardiogram evaluated by a medical physician or cardiologist for surgical clearance. Preferentially, patients who smoke will have gone at least 2 weeks without smoking before the day of surgery. In addition, in the event of a STSG, these same patients should be prepared to refrain from smoking during the postoperative follow-up, and wound care process. Smoking has been proven to decrease healing rates, increasingly so in the setting of a patient with diabetes mellitus (30).

Tight glucose control is recommended in preoperative evaluation as chronic hyperglycemia is linked with increased postoperative rates of complications (5,21,37,38). Surgical literature indicates optimal hemoglobin A_{1c} (HbA_{1c}) target between 6.5% and 9% to decrease the risk of postoperative morbidity and mortality (25). Real-time blood glucose will be evaluated in the perioperative setting, and although corrections and monitoring will be made during the operative course, physician verification that a patient's blood glucose is well managed is imperative in all phases of surgical preparation, surgical procedure, and the postoperative course.

Review of systems should reveal other areas of skin breakdown and possible additional sites of infection. To reduce the risk of introducing new infection to the carefully prepared STSG site, all patients will ideally be free of other areas of soft tissue infection at the time of the procedure.

Laboratory results may reveal additional points of optimization prior to surgery including infection control, anemia, or anticoagulation risks such as decreased liver function (1). Any evidence of systemic infection must be addressed before a patient is scheduled for a STSG procedure and should be confirmed with laboratory studies and clinical evaluation. Patients with diabetes mellitus often present with persistently decreased hemoglobin and hematocrit ratios, and simple monitoring for anemia should take place. Anemia can pose a critical complication not only during the course of the procedure but also postoperatively.

Patients on anticoagulation therapy and those with platelet dysfunction secondary to other diseases, such as liver disease or end-stage renal disease, will present an increased risk of postoperative bleeding. Physician knowledge of anticoagulation status is vital to decrease the incidence of bleeding at the donor site and decrease the risk of hematoma formation at the skin graft to recipient site interface. Bleeding risks and all anticoagulation therapies should be addressed and either altered or discontinued appropriately before surgery.

An often overlooked yet critical laboratory value for the promotion of wound healing is the patient's nutrition status. Nutrition status has been found to be directly correlated with healing of DFUs (7). If questionable, nutrition status should be addressed with a clinical dietitian and followed until the patient reaches a stable clinically acceptable level.

WOUND SIZE AND EFFECTS OF ANATOMIC LOCATION

Due to the complexity of procedure, potential complications, and costs of STSG application to DFU, its use on small ulcerations is less practical. Efforts should be made for small wounds to heal by secondary intention with appropriate offloading, wound care, and patient health optimization.

Very large diabetic foot wounds, those with surface area greater than 80 cm² are less likely to completely heal with STSG and have reduced total area of graft success, compared to moderately sized wounds (32). The greater the cross-sectional area of the wound, the more likely patients will experience difficulty healing or advance to amputation. Other confounding factors that negatively affect wound healing include ischemia, wound depth, and the presence of infection (23).

Typically, STSG application to weight bearing surfaces of the plantar foot is poorly recommended. However, recent findings demonstrate good outcome with the placement of STSG over problematic wounds such as the plantar foot, amputation sites, and the heel (17,32).

WOUND BED PREPARATION

Wound bed preparation for the STSG application on the diabetic foot wound is the longest phase of patient care, second only to patient follow-up. Because infection may prove catastrophic in the STSG process, both clinical picture and laboratory results must confirm the absence of infection before considering the application of a STSG to a DFU.

Second, areas of large soft tissue deficit should be allowed to fill completely with granular tissue. This is the "vertical" phase of wound healing (Fig. 10.2). High-quality wound care with adjunctive therapies such as negative pressure wound therapy (NPWT) in conjunction with biologic wound products may be used during this phase to facilitate the advancement of healthy granular tissue into the deficit. Ideally, this process would also decrease the area of defect requiring the application of skin graft (Fig. 10.3).

Wound bed preparation as it continues into the operating room focuses on removing all areas of superficial detritus tissue, any areas with exudative films, or small areas of tissue necrosis to result in an optimized recipient site for graft fixation. All nonviable tissue should be eliminated. Any number of medical instrumentation can facilitate this; however, the authors prefer the use of dermal curettes and hydrosurgical débridement. Hydrosurgical débridement, with the use of the VERSAJET device (Smith & Nephew, London, United Kingdom), uses a high-pressure jet of saline to utilize both Bernoulli and Venturi effects to first lift and then removes superficial tissue from a wound for faster and clean débridement. All areas of remaining visible fibrotic tissue or bone should be carefully addressed and removed because they inhibit skin graft incorporation. If undermining is present, it should be resected to present clean shallow wound margins.

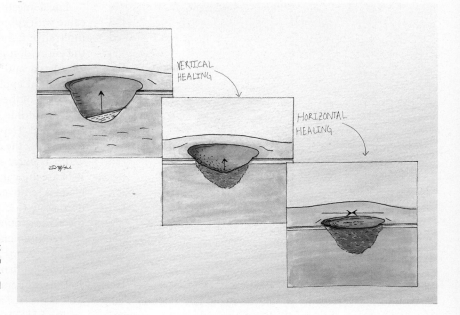

FIGURE 10.2 Wound healing consists of 2 phases: (a) vertical healing at the base of the wound with healthy granular tissue and (b) horizontal healing by epithelialization of the wound surface and gradual decreasing surface area.

The last step in wound bed preparation preferred by the authors is the subtle agitation of the recipient site with the use of sterile scrub brush. This is immediately followed by copious irrigation, often utilizing pulse lavage. The completion of these steps should reveal a healthy red granular tissue base with shallow margins, devoid of fibrous tissue or significant defect, and evidently well perfused.

DETAILED SURGICAL TECHNIQUES

Donor Sites

Theoretically, any area of skin with sufficient surface area to facilitate harvesting that is free from substantial irregularity may be a donor for STSG. The earliest donor sites included

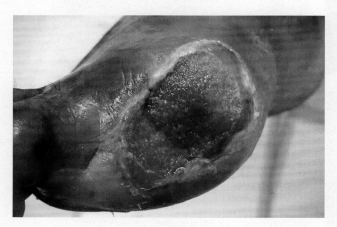

FIGURE 10.3 An example of a recipient wound bed ready for the application of a STSG. Please note the healthy-appearing and granular wound bed to an area of prior partial first ray amputation demonstrating clinical evidence of perfusion without evidence of local soft tissue infection, is of moderate size and has delayed progress in horizontal healing.

the buttocks, and an ideal location on young individuals also includes the scalp of the head. Of additional importance is the knowledge that previous STSG donor sites that have completely healed without hypertrophic scarring or keloid formation are also acceptable as repeat donor sites.

For the purpose of DFU, a STSG is commonly harvested from a location that provides intraoperative convenience and is of minimal conspicuity. The most common donor sites include the thigh, leg, and foot. The authors' preference is from the upper anterior thigh, above the shorts line. In most situations, this area has been found to provide more than adequate surface area for repetitive passes of a dermatome to supply coverage of even the largest DFU. In addition, it has been found that by concentrating on the anterior middle aspect of the thigh, discomfort from pressure or friction caused by harvesting grafts from other locations such as the posterior or inner thigh can be reduced.

The resulting wound at the donor site from harvesting a STSG progresses to healing spontaneously, frequently without significant complication. Due to the increased vascularity and increased proximity to the center of the body, this donor site is noted to heal well within a matter of weeks even in the diabetic population. The consideration of propensity toward donor site healing may significantly alter preoperative planning and postoperative course and should be discussed thoroughly with each patient.

Split-Thickness Skin Graft Harvesting and Preparation

Before the patient's extremity is prepped, the planned area of harvest should be shaved with a generous margin with operative clippers. Then, sterile prepping of physician's choice to the level of the groin is performed on the extremities that will be involved in the procedure. The appropriate draping is then performed.

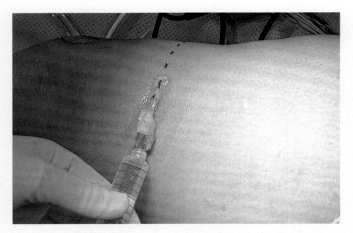

FIGURE 10.4 Local subcuticular infiltration of anesthetic to the donor site area provides anesthesia, augments hemostasis, and may increase dermatome precision.

Wound measurements should be made and documented. The donor site is then marked appropriately with a surgical marker to demonstrate the dimensions required to sufficiently cover the defect. During this step, familiarity with the any meshing or pie-crusting technique that is anticipated will facilitate appropriate adjustment to the donor site planning. This facilitates accuracy while ensuring sufficient graft harvesting and decreasing graft excess and therefore donor site wound area.

Local anesthetic, typically 1% lidocaine or 0.25% bupivacaine with epinephrine is injected just under the dermis in an infiltrative fashion sufficient to create a uniform whealing of the entire donor site tissue (Fig. 10.4). This method facilitates anesthesia and decreases donor site bleeding; however, the procedural application is for the skin wheal to augment the precision of the passing dermatome.

Dermatome settings including depth and width are then confirmed. Depth typically ranges from 0.012 to 0.018 in. In most cases, the authors prefer 0.016 depth. Interestingly, blade width is currently measured in inches in the United States. Because this can become confusing, it is recommended that the blade is removed from the dermatome, and be placed over the donor site to evaluate for appropriateness. In most instances, the blade should be minimally larger than the expected donor site requirement. Once confirmed and secured onto the dermatome, a no. 15 blade is passed between the guide and the blade to confirm uniformity and adequate fixation. Next, mineral oil is liberally applied to the marked donor site wheal as well as the face and blade of the electric dermatome (Fig. 10.5).

The STSG is then harvested with the electric dermatome by placing the activated dermatome deliberately onto the beginning of the donor site area and, while firmly applying pressure and maintaining a dermatome face with the tissue, advancing the dermatome over the entirety of the required donor site length. This should be performed in a single consistent pass maintaining the dermatome at a 45-degree angle to the skin (Fig. 10.6).

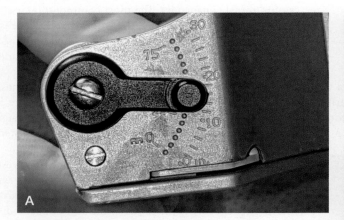

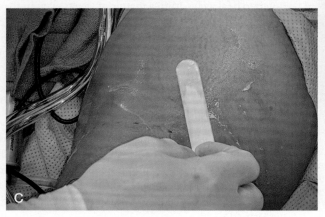

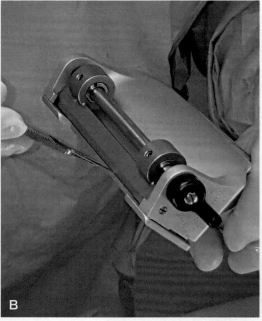

FIGURE 10.5 Appropriate dermatome settings are confirmed. Depth typically ranges from 0.012 to 0.018 in. **(A)**. A surgical blade is used to verify uniformity of depth and adequate dermatome blade and guide fixation **(B)**. Mineral oil is liberally applied to the face of the dermatome and donor site **(C)**.

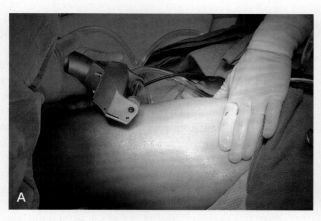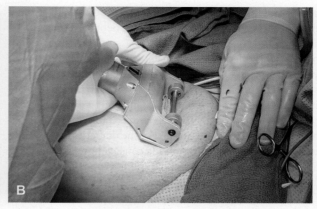

FIGURE 10.6 Apply the activated dermatome deliberately to the skin at the beginning of the donor site area **(A)**. Harvesting should be performed in a single consistent pass maintaining the dermatome at a 45-degree angle to the skin **(B)**.

When reaching the terminus of the anticipated donor site, the dermatome must be lifted off the tissue at a slight angle as opposed to an abrupt stop. An assistant is used during the harvesting process to lift the STSG from the dermatome recess as it is shaved, and therefore decrease the risk of bunching or undesired damaging of harvested tissue. The harvested STSG will then be applied to a meshing plate, if applicable, or other hard surface to facilitate pie crusting and transferred to the surgical back table. Saline should be applied to the harvested STSG to maintain expanded shape and hydration.

The donor site may then be dressed according to physician preference. Typical dressings include a 3% bismuth tribromophenate petrolatum gauze directly over the donor site that can be sutured in place to reduce motion. This dressing is then secured with a manually fenestrated transparent film dressing such as Tegaderm (3M, Hebron, KY).

The authors also prefer the application of platelet-rich plasma (PRP) directly applied to the wound site. PRP is acquired from the patient's blood preoperatively and applied intraoperatively by a specialized team. PRP and dressings typically remain intact for the duration of a week or longer based on follow-up evaluations (Fig. 10.7). A study by Miller et al. (22) evaluated postoperative donor site pain in patients under-going additional STSG and receiving PRP dressings after having been treated with traditional dressings during prior STSG procedures. This study reported reduction in perceived pain of approximately 60% with the application of PRP compared to traditional dressings on subsequent STSG donor sites (22).

Upon procedure completion in entirety, the donor site will then be dressed with additional gauze and army battle dressing (ABD) for absorption and secured in place with a layer of cast padding and light compression wrap.

Split-Thickness Skin Graft Meshing versus Pie-Crusting Technique

After delivery of the STSG to the surgical back table, the harvested STSG can then be expanded by meshing utilizing a surgical meshing system such as the Brennen mesher (Mölnlycke Health Care Ltd, Gothenburg, Sweden) or Zimmer mesher (Zimmer Biomet, Columbus, OH). A mesher processes STSGs by making small perforations, or slits into the graft, thus allowing the tissue to expand by degrees before application over the recipient site. Considerations should be made when choosing to mesh a STSG that increased healing by secondary intention will be required to fill the multitudinous perforations, and, as

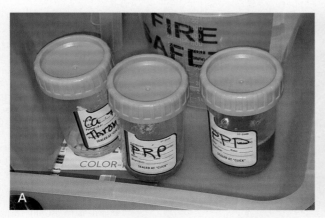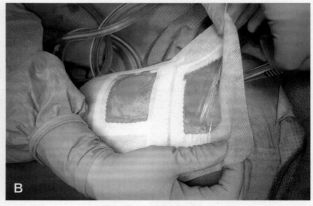

FIGURE 10.7 Platelet-rich plasma (PRP) is acquired and isolated preoperatively by the specialty team **(A)**. The PRP is applied directly over the donor site and secured by the specialist team **(B)**.

previously stated, meshed STSG can be found visually unappealing. Meshing a STSG has a significant benefit of increasing surface area for coverage provided by a single graft (6). The perforations provided by meshing allow for the escape of fluids and decrease the risk of seroma or hematoma (8,14). Meshing increases microscopic exposure to vessels within the STSG and facilitate vascular ingrowth (14). STSG meshing also increases graft plasticity allowing for increased manipulation into areas of irregular shape (8). In the context of the diabetic patient, this technique has been shown to provide consistent results and acceptable appearance when applied to DFU (28) (Fig. 10.8).

Pie crusting is the method of manually making slits into the STSG with sharp instrumentation. This can be used on grafts that do not require size augmentation and still allow drainage and increased plasticity. Healing rates have been reported as equivalent when comparing meshed skin graft versus piecrusted STSG in DFU (28).

SECURING THE SPLIT-THICKNESS SKIN GRAFT

Intraoperative securing of STSG to the recipient site is typically achieved via the use of 4-0 chromic gut suture or via the use of surgical staples. Chromic gut has the benefit of being absorbable; however, it has the increased risk of inflammatory response and possibility of serving as a nidus for infection.

The authors also often use staples that can be applied faster, create less inflammatory response, and can be easily removed

prior to the typical 2 to 3 weeks if necessary. However, in patients with intact protective sensation, an absorbable suture may be preferable.

Traditional bolster dressings of moist saline secured in place with sutures have largely fallen out of favor. An increasingly utilized dressing for securing STSG is NPWT. The use of NPWT has been shown to improve graft take with decrease in seroma and hematoma formation (4,12). NPWT can be applied with increased ease of applications in anatomically difficult areas such as the foot. NPWT can also serve to increase the amount of oxygenation at the recipient graft interface and allows for continuous removal of exudate, ultimately allowing for improved STSG quality and epithelization (24). The NPWT is applied with the use of white vacuum-assisted closure (VAC) foam (V.A.C. WhiteFoam Dressings, Kinetic Concepts, Inc., San Antonio, TX) directly in contact with the STSG. White VAC foam is a polyvinyl alcohol dressing that has been premoistened with sterile water and designed to be less adherent to facilitate use for STSG. The white foam serves as the nonadherent layer and allows for more comfortable dressing change while ensuring the graft is not disturbed from the recipient site during changes. The white foam is an immediate graft covering, which is then covered with traditional black Granufoam (V.A.C. GranuFoam, Kinetic Concepts, Inc., San Antonio, TX) and secured in place in the usual NPWT fashion. The typical postoperative settings are usually 125 mmHg or lower of continuous pressure. NPWT is left intact and undisturbed until patient follow-up between 5 and 7 postoperative days.

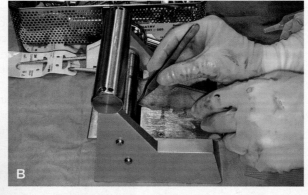

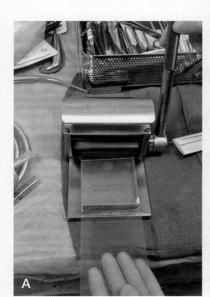

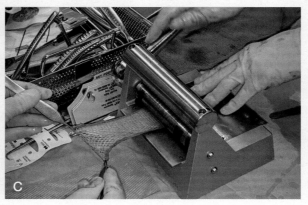

FIGURE 10.8 A Zimmer mesher is available with varying meshing options. A mesh carrier is required and must be faced with the grooves in contact with the graft when passing through the instrument **(A)**. A Brennen mesher does not allow varying meshing capacity; however, it does not utilize a carrier and therefore does not dictate graft length **(B)**. Utilizing the Brennen mesher, the graft tissue is manually fed and further secured during output of the meshing process **(C)**.

POSTOPERATIVE COURSE

STSG application is typically performed on the stable, noninfected diabetic foot wound, in an outpatient setting. Initial dressings remain in place for a period of 5 to 7 days, after which the graft is inspected in a clinical setting. If using NPWT for securing the STSG recipient site, evaluation for signs of infection or areas of maceration significant enough to alter the course of care need to be assessed in an expedited manner. If a healthy-appearing graft and periwound tissue is noted, NPWT can be reapplied for an additional 5 to 7 days. In the event of concern for graft infection or severe periwound maceration, the NPWT should be discontinued at the first postoperative visit. Further dressings should consist of a topical nonadherent dressing directly to the STSG to remain in place for approximately 10 to 14 days with topical wet to dry dressings of 0.25% sodium hypochlorite (Dakin's ½ solution) or 1% to 5% acetic acid. These dressings should follow the removal of any application of NPWT where the graft or surrounding tissue has a greater than physiologic moisture level. Residual deficit or areas of graft failure should continually be treated with high-quality wound optimization and care.

Staple removal consideration may be made when the STSG appears generally well adhered and of physiologic hydration. Wound dressings should be applied per the surgeon's preference and comfort level.

After STSG healing, the physician should promote hydration of the adhered graft and all juvenile epithelium with a topical moisturizer of choice because STSGs do not often transfer dermal appendages that provide moisture and protection to the skin. Efforts for protection of all areas of vulnerable prominences or new tissue coverage should be maximized during tissue maturation and remodeling (Figs. 10.9 and 10.10).

COMPLICATIONS

A STSG is at risk for failure from many aspects including hematoma or seroma formation, infection, shear forces, and unknown causes. Proper dressing application is the forefront modality to reduce the formation of hematoma and seroma. The appropriate dressing serves to decrease the incidence of fluid buildup and stabilize graft-to-recipient site interface. As previously discussed, the use of NPWT is an ideal postoperative dressing for these reasons.

All skin grafts are subject to bacterial infection and colonization. STSGs are particularly vulnerable to *Pseudomonas aeruginosa* colonization, with catastrophic outcomes (9,11). Acetic acid and Dakin's solution have been proven effective and inexpensive methods in the controlling and elimination of *Pseudomonas* species colonization (27,35). NPWT inhibits the invasion and proliferation of *Pseudomonas aeruginosa* in wounds, which is further indication to its use in this setting (16,18).

Shear forces disrupt the early process of wound healing and angiogenesis and alter adherence proteins. The application of a

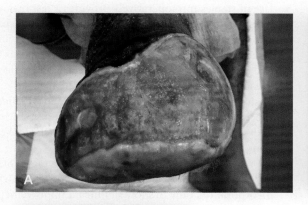
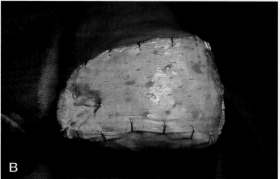
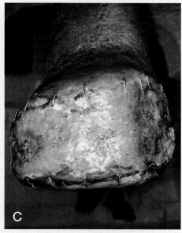

FIGURE 10.9 Clinical picture of a 49-year-old male with type 2 diabetes mellitus 4 months after a right foot transmetatarsal amputation complicated by wound dehiscence presented with a healthy-appearing wound and a lateral located circular focal area of yellow fibrotic tissue. **A.** Split-thickness skin graft (STSG) was applied, and a pie-crusting meshing technique is utilized. The STSG was secured with staples at the recipient area **(B)**. The STSG site approximately 3 weeks postoperatively demonstrating significant wound epithelialization with marginal areas of decreased graft "take." Note the decreased graft take in the area of fibrosis. Further focus of care needs to be shifted toward graft moisturization and protection with high-quality wound care to promote the further epithelialization of any remaining open wounds **(C)**.

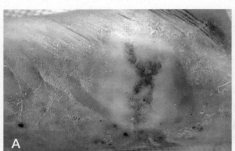
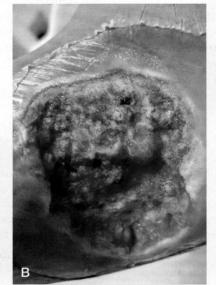
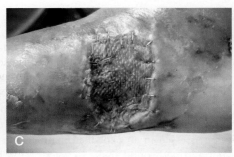
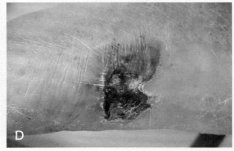

FIGURE 10.10 Clinical picture of a 67-year-old male with type 2 diabetes mellitus and end-stage renal disease presented with localized area of soft tissue swelling, erythema, increased warmth, and fluctuance without crepitus to the right plantar midfoot **(A)**. After soft tissue incision and drainage, infection control, and the application of negative pressure wound therapy, the wound progressed to healthy granular tissue with minimal areas of exposed fascial tissue **(B)**. One week after STSG application utilizing the pie-crusting technique and secured by stapling **(C)**. Approximately 4 months postoperatively, the wound demonstrates complete epithelialization with graft discoloration and superficial xerosis. The focus of care needs to be shifted toward graft moisturization and protection because it is in an area subject to high pressures **(D)**.

well-padded posterior splint is often utilized in the protection of the vulnerable STSG recipient site interface from shear forces.

Revision surgery due STSG failure should proceed with caution. Thorough investigation should identify the most likely cause of previous STSG failure. The problem should be remedied when possible, and the surgeon should have a clear plan and strategy to decrease the chance of recurrent graft failure. Revision surgery can be avoided if the majority of the graft is incorporated. Smaller areas of graft failure can be allowed to heal in by secondary intention, and application of orthobiologics can be considered to assist in wound healing.

CLINICAL TIPS AND PEARLS

- Preoperative patient optimization is crucial. A patient's vascular, renal, glycemic, and overall systemic status should be inspected and optimized to increase the chance of skin graft incorporation.
- Preoperative wound bed preparation should provide an ulceration that is clear of infection, with minimal depth and granular wound base.
- A portable NPWT machine should be ordered in advance if used as a bolster dressing, thereby preventing intraoperative or postoperative delays.
- The electric dermatome should be held at a 45-degree angle to the skin with sufficient pressure to prevent skipping and uneven STSG harvest.

- Use of staples intraoperatively provides a fast means of securing a STSG with fast and easy removal should complications arise.
- Adequate protection of the STSG recipient site is crucial, and application of a posterior splint can assist in decreasing shear forces and off-loading the affected area.
- Postoperative recipient site inspection for *Pseudomonas* species colonization can require frequent dressing changes with acetic acid or Dakin's solution to help prevent skin graft failure.
- A practitioner should be patient in achieving STSG incorporation. Often, a STSG may appear to be failing with little incorporation, only to show significant improvement at the next clinical visit.
- The highest level of wound prevention strategies should be utilized after wound epithelialization to increase the longevity of STSG after application.

Conclusion

A surgeon's thorough understanding of the indication and application of STSG is crucial. As the prevalence of diabetes mellitus continues to rise, an increased number of patients will require reconstructive procedures to cover large skin deficits and provide wound closure surgery rather than healing by secondary intention. The use of STSG allows for an effective means of treatment for DFUs and provides the possibility of large wound coverage in diabetic patients that are not amenable to or have already failed traditional wound care modalities. By reducing wound surface area, a patient may proceed to healing at a faster rate allowing patient transition into wound remission. Once in a state of remission, modalities such as graft moisturization and protective footwear should be implemented to promote graft health and decrease rate of wound recurrence (3). Ultimately, the proper preoperative optimization, intraoperative technique, and postoperative care with STSG application can allow patients with diabetes mellitus to return to their regular daily activities faster and increase their quality of life.

References

1. Abu-Rumman PL, Armstrong DG, Nixon BP. Use of clinical laboratory parameters to evaluate wound healing potential in diabetes mellitus. J Am Podiatr Med Assoc 2002;92:38–47.
2. Anderson JJ, Wallin KJ, Spencer L. Split thickness skin grafts for the treatment of non-healing foot and leg ulcers in patients with diabetes: a retrospective review. Diabet Foot Ankle 2012;3.
3. Armstrong DG, Boulton AJM, Bus SA. Diabetic foot ulcers and their recurrence. N Engl J Med 2017;376:2367–2375.
4. Blackburn JH II, Boemi L, Hall WW, et al. Negative-pressure dressings as a bolster for skin grafts. Ann Plast Surg 1998;40:453–457.
5. Capes SE, Hunt D, Malmberg K, et al. Stress hyperglycaemia and increased risk of death after myocardial infarction in patients with and without diabetes: a systematic overview. Lancet 2000;355:773–778.
6. Davison PM, Batchelor AG, Lewis-Smith PA. The properties and uses of non-expanded machine-meshed skin grafts. Br J Plast Surg 1986;39:462–468.
7. Demling RH, DeSanti L. The stress response to injury and infection: role of nutritional support. Wounds 2000;12:3–14.
8. Glogau RG, Stegman SJ, Tromovitch TA. Refinements in split-thickness skin grafting technique. J Dermatol Surg Oncol 1987;13:853–858.
9. Griffiths RW. Bacterial colonisation of leg ulcers and its effect on the success rate of skin grafting. Plast Reconstr Surg 1989;84:383.
10. Hauben DJ, Baruchin A, Mahler A. On the history of the free skin graft. Ann Plast Surg 1982;9:242–245.
11. Høgsberg T, Bjarnsholt T, Thomsen JS, et al. Success rate of split-thickness skin grafting of chronic venous leg ulcers depends on the presence of pseudomonas aeruginosa: a retrospective study. PLoS One 2011;6:e20492.
12. Isaac AL, Rose J, Armstrong DG. Mechanically powered negative pressure wound therapy as a bolster for skin grafting. Plast Reconstr Surg Glob Open 2014;2:e103.
13. Ketchum LD. An historical account of the development of the calibrated dermatome. Ann Plast Surg 1978;1:608–611.
14. Knight SL, Moorghen M. Configurational changes within the dermis of meshed split skin grafts: a histological study. Br J Plast Surg 1987;40:420–422.
15. Krause F. Ueber die Transplantation grosser ungestielter Hautlappen. Verh Dtsch Ges Chir 1893;22:46–51.
16. Lalliss SJ, Stinner DJ, Waterman SM, et al. Negative pressure wound therapy reduces pseudomonas wound contamination more than Staphylococcus aureus. J Orthop Trauma 2010;24:598–602.
17. Lew EJ, Sauciuc V, Armstrong DG. Pearls and pitfalls of split thickness skin grafting the diabetic foot ulceration. J Wound Technol 2014;26:16–21.
18. Liu Y, Zhou Q, Wang Y, et al. Negative pressure wound therapy decreases mortality in a murine model of burn-wound sepsis involving Pseudomonas aeruginosa infection. PLoS One 2014;9:e90494.
19. Mahmoud SM, Mohamed AA, Mahdi SE, et al. Split-skin graft in the management of diabetic foot ulcers. J Wound Care 2008;17:303–306.
20. McCartan B, Dinh T. The use of split-thickness skin grafts on diabetic foot ulcerations: a literature review. Plast Surg Int 2012;2012:715273.
21. Mesotten D, Van den Berghe G. Clinical potential of insulin therapy in critically ill patients. Drugs 2003;63:625–636.
22. Miller JD, Rankin TM, Hua NT, et al. Reduction of pain via platelet-rich plasma in split-thickness skin graft donor sites: a series of matched pairs. Diabet Foot Ankle 2015;6:24972.
23. Mills JL Sr, Conte MS, Armstrong DG, et al. The Society for Vascular Surgery Lower Extremity Threatened Limb Classification System: risk stratification based on wound, ischemia, and foot infection (WIfI). J Vasc Surg 2014;59:220–234.
24. Moisidis E, Heath T, Boorer C, et al. A prospective, blinded, randomized, controlled clinical trial of topical negative pressure use in skin grafting. Plast Reconstr Surg 2004;114:917–922.
25. Nicholas J, Charlton J, Dregan A, et al. Recent HbA1c values and mortality risk in type 2 diabetes. Population-based case-control study. PLoS One 2013;8:e68008.
26. Padgett EC. Skin grafting in severe burns. Am J Surg 1939;43:626–636.
27. Phillips I, Lobo AZ, Fernandes R, et al. Acetic acid in the treatment of superficial wounds infected by Pseudomonas aeruginosa. Lancet 1968;1:11–14.
28. Puttirutvong P. Meshed skin graft versus split thickness skin graft in diabetic ulcer coverage. J Med Assoc Thai 2004;87:66–72.
29. Ramanujam CL, Han D, Fowler S, et al. Impact of diabetes and comorbidities on split-thickness skin grafts for foot wounds. J Am Podiatr Med Assoc 2013;103:223–232.
30. Ramanujam CL, Stapleton JJ, Kilpadi KL, et al. Split-thickness skin grafts for closure of diabetic foot and ankle wounds: a retrospective review of 83 patients. Foot Ankle Spec 2010;3:231–240.
31. Reverdin JL, Ivy RH. The classic reprint greffe epidermique—experience faite dans le service de m. le docteur guyon, a l'hôpital necker. Plast Reconstr Surg 1968;41:79–81.
32. Rose JF, Giovinco N, Mills JL, et al. Split-thickness skin grafting the high-risk diabetic foot. J Vasc Surg 2014;59:1657–1663.
33. Rudolph R. Inhibition of myofibroblasts by skin grafts. Plast Reconstr Surg 1979;63:473–480.
34. Santema TB, Poyck PP, Ubbink DT. Skin grafting and tissue replacement for treating foot ulcers in people with diabetes. Cochrane Database Syst Rev 2016;(2):CD011255.
35. Sloss JM, Cumberland N, Milner SM. Acetic acid used for the elimination of Pseudomonas aeruginosa from burn and soft tissue wounds. J R Army Med Corps 1993;139:49–51.
36. Urban G. Ueber die Hautverpflanzung nach Thiersch. Dtsch Z Chir 1892;34:187–237.
37. van den Berghe G, Wouters P, Weekers P, et al. Intensive insulin therapy in critically ill patients. N Engl J Med 2001;345:1359–1367.
38. Wass CT, Lanier WL. Glucose modulation of ischemic brain injury: review and clinical recommendations. Mayo Clin Proc 1996;71:801–812.
39. Wolfe JR. On a new method of performing plastic operations. Br Med J 1881;1:426–427.

CHAPTER 11

Lower Extremity and Foot Angiosome Considerations for Vascular and Plastic Surgical Reconstruction of the Diabetic Foot

Alexandru V. Georgescu • Ileana R. Matei • Michel Saint-Cyr • Manuel Llusá-Pérez

INTRODUCTION

Soft tissue reconstruction of lower extremity defects is challenging, especially in the diabetic foot, while surgeons around the world are still developing advanced surgical techniques for closure of the most difficult diabetic lower extremity wounds (19,20,36,44). The plastic reconstructive surgical techniques need to be based on very reliable and reproducible vascular studies (38) in order to achieve a successful functional and durable outcome based on the soft tissue defect's needs and patient's soft tissue resources.

The anatomic and functional characteristics of the lower extremity and foot make these areas of the human body some of the most vulnerable areas from a vascular point of view in the diabetic population. Surgical experience and vast knowledge of the blood supply in these areas play an essential role in planning and performing the plastic reconstruction and soft tissue coverage of the diabetic foot.

GROSS VASCULAR ANATOMY OF THE LOWER EXTREMITY AND FOOT

The main arteries of the lower extremity and foot are the anterior tibial artery (ATA), posterior tibial artery (PTA), and peroneal artery (PA), as they originate from the popliteal artery (Fig. 11.1). After passing through the adductor hiatus, the femoral artery becomes the popliteal artery. The popliteal artery is located in the region of the popliteal fossa, deep and medial to the popliteal vein. This artery sends off a series of collateral branches that form the articular arterial network of the knee anteriorly. There are 2 superior branches, 2 inferior branches, and a middle branch, in addition to the sural artery. There are 2 sural arteries, one on each side, which are distributed on the triceps surae. The popliteal artery passes under the

tendinous arch of the soleus and bifurcates into the ATA and the tibioperoneal trunk (Fig.11.1). The tibioperoneal trunk in turn bifurcates into the PTA and PA arteries. These 3 arteries distribute in the leg compartments: the PTA and PA in the posterior compartment and the ATA in the anterior compartment (Fig. 11.2). Any of these arteries could present with anatomic variations, with the PA being the most frequent. The PA could have an origin from the PTA in 90% of the cases and can also arise from the ATA or directly from the popliteal artery in 1% of the cases. In some clinical case scenarios, the PTA does not exist and the only arterial trunk is the peroneal vessel named as *peronea arteria magna* (peroneal magnus artery).

Anterior Tibial Artery

The ATA originates at the level of the popliteal muscle in the posterior region of the knee, passes below it, and crosses the interosseous membrane to enter the anterior compartment of the leg. From the ATA arises the anterior recurrent tibial artery, which ascends to anastomose with the arterial articular network of the knee. The ATA descends in the anterior compartment between the anterior tibial and the extensor digitorum longus muscles. Distally, it is located medially between the anterior tibial and the extensor hallucis longus muscles. At the level of the malleoli, it sends off 2 branches, 1 for each malleolus, which are named the anterior medial and lateral malleolar arteries and form part of the medial and lateral malleolar networks, respectively.

After passing under the extensor retinaculum of the foot, the ATA is called the dorsal artery of the foot (dorsalis pedis artery). It is located between the tendons of the extensor digitorum longus and extensor hallucis longus, where its pulse can be felt (22,43). There are different anatomic variations of the dorsalis pedis artery at this level; in 3% of cases, the dorsalis pedis artery presents as a continuation of the PA, and in 2% of cases, it could arise from the ATA, but that is in the position of

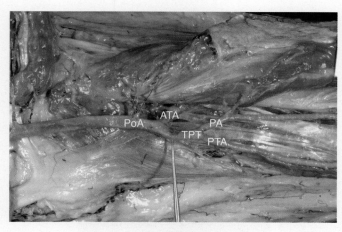

FIGURE 11.1 Anatomic specimen view of the popliteal artery and its division to the tibioperoneal trunk and anterior tibial artery at the posterior compartment of the upper leg. *ATA*, anterior tibial artery; *PA*, peroneal artery; *PoA*, popliteal artery; *PTA*, posterior tibial artery; *TPT*, tibioperoneal trunk.

the perforating terminal branch of the PA (at the tibiofibular joint level). In 10% of cases, the dorsalis pedis artery could be absent or have a very small diameter (15,25).

The dorsalis pedis artery gives off the medial tarsal artery, distributed over the medial border of the foot, and the lateral tarsal artery, which courses from the talar region toward the lateral border of the foot under the lesser toe extensor muscles. The medial and lateral tarsal arteries communicate with each other through the arcuate artery, forming a dorsal arterial arch. From this arch originate the dorsal metatarsal arteries (Fig. 11.3), which are located in the interosseous spaces between the toes. At the level of the metatarsophalangeal joints, these arteries each bifurcate into 2 dorsal digital arteries that course toward both sides of the toes in each interosseous space. The lateral border of the fifth toe is vascularized by an artery that originates in the same arcuate artery, whereas the medial border of the great toe is vascularized by plantar arteries (1,30,43). The deep plantar artery (Fig. 11.4) is

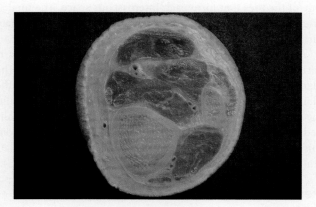

FIGURE 11.2 Anatomic specimen view of a transverse section in the distal leg showing the 3 different compartments, that is, anterior, lateral, and posterior. Inside the anterior compartment, there are the anterior tibial artery and veins, whereas inside the deep posterior compartment, there are the posterior tibial and peroneal arteries and veins.

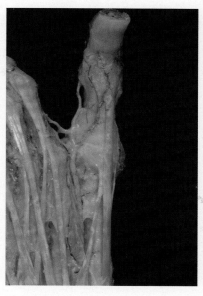

FIGURE 11.3 Anatomic specimen dorsal view of the forefoot, hallux, and toes. Arterial system injected with black latex. The first dorsal metatarsal artery courses in different ways in relation to the interosseous muscle, but it is more constant at the level of the metatarsal heads, localized superficially to the transverse ligament. After that point, it divides into 2 dorsal digital arteries that run on the sides of the hallux and second toe.

a perforating artery that connects the dorsal metatarsal arteries with the deep plantar arch through the first interosseous space.

The first dorsal metatarsal artery courses in different ways in relation to the interosseous muscle (anatomic variations in a superficial or deep type depending on their relationship to the first interosseous muscle or even could be absent), but it is more constant at the level of the metatarsal heads, localized superficially to the transverse ligament. After that point, it divides into 2 dorsal digital arteries that run on the sides of the hallux and second toe. The first dorsal metatarsal artery and the deep plantar artery (communicating branch of the dorsalis pedis artery to the first plantar metatarsal artery) have a proximal level communication and also a distal communication localized superficially to the transverse ligament, just after it divides into 2 dorsal digital arteries that run on the sides of the hallux and second toe; this latter branch communicates with the plantar digital arteries (1,43) (Fig.11.4).

Posterior Tibial Artery

The PTA is distributed in the posterior compartment of the leg, between the superficial and deep groups. Shortly after its origin, the nutrient artery of the tibia branches off. Along its course, the PTA becomes more medial as it travels toward the tarsal tunnel. At the level of the medial malleolus, the medial malleolar branches help form the medial malleolar network.

The tarsal tunnel is formed by the distal tibial epiphysis, the talus, and the calcaneus, which are joined by the medial collateral ligament. This tunnel is covered by the flexor retinaculum. The tendinous floor of this region is formed by the tendons of the flexor digitorum longus and the posterior tibial

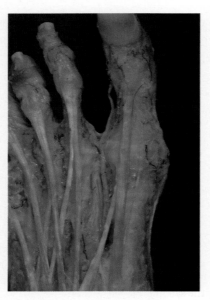

FIGURE 11.4 Anatomic specimen dorsal view of the forefoot, hallux, and toes. Arterial system injected with black latex. Observe the first dorsal metatarsal artery and the deep plantar artery (communicating branch of the dorsalis pedis artery to the first plantar metatarsal artery) at a proximal level and a distal communication localized superficially to the transverse ligament, just after it divides into 2 dorsal digital arteries that run on the sides of the hallux and second toe; this latter branch communicates with the plantar digital arteries.

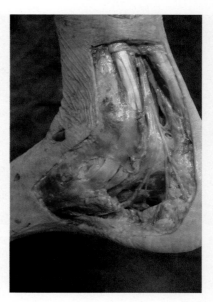

FIGURE 11.6 Anatomic specimen view of dividing the deep fascia and flexor retinaculum (separated with *blue stitches*), the posterior tibial artery and veins are identified between the flexor digitorum longus and flexor hallucis longus tendons. Under the origin of the abductor hallucis muscle (resected for demonstration), the main posterior tibial artery divides into medial and lateral plantar arteries. The posterior tibial nerve is located posterior and medial to the vessels.

muscle with their tendon sheaths. The neurovascular contents are the PTA, posterior tibial vein, and posterior tibial nerve that distribute in the sole of the foot (Fig. 11.5). In the tarsal tunnel, the PTA bifurcates into the medial and lateral plantar arteries (Fig. 11.6). The medial plantar artery bifurcates into a deep branch that course between the abductor hallucis and the flexor hallucis brevis muscles of the great toe toward the first interosseous space, whereas the superficial branch follows the medial border of the foot to the great toe. The lateral

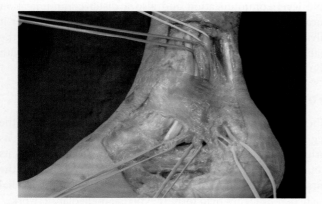

FIGURE 11.5 Anatomic specimen view of the tibial neurovascular bundle at the ankle level. *Orange slings* mark the posterior tibial artery under the flexor retinaculum and its division in the medial and lateral artery coursing deep to the abductor hallucis muscle. *Lime-green slings* mark the posterior tibial nerve and, at the right corner, the cutaneous calcaneal branch.

plantar artery courses obliquely in the plane between the flexor digitorum brevis muscles of the toes and the quadratus plantaris muscle toward the lateral region of the foot (21,59). Both arteries anastomose with each other at the midlevel of the metatarsals, forming the deep plantar arch. From this arch originate the plantar metatarsal arteries, which course in the interosseous spaces of the foot and are continued by the common plantar digital arteries. In addition, a pair of perforating branches course toward the dorsum of the foot (1,30,43). Near the metatarsophalangeal joints, the common digital arteries bifurcate into the proper digital arteries, which extend on each side of the toes that form each interosseous space. The medial artery of the great toe and the lateral of the fifth toe originate directly from the deep plantar arch.

A superficial anastomosis between the plantar arteries is variably present and is called the superficial plantar arch. The plantar arterial system is formed from the union between the plantar arch (continuation of the lateral plantar artery) and the deep plantar artery (communicating branch of the dorsalis pedis artery). The first plantar metatarsal artery comes from this system and divides on plantar digital arteries for the lateral part of the hallux and medial part of the second toe (25).

Peroneal Artery

The PA is located behind the fibula and courses distally toward the calcaneus. At the level of the fibular diaphysis, the nutrient artery of the fibula branches from the PA. Distally, a communicating branch from the PA connects with the PTA. Immediately distal to this branch, the PA produces the perforating branch, crosses the interosseous membrane, and distributes over the lateral malleolus and the dorsum of the foot. Near the lateral malleolus, it sends off the lateral malleolar branches, which anastomose with those of the ATA. Finally, the calcaneal branches help form the calcaneal network in the posterior aspect of this bone.

SKIN VASCULARIZATION OF THE LOWER EXTREMITY AND FOOT

Currently, it is well known that the vascular supply of the skin is provided by perforator vessels with a specific pattern for each region of the human body (55). A vast knowledge of the particular vascular supply in different regions, that is, in the lower extremity and foot, not only will help the planning and performing of the diabetic foot reconstruction but also will offer to the reconstructive surgeon a potential alternative option in cases of revisional surgery.

The skin vascularization studies started early on with the first known one being the Manchot's (32) anatomic description of vascularization, forgotten and later reappraised in Salmon's (48) work, and finally reacknowledged in 1983 (33). During World War I, many surgeons such as Esser (14) and Davis (13) described and utilized flaps to reconstruct war-related wounds. Esser (14) and then Milton (37) demonstrated that flaps are completely dependent on a viable vascular source to survive. In 1971, Antia and Buch (3) proved the importance of the vascular pedicle by transferring a free revascularized dermal-fat flap prior to the development of the microscope.

In 1975, Behan and Wilson (5) described the "angiotome" 2-dimensional concept as "the area of skin that can be cut as a flap which is supplied by an axial vessel but may be extended by its communication with branches of an adjacent vessel" (5,39). Cormack and Lamberty (12) excellently described the anatomy of the skin vascularization throughout the body and presented the flap design in relation with this vascularization. These authors also introduced an innovative description of the possible types of vascular territories of the body, using the terms "anatomical, dynamic, and potential," which could be used as a single source vessel to base a skin flap (11).

Angiosome Concept

In 1987, Taylor and Palmer (55) described more than 300 perforators over the entire human body and defined the 3-dimensional concept of "angiosome," which should be considered as a composite block of tissues supplied by a single vessel. This unit contains skin and the underlying connective tissue, muscle, nerve, and bone. Their conclusions were fundamental in achieving a better understanding of tissue vascularization. They found that the vessels accompany the connective tissue structure over the entire body and are traveling from the fixed toward the mobile areas by creating a continuous vascular network. The territories can be linked usually through choke anastomoses and sometimes by true anastomoses. Taylor and Palmer described 40 angiosomes but accepted that those could

be divided into smaller territories that they later described (53,55). The 3-dimensional concept was demonstrated by using not only their experiments but also their clinical experience in harvesting flaps composed of skin and the subjacent tissues. Their special injection radiography techniques showed that there are 2 anastomotic networks, 1 between cutaneous arteries (subdermal or dermal) and another uniting the cutaneous arteries with the profound ones. The skin territories do not have exactly the same delineation in different populations, but statistically, they could describe some reliably sound margins, noting also the hypo- and hypervascularized areas. Regarding the lower extremity and foot, they described the following territories:

- For the *leg*, the skin vascularization was divided between the ATA, PTA, PA, some branches from the gastrocnemius muscle arteries, 2 small areas supplied by the saphenous artery (satellite artery of the short saphenous vein), and, respectively, by the satellite artery of the great saphenous vein.
- The territories of the ATA, PTA, and PA continue distally in the *ankle* and foot instep region.
- The *dorsum of the foot* is supplied mainly by the dorsalis pedis artery, with the exception of a small region on the lateral foot aspect, which is vascularized by the PA.
- For the *plantar aspect of the foot*, the authors described 2 main territories, supplied by the medial and lateral plantar arteries, complemented by small regions vascularized by the PTA and the dorsalis pedis artery.

Some studies realized on the delay flap procedures and showed the dilation of the choke anastomoses by creating true anastomoses between adjacent angiosomes (9,39). The importance of the angiosome concept is reflecting not only in defining the amount of tissue that can belong to a flap but also in well planning the area to be surgically débrided in a vascularly compromised foot. In cases of ulcerations secondary to an arterial obstruction, all of the angiosomes dependent to the occluded artery should be excised in order to avoid complications and obtain a satisfactory result (Fig. 11.7).

Perforasome Concept

Based on the angiosome concept, it was possible to describe and perform the first perforator flap by Koshima and Soeda (28) in 1989, which opened the era of perforator flaps. Twenty years later, after an increasing use of perforator flaps, it appeared the necessity of a better assessment of the vascular structure of these flaps. Saint-Cyr et al. focused their studies not only on the source vessel but also on the perforator itself (46,47,49). The authors injected the largest perforator artery of specific flaps with contrast substance and scanned through 32 or 64 slices of computed tomography angiography, as they were able to identify the amount of tissues that were vascularly dependent to this perforator. They defined such a territory blood supplied by a single perforator as "perforasome" (47) (Fig. 11.8). According with other authors, the territory vascularized by a single perforator is named "perforator angiosome" (45) or "cutaneous angiosome" (54).

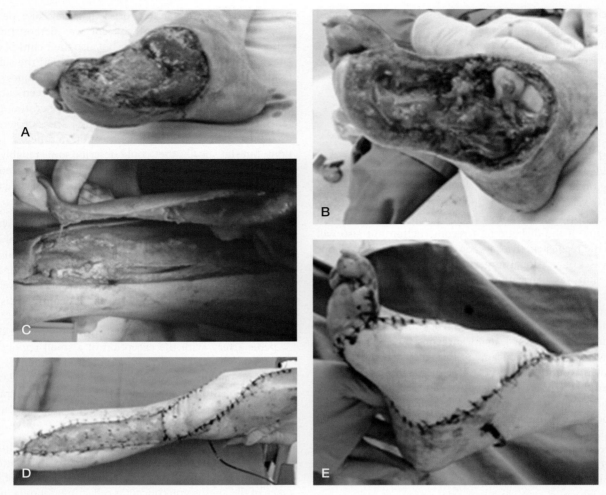

FIGURE 11.7 Preoperative clinical picture of an open nonhealing diabetic foot wound after a partial foot amputation **(A)** followed by adequate surgical débridement based on the angiosome concept **(B)**. Note the harvesting of a propeller perforator flap based on a peroneal perforator **(C)**, application of a split-thickness skin graft at the donor site **(D)**, and postoperative outcomes **(D,E)**.

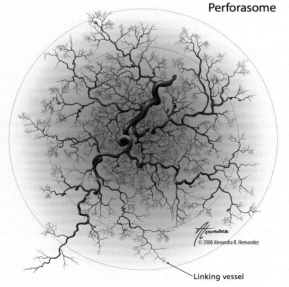

Perforasome

FIGURE 11.8 Schematic representation of a perforasome. (© Alexandra B. Hernandez of Gory Details Illustration.)

Four main principles derive from the perforasome concept:

1. Linking vessels connect the neighboring perforasomes. There are 2 different types of linking vessels (Fig. 11.9):
   - Direct, which are *macroscopic vessels* realizing a direct bridge between 2 branches of adjacent perforators (Fig. 11.10)
   - Indirect, which are equivalent to the choke vessels described by Taylor et al. (54,55) and constitute for the *microscopic subdermal network* (Fig. 11.10)
2. Due to the axial orientation of the linking vessels in the lower leg, the design of flaps in this region should be also axial.
3. The perforasome dependent to a specific perforator is filled before the neighboring perforasomes dependent to adjacent source arteries.
4. If a perforator is located close to a joint or under nonmobile skin, the blood flow through linking vessels is going in distal direction; if the perforator is located relatively centrally between 2 joints, the blood flow is multidirectional.

PERFUSION IN MULTIPLE PERFORASOMES VIA LINKING VESSELS

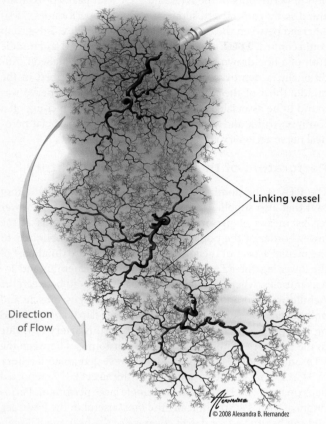

FIGURE 11.9 Schematic representation of the linking vessels between neighboring perforasomes. (© Alexandra B. Hernandez of Gory Details Illustration.)

Respecting these principles and ensuring as many as possible linking vessels in a flap will enhance the flap blood supply and its viability.

PERFORATOR FLAPS BASED ON THE ANGIOSOME AND PERFORASOME CONCEPTS FOR DIABETIC LOWER EXTREMITY AND FOOT RECONSTRUCTION

Perforator flaps in the lower extremity and foot, used as local or regional flaps, enable reconstruction of a variety of defects

with the advantage of minimal donor site morbidity and avoidance of microvascular anastomosis (49), which generates their nomination as *microsurgical non-microvascular flaps* (16–18,35,56).

Perforators of the Anterior Tibial Artery

As previously mentioned, the ATA arises from the popliteal artery and travels in the anterior compartment of the lower leg. Proximally, it travels between the tibia and tibialis anterior muscles; while as it migrates more laterally and distally, it travels between the tendons of the extensor hallucis longus and extensor digitorum longus. During this course, perforators branch off and travel along the intramuscular septa in a linear direction supplying the fascia and overlying skin (41). In an anatomic and clinical study about perforators of the lower leg, Schaverien and Saint-Cyr (49) found that perforators emerged from the crural fascia in 4 longitudinal rows within the intermuscular septa. Perforators of the ATA were the most numerous perforators compared to the other main arteries which were in accordance with other authors (7,34). Schaverien and Saint-Cyr (49) found a mean number of 9.9 ± 4.4 perforators per leg. Other authors reported mean numbers of 6 to 14 (57), 6 to 10 (10), 6.2 (40), 19 ± 2 (34), 6.6 ± 2.4 (41), and 6.3 (7) perforators per leg. However, these perforators were found to have the smallest diameter compared to the other main arteries but showed an increase of diameter from distal to proximal (49). The diameter of perforators varied between 0.5 and 1.0 mm (49), 0.3 and 0.8 mm (10), 0.81 mm (40), 0.52 and 2.49 mm (34), and 0.75 mm (7). In general, perforators of the lower leg were found to accumulate within 3 distinct intervals of 5-cm length. The distribution of reliable perforators emerging from the ATA was found within 2 5-cm intervals (Fig. 11.11) (49). The proximal accumulation could be found within 21 and 26 cm distance from the bimalleolar line. The distal accumulation was found between 4- and 9-cm distance of this line (49). Even if the distal perforators are small enough (49), they can be able to ensure the blood supply of a flap to cover small to medium defects in the distal lower leg and malleolar regions (16,18).

In the septum between the tibia and anterior tibial muscle, 93% of studied legs had at least 1 perforator and in this septum can generally be found 23% of all the perforators emerging from the ATA (Fig. 11.12) (49). Perforators within this septum had a mean distance to the artery of 3.7 ± 1.3 cm. In the septum between the extensor digitorum longus and peroneus longus, 80% of specimens carried at least 1 perforator and in

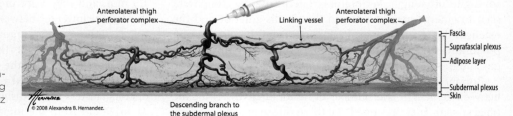

FIGURE 11.10 Schematic representation of direct and indirect linking vessels. (© Alexandra B. Hernandez of Gory Details Illustration.)

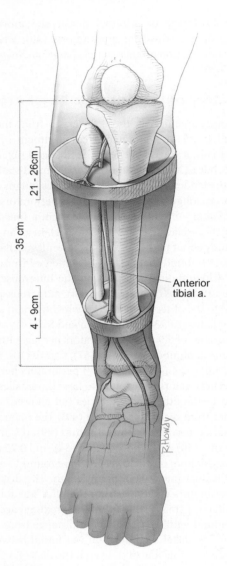

FIGURE 11.11 Localization of reliable perforators from the anterior tibial artery (49).

this septum can be found 22% of all the perforators from the ATA (Fig. 11.12), whereas the mean distance to the artery is 2.6 ± 1.5 cm (49).

Martin et al. (34) detected a cluster with 3 accumulations of perforators at 28%, 59%, and 83% of the leg length, which was defined as the length of the tibia measured from the lateral malleolus to the plateau of the tibia. The majority of perforators from the proximal group emerged between the tibialis anterior and the tibia, and the tibialis anterior and the extensor digitorum longus. Perforators from the middle group were seen to emerge mainly between the tibialis anterior and the extensor digitorum longus. Perforators from the distal group predominantly emerged between the extensor digitorum longus and the peroneus longus (34).

Boriani et al. (7) showed that there exists a correlation between leg length and number of perforating vessels for the tibial system. They presumed that this is due to neoangiogenesis

during growth at the level of metaphyseal plates. The distribution of perforators of the ATA and PTA with peaks proximally and distally, respectively, supports this. Most perforators (75%) emerged between the extensor and fibular muscles. This group could confirm a peak of perforators in the upper 3rd and middle 10th of a line drawn between the knee joint and malleoli. Additionally, a neurovascular pattern has been described in the middle third of the tibia. The superficial peroneal nerve was found to be associated with 2 or 3 perforators, branching off a common trunk and supplying the nerve, the superficial peroneal nerve accessory artery (7).

Perforators of the Posterior Tibial Artery

The PTA is the dominant source of blood supply to the foot (49) that also supplies the posteromedial surface of the lower leg by means of perforating branches (31). It begins at the lower border of the popliteal muscle and courses obliquely to the medial aspect of the lower leg (52). In the proximal part of the lower leg, the PTA is covered by the gastrocnemius and soleus muscles, whereas in the distal part, it is found between the Achilles tendon and the flexor digitorum longus muscle and only covered by skin and fascia (31). A large flap territory based on a single perforator can be raised from this artery (23) due to the existence of numerous arterial anastomoses between the PTA and the PA (31). Tang et al. (52) revealed a flap territory of 34 ± 12 cm² per perforator and Koshima et al. (27) reported flaps up to 19 × 13 cm based on a single large perforator. Perforators of the PTA are clinically the most useful in the lower leg and can be utilized for defect coverage of the heel, medial malleolus, Achilles tendon, and distal two-thirds of the tibia (49).

Whetzel et al. (57) defined 2 septa in which perforators of the PTA typically course: septum 6 (which is between the tibia and the flexor digitorum longus muscle) and septum 5 (which is between the flexor digitorum longus and the soleus muscles). The majority of perforators from the posterior tibial system are usually septocutaneous perforators (7), which emerge in the septum between the flexor digitorum longus and soleus muscles (septum 5) in 64%. Septocutaneous perforators emerging between the flexor digitorum longus muscle and tibia (septum 6) have been found in 12%, and musculocutaneous perforators proceeding through the soleus muscle have been detected in 24% (7). The average number of perforating vessels per leg varies between 2.3 (51) and 8.4 (34) on which most authors describe numbers around 4 (7,10, 49). In a clinical and cadaveric study, Schaverien and Saint-Cyr (49) found that perforators of the PTA were constantly the largest in the lower leg. They were accompanied by venae comitantes, which is in accordance with other authors (2,10,31,57). Their caliber varied between 1 and 1.5 mm, and they were predominantly found in the middle third of the lower leg between the flexor digitorum longus and soleus. Other authors reported calibers that ranged between 0.82 (7) and 1.5 mm (10). The largest vessels were found in the proximal two-thirds of the tibia. At this location, the majority of perforators followed a septocutaneous course (49). Three distinct clusters with a distance of 4 to 9 cm, 13 to 18 cm, and 21 to 26 cm from the intermalleolar line could be detected,

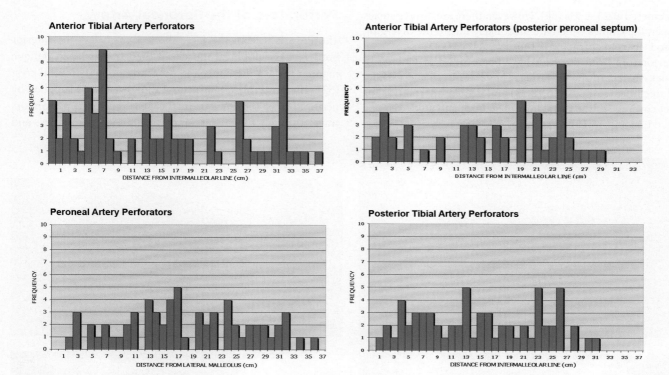

FIGURE 11.12 Graphic representations of the distribution of perforators in the lower leg (49): perforators from the anterior tibial artery in the septum between the tibia and tibialis anterior muscle *(above left)*, perforators from the anterior tibial artery in the septum between the extensor digitorum longus and peroneus longus muscles *(above right)*, perforators from the peroneal artery *(below left)*, and perforators from the posterior tibial artery *(below right)*.

which contained 23% of perforators, respectively (Fig. 11.13). The mean number of perforators per leg was 4.9 ± 1.7 with a distance of 3.2 ± 1.8 from the source artery (49).

As shown with the ATA, a correlation between leg length and number of perforating vessels has been detected for the PTA as well. The clinical implication of this phenomenon is that with increasing limb length and thus increasing number of perforators, the safety of a single-based perforator flap decreases (7). In an anatomic study, Boriani et al. (7) investigated the distribution of perforators of 22 lower extremities with a standardization based on limb length. Regarding the distribution of perforating vessels along the posterior tibial axis, 2 peaks of density were detected (Fig. 11.12) (49). The first peak was found between the beginning of the fourth tenth and the ending of the sixth tenth. The second one was found in the eighth tenth, especially in the supramalleolar area (7). These findings are consistent with Liu et al. (31) who described a peak of perforating vessels in the distal part of the lower leg. Whetzel et al. (57) demonstrated that 95.5% of the perforators emerging from the septum between the flexor digitorum longus and soleus were found in the distal six-tenths of the tibia. In this septum, the majority of perforators have been detected, which is in accordance with other authors (7). In a computed tomography angiography study about the localization of cutaneous perforators of the lower leg, Martin et al. (34) found 2 distinct clusters for the PTA. The proximal group was found at 56 ± 12% of the leg measured from the lateral malleolus, and the distal group

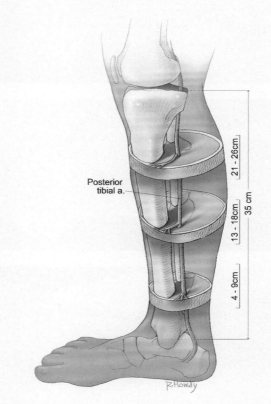

FIGURE 11.13 Localization of reliable perforators from the posterior tibial artery (49).

was centered at 23 ± 7% (34). However, there are discrepancies between the studies which are most likely due to the diverging methods used to characterize those vessels (34).

Perforators from the PTA have been found to emerge in distinct clusters in the lower leg. They have been successfully used in clinical settings (16,18,29) and display alternatives for defect coverage of the distal lower leg, heel, and ankle regions (Figs. 11.14 and 11.15).

Perforators of the Peroneal Artery

The PA arises from the PTA about 3 cm below the inferior border of the popliteal muscle. It then travels in an oblique manner toward the fibula and descends along its medial crest (52). The posterolateral aspect of the lower leg is supplied by perforators of the PA (7). In the proximal part, perforators travel through the soleus or peroneus longus muscles, and

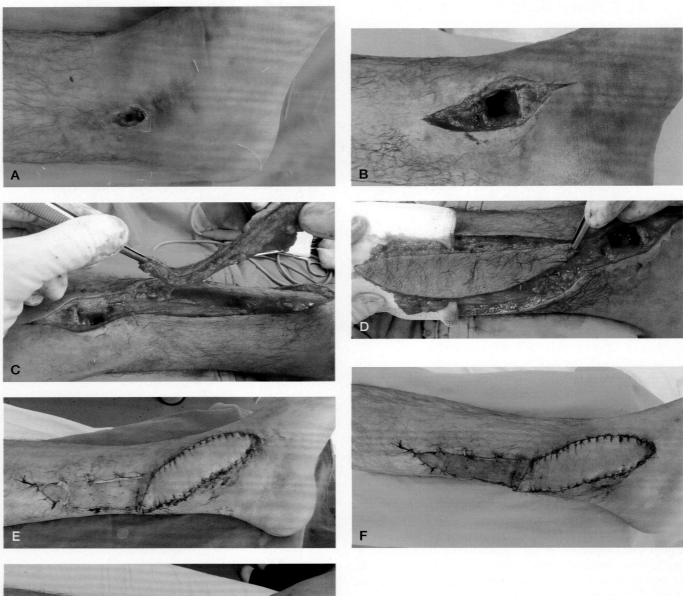

FIGURE 11.14 Preoperative clinical picture of a chronic medial malleolus ulceration with osteomyelitis in a diabetic patient **(A)** followed by surgical débridement **(B)**, propeller perforator flap harvesting and elevation based on a perforator from the posterior tibial artery **(C)**, and insetting by also harvesting supplementary adipofascial tissue to cover the osseous defect **(D)**. Clinical outcomes at postoperative day 1 **(E)**, day 5 **(F)**, and day 14 **(G)**.

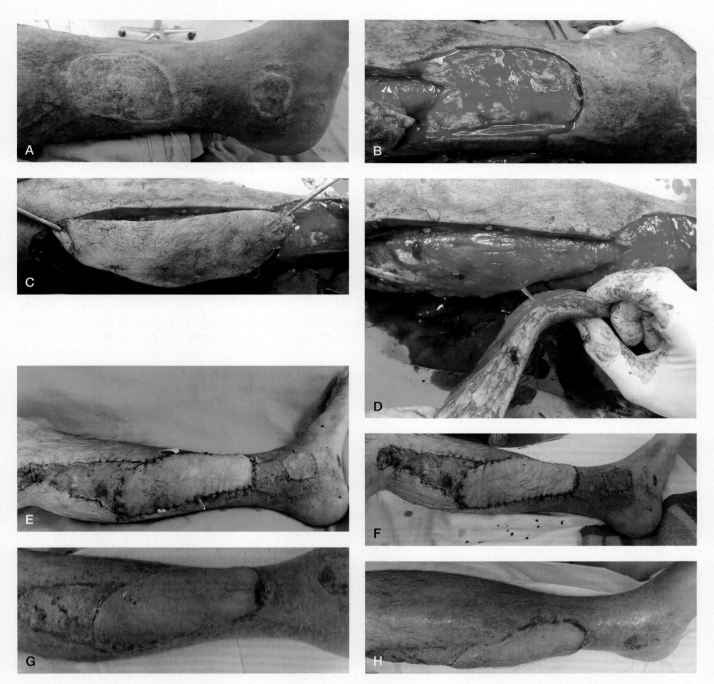

FIGURE 11.15 Preoperative clinical picture of chronic venous stasis ulcerations in a diabetic patient **(A)** followed by surgical débridement **(B)**, propeller perforator flap harvesting **(C)** and elevation based on a perforator from the middle portion of the posterior tibial artery **(D)**, and insetting at the proximal main medial soft tissue defect of the leg **(E)**, whereas a split-thickness skin graft was utilized to cover the smaller soft tissue defect distally **(E)**. Clinical outcomes at postoperative day 2 **(E)**, day 4 **(F)**, and day 21 **(G,H)**.

more distally, they travel in the septum between the flexor hallucis longus and peroneus brevis muscles. Perforators of the PA seem to predominate in the middle third of the fibula. A distinct cluster 13 to 18 cm proximal to the lateral malleolus has been detected (Fig. 11.16) (49). Within this cluster, 28% of all PA perforators were found. Ninety-three percent of lower leg studies had a perforator within this region (49).

According to Boriani et al. (7), 38% of PA perforators are musculocutaneous perforators. The remaining 62% have been found to emerge in the septum between the muscles of the posterior compartment (7). In a systematic review about PA perforators, Iorio et al. (24) found that the peak density of septocutaneous perforators was found in an interval of 0.6 along the axis of the fibula measured from the proximal fibular head

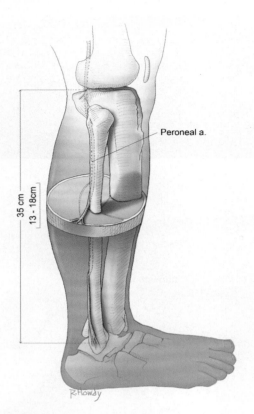

FIGURE 11.16 Localization of reliable perforators from the peroneal artery (49).

to the lateral malleolus. A 19 ± 1% of total perforators were present in this interval. The probability to find a perforator in this interval was calculated with 79.1 ± 2.1%. The highest density of musculocutaneous perforators was found in an interval of 0.4; the frequency of perforators was 18.9 ± 1.4% (24). Unlike the tibial vascular systems, no relation between leg length and number of perforators was found for the peroneal vascular system. This phenomenon is most likely caused due to the fact that perforators of the PA concentrate far away from the growth cartilages (7). Regarding the amount of perforators, Schaverien and Saint-Cyr (49) reported numbers around 4.4 ± 2.3 per leg (Fig. 11.12), which is consistent with other authors (6,42,50,57,58,60). The diameter of PA perforators varies between 0.5 and 1.5 mm, and the distance to the source artery averages out 3.7 ± 1.7 mm.

The technically demanding dissection of PA perforators down to the source artery and the location of reliable perforators set limits to the clinical usability (49). Despite this fact, because the PA is the last artery remaining permeable in the diabetic foot, its perforators, and especially the one emerging in the interval 5 to 8 cm above the lateral malleolus represents a very reliable vascular source for flaps to cover the distal lower extremity and foot (Figs. 11.7 and 11.17).

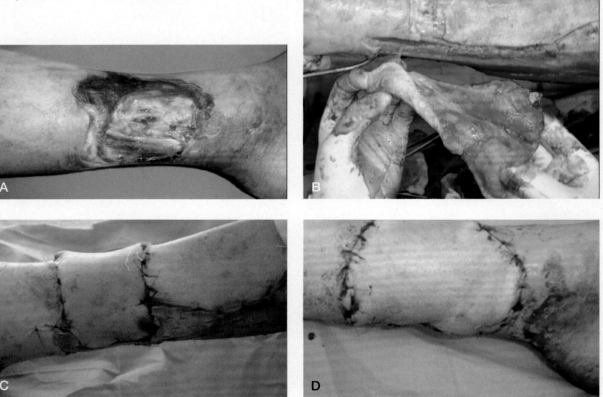

FIGURE 11.17 Preoperative clinical picture of a chronic nonhealing ulceration over the anterior, medial, and posterior aspect of the distal lower extremity **(A)** followed by surgical débridement and a propeller perforator flap harvesting and elevation based on a distal perforator of the peroneal artery and crossing over the distal lower extremity to cover the soft tissue defect **(B)**. Lateral **(C)** and medial **(D)** clinical pictures at postoperative day 7.

The terminal branches of all described main arteries give perforators or finish themselves as perforators able to provide blood supply in very useful flaps to cover the ankle and foot. These perforators respect the same rules of the angiosome/perforasome concept, but for some of them, their distribution and territories have not been studied in great detail. These perforators can successfully supply flaps such as the anteromedial and anterolateral malleolar flaps from the ATA (26); posteromedial malleolar flap from the PTA (26); posterolateral malleolar flap (26), lateral calcaneal flap (4,8,26), and lateral supramalleolar flap from the PA (26); and forefoot plantar flaps from the deep plantar arch resulted from the anastomosis between the deep plantar artery (ATA) and medial and lateral plantar arteries (PTA) (56).

TIPS AND PEARLS OF UTILIZING PERFORATOR FLAPS IN THE DIABETIC LOWER EXTREMITY AND FOOT

- The most important source of perforators in the lower leg is the PTA, but the PA represents the most resistant artery in vascular compromised diabetic lower extremity.
- The number of perforators in a flap is less important than the quality and number of choke/linking vessels.
- Respecting the axiality in designing flaps and maintaining the patient's blood pressure as close as possible to the original one, will allow the opening of more choke/linking vessels which permits the harvesting of larger flaps.
- As central as the perforator enters the flap, the more the vascularized flap will be due to the multidirectional blood flow.

Conclusion

Even with the reputation of a demanding anatomic region, in the lower extremity and foot, there are enough vascular resources able to provide adequate blood supply for flaps to cover defects. The respect of the aforementioned principles and new knowledge in the vascular anatomy and functionality represents a great source of information to utilize local resources as perforator flaps in these demanding areas of reconstruction.

Acknowledgment

Alexandra Hernandez, M.A., of Gory Details Illustration.

References

1. Alagoz MS, Orbay H, Uysal AC, et al. Vascular anatomy of the metatarsal bones and the interosseous muscles of the foot. J Plast Reconstr Aesthet Surg 2009;62:1227–1232.
2. Amarante J, Costa H, Reis J, et al. A new distally based fasciocutaneous flap of the leg. Br J Plast Surg 1986;39:338–340.
3. Antia NH, Buch VI. Transfer of an abdominal dermo-fat graft by direct anastomosis of blood vessels. Br J Plast Surg 1971;24:15–19.
4. Argenta LC. Lateral calcaneal artery skin flap. In: Strauch B, Vasconez LO, Herman CK, et al., eds. Grabb's encyclopedia of flaps: head and neck. 4th ed. Philadelphia: Wolters Kluwer, 2016:1472–1474.
5. Behan FC, Wilson JSP. The principle of the angiotome: a system of linked axial pattern flaps. In: Marchac D, Hueston JT, eds. Transactions of the sixth international congress of plastic and reconstructive surgery. Paris, France: Masson, 1975:6.
6. Beppu M, Hanel DP, Johnston GH, et al. The osteocutaneous fibula flap: an anatomic study. J Reconstr Microsurg 1992;8:215–223.
7. Boriani F, Bruschi S, Fraccalvieri M, et al. Leg perforators and leg length: an anatomic study focusing on topography and angiogenesis. Clin Anat 2010;23:593–605.
8. Burusapat C, Tanthanatip P, Kuhaphensaeng P, et al. Lateral calcaneal artery flaps in atherosclerosis: cadaveric study, vascular assessment and clinical applications. Plast Reconstr Surg Glob Open 2015;3:e517.
9. Callegari PR, Taylor GI, Caddy CM, et al. An anatomic review of the delay phenomenon. I. Experimental studies. Plast Reconstr Surg 1992;89:397–407.
10. Carriquiry C, Aparecida Costa M, Vasconez LO. An anatomic study of the septocutaneous vessels of the leg. Plast Reconstr Surg 1985;76:354–363.
11. Cormack GC, Lamberty BG. Cadaver studies of correlation between vessel size and anatomical territory of cutaneous supply. Br J Plast Surg 1986;39:300–306.
12. Cormack GC, Lamberty BGH, eds. The arterial anatomy of skin flaps. London, United Kingdom: Churchill Livingstone, 1986.
13. Davis JS. Plastic surgery. Its principles and practice. Philadelphia: Blakiston, 1919.
14. Esser JFS. General rules used in simple plastic work on Australian war-wounded soldiers. Surg Gynecol Obstet 1917;34:737.
15. Garcia-Pumarino R, Moraleda E, Aburto A, et al. Vascular anatomy of the dorsum of the foot. Plast Reconstr Surg 2010;126:2012–2018.
16. Georgescu AV. Propeller perforator flaps in distal lower leg: evolution and clinical applications. Arch Plast Surg 2012;39:94–105.
17. Georgescu AV, Matei I, Ardelean F, et al. Microsurgical nonmicrovascular flaps in forearm and hand reconstruction. Microsurgery 2007;7:384–394.
18. Georgescu AV, Matei IR, Capota IM. The use of propeller perforator flaps for diabetic limb salvage: a retrospective review of 25 cases. Diabet Foot Ankle 2012;3.
19. Ger R. The operative treatment of the advanced stasis ulcer. A preliminary communication. Am J Surg 1966;111:659–663.
20. Hallock GG. Lower extremity muscle perforator flaps for lower extremity reconstruction. Plast Reconstr Surg 2004;114:1123–1130.
21. Hamada N, Ikuta Y, Ikeda A. Arteriographic study of the arterial supply of the foot in one hundred cadaver feet. Acta Anat (Basel) 1994;151:198–206.
22. Huber JF. The arterial network supplying the dorsum of the foot. Anat Rec 1941;80:373–391.
23. Hung LK, Lao J, Ho PC. Free posterior tibial perforator flap: anatomy and a report of 6 cases. Microsurgery 1996;17:503–511.
24. Iorio ML, Cheerharan M, Olding M. A systematic review and pooled analysis of peroneal artery perforators for fibula osteocutaneous and perforator flaps. Plast Reconstr Surg 2012;130:600–607.
25. Keen JA. A study of the arterial variations in the limbs, with special reference to symmetry of vascular patterns. Am J Anat 1961;108:245–261.

26. Koshima I, Itoh S, Nanba Y, et al. Medial and lateral malleolar perforator flaps for repair of defects around the ankle. Ann Plast Surg 2003;51:579–583.

27. Koshima I, Moriguchi T, Ohta S, et al. The vasculature and clinical application of the posterior tibial perforator-based flap. Plast Reconstr Surg 1992;90:643–649.

28. Koshima I, Soeda S. Inferior epigastric artery skin flaps without rectus abdominis muscle. Br J Plast Surg 1989;42:645–648.

29. Lecours C, Saint-Cyr M, Wong C, et al. Freestyle pedicle perforator flaps: clinical results and vascular anatomy. Plast Reconstr Surg 2010;126:1589–1603.

30. Lee JH, Dauber W. Anatomic study of the dorsalis pedis-first dorsal metatarsal artery. Ann Plast Surg 1997;38:50–55.

31. Liu K, Li Z, Lin Y, et al. The reverse-flow posterior tibial artery island flap: anatomic study and 72 clinical cases. Plast Reconstr Surg 1990;86:312–316.

32. Manchot C. Die hautarterien des menschlichen körpers. Leipzig, Germany: FCW Vogel, 1889.

33. Manchot C. The cutaneous arteries of the human body. New York: Springer-Verlag, 1983.

34. Martin AL, Bissell MB, Al-Dhamin A, et al. Computed tomographic angiography for localization of the cutaneous perforators of the leg. Plast Reconstr Surg 2013;131:792–800.

35. Matei I, Georgescu A, Chiroiu B, et al. Harvesting of forearm perforator flaps based on intraoperative vascular exploration: clinical experiences and literature review. Microsurgery 2008;28:321–330.

36. McGregor IA, Morgan G. Axial and random pattern flaps. Br J Plast Surg 1973;26:202–213.

37. Milton SH. The tubed pedicle flap. Br J Plast Surg 1969;22:53–59.

38. Morris SF, Miller BJ, Taylor GI. Vascular anatomy of the integument. In: Blondeel PN, Morris SF, Hallock GG, et al., eds. Perforator flaps: anatomy, technique and clinical applications. St. Louis: Quality Medical Publishing Inc, 2006:25.

39. Morris SF, Taylor GI. The time sequence of the delay phenomenon: when is a surgical delay effective? An experimental study. Plast Reconstr Surg 1995;95:526–533.

40. Pan WR, Taylor GI. The angiosomes of the thigh and buttock. Plast Reconstr Surg 2009;123:236–249.

41. Panagiotopoulos K, Soucacos PN, Korres DS, et al. Anatomical study and colour Doppler assessment of the skin perforators of the anterior tibial artery and possible clinical applications. J Plast Reconstr Aesthet Surg 2009;62:1524–1529.

42. Papadimas D, Paraskeuopoulos T, Anagnostopoulou S. Cutaneous perforators of the peroneal artery: cadaveric study with implications in the design of the osteocutaneous free fibular flap. Clin Anat 2009;22:826–833.

43. Perliński L. Variation of the course and the division of dorsalis pedis artery in man. Folia Morphol (Warsz) 1981;40:141–148.

44. Pontén B. The fasciocutaneous flap: its use in soft tissue defects of the lower leg. Br J Plast Surg 1981;34:215–220.

45. Rozen WM, Ashton MW, Le Roux CM, et al. The perforator angiosome: a new concept in the design of deep inferior epigastric artery perforator flaps for breast reconstruction. Microsurgery 2010;30:1–7.

46. Saint-Cyr M, Schaverien M, Arbique G, et al. Three- and four-dimensional computed tomographic angiography and venography for the investigation of the vascular anatomy and perfusion of perforator flaps. Plast Reconstr Surg 2008;121:772–780.

47. Saint-Cyr M, Wong C, Schaverien M, et al. The perforasome theory: vascular anatomy and clinical implications. Plast Reconstr Surg 2009;124:1529–1544.

48. Salmon M. Arteres de la peau. Paris, France: Mason et Cie, 1936.

49. Schaverien M, Saint-Cyr M. Perforators of the lower leg: analysis of perforator locations and clinical application for pedicled perforator flaps. Plast Reconstr Surg 2008;122:161–170.

50. Schusterman MA, Reece GP, Miller MJ, et al. The osteocutaneous free fibula flap: is the skin paddle reliable? Plast Reconstr Surg 1992;90:787–793.

51. Tanaka K, Matsumura H, Miyaki T, et al. An anatomic study of the intermuscular septum of the lower leg; branches from the posterior tibial artery and potential for reconstruction of the lower leg and the heel. J Plast Reconstr Aesthet Surg 2006;59:835–838.

52. Tang M, Mao Y, Almutairi K, et al. Three-dimensional analysis of perforators of the posterior leg. Plast Reconstr Surg 2009;123:1729–1738.

53. Taylor GI. The angiosomes of the body and their supply to perforator flaps. Clin Plast Surg 2003;30:331–342.

54. Taylor GI, Corlett RJ, Dhar SC, et al. The anatomical (angiosome) and clinical territories of cutaneous perforating arteries: development of the concept and designing safe flaps. Plast Reconstr Surg 2011;127:1447–1459.

55. Taylor GI, Palmer JH. The vascular territories (angiosomes) of the body: experimental study and clinical applications. Br J Plast Surg 1987;40:113–141.

56. Valentin GA, Rodica MI, Manuel L. Plantar flaps based on perforators of the plantar metatarsal/common digital arteries. J Reconstr Microsurg 2014;30:469–474.

57. Whetzel TP, Barnard MA, Stokes RB. Arterial fasciocutaneous vascular territories of the lower leg. Plast Reconstr Surg 1997;100:1172–1183.

58. Wolff KD. The supramalleolar flap based on septocutaneous perforators from the peroneal vessels for intraoral soft tissue replacement. Br J Plast Surg 1993;46:151–155.

59. Yamada T, Gloviczki P, Bower TC, et al. Variations of the arterial anatomy of the foot. Am J Surg 1993;166:130–135.

60. Yoshimura M, Shimada T, Hosokawa M. The vasculature of the peroneal tissue transfer. Plast Reconstr Surg 1990;85:917–921.

CHAPTER 12

Local Random Flaps for Soft Tissue Coverage of the Diabetic Foot

Peter A. Blume • Ashley A. Bruno • Amber Rose Morra

INTRODUCTION

Successful surgical reconstruction of diabetic foot pathology is one of the biggest challenges surgeons face. Although there are a variety of surgical treatments, local random flaps for soft tissue coverage of the diabetic foot are a reliable option. In the mid-19th century, Gillies and Millard described the art of plastic surgical reconstruction (51). During that time, local flaps began to gain popularity for healing diabetic foot soft tissue defects, as they aimed to target the isolated pathology without sacrificing healthy tissue. Over the next several years, the research on local flaps expanded and new technique options and success rates were established. Current research suggests flaps are especially useful for reconstruction of the plantar aspect of the foot because skin grafting is not optimal as a reconstructive option for weight bearing areas (49,50,127). In the surgical reconstruction of diabetic foot pathology, 90% of cases are treated with simple operative techniques, whereas 10% require complex flap reconstruction to adequately address and treat the diabetic patient (36).

PREOPERATIVE CONSIDERATIONS AND SURGICAL EVALUATION

When deciding on the use of local flaps for the treatment of diabetic foot pathologies, several factors must be considered. Prior to surgical intervention, preoperative planning is necessary to include evaluation of the size and depth of ulceration/defect and management of infection (3,6–8). Other key considerations include location, quality, vascularity, thickness, function, color, texture, and turgor of the tissue (49,50). Local skin flaps should be evaluated for tissue mobility and elasticity; otherwise, the flap could be under tension after relocation. Additionally, the composition of the skin at the donor site should be equal or greater in durability than the recipient site.

Medical Comorbidities

Patient past medical history and comorbidities are one the most important preoperative considerations. Comorbidities such as diabetes mellitus, hypertension, peripheral arterial disease, venous insufficiency, anemia, neuropathy, malnutrition, renal disease, hemodialysis, infection, history of abnormal scarring, bleeding abnormalities, age, musculoskeletal abnormalities, and use of tobacco should all be addressed preoperatively and optimized if possible (9,10).

Current research indicates that hemoglobin A_{1c} levels over 8% are associated with delayed wound healing, as is the hypoxia environment caused by tobacco use. Additionally, when evaluating a diabetic patient for a potential local flap preoperatively, it is important to consider kidney function because end-stage renal disease patients often have decreased fibroblast function which corresponds to delayed wound healing (10,33,68,91). Also, although patient's age is not a relative contraindication for flap closure, research shows that insensate patients $\leq$40 years of age have better outcomes when compared to patients over 40 with regard to flaps on the sole of the foot (25).

In addition to all of the preceding factors, the patient's occupation and capacity to deal with lost time from work and economic impact should be considered. The patient's expectations regarding the outcome of the surgery, possibility of additional surgeries, and potential risks (e.g., amputation) should be taken into account.

Vascular Assessment

Vascular insufficiency is often detrimental to flap success. When insufficiency is suspected preoperatively, a vascular surgery consultation is strongly recommended. Parameters to consider vascular consultation include ankle-brachial index (ABI) of <0.7, toe-brachial index (TBI) <40 mmHg, or transcutaneous oxygen tension ($TcPo_2$) levels <30 mmHg. Abnormal noninvasive vascular studies are a direct predictability for wound healing (11,12,18).

Diabetic patients usually have multiple medical comorbidities, and as such, it is not uncommon for them to have calcified vessels. This vessel calcification results in vascular noninvasive testing with falsely elevated ABIs (>1.3). For this reason, TBI is a more reliable indicator of pedal flow because the small vessels of the toes are generally spared of calcification (13–22).

Functional photoplethysmography (fPPG) is a noninvasive automated device using a cuffless functional test for assessing peripheral arterial disease (PAD) without the operator dependency issues associated with resting ankle-brachial pressure index (RABPI). fPPG may prove to be superior to RABPI and may be useful as a simple screening tool for early detection of PAD (23). If inconclusive, then duplex scanning, contrast arteriography, or gadofosveset-enhanced magnetic resonance angiography may be necessary (27). Hyperspectral imaging is a new technique that evaluates for tissue oxygenation by using scanning spectroscopy targeted to wavelengths for the absorption peaks of oxyhemoglobin and deoxyhemoglobin. This helps construct spatial maps of the foot and lower extremity and has been shown to help identify changes in microcirculation in diabetic patients (11,24,92). If inadequate perfusion is found, a vascular surgical procedure may be performed to increase peripheral perfusion.

Wound Bed Assessment

Addressing underlying osseous pathology and control of both infections and wound bed bioburden must be addressed prior to flap reconstruction. These factors have all been shown to increase risk of flap failure (1). Flaps should never be raised or advanced in patients with active acute infections. Instead, proper protocol should include effective incision and drainage procedures, débridement, resection of infective tissue and bone, copious lavage, and additional infection-reducing surgery. In cases where infection may be suspected or previous infection has been documented, it is important to examine the microbiology cultures and sensitivities, as well as the pathology results. In doing so, the guidance of infectious disease experts is also useful in the management of antibiotic therapy as well as therapy duration. Additionally, vancomycin prophylaxis should be considered in patients with a history of methicillin-resistant *Staphylococcus aureus* for upward of 5 days prior and up to 2 weeks after surgery. Similarly, patients with a history of vancomycin-resistant *Enterococci* should also be effectively prophylaxed to help increase flap success (13,17).

LOCAL RANDOM FLAP INDICATIONS AND CONTRAINDICATIONS

The main indications for local random flaps in the diabetic foot are to provide long-term viability by offering tissue coverage for exposed tendon, muscle, and bone; defect filling; failed primary and secondary closure; skin graft failure; coverage for weight bearing surfaces; increased durability; reducing scar formation; and esthetically appealing. The main contraindications for local random flaps in the diabetic foot are gross contamination and infection, PAD with micro- and/or macrovascular disease, minimal tissue expansibility, extensively large soft tissue defects, scar contracture, and poor patient compliance.

LOCAL FLAPS

There are several different surgical options and techniques that are useful for providing diabetic wound closure. Generally, a treatment algorithm, or reconstructive wound closure ladder, is utilized to determine the appropriate treatment (Fig. 12.1). Grafts and flaps are commonly used in treatment algorithms with a high success rate.

A flap is defined as a piece of tissue used for transplantation that is vascularized by a pedicle or stem (2). A flap can be categorized by its blood supply, shape, anatomic donor location, eponym, tissue type, or movement pattern. For example, a local flap indicates that the tissue is adjacent to the area needed for coverage. Local flaps include the epidermis, dermis, and subcutaneous tissue and may also include underlying fascia, muscle, or both.

Local skin flaps are further classified based on blood supply as either random or axial. An axial flap is supplied by a known blood vessel or via direct cutaneous arteries. In comparison, a local random flap has no dominant blood supply and instead receives supply diffusely from the dermal and subdermal vascular plexus (3). This intrinsic blood supply is ideal for covering defects containing exposed bone or tendon as well as defects that do not have the vascular supply sufficient enough to support a skin graft (1,4,5). This chapter separates the various types of local flaps according to movement as shown in Table 12.1.

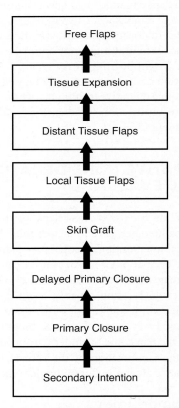

FIGURE 12.1 The "reconstructive wound closure ladder" is a treatment algorithm commonly utilized by surgeons to assess appropriate treatment options for complex wounds.

TABLE 12.1

Types of Local Random Flaps

Advancement Flaps	Rotation Flaps	Transposition Flaps
Single advancement	Single rotation	Single lobe
Double advancement	Satterfield-Jolly	Bilobed
V-Y	Double rotation	Z-plasty
Double V-Y	Biwinged	Double opposing Z-plasty
Y-V plasty		Rhomboid or Limberg Flap of Dufourmentel Double-Z rhomboid 30-Degree transposition flap

Local Flap Surgical Planning

Whenever possible, incision lines for pedal flaps should be parallel to the lines of minimal relaxed tension or relaxed skin tension lines (RSTL). This helps to create minimal transverse forces, which can ultimately impede healing (57–59). Ignoring the RSTL can lead to increased motion at flap site and subsequently hypertrophic scarring and delayed healing (59). Examining the lines of maximal extensibility (LME) is also useful when creating flaps because the LME help indicate where the skin is most pliable. Because skin flaps rely on the movement of skin, it is necessary to plan these flaps so that the direction of desired movement of the flap corresponds to the LME (79).

Knowledge of pedal vascular anatomy allows for safe incisions providing sufficient blood flow for healing. This allows the surgeon to assess whether the flap can be harvested successfully or whether revascularization will give the best chance to heal existent defects (22,90,104). Flaps should be positioned to maximize the vascularity of the flap. For example, flaps placed in the proximal plantar area of the foot should be based either medially or laterally and should only be based medially if the heel sensation is intact (42). Large rotation flaps on the plantar surface of the foot should also be based medially to take advantage of the blood supply from the superficial branch of the medial plantar artery (29,43). Flap elevation and rotation can be designed in anticipation of the increased mobility achieved because of osseous resection and undermining (52,54,55). LME and RSTL may be partially or entirely overlooked when concomitant bone surgery is performed.

Local Flap Blood Supply

In general, the blood supply of the skin comes from 1 of 3 sources: a cutaneous artery, musculocutaneous perforating arteries, or fasciocutaneous arteries. Furthermore, Taylor et al. (121) first introduced the concept of angiosomes, which

is a cutaneous territory fed by a source artery and drained by specific veins. Although each angiosome covers a specific area, adjacent angiosomes communicate by true anastomoses of caliber vessels or "choke" vessels. These small choke vessels are reduced caliber connecting branches that are usually closed (119). However, when a particular angiosome becomes compromised, choke vessels open, allowing the neighboring angiosome to support and feed the compromised angiosome. It is important to note that an angiosome can only support a directly adjacent neighbor. If an angiosome needs to support a nonadjacent neighbor, intervention is necessary to allow 2 consecutive sets of choke vessels to open.

Understanding the angiosomes of the foot and ankle is especially useful in surgery and wound healing to ensure successful results. The foot and ankle have 6 distinct angiosomes that originate from 3 main arteries: the anterior tibial, posterior tibial and peroneal arteries (Fig. 12.2). These 3 major arteries supplying the foot and ankle have several arterial–arterial connections, which creates redundant pedal blood flow. The anterior tibial artery supplies the anterior ankle and the dorsum of the foot. The posterior tibial artery supplies portions of the plantar foot and medial ankle, whereas the peroneal artery supplies the lateral border of the ankle and heel (31,120,121).

The anterior tibial artery, along with its continuation as the dorsalis pedis, is responsible for supplying the complete dorsal forefoot (Fig. 12.3). The anterior tibial artery extensively contributes to the anterior angiosome concept by providing the medial and lateral malleolar arteries, medial and lateral tarsal

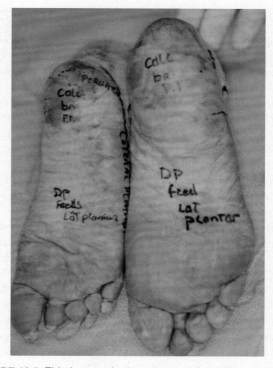

FIGURE 12.2 This image depicts the pedal angiosomes distribution after fresh cadaver specimens were injected with polymethylmethacrylate dye.

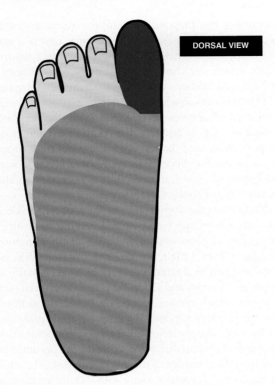

DORSAL VIEW

PLANTAR VIEW

FIGURE 12.3 The anterior angiosome—dorsal view. The *orange* shows the angiosome supplied by the anterior tibial artery and its branches to the dorsal aspect of the foot. The *purple* shows the blood supply to the hallux and its dual supply from the anterior angiosome and the posterior angiosome. The lateral plantar artery (from the posterior angiosome) supplies the remaining neutral colored portion of the foot.

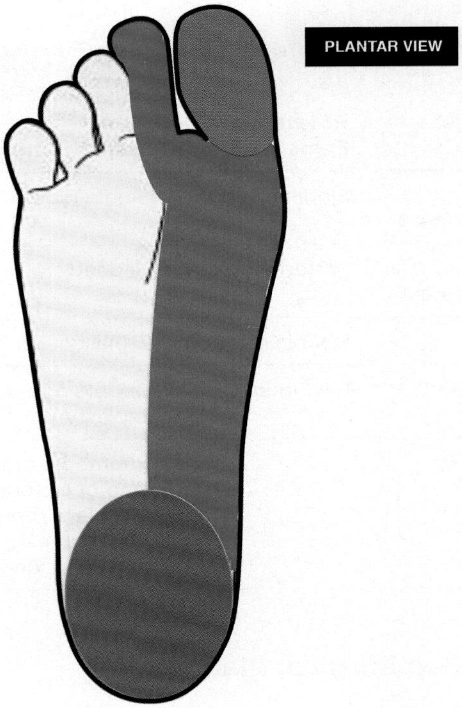

FIGURE 12.4 The posterior angiosome—plantar view. The posterior angiosome is supplied by the posterior tibial artery and its main branches. The *green* image depicts the angiosome to the plantar hallux that is supplied by the medial plantar artery via the deep branch. The *red* shows the medial plantar artery angiosome, whereas the *blue* shows the angiosome supplied by the medial calcaneal artery. The lateral plantar artery supplies the remaining neutral colored portion of the foot.

arteries, and the arcuate artery. Additionally, the hallux is supplied by anterior angiosomes via the first dorsal metatarsal artery and receives redundant flow by the posterior angiosomes (34,43,120).

The 3 branches of the posterior tibial artery each feed different angiosomes (Figs. 12.4 and 12.5). The medial calcaneal artery supplies the medial malleolus and the medial planter heel. The medial plantar artery supplies the medial plantar instep and has a deep branch that contributes to the supply of the hallux, along with the supply from the anterior angiosomes. The lateral plantar artery supplies the lateral plantar foot and forefoot (120,121).

The peroneal artery bifurcates at the malleolus level into the anterior perforating and the lateral calcaneal branch, which again supply specific angiosomes (Fig. 12.6). The anterior branch supplies the angiosome of the anterior lateral ankle, whereas the lateral calcaneal branch supplies the lateral heel angiosome (120,121).

As mentioned previously, the pedal angiosomes often overlap each other and provide extensive vascularization to certain areas. One example of this, as examined by Hidalgo and Shaw (59), is the area overlying the distal two-thirds of the plantar fascia. This area is known as the "watershed area" because it receives blood supply from multiple sources, such

as the proximal plantar subcutaneous plexus, the medial and lateral plantar arteries, and branches of the deep plantar artery (59). Hidalgo and Shaw (59) also demonstrated that the lateral plantar surface of the midfoot receives its blood supply from branches of the dorsalis pedis artery found at the lateral aspect of the foot and branches of the lateral plantar artery. Other authors demonstrated a clear line of demarcation at the sole of the foot intersecting the lateral dorsal skin (43). Another example of overlapping flow is the area of the plantar foot distal to the plantar fascia, which receives blood supply from an arch formed by the dorsalis pedis artery and lateral plantar artery (45). Also, although the dorsalis pedis artery and first dorsal metatarsal artery provide the majority of the blood supply to the dorsum of the foot, the distal aspect of the anterior tibial, peroneal artery, dorsal arterial rete, and marginal anastomotic branches along the medial and lateral aspects of the foot may also provide supply to the dorsum of the foot (46). Although there are several areas of redundant flow, there are also areas of decreased flow, namely the skin covering the extensor digitorum brevis, which has the poorest blood supply (104).

Even though sufficient blood supply and knowledge of angiosomes are crucial in flap success, appropriate technique is

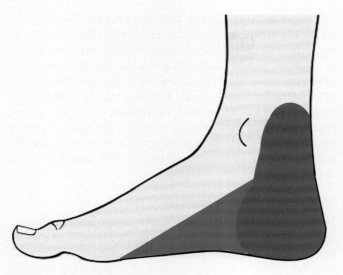

FIGURE 12.5 The posterior angiosome—medial view. The *red* shows the medial plantar artery angiosome, whereas the *blue* shows the angiosome supplied by the medial calcaneal artery.

also necessary. One of the most important surgical theories is the "delay procedure." This theory is based on the concept of gradually exposing a flap of skin to an environment of decreased blood flow to allow the flap to survive in such an environment. The delay procedure is performed by surgically disrupting the vessels around the proposed flap or by elevating the original flap of skin and suturing it back to its original position. When the blood flow is disrupted, the flap undergoes ischemic changes. Metabolism is converted from aerobic to anaerobic, lactic acid and carbon dioxide is produced, and the tissue pH changes to a more acidic environment. As a result, the blood vessels in the flap dilate, and the preexisting choke vessels between adjacent perforators dilate, especially along

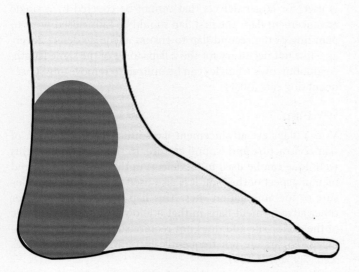

FIGURE 12.6 The peroneal angiosome—lateral view. The *pink* represents the angiosome supplied by the peroneal artery and its main branches.

the axis of the flap (1,21,31–35,120). In addition to changes in blood flow, the delay technique creates a local sympathectomy that also causes vasodilation secondary to the decrease in sympathetic tone (32,36). After approximately 2 to 3 weeks, the major beneficial effects of the delay procedure are seen and the flap can be transposed or another delay procedure can be performed (36). For maximal flap survival, it is best to progressively undermine and ligate perforators of a flap while leaving the tip attached until the final elevation and relocation. Additionally, the more choke vessels present in a particular flap, the less pressure there is available for flow at the distal aspect of the flap, which helps to decrease necrosis (26).

The delay phenomenon can add at least 1 additional anatomic vascular territory to the length of a flap (31,32,35). Without the use of a surgical delay, the first territory in a random area of a flap can be accessed with ease; however, necrosis tends to occur in a flap when an attempt is made to capture the next or subsequent angiosome (1,21,29–35). As such, the survival of a length of a flap is inversely proportional to the distance between the artery at the base of the flap and the next perforator territory (90). An alternative to the surgical delay procedure is to perform soft tissue expansion to increase the size of the flap while helping to augment the vascular territory (39).

The soft tissue surrounding the vascular supply is also important to consider when creating flaps. Blood vessels conform to the connective tissue framework. Specifically, if the connective tissue is rigid, then the vessels embrace its surface, whereas if the connective tissue is loose, the vessels travel within it. Blood vessels radiate from the fixed areas where tissues are anchored into more mobile areas. Additionally, blood vessels also radiate from concavities and converge on convexities (26,31,32,34). Increased mobility between tissue planes help increase the size of flaps that are available for transfer (26). The safest design of a flap is when the axis of the flap is placed along the direction of the LME (31).

A major misconception regarding blood flow and flaps was that skin flap dimensions must be based on length-to-width ratios. The accepted ratios of length to width had been defined as 3:1 in the face, 2:1 on the trunk, and 1:1 on the extremities. Milton demonstrated that the presence of an artery at the base of a flap determined its success and not the length-to-width ratio (40,41,88).

INTRAOPERATIVE PEARLS FOR LOCAL FLAP CLOSURE

There are 4 main factors to consider when choosing a surgical incision placement. First, the surgical incision has to provide adequate exposure. Second, there needs to be adequate blood supply on either side of the incision for both the incision and flap to heal normally. Third, the surgical incision should attempt to spare the sensory and motor nerves. Fourth and finally, the surgical incision, when placed perpendicular to the skin tension lines, carries the risk of causing scar contracture (29). Although all 4 factors should be honored, there are occasions when some have to be overlooked, but ideally, the choice for incision should be a balance of all 4 factors.

When dissecting and handling skin flaps, it is critical to employ atraumatic technique to preserve blood supply and skin viability. This technique involves the use of bipolar cautery, sharp dissection, the use of skin hooks or fine-toothed forceps, and delicate handling of the flap. Care should be taken to avoid compromising the flap's blood supply by traumatizing the base or distorting the base during movement. Additionally, skin flaps should be raised by undermining below the subdermal plexus of vessels in the subcutaneous plane to help increase tissue viability. However, undermining also increases dead space and thus increases the chance of hematoma/seroma formation. Meticulous hemostasis prior to suturing avoids such formation (36,62).

When closing the surgical incision and suturing the flap into place, deep sutures should be avoided if possible to prevent tissue reaction and preserve plexus viability. When closing the surgical incision, larger bites suture technique should be taken on the side of the flap in order to prevent flap override. In all flaps, sutures should be placed "from island to shore," starting in the flap and ending in the adjacent skin. The key sutures that bear the greatest tension and align the flap should be placed near the tip of the flap with subsequent sutures placed obliquely to help alleviate tension and malalignment. After final suturing, the flap should be evaluated for excessive tension and adequate vascularity. If a flap cannot be inset with 4-0 nylon suture or suture of lesser strength, then most likely there is too much tension on the flap and a delay procedure may be prudent.

During the movement of skin flaps, cones of skin may be created, which can be inverted or everted. When everted, they are commonly referred to as a "dog ear" and can be corrected using Burrow's triangles. Burrow's triangles excise the excess skin to allow for optimum mobility of the flap while correcting the buckling of the adjacent tissues. It is important not to back cut the flap when excising a dog ear because it may compromise the blood flow to the flap (44,60,62,66).

Ideally, the surgeon should wait 15 minutes prior to closing for evaluating the tension to allow for normal skin relaxation (4). Various methods are employed to evaluate flap viability and include subjective assessments, such as observation of color, capillary blanching and refill, warmth of the flap, and bleeding from stab wounds. Warmth of a flap is not considered to be a reliable method for assessing flap viability (44). For flaps >1:1 ratio of length to width, a Doppler or other technique should be employed to ensure adequate vascularity into the flap (13,52).

DETAILED SURGICAL LOCAL FLAP TECHNIQUES

Advancement Flaps

Advancement flaps are local random flaps in which the tissue is advanced in a linear, single direction. Although difficult in the foot, they are best used in areas of the foot with adequate soft tissue laxity in order to allow for primary closure of the donor and recipient site without resulting in the formation of dog ears (33,82,89). Ideal placement should be perpendicular to the RSTL and advancement should be parallel to the LME (93). Flap blood supply is dependent on the local perforators. Minimal undermining should be performed in order to prevent flap necrosis. Once inset, the tension is then distributed equally along the entire length of the flap using the "running pleated" suture (84). There are several variations including the single or double advancement flaps, the V-Y, double V-Y, and the Y-V flap.

Single Advancement Flap

The single advancement flap advances skin from a single side, into the area of the defect. It can be utilized for defects that are large and would require significant tension to close primarily. This flap works well for skin closure of defects along the plantar aspect of the foot, particularly at the level of the metatarsal heads after excision of a wound or lesion (60). It is also useful in defects of up to 1 cm on the plantar heel. When used plantarly, the single advancement flap should be based medially or laterally to avoid venous congestion of the flap (87). When this is done, the resulting incision line lies outside of the weight bearing region.

Surgical technique involves 2 parallel incisions extending away from the defect, creating a flap that is of similar depth to that of the defect. The incisions should be made perpendicular to the RSTL or parallel to the LME. The length of the incisions should be adequate to provide enough mobility for the flap to advance into the defect while minimizing tension (83,86).

Double Advancement Flap

The double advancement flap, also known as "H-plasty," consists of 2 single advancement flaps from opposing sides which are advanced toward each other into the area of the defect. It is used for larger defects that cannot be covered by a single advancement flap. The first flap should be fully raised prior to planning of the second flap to ensure adequate defect coverage. It is not necessary for the 2 flaps to be of the same length. Again, Burrow's triangles can be utilized to remove any subsequent dog ears (30,44).

V-Y Flap

V-to-Y flaps are advancement flaps utilized for reduction of scar contracture and wound closure. In the diabetic foot, this technique can be used to fill defects in the posterior heel and plantar aspect of the foot. It is also used as an adjunct for closure of toe amputation sites. This flap is advantageous over other advancement flaps in that it allows for primary closure of the donor site and does not require subsequent skin grafting. Dog ears are not frequently encountered in this flap as well (7,9,76,101,109).

The flap consists of a V-type incision with a 30-degree apex facing furthest away from the wound. The length of the V should be 2 to 3 times the defect diameter, and the widest point

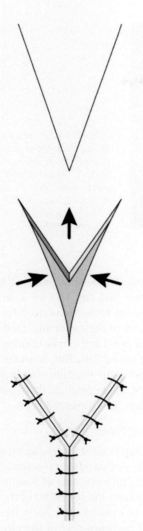

should be equal to the largest area of the defect (3,76,97). Undermining along the edges can help increase tissue mobilization. Once advanced, the resultant incision is transformed into a "Y" shape, with the base of the V filling the wound (Fig. 12.7).

Double V-Y Flap

A double V-to-Y flap, also known as a "double kite flap," is useful when a defect is >2 cm and may be used to close defects as large as 3 to 4 cm (4). In the foot, these flaps have been utilized for open wounds or excision of lesions plantar to the metatarsal heads as well as in the plantar heel (1,60,92,97,100). Similarly, this technique is advantageous because it allows for primary closure of the donor sites and avoids tissue distortion (13,38). This technique is the same as the single V-Y flap; however, a second identical flap is designed on the opposite side of the defect. Each flap is elevated in the same manner and advanced toward each other to cover the defect (Fig. 12.8).

Y-V Plasty

The Y-V flap is similar technique to the V-Y flap; however, it releases tension perpendicular to the "Y" incision and increases tension in line with direction of advancement. It is often performed over the dorsum of the foot to alleviate scar/burn contracture or toe contracture. A disadvantage of this flap includes the creation of dog ears at the base of the flap as there is increased tension created with advancement (Fig. 12.9) (86).

Rotation Flaps

Rotation flaps are those that pivot around a point and move through an arc. This arc rotation allows for redistribution of tension from the site of the primary defect to the donor site. Rotation flaps can be used to repair defects with convex surfaces where the tension lines are curved (33). In the diabetic foot, this flap is used to correct larger defects, particularly on the plantar heel (100). It is also useful in Charcot neuroarthropathy foot reconstruction, allowing for wide plantar exposure of the involved subluxed or dislocated joints (101). These flaps can be suprafascial, fasciocutaneous, myocutaneous, or

FIGURE 12.7 V-Y flap along the direction of the lines of maximal extensibility (LME). The width of the extended V-to-Y flap is greater than the width of the defect because of the presence of an extension of the flap on one or both sides of the defect. (With permission from Blume PA, Key JJ. Local random flaps for soft tissue coverage of the diabetic foot. In: Zgonis T, ed. Surgical reconstruction of the diabetic foot and ankle. Philadelphia: Lippincott Williams & Wilkins, 2009:147.)

FIGURE 12.8 A preoperative picture of an ischemic and infected right second toe **(A)**, followed by an amputation at the metatarsophalangeal joint level **(B)** and closure by a double V-Y flap **(C)**. *(continued)*

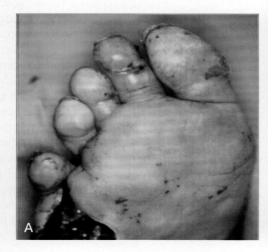
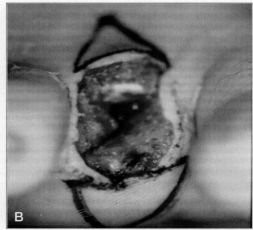

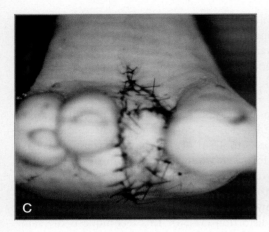

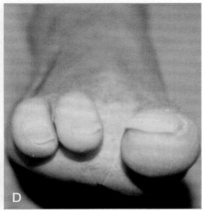

FIGURE 14.8 *(Continued)* **D.** A final clinical postoperative outcome. (With permission from Blume PA, Key JJ. Local random flaps for soft tissue coverage of the diabetic foot. In: Zgonis T, ed. Surgical reconstruction of the diabetic foot and ankle. Philadelphia: Lippincott Williams & Wilkins, 2009:148.)

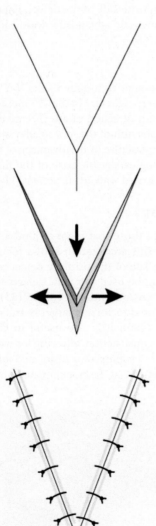

FIGURE 12.9 Y-V plasty that is the opposite of the V-Y flap by increasing tension in line with the Y-to-V flap and releasing tension perpendicular to the flap. (With permission from Blume PA, Key JJ. Local random flaps for soft tissue coverage of the diabetic foot. In: Zgonis T, ed. Surgical reconstruction of the diabetic foot and ankle. Philadelphia: Lippincott Williams & Wilkins, 2009:149.)

a combination (59). The level at which the flap is dissected determines whether this flap will be axial or random. Disadvantages of this flap include the need for skin grafting and subsequent elevation of the donor site. Dog ears are also often created at the pivot point and can be eliminated by performing a backcut into the raised flap. This, however, does increase the risk of compromising the vascular supply to the flap (30,37). These flaps include single rotation flaps, Satterfield-Jolly flap, double rotation flaps, and biwinged flaps.

Single Rotation Flap

A single rotation flap is ideal for triangular shaped defects but can also be used for circular defects. A semicircle extends from the defect and arcs into the area of healthy tissue (30). As a general rule, the greater the curvature of the arc, the more flap mobilization can be created (98). For a triangular defect, the base of the defect becomes part of the circumference of this semicircle (Fig. 12.10).

The length of the flap semicircle should measure 5 to 8 times the width of the defect or have an area of 3 to 4 times the area of the defect to minimize the donor site defect (33,66). The narrower the triangular defect, the less distance the flap will need to move (102); therefore, the defect should be excised with as narrow a triangle as possible. The flap is carefully raised at the desired level and is rotated about the circumference of the circle and into the defect. Although the major movement of the flap is in the arc of flap rotation, the adjacent tissues can also be mobilized in the opposite direction of the flap. Care should be taken to avoid over rotation of the base of the flap because this can choke the vascular supply, leading to flap failure.

The key sutures are placed on the shorter side of the flap, and subsequent sutures are placed using the "rule of halves." Dog ears tend to be present at the base of the flap, and Burrow's triangles may be created to allow for better inset (Fig. 12.11). The use of a back cut at the pivot point of the flap can alternatively be performed but is controversial. Although it allows for additional mobility and therefore reduced tension of the flap, it can also potentially jeopardize the integrity of the vascular supply to the flap (4,36). One way to avoid this is to use a Doppler to locate the perforators (4,52). As previously mentioned, in the

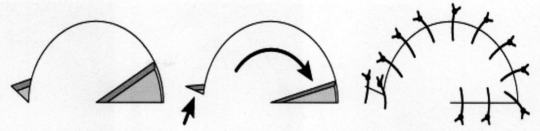

FIGURE 12.10 A single rotation flap being used to close a triangular defect. Note that the flap is shaped semicircular and rotates about a pivot point. Dog ears tend to be present at the base of the flap, and Burrow's triangles *(black arrow)* may be created to allow for better inset. (With permission from Blume PA, Key JJ. Local random flaps for soft tissue coverage of the diabetic foot. In: Zgonis T, ed. Surgical reconstruction of the diabetic foot and ankle. Philadelphia: Lippincott Williams & Wilkins, 2009:150.)

plantar foot, the donor site is often too large to close primarily and may require skin grafting with subsequent elevation and hospital stay (Fig. 12.12).

Satterfield-Jolly Rotation Flap

The Satterfield-Jolly flap is a variant of the single rotation flap specifically used for plantar metatarsal head lesions. Ideally, when planning the flap, the tissue should be rotated from a distal point to a more proximal position to allow for shortening that occurs with rotation. The technique consists of a transverse incision made along the plantar margin of the sulcus, following the natural arc. Metatarsal length can dictate whether the incision is placed medially or laterally, although most frequently, the incision is made from medial to lateral.

The ulceration or lesion is then excised by taking a triangular portion of tissue with the base being part of the initial transverse incision and the apex directed proximally. The length of the triangle should be 4 to 5 times as long as it is wide. Please note that the incision along the sulcus should also be 4 to 5 times of the width of the base of this triangle in order to compensate for the inelasticity of the plantar skin. The leading edge of the flap should be undermined; however, the donor site should not. Burrow's triangles are often necessary to prevent dog ears, with the bases along the original transverse incision and the apices pointed interdigitally in the sulcus. All triangular incisions, if possible, should be made between weight bearing surfaces. The flap is then sutured into the defect, whereas the interdigital triangles are closed with apical

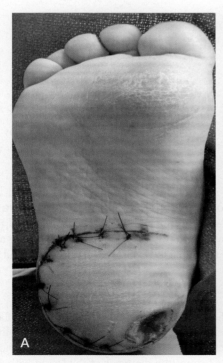
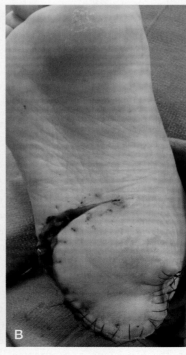
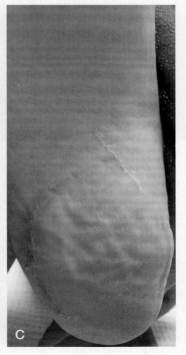

FIGURE 12.11 A delayed single rotation flap at the initial heel ulcer débridement **(A)**, raising the flap **(B)**, followed by a delayed closure. **C.** A final clinical postoperative outcome. (With permission from Blume PA, Key JJ. Local random flaps for soft tissue coverage of the diabetic foot. In: Zgonis T, ed. Surgical reconstruction of the diabetic foot and ankle. Philadelphia: Lippincott Williams & Wilkins, 2009:151.)

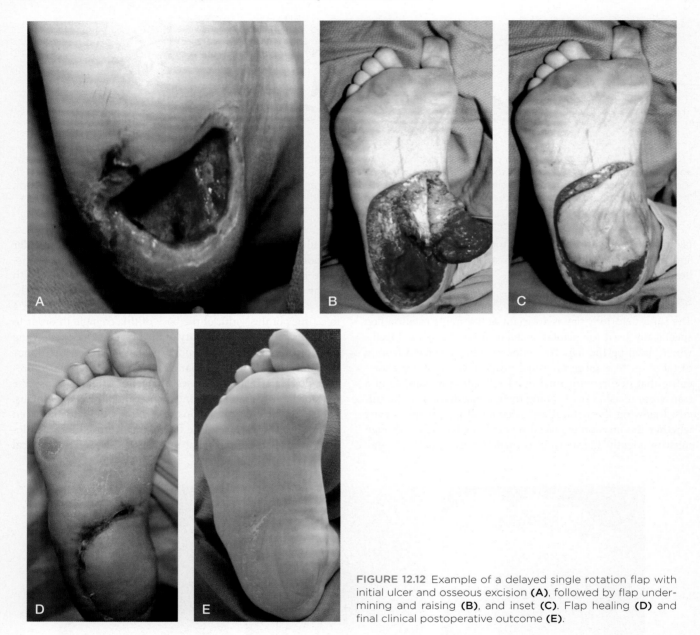

FIGURE 12.12 Example of a delayed single rotation flap with initial ulcer and osseous excision **(A)**, followed by flap undermining and raising **(B)**, and inset **(C)**. Flap healing **(D)** and final clinical postoperative outcome **(E)**.

stitches to prevent skin necrosis (99,105). Advantages of this flap include a non–weight-bearing scar with primary closure of both the donor site and flap.

Double Rotation Flap

The double rotation flap, also known as "O-to-Z" flap, involves 2 arched incisions on opposite sides of a defect. In the foot, it can be utilized on any area to excise a lesion or ulceration (105). It can also be used in lieu of a standard elliptical-shaped closure of wounds. The ulceration or lesion is excised in a circular "O" type fashion, with 2 arcs placed tangentially from the circle and on opposite sides of the defect. The 2 incisions should also be arched in opposite directions. Each arc length should be longer than the original defect; however, both incisions do not need to be of equal length. The 2 flaps are

subsequently raised using atraumatic technique and are approximated so that the short arms of the flaps are sutured together in order to fill the defect. This central arm of the "Z" holds the greatest amount of suture tension. The long arms of the 2 flaps are then able to be sutured, creating the final 2 arms of the "Z."

Biwinged Flap

A variant of the double rotation flap is the "biwinged" flap used for circular defects. The round defect is bisected in a line that is in the direction of RSTL. The length of this line should be approximately 3 times the diameter of the lesion with 2 equal triangles drawn on opposite sides of the defect. The triangles should also be drawn on opposite sides of the bisecting line with the bases of each triangle measuring one-fourth to one-half the

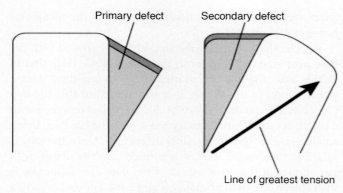

Primary defect   Secondary defect

Line of greatest tension

FIGURE 12.13 A transposition flap that moves over adjacent intact skin to close a defect and combines the use of both rotation and advancement techniques. (With permission from Blume PA, Key JJ. Local random flaps for soft tissue coverage of the diabetic foot. In: Zgonis T, ed. Surgical reconstruction of the diabetic foot and ankle. Philadelphia: Lippincott Williams & Wilkins, 2009:152.)

diameter of the lesion. The flaps are then raised to the subcutaneous tissue level and approximated and sutured together, forming a "lazy S" shape. Similarly, suture tension is greatest at the central aspect of the incision (61,95).

Transposition Flaps

Transposition flaps combine the use of both rotation and advancement to mobilize adjacent skin in order to close a defect (Fig. 12.13). They tend to have a narrower base compared to a rotation flap and require less flap surface area than a rotational flap in order to cover a defect of the same size. Similar to rotation flaps, transposition flaps redistribute tension away from the primary defect and into the donor site (33,106). Transposition flaps, however, are more likely to require split-thickness skin grafting to close the donor site, particularly when used in the pedal arch (Fig. 12.14). There are several types of transposition flaps, including the single-lobe flap, bilobed flap, Z-plasty, rhomboid flap, flap of Dufourmentel, double-Z rhomboid flap, and the 30-degree transposition flap (20,63,71,125).

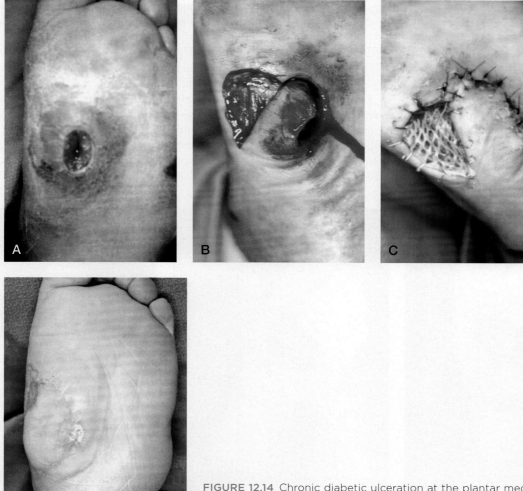

FIGURE 12.14 Chronic diabetic ulceration at the plantar medial aspect of the foot **(A)** closed with a transposition flap created after wound excision **(B)**. After the flap was inset into the original defect, a split-thickness skin graft was used to cover the donor site **(C)**. **D.** Final clinical postoperative outcome.

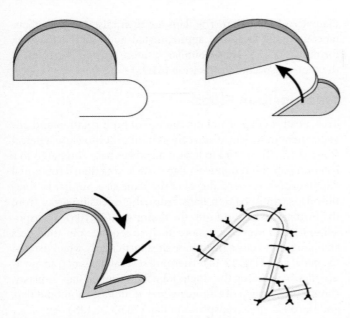

FIGURE 12.15 The single-lobe flap, also known as the "Schrudde" or "slide-swing plasty," may be used to close circular, oval, and semicircular defects. (With permission from Blume PA, Key JJ. Local random flaps for soft tissue coverage of the diabetic foot. In: Zgonis T, ed. Surgical reconstruction of the diabetic foot and ankle. Philadelphia: Lippincott Williams & Wilkins, 2009:153.)

Single-Lobe Flap

The single-lobe flap, also known as the "slide-swing plasty" or "Schrudde" flap, may be used to close circular, oval, and semicircular defects (Fig. 12.15). In the foot, it has been described for removal of small digital lesions such as mucoid cysts and intractable keratoses (22,108). In the diabetic foot, it serves to

cover excised wounds, particularly plantar to the metatarsal heads (1,3,22,60,101).

For circular defects, a lobe-shaped flap is created with the base positioned 90 degrees to the defect (108). Note that in thicker skin, the flap can shorten by up to one-third during transposition in which case it is recommended that the flap pivot less than 90 degrees (107,109). The flap is designed with a length-to-width ratio of roughly 3:1, with the flap itself being smaller in size than the original defect (33). Once the lobe is raised at the desired level, it is sutured into the defect, with key sutures at the distal aspect of the flap. The donor site is then able to be closed primarily (Fig. 12.16). For oval defects, a similar flap is designed; however, the base of the flap is placed at a 60-degree angle to the defect (84).

Single-lobe flaps are advantageous because they can close large defects, and the broad base of the flap provides good vascularity. Additionally, because the lobe is designed to close both oval and circular defects, it avoids creation of deficits in healthy tissue that other geometric flaps, such as the rhomboid flap, create (102,106). Disadvantages of the single-lobe flap include shortening that can occur in thicker skin and the potential for increased tension for simple closure. If this occurs, an additional lobe may be created to redistribute the tension.

Bilobed Flap

The bilobed flap consists of 2 flaps that share a common pedicle in order to fill a defect (Fig. 12.17). In the diabetic foot, it is used to close defects on the plantar surface of the forefoot and rearfoot but has also been described for excising toe lesions overlying the interphalangeal joints (47,53,60,69,87,103,118). It allows for greater movement of skin over a larger area than the single transposition flap, being used for defects measuring 1 to 3 cm in diameter (56,111,113). The bilobed flap utilizes

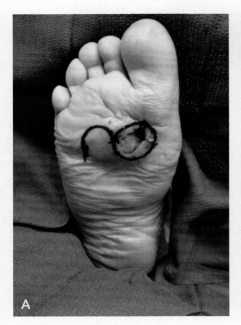
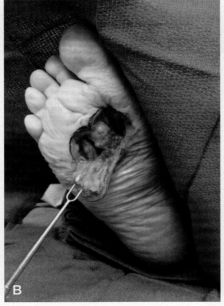
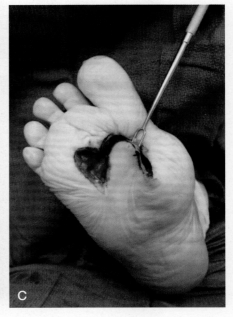

FIGURE 12.16 Intraoperative picture of a circular excision for a plantar ulceration **(A)** and transposition of adjacent single-lobe flap **(B,C)**, with primary closure at the donor site **(D)** and postoperative outcome **(E)**. *(continued)*

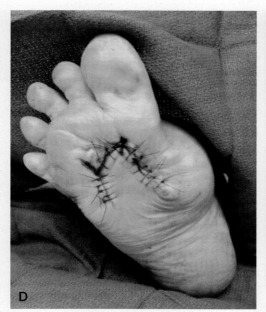
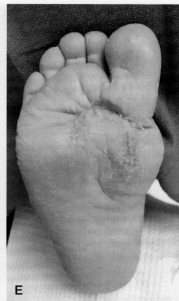

FIGURE 12.16 *(Continued)*

the "Robin Hood" principle of borrowing from the rich laxity of neighboring skin and transposing it to a relatively poor area of inelastic skin (112).

Classically, the first lobe is created 90 degrees from the circular defect and the second lobe is made 90 degrees to the first, but this is not always required (60,106,109). Some authors describe varying angles, ranging from 45 to 90 degrees to each other. In the plantar foot, it is discouraged to make angles any greater than 60 degrees (53,113). The size of the first lobe is generally 75% of the width of the original defect, whereas the second lobe is generally 50% of the width of the original defect (60,114). Flap size has also been described as having the first lobe being 20% smaller than the original defect and the second lobe being 20% smaller than the size of the first lobe (102,112). The flaps are then raised using atraumatic technique, taking care to undermine only the base where rotation occurs. The first lobe is meant to close the original defect, whereas the second lobe closes the first lobe's donor site. The second lobe's defect is then closed primarily (Fig. 12.18). The 2 frenula of the lobes should be sutured first, followed by

the lobes. Some authors feel that it is easier to suture the second lobe into its defect first, followed by the first lobe into the original defect (115). The second lobe's donor site can then be closed primarily.

Huang et al. (63) described a variation of the bilobed flap, meant to decrease dog ear formation and distortion. The authors suggested rotating each lobe only 45 degrees with the length of the second lobe being extended. A Burrow's triangle is then incorporated in the original flap design (56). The trilobed flap has also been described in order to reduce resultant dog ears; however, it comes at the cost of mobilizing more skin (109).

Bilobed flap advantages include the ability to close lesions over areas of limited skin mobility with each flap smaller than the original defect (56,111). Disadvantages include the length of the incisions as well as the varying directions required of each flap (109,116).

Z-Plasty

The Z-plasty is a type of transposition flap where a "Z"-shaped incision is made, resulting in 2 triangular flaps which are

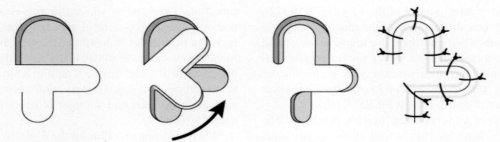

FIGURE 12.17 The bilobed flap consists of two flaps that are separated by an angle and share a common pedicle. (With permission from Blume PA, Key JJ. Local random flaps for soft tissue coverage of the diabetic foot. In: Zgonis T, ed. Surgical reconstruction of the diabetic foot and ankle. Philadelphia: Lippincott Williams & Wilkins, 2009:155.)

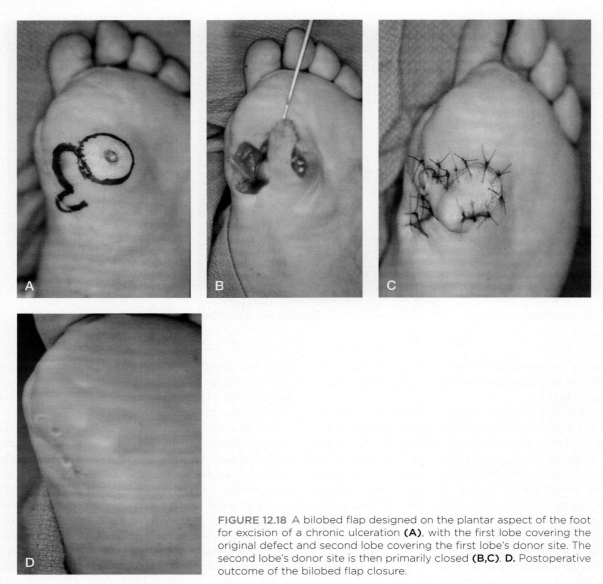

FIGURE 12.18 A bilobed flap designed on the plantar aspect of the foot for excision of a chronic ulceration **(A)**, with the first lobe covering the original defect and second lobe covering the first lobe's donor site. The second lobe's donor site is then primarily closed **(B,C)**. **D.** Postoperative outcome of the bilobed flap closure.

transposed (Fig. 12.19). It is frequently used for lengthening scar contracture, breaking up linear scars, rearranging the contour of soft tissues, and for construction and widening of web spaces (3,62). It can also be used for correcting congenital fifth toe contractures and reconstructing burn scar contractures on the dorsal and plantar aspects of the foot (117,119,122). Similarly, this flap can also be used as an adjunct to improve movement of another flap and therefore improve the overall cosmesis of the foot (36,52). The Z-plasty should only be used if the area in question has sufficient skin laxity perpendicular to the direction of contracture. It should not be used if the scar or area of contracture does not cross the RSTL (62).

Symmetry is very important for incision planning. The lateral and central limb lengths as well as the angles must all be equal to each other for ease of transposition into the donor sites. This design will result in two 30-60-90-degree triangles (3). The length gained by performing the Z-plasty

is determined by both the length of the incisions as well as the angles between the incisions. Although a 90-degree angle will theoretically result in 120% increase in central limb length, it creates 10 times more tension and would likely result in dehiscence or contracture in the opposite direction. Conversely, when the angles are too acute, it not only causes less central arm lengthening but also can increase the risk of ischemia at the tips of the flaps (118). Ideally, a 60-degree Z-plasty is the best balance of lengthening and tension, creating 75% gain in length (36,119). If the surrounding skin is extremely taut, then a smaller angle, such as 45 degrees, and a longer central incision should be used (Table 12.2).

When planning incisions for the Z-plasty, the central line of the "Z" will be made longitudinally over the line of contracture or over the area to be lengthened. The other 2 incisions are then made from each end of the central line at either 45- or

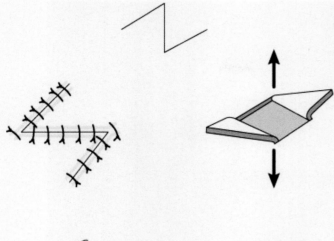

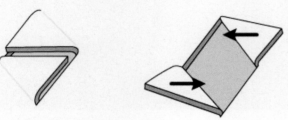

TABLE 12.2

Percentage Increase of Central Arm Length of Z-Plasty Based on Angle Size

Angle of Central Limb to Lateral Limb (degrees)	Increase of Central Limb Length (%)
30	25
45	50
60	75
75	100
90	120

FIGURE 12.19 The Z-plasty with 2 triangular flaps being transposed by using a Z-shaped incision. The Z-plasty is a useful technique for lengthening a linear scar contracture and realigning a scar within the lines of maximal extensibility (LME). (With permission from Blume PA, Key JJ. Local random flaps for soft tissue coverage of the diabetic foot. In: Zgonis T, ed. Surgical reconstruction of the diabetic foot and ankle. Philadelphia: Lippincott Williams & Wilkins, 2009:157.)

60-degree angles and all of equal length. These arms should ideally be parallel to the RSTL. The flaps are then carefully raised below the subdermal plexus, including the subdermal vascular plexus, taking care to avoid undermining the tips of the flaps (3,98). An imaginary line connecting the 2 noncentral incisions becomes the new central line of the final Z after the flaps have been transposed. The key sutures should be first placed in the midpoint of the new central arm, with subsequent sutures at the base of the flaps (Fig. 12.20). Oblique sutures should be used to advance the tip of each flap, with apical stitches used to inset the apices.

If excess tension is created across the new central limb of the Z-plasty, or if the original design was slightly larger than desired,

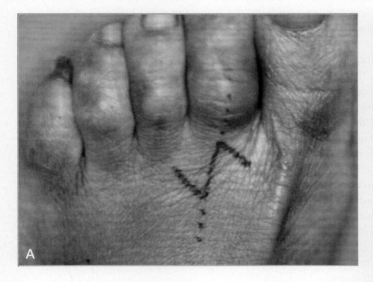

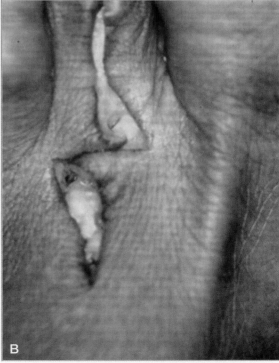

FIGURE 12.20 A Z-plasty is shown over a contracted second toe **(A)**, followed by transposition of the flaps **(B)** and arthrodesis of the proximal interphalangeal joint **(C)**. *(continued)*

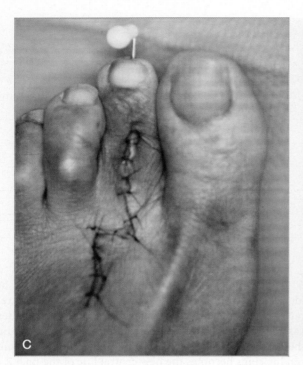
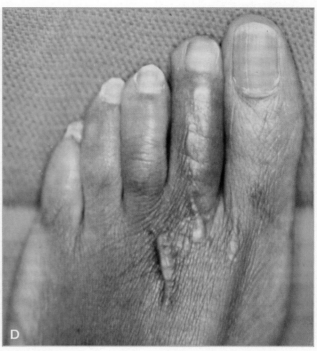

FIGURE 12.20 *(Continued)* **D.** Final clinical postoperative outcome. (With permission from Blume PA, Key JJ. Local random flaps for soft tissue coverage of the diabetic foot. In: Zgonis T, ed. Surgical reconstruction of the diabetic foot and ankle. Philadelphia: Lippincott Williams & Wilkins, 2009:157.)

then a "mini Z-plasty" can be performed to correct problems resulting from poor planning (85,119). With the mini Z-plasty, 2 lines are extended out from the central arm of the larger Z and made parallel to its outer limbs. The length of these new limbs should be less than half of the length of the larger limbs and should be placed within the central one-third of the central arm of the larger Z. It is important that the incisions should be made just through the dermal layer (85).

There is debate whether one large Z-plasty is more advantageous over multiple smaller consecutive Z-plasties (Fig. 12.21). Proponents of the large Z-plasty argue that the larger flaps have better blood supply and result in less central axis tension as compared to multiple Z-plasties (3,62). However, in the digits, larger Z-plasties may constrict the digit horizontally, thus compromising the vascular supply to the digit; therefore, in the digit, it may be better to use multiple Z-plasties (36,60).

The double opposing Z-plasty can be used when the anatomy or vascularity of the area does not permit the use of a large single Z-plasty (62,69). In the foot, it is useful in releasing scar contracture and for desyndactylization of toes (96). Two Z-plasties are designed so that the central arm of the Z is along the same line. The 2 Z-plasties are then created such that 1 "Z" is backward and 1 is forward, in relation to each other. The flaps are then elevated and transposed in a manner similar to single Z-plasties.

Rhomboid or Limberg Flap

The rhomboid or Limberg flap (Fig. 12.22) is a versatile flap that allows for closure of a primary defect with reduced

suture line tension (24,28). It can be used to close a rhomboid-shaped defect but more typically is used for larger circular defects (25,29,30). The rhomboid flap is frequently used in the foot for closure of wounds. It allows for correction of an isolated metatarsal head lesion with simultaneous access to the bone for any necessary procedure such

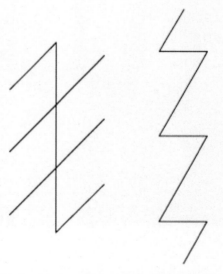

FIGURE 12.21 A schematic diagram showing multiple Z-plasties with post-transposition outcome. (With permission from Blume PA, Key JJ. Local random flaps for soft tissue coverage of the diabetic foot. In: Zgonis T, ed. Surgical reconstruction of the diabetic foot and ankle. Philadelphia: Lippincott Williams & Wilkins, 2009:158.)

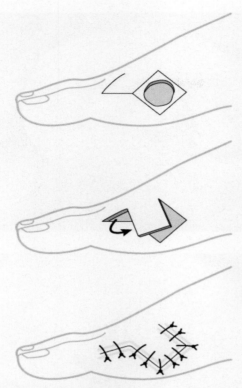

FIGURE 12.22 The rhomboid or Limberg flap is typically used to close a rhomboid-shaped defect but may be used to close circular defects. A flap of exactly the same shape and size as the defect is raised and transposed 60 degrees into the defect. Although the flap covers the original defect 100%, it only closes half of the total defect; the remaining defect is closed primarily. (With permission from Blume PA, Key JJ. Local random flaps for soft tissue coverage of the diabetic foot. In: Zgonis T, ed. Surgical reconstruction of the diabetic foot and ankle. Philadelphia: Lippincott Williams & Wilkins, 2009:162.)

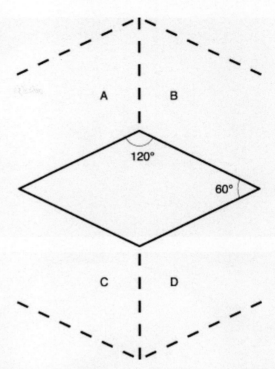

FIGURE 12.23 The versatility of the rhomboid flap is shown on this schematic diagram. Two parallel lines are drawn in the same direction as the lines of maximal extensibility (LME) or perpendicular to the relaxed skin tension lines (RSTL). These are drawn tangential to the defect. Two additional lines are drawn that complete the design of an equilateral parallelogram or rhombus with 60- and 120-degree angles. Hereafter, 4 possible rhomboid flaps can be drawn and used to close the primary defect. (With permission from Blume PA, Key JJ. Local random flaps for soft tissue coverage of the diabetic foot. In: Zgonis T, ed. Surgical reconstruction of the diabetic foot and ankle. Philadelphia: Lippincott Williams & Wilkins, 2009:163.)

as condylectomy, ostectomy, or metatarsal head resection. Although this flap may be used for plantar lesions, it can also be used on the dorsum of the foot though greater mobility is required for closure (42). The rhomboid flap has also been described for plantar closure of desyndactylization (44,48,124,129).

The primary defect is converted to a four-sided parallelogram with arms of equal length drawn tangentially to the defect with angles of 60 and 120 degrees (30,128). This allows for the possibility of 4 different flaps to be raised from 1 rhomboid (Fig. 12.23). Two of the parallel lines should be drawn in the same direction as the LME. An incision of equal length of the rhomboid should be extended perpendicularly from 1 of the 120-degree sides. A second incision is then extended from here, angled at 60 degrees from this newly made incision and parallel to 1 of the arms of the proximal arms of the rhombus. The flap is then lifted and rotated 60 degrees into the defect, with the donor site closed primarily (Figs. 12.24 and 12.25). The flap redistributes and redirects tension from the donor site to the recipient site in 90 degrees (33,60,128).

Flap of Dufourmentel

The flap of Dufourmentel is more versatile than the Limberg flap because it can be used for rhombic defects of any acute angle, not just those of 60 and 120 degrees. Although more difficult than the classic Limberg flap, it is especially useful for rhombic defects with an acute angle of 60 to 90 degrees, or when excision of additional skin to create a more acute angle is undesirable. If the acute angle is <60 degrees, then the flap becomes wider than the primary defect and the use of the flap is not advantageous (46,77).

First, the defect is excised in the shape of a rhombus or an equilateral parallelogram. The short diagonal of the rhombus is extended from the tip of 1 of the less acute sides. From that same point, 1 of the sides of the defect is also extended. The angle formed by these 2 lines is then bisected by a line equal in length to the sides of the rhombus and the corresponding line forms 1 of the sides of the flap. The final side of the flap is incised equal in length to all the other sides of the rhombus but parallel to the long axis of the defect. Similarly, as with the Limberg flap, the use of calipers may facilitate the design, although the addition of a protractor may also be helpful (46).

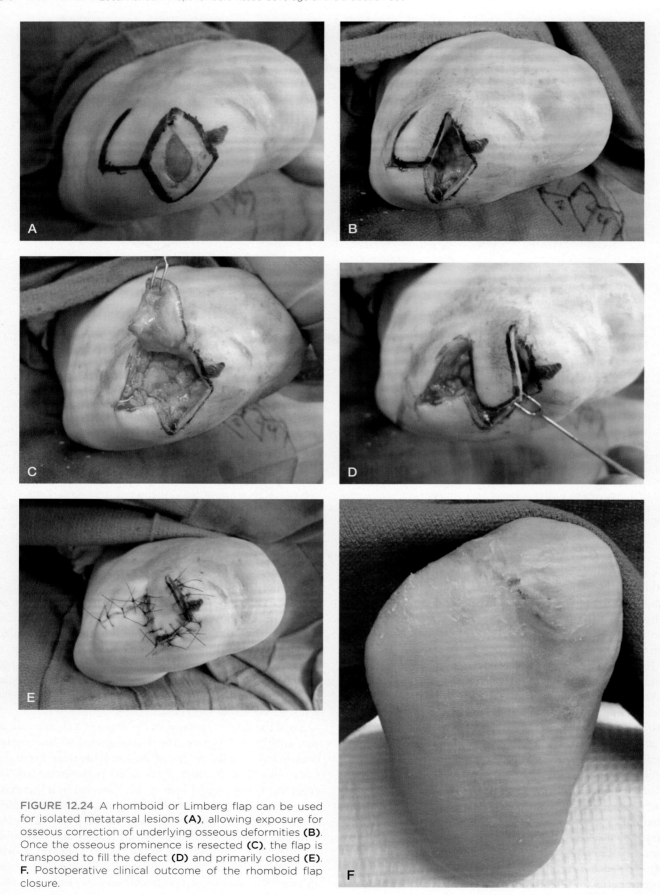

FIGURE 12.24 A rhomboid or Limberg flap can be used for isolated metatarsal lesions **(A)**, allowing exposure for osseous correction of underlying osseous deformities **(B)**. Once the osseous prominence is resected **(C)**, the flap is transposed to fill the defect **(D)** and primarily closed **(E)**. **F.** Postoperative clinical outcome of the rhomboid flap closure.

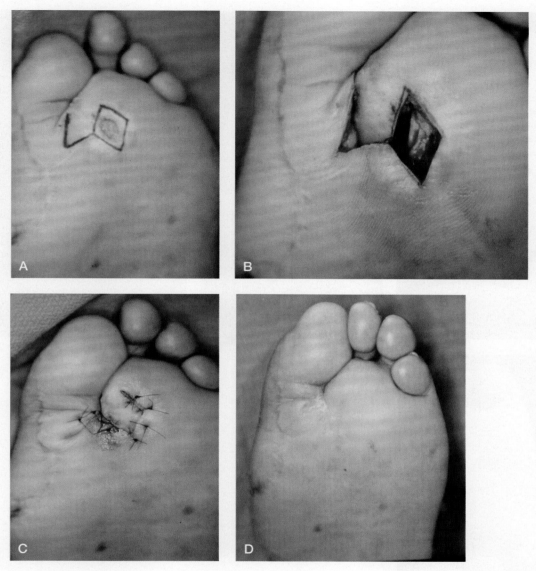

FIGURE 12.25 An example of a rhomboid flap for a diabetic plantar ulceration **(A)**, with excision of the defect and flap creation **(B)**. The flap is then inset and primarily closed **(C)**. **D.** Final clinical postoperative outcome.

Double-Z Rhomboid Flap

The double-Z rhomboid flap implements the classic rhomboid flap with 2 Z-plasties. In the foot, it can be used for fifth metatarsal head pathologies as well as different forefoot and rearfoot conditions. It can be used in the plantar foot because the transposition of the Z-flaps allows for creation of a non–weight-bearing incision if planned appropriately. Surgical technique involves creation of a rhomboid shape around the defect to be excised. Two of the parallel lines should be parallel to the direction of the RSTL, whereas the other 2 parallel lines are placed to create 120- and 60-degree angles (70,121,122). Two Z-plasties are then drawn on opposing sides of the rhombus, with the central arms being extensions of 2 of the parallel lines from the rhombus (Figs. 12.26 and 12.27). The flaps are then lifted similarly to the Z-plasty and are inset (60,121,123).

Thirty-Degree Transposition Flap

A variation of the rhomboid flap, the 30-degree transposition flap contains a 30-degree angle at the distal end of the typical rhomboid flap. It was found that a 30-degree angulation will not cause cosmetically significant bulges that plague the typical rhomboid flap (84,126). Because one drawback of using a 30-degree distal angle is a significantly increased incision length, the 30-degree angle is typically combined with an "M-plasty," which shortens the rhomboid shape.

The distal end of the flap is designed parallel to the RSTL. The final edge of the flap is at a 30-degree angle to the distal end of the flap. The flap is transposed in a similar fashion to the rhomboid flap. The sides of the M-plasty are advanced into the side of the defect. Although more difficult than the classic Limberg flap, it has the advantages of dispersing tension more evenly around the flap, thereby closing with less tension (84).

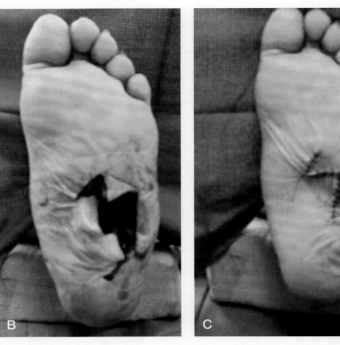

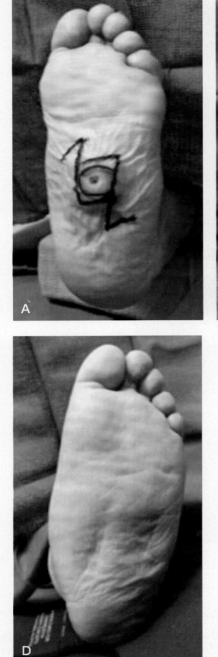

FIGURE 12.26 A double-Z rhomboid flap uses the technique of 2 Z-plasties to correct the soft tissue defect **(A)**. The defect is excised **(B)** and flaps are transposed **(C)**, with no skin tension postoperatively **(D)**.

POSTOPERATIVE CARE

The postoperative care of each local flap is extremely important and requires close observation. Each patient who undergoes reconstruction heals at his or her own pace, so one should avoid premature suture removal (63). Bandages over skin flaps should be loose and well-padded and must allow for normal postoperative edema. Bandages that are too tight might alter blood flow within the flap. Venous congestion is a common sequela of tight bandages. Patients must be restricted to bed rest, non–weight-bearing of the affected lower extremity, and strict nondependency of the lower extremity for 1 to 2 weeks. After that period of strict bed rest, dependency of the lower extremity by sitting and dangling may be permitted (60).

Some authors feel that compressive wraps, such as Unna boots or elastic stockings, are essential in the early ambulatory period. They may be replaced by fitted elastic stockings or light bandages after the wounds are stable and the edema has been resolved. Proper footwear that redistributes weight away from the operative site should be used until the wound has healed completely to avoid recurrent ulceration or dehiscence of the surgical site (60,64).

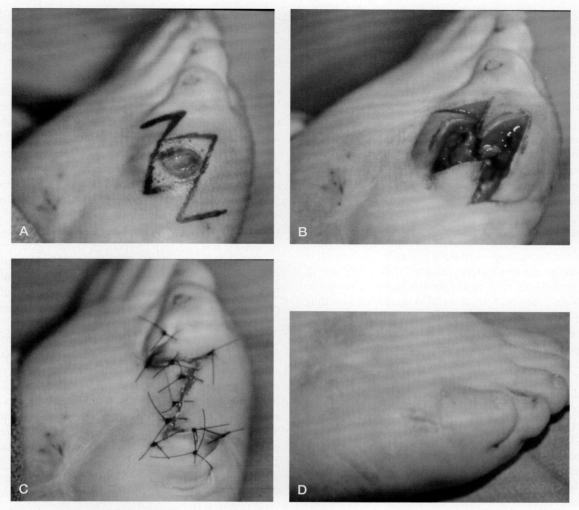

FIGURE 12.27 An example of a double-Z rhomboid flap on the lateral aspect of the foot **(A)**. The defect is excised **(B)**, and flaps are transposed and primarily closed **(C)**. **D.** Final clinical postoperative outcome of the double-Z rhomboid flap closure.

Wet-to-dry dressings, championed in the past and useful on initial débridement of the wound, impede normal healing by removing healthy neoepithelium and granulation tissue every time the cotton dressing is ripped off the wound (17). The use of moist dressings on clean, granulating wounds improves the wound environment. The dressings not only provide protection against further bacterial contamination but also maintain moisture balance, optimize the wound pH, absorb fibrinous fluids, and reduce local pain. A variety of dressings are currently available that can be targeted to specific characteristics of the wound. However, moist normal saline dressings are probably sufficient for the majority of wounds. These inexpensive dressings are highly absorptive of exudative drainage and maintain the moist environment (3,64,65).

Postoperative evaluation of the viability of a flap may be performed by assessing bleeding from small stab or puncture wounds (66). Using an 18-gauge needle or a no. 11 scalpel blade, the flap is penetrated. Absence of bleeding from the resultant wound may indicate arterial failure of the flap, whereas delayed bright red bleeding can indicate some degree of arterial spasm.

Cyanotic bleeding that promptly converts to bright red blood can indicate some amount of venous congestion. Conversely, normal arterial perfusion will display brisk, bright red bleeding. In 1 study, intraoperative application of 60% dimethyl sulfoxide solution onto the entire flap, followed by application every 2 hours for the first 48 hours postoperatively, and then every 4 hours during postoperative days 3 through 10 was shown to help reduce ischemia to the skin flap by >36% (67).

COMPLICATIONS

Extrinsic postoperative complications are confirmations of both intraoperative suspicions and judgmental errors and can be divided into preoperative, intraoperative, and postoperative causes (66).

Preoperative Local Flap Complications

Preoperative flap complications can include poor flap design, which may result in an inadequate donor size or a flap that is not mobile enough to reach the defect. In addition, medical comorbidities can lead to indirect and direct flap complications. Diabetic patients, especially those with elevations at hemoglobin A_{1c}, are known to have a reduced healing capacity (34). More specifically, every 1% increase in hemoglobin A_{1c} is associated with a daily wound-area healing rate decrease of 0.028 cm²/day (68). Preoperative nutritional levels, including albumin, serum protein, and total lymphocyte counts are important parameters that must be evaluated prior to surgery. Patients who are active smokers are found to have an increased risk for complications in skin flap surgery (5,69). Hypertension, anemia, and the presence of an infection can also lead to flap complications.

Intraoperative Local Flap Complications

Intraoperative flap complications are usually the result of poor technique or insufficient surgical skills. The use of traumatic techniques, such as improperly grabbing or pinching the tissue, excessive retraction of skin and surrounding tissues, or the use of aggressive monopolar cautery dissection should be avoided. Incisions should be made with the blade perpendicular to the skin, and the incision should be made with 1 single movement. Multiple strokes lead to small pockets of dead space and ischemia along the incision line. Care should be taken not to kink or twist the pedicle or base of the flap during the procedure. Undermining of the flap should only be used when it is necessary for flap mobility and must be kept to a minimum (3,80). Excessive undermining reduces the vascularity of the flap and may lead to flap failure. Poor wound bed preparation is a common cause of failure because grafts and flaps rely on the vascularity of wound beds.

Postoperative Local Flap Complications

Postoperative complications resulting in compromised vascularity to the flap include infection, tight bandages, shearing forces, flap tension due to a hematoma/seroma, venous congestion, edema, or kinking of the flap's pedicle. These factors all prevent ideal contact between the graft/flap and wound bed, which ultimately inhibit revascularization (13,51,81). Additionally, patient noncompliance, such as premature dependency of the lower extremity or early weight bearing, will most likely lead to flap failure.

Intrinsic postoperative complications are functions of the physiology of flaps and metabolic, hemodynamic, and neurologic changes that occur during the elevation and transplantation of the flap. The ischemic insult occurring secondary to flap elevation creates havoc at the local metabolic level. When there is inadequate oxygen supply, tissues convert to anaerobic metabolism, and oxygen, glucose, and adenosine triphosphate levels drop dramatically (60,66). Subsequently, carbon dioxide and lactic acid levels rise, as does the production of toxic superoxide radicals (82). Hemodynamic changes in skin flaps were studied by Palmer et al. (94) using radioactive isotopes. They determined that flow at the base of a pedicle flap

remained at 100%, but that flow at the tip of the flap decreased to 18% on the first postoperative day. The flow gradually increased to 65% in the first week and 75% to 90% in 2 weeks postoperatively (94).

Necrosis of a flap typically occurs in the zone of choke vessels that connect adjacent arterial territories (3,33–36,38–46). The survival length of each flap is dependent on the distance between the perforator at the base of the flap and the next dominant perforator along the length of the flap. Excessive wound tension can cause disruption of the wound, crosshatching stitch marks, widening and thickening of scars, and necrosis of the flap (62). Tension may be inherent to an inaccurate flap design, poor choice of flap, inappropriate closure, or the result of underlying hematoma or edema. Adequate skin closure can also help prevent necrosis. Anatomic reapproximation of the deep layers helps remove extensive tension from the skin (55). Tension on flaps for foot reconstruction can often be avoided when concomitant bone reconstruction is considered. Flap necrosis caused by inadequate blood supply is a common postoperative complication in reconstructive surgery (110).

It is critical to monitor flap viability with objective tests including capillary refill, warmth of the flap, Doppler ultrasound, tissue pH, $TcPo_2$, differential thermometry, plethysmography, angiography, and fluorescein dye. Fluorescein dye is considered by some to be the most useful in assessing viability of the flap both preoperatively and postoperatively. The 1.5 mg/kg of fluorescein dye is injected intravenously with peak serum concentrations usually obtained within 20 minutes (51,68,72,73,78). The flap can then be examined with the use of a Wood's lamp. Although an excellent method for evaluating flap circulation, it may underestimate flap survival (4,60). If the flap appears to be under extensive tension, is dusky or white, or does not have an adequate capillary fill time, then sutures should be removed and the cause needs to be determined.

Because there are many causes for postoperative flap ischemia, research has been performed to identify therapeutic targets within the body to enhance blood vessel growth and flap survival. For example, adipose-derived mesenchymal stem cells, found within the adipose tissue have been shown to possess angiogenic potential, by selectively inducing neovascularization, and increasing the viability of random pattern skin flaps. Histologic examination has also demonstrated a statistically significant increase in capillary density. The mechanism by which this works is believed to be the result of direct differentiation of adipose-derived stem cells into endothelial cells and the indirect effect of angiogenic growth factor released from adipose-derived stem cells (74,130). Vascular endothelial growth factor (VEGF) also plays an important role in inducing angiogenesis by increasing ischemic flap neovascularization and augmenting the surviving areas. In 1 murine study, VEGF-transduced mesenchymal stem cells expressed VEGF highly both in vitro and in vivo. The mesenchymal stem cells that were transplanted into ischemic mouse flaps survived and incorporated into the capillary networks of these flaps. The capillary density and the blood perfusion of these flaps were significantly higher than those in the control groups (75).

Another postoperative issue that may be encountered is the potential for flap infection. Generally, if the bacterial count on the flap is greater than 100,000 organisms per gram, there is a statistically significant probability the graft will not take. However, certain organisms such as group A beta hemolytic *Streptococcus* and *Pseudomonas aeruginosa* can cause graft infection in much smaller quantities (50,76). In the presence of infection and cellulitis, oral or intravenous antimicrobial therapy should be initiated on the basis of the suspected pathogen and clinical findings. After the bacterial infection has been controlled, small wounds usually can be excised and closed primarily. Large open wounds, however, are treated with a staged approach, with frequent surgical débridements and establishment of granulation base. The clean wounds can then be closed with healthy tissue, with the use of local or free-flap coverage and soft tissue repair. Any remaining extrinsic or intrinsic pressures can be reduced with the postoperative use of orthoses (19).

REVISIONAL SURGERY

In the event that a local random flap fails, it is important to understand the underlying cause of flap failure. If underlying infection is the cause of failure, treatment involves surgical débridement of infected or nonviable soft tissue and bone with copious irrigation. Cultures can be obtained and antibiotic therapy can be initiated with local wound care. If the flap fails without local infection, the failed portion of the flap can be surgically débrided with application of a negative pressure wound therapy or biologic dressing over the exposed tissue. If vascular insufficiency is suspected, consultation to a vascular surgeon may be warranted.

Conclusion

In conclusion, local flap reconstruction of pedal defects can be accomplished with a variety of different techniques. Although each flap has its own unique set of indications, there are several key factors that must be considered to increase flap success. Patient health should be optimized, specifically adequate vascular workup and absence of infection prior to surgical planning. The important operative factors to consider are flap placement, atraumatic surgical techniques, minimal tension with small diameter suture, and avoidance of deep sutures. Postoperatively, strict non–weight-bearing and lower extremity elevation will be beneficial to preventing venous congestion and subsequent flap failure. It is important to remember that local flaps utilized for closure of foot defects should be located within the higher level of any treatment algorithm. The diversity, versatility of the flaps, as well as the reproducibility and functional outcomes indicate the numerous benefits of local random flaps in the successful treatment of diabetic foot pathology.

References

1. Akhtar S, Ahmad I, Khan AH, et al. Modalities of soft-tissue coverage in diabetic foot ulcers. Adv Skin Wound Care 2015;28: 157–162.
2. Alnaeb ME, Boutin A, Crabtree VP, et al. Assessment of lower extremity peripheral arterial disease using a novel automated optical device. Vasc Endovascular Surg 2007;41:522–527.
3. Aoki R, Pennington DG, Hyakusoku H. Flap-in-flap method for enhancing the advancement of a V-Y flap. J Plast Reconstr Aesthet Surg 2006;59:653–657.
4. Aranmolate S, Attah AA. Bilobed flap in the release of postburn mentosternal contracture. Plast Reconstr Surg 1989;83:356–361.
5. Archer KA, Lembo T Jr, Haber JA. Protein S deficiency and lower-extremity arterial thrombosis: complicating a common presentation. J Am Podiatr Med Assoc 2007;97:151–155.
6. Ashbell TS. The rhomboid excision and Limberg flap reconstruction in difficult tense-skin areas. Plast Reconstr Surg 1982;69:724.
7. Askar I. Double reverse V-Y-plasty in postburn scar contractures: a new modification of V-Y-plasty. Burns 2003;29:721–725.
8. Asken S. A modified M-plasty. J Dermatol Surg Oncol 1986;12: 369–373.
9. Atasoy E, Ioakimidis E, Kasdan ML, et al. Reconstruction of the amputated finger tip with a triangular volar flap. A new surgical procedure. J Bone Joint Surg Am 1970;52A:921–926.
10. Attinger C. Soft-tissue coverage for lower-extremity trauma. Orthop Clin North Am 1995;26:295–334.
11. Attinger CE. Use of soft tissue techniques for salvage of the diabetic foot. In: Kominsky S, ed. Medical and surgical management of the diabetic foot. St. Louis: Mosby, 1994:323–366.
12. Attinger C, Bulan EJ, Blume PA. Pharmacological and mechanical management of wounds. In: Mathes SJ, ed. Plastic surgery, vol 1. St. Louis: Elsevier, 2006:863–899.
13. Attinger C, Cooper P, Blume P. Vascular anatomy of the foot and ankle. In: Jurkiewicz MJ, Culbertson JH, eds. Operative techniques in plastic and reconstructive surgery. Los Angeles: General Publishing Group, 1996:183–198.
14. Attinger C, Cooper P, Blume P, et al. The safest surgical incisions and amputations applying the angiosome principles and using the Doppler to assess the arterial-arterial connections of the foot and ankle. Foot Ankle Clin 2001;6:745–799.
15. Attinger CE, Evans KK, Bulan E, et al. Angiosomes of the foot and ankle and clinical implications for limb salvage: reconstruction, incisions, and revascularization. Plast Reconstr Surg 2006;117(7 suppl):261–293.
16. Barret JP, Herndon DN, McCauley RL. Use of previously burned skin as random cutaneous local flaps in pediatric burn reconstruction. Burns 2002;28:500–502.
17. Becker H. The rhomboid-to-W technique for excision of some skin lesions and closure. Plast Reconstr Surg 1979;64:444–447.
18. Benitez E, Sumpio BJ, Chin J, et al. Contemporary assessment of foot perfusion in patients with critical limb ischemia. Semin Vasc Surg 2014;27:3–15.
19. Bhattacharya V, Bhattacharya S. Grafts and flaps for the lower limb. In: Khanna AK, Tiwary SK, eds. Ulcers of the lower extremity. New Delhi, India: Springer Publishing, 2016:423–444.
20. Blake BP, Simonetta CJ, Maher IA. Transposition flaps: principles and locations. Dermatol Surg 2015;41(suppl 10):255–264.

21. Blume PA, Donegan R, Schmidt BM. The role of plastic surgery for soft tissue coverage of the diabetic foot and ankle. Clin Podiatr Med Surg 2014;31:127–150.

22. Blume PA, Moore JC, Novicki DC. Digital mucoid cyst excision by using the bilobed flap technique and arthroplastic resection. J Foot Ankle Surg 2005;44:44–48.

23. Blume PA, Paragas LK, Sumpio BE, et al. Single-stage surgical treatment of noninfected diabetic foot ulcers. Plast Reconstr Surg 2002;109:601–609.

24. Borges AF. Choosing the correct Limberg flap. Plast Reconstr Surg 1978;62:542–545.

25. Borges AF. The rhombic flap. Plast Reconstr Surg 1981;67:458–466.

26. Borges AF. The W-plastic versus the Z-plastic scar revision. Plast Reconstr Surg 1969;44:58–62.

27. Bosch E, Kreitner KF, Peirano MF, et al. Safety and efficacy of gadofosveset-enhanced MR angiography for evaluation of pedal arterial disease: multicenter comparative phase 3 study. AJR Am J Roentgenol 2008;190:179–186.

28. Bray DA. Clinical applications of the rhomboid flap. Arch Otolaryngol 1983;109:37–42.

29. Brobyn TJ, Cramer LM, Hulnick SJ, et al. Facial resurfacing with the Limberg flap. Clin Plast Surg 1976;3:481–490.

30. Budd ME, Hovsepian R, Basseri B, et al. Flaps. In: Guyuron B, Eriksson E, Persing JA, et al., eds. Plastic surgery: indications and practice. Philadelphia: Saunders Elsevier, 2009:67–78.

31. Callegari PR, Taylor GI, Caddy CM, et al. An anatomic review of the delay phenomenon: I. Experimental studies. Plast Reconstr Surg 1992;89:397–407.

32. Chang TJ, Stanifer EG, Jimenez AL. Plastic repair techniques: skin plasties and local flaps. In: Tucker GA, ed. Reconstructive surgery of the foot and leg update 93. Tucker, GA: Podiatry Institute, 1993:52–65.

33. Chasmar LR. The versatile rhomboid (Limberg) flap. Can J Plast Surg 2007;15:67–71.

34. Christman AL, Selvin E, Margolis DJ, et al. Hemoglobin A1c predicts healing rate in diabetic wounds. J Invest Dermatol 2011;131:2121–2127.

35. Clemens MW, Attinger CE. Angiosomes and wound care in the diabetic foot. Foot Ankle Clin 2010;15:439–464.

36. Clemens MW, Attinger CE. Functional reconstruction of the diabetic foot. Semin Plast Surg 2010;24:43–56.

37. Coban YK, Aytekin AH, Tenekeci G. Skin graft harvesting and donor site selection. In: Spear M, ed. Skin grafts—indications, applications and current research. Rijeka, Croatia: InTech, 2011.

38. Colen LB, Replogle SL, Mathes SJ. The V-Y plantar flap for reconstruction of the forefoot. Plast Reconstr Surg 1988;81:220–228.

39. Crawford ME, Dockery GL. Use of Z-skin plasty in scar revisions and skin contractures of the lower extremity. J Am Podiatr Med Assoc 1995;85:28–35.

40. Daniel RK, Kerrigan CL. Principles and physiology of skin flap surgery. In: McCarthy JG, ed. Plastic surgery general principles. Philadelphia: Saunders, 1990:275–328.

41. Dayton PD, Griffiths T. Biwinged excision for round pedal lesions. J Foot Ankle Surg 1996;35:244–249.

42. Di Santis EP, Elias BLF, Andraus IN, et al. Rhomboid flap: an option to many anatomical regions. J Adv Plast Surg 2015;1:14–18.

43. Dockery GL. Single-lobe rotation flaps. J Am Podiatr Med Assoc 1995;85:36–40.

44. Dockery GL, Christensen JC. Principles and descriptions of design of skin flaps for use on the lower extremity. Clin Podiatr Med Surg 1986;3:563–577.

45. Dockery GL, Crawford ME. Lower extremity soft tissue & cutaneous plastic surgery. Philadelphia: Saunders, 2006.

46. Dufourmentel C. Closure of limited loss of cutaneous substance. So-called "LLL" diamond-shaped L rotation-flap [in French]. Ann Chir Plast 1962;7:60–66.

47. Esser JFS. Gestielte lokale nasenplastik mit zweizipfligem lappen deckung des sekundaren detektes vom ersten zipfel durch den zweiten. Dtsch Z Chir 1918;143:385–390.

48. Frick L, Fraisse B, Wavreille G, et al. Results of surgical treatment in simple syndactily using a commissural dorsal flap. About 54 procedures [in French]. Chir Main 2008;27:76–82.

49. Frykberg RG, Zgonis T, Armstrong DG, et al. Diabetic foot disorders: a clinical practical guideline (2006 revision). J Foot Ankle Surg 2006;45(suppl 5):1–66.

50. Gidumal R, Carl A, Evanski P, et al. Functional evaluation of nonsensate free flap to the sole of the foot. Foot Ankle 1986;7:118–123.

51. Gillies HD, Millard DR Jr. The principles and art of plastic surgery. Boston: Little, Brown, 1957:5.

52. Golomb FM. Closure of the circular defect with double rotation flaps and Z-plasties. Plast Reconstr Surg 1984;74:813–816.

53. Hamilton K, Wolfswinkel EM, Weathers WM, et al. The delay phenomenon: a compilation of knowledge across specialties. Craniomaxillofac Trauma Reconstr 2014;7:112–118.

54. Han KD, Colen L, Attinger, CE. Intrinsic foot and ankle flaps. Tech Foot Ankle Surg 2013;12:63–73.

55. Hanft JR, Blume PA, Dardik P, et al. A pilot clinical study for the treatment of diabetic foot ulcers with an injectable bioactive co-polymer (abstract). Presented at: Symposium on Advanced Wound Care and the 15th Annual Medical Research Forum on Wound Repair; April 2005; San Diego, CA.

56. Heinz TR. Local flaps for hindfoot reconstruction. In: Jurkiewicz MJ, Culbertson JH, eds. Operative techniques in plastic and reconstructive surgery. Los Angeles: General Publishing Group, 1996:157–164.

57. Heit YI, Lancerotto L, Mesteri I, et al. External volume expansion increases subcutaneous thickness, cell proliferation, and vascular remodeling in a murine model. Plast Reconstr Surg 2012;130:541–547.

58. Heniford BW, Bailin PL, Marsico RE Jr. Field guide to local flaps. Dermatol Clin 1998;16:65–74.

59. Hidalgo DA, Shaw WW. Anatomic basis of plantar flap design. Plast Reconstr Surg 1986;78:627–636.

60. Hirshowitz B, Karev A, Levy Y. A 5-flap procedure for axillary webs leaving the apex intact. Br J Plast Surg 1977;30:48–51.

61. Hirshowitz B, Kaufman T, Amir I. Biwinged excision for closure of rounded defect. Ann Plast Surg 1980;5:372–380.

62. Hirshowitz B, Mahler D. T-plasty technique for excisions in the face. Plast Reconstr Surg 1966;37:453–458.

63. Huang SR, Li XY, Wang H, et al. The use of local flap in repairing deeply burned wound of extremities [in Chinese]. Zhonghua Wai Ke Za Zhi 2005;43:182–184.

64. Ignatiadis II, Tsiampa VA, Papalois AE. A systematic approach to the failed plastic surgical reconstruction of the diabetic foot. Diabet Foot Ankle 2011;2.

65. Imanishi N, Kish K, Chang H, et al. Anatomical study of cutaneous venous flow of the sole. Plast Reconstr Surg 2007;120: 1906–1910.

66. Jackson IT. Local flaps in head and neck reconstruction. New York: Mosby, 1985.

67. Jang YJ, Park MC, Hong YS, et al. Successful lower extremity salvage with free flap after endovascular angioplasty in peripheral arterial occlusive disease. J Plast Reconstr Aesthet Surg 2014;67: 1136–1143.

68. Janis JE, Kwon RK, Lalonde DH. A practical guide to wound healing. Plast Reconstr Surg 2010;125:230e–244e.

69. Jose RM, Timoney N, Vidyadharan R, et al. Syndactyly correction: an aesthetic reconstruction. J Hand Surg Eur Vol 2010;35: 446–450.

70. Katoh H, Nakajima T, Yoshimura Y. The double-Z rhomboid plasty: an improvement in design. Plast Reconstr Surg 1984;74:817–824.

71. Keser A, Sensöz O, Mengi AS. Double opposing semicircular flap: a modification of opposing Z-plasty for closing circular defects. Plast Reconstr Surg 1998;102:1001–1007.

72. Kinsella JB, Rassekh CH, Wassmuth ZD, et al. Smoking increases facial skin flap complications. Ann Otol Rhinol Laryngol 1999;108:139–142.

73. Kouba DJ, Miller SJ. "Running pleated" suture technique opposes wound edges of unequal lengths. Dermatol Surg 2006;32: 411–414.

74. Larrabee WF Jr. Design of local skin flaps. Otolaryngol Clin North Am 1990;23:899–923.

75. Lesavoy MA. Local incisions and flap coverage. In: McCarthy JG, ed. Plastic surgery general principles. Philadelphia: Saunders, 1990:4441–4458.

76. Li JH, Xing X, Li P, et al. Transposition movement of V-Y flaps for facial reconstruction. J Plast Reconstr Aesthet Surg 2007;60:1244–1247.

77. Lister GD, Gibson T. Closure of rhomboid skin defects: the flaps of Limberg and Dufourmentel. Br J Plast Surg 1972;25: 300–314.

78. Lohman RF, Langevin CJ, Bozkurt M, et al. A prospective analysis of free flap monitoring techniques: physical examination, external Doppler, implantable Doppler, and tissue oximetry. J Reconstr Microsurg 2013;29:51–56.

79. LoPiccolo MC. Rotation flaps—principles and locations. Dermatol Surg 2015;41(suppl 10):247–254.

80. Lu F, Mizuno H, Uysal CA, et al. Improved viability of random pattern skin flaps through the use of adipose-derived stem cells. Plast Reconstr Surg 2008;121:50–58.

81. Maciel-Miranda A, Morris SF, Hallock GG. Local flaps, including pedicled perforator flaps: anatomy, technique, and applications. Plast Reconstr Surg 2013;131:896e–911e.

82. Manson PN, Anthenelli RM, Im MJ, et al. The role of oxygen-free radicals in ischemic tissue injury in island skin flaps. Ann Surg 1983;198:87–90.

83. Marcinko DE. Plastic surgery in podiatry (simplified illustrated techniques). J Foot Surg 1988;27:103–110.

84. Maruyama Y, Iwahira Y, Ebihara H. V-Y advancement flaps in the reconstruction of skin defects of the posterior heel ad ankle. Plast Reconstr Surg 1990;85:759–764.

85. McCarthy JG. Introduction of plastic surgery. In: McCarthy M, ed. Plastic surgery general principles. Philadelphia: Saunders, 1990:55–68.

86. McGregor AD, McGregor IA. Fundamental techniques of plastic surgery and their surgical applications. New York: Churchill Livingstone, 2000.

87. Miller CJ. Design principles for transposition flaps: the rhombic (single-lobed), bilobed, and trilobed flaps. Dermatol Surg 2014;40(suppl 9):43–52.

88. Milton SH. Pedicled skin-flaps: the fallacy of the length:width ratio. Br J Surg 1970;57:502–508.

89. Morain WD, Dellon AL, MacKinnon SE, et al. Current concepts in plastic surgery for the diabetic. Adv Plast Reconstr Surg 1987;4:1–36.

90. Morris SF, Taylor GI. Predicting the survival of experimental skin flaps with a knowledge of the vascular architecture. Plast Reconstr Surg 1993;92:1352–1361.

91. Nishimura K, Blume P, Ohgi S, et al. The effect of different regimen stretch on human dermal fibroblasts. J Surg Res 2006;130: 331–332.

92. Nuovong A, Hoogwerf B, Mohler E, et al. Evaluation of diabetic foot ulcer healing with hyperspectral imaging of oxyhemoglobin and deoxyhemoglobin. Diabetes Care 2009;32:2056–2061.

93. Ono I, Gunji H, Sato M, et al. Use of the oblique island flap in excision of small facial tumors. Plast Reconstr Surg 1993;91: 1245–1251.

94. Palmer B, Jurell G, Norberg KA. The blood flow in experimental skin flaps in rats studied by means of the 133 xenon clearance method. Scand J Plast Reconstr Surg 1972;6:6–12.

95. Papel ID, ed. Facial plastic and reconstructive surgery. 2nd ed. New York: Thieme Medical, 2002.

96. Park S, Eguchi T, Tokioka K, et al. Reconstruction of incomplete syndactyly of the toes using both dorsal and plantar flaps. Plast Reconstr Surg 1996;98:534–537.

97. Pribaz JJ, Chester CH, Barrall DT. The extended V-Y flap. Plast Reconstr Surg 1992;90:275–280.

98. Price NM. Closure of surgical wounds using contiguous island flaps (double V to Y procedure). Ann Plast Surg 1979;3:321–325.

99. Pyka RA, Coventry MB. Avascular necrosis of the skin after operations on the foot. J Bone Joint Surg Am 1961;43-A: 955–960.

100. Rand-Luby L, Pommier RF, Williams ST, et al. Improved outcome of surgical flaps treated with topical dimethylsulfoxide. Ann Surg 1996;224:583–589.

101. Roukis TS, Schweinberger MH, Schade VL. V-Y fasciocutaneous advancement flap coverage of soft tissue defects of the foot in the patient at high risk. J Foot Ankle Surg 2010;49:71–74.

102. Sahin C, Ergun O, Kulahci Y, et al. Bilobed flap for web reconstruction in adult syndactyly release: a new technique that can avoid the use of skin graft. J Plast Reconstr Aesthet Surg 2014;67:815–821.

103. Sanchez-Conejo-Mir J, Bueno Montes J, Moreno Gimenez JC, et al. The bilobed flap in sole surgery. J Dermatol Surg Oncol 1985;11:913–917.

104. Sarrafian SK. Anatomy of the foot and ankle: descriptive, topographic, functional. 2nd ed. Philadelphia: Lippincott Williams & Wilkins, 1993:329.

105. Satterfield VK, Jolly GP. A new method of excision of painful plantar forefoot lesions using a rotation advancement flap. J Foot Ankle Surg 1994;33:129–134.

106. Schrudde J, Petrovici V. The use of slide-swing plasty in closing skin defects: a clinical study based on 1,308 cases. Plast Reconstr Surg 1981;67:467–481.

107. Seyhan A. Mini Z in Z to relieve the tension on the transverse closure after Z-Plasty transposition. Plast Reconstr Surg 1998;101:1635–1637.

108. Shaw WW, Hidalgo DA. Anatomic basis of plantar flap design: clinical applications. Plast Reconstr Surg 1986;78:637–649.

109. Sheridan AT, Humzah D. V-Y-S-plasty closure of circular defects. Australas J Dermatol 2000;41:260–261.

110. Soltanian H, Garcia RM, Hollenbeck ST. Current concepts in lower extremity reconstruction. Plast Reconstr Surg 2015;136:815e–829e.

111. Stedman's medical dictionary. 26th ed. Baltimore: Lippincott Williams & Wilkins, 1995:660.

112. Sumpio BE, Blume PA. Contemporary management of foot ulcers. In: Pierce WH, Matsumura JS, Yao JST, eds. Trends in vascular surgery. Chicago: Precept Press, 2002:277–290.

113. Sumpio BE, Blume PA. Treatment of foot ulcers. N Engl J Med 2001;344(2):correspondence.

114. Sumpio BE, Paszkowiak J, Aruny J, et al. Lower extremity ulceration. In: Creager MA, Dzau VJ, Loscalzo J, eds. Vascular medicine, a companion to Braunwald's heart disease. Philadelphia: Saunders, 2006:880–893.

115. Sumpio BE, Paszkowiak JJ, Blume PA. Vascular ulcers. In: Creager J, Olin J, eds. Vascular medicine. St. Louis: Mosby, 2006:880–893.

116. Sumpio BE, Schroeder SM, Blume PA. Etiology and management of foot ulcerations. In: Lee BY, ed. The wound management manual. New York: McGraw-Hill, 2005:126–133.

117. Sungur N, Kankaya Y, Gursoy K, et al. A local flap that never disappoints: V-Y rotation advancement flap. Ann Plast Surg 2013;71:575–580.

118. Sutton AE, Quatela VC. Bilobed flap reconstruction of the temporal forehead. Arch Otolaryngol Head Neck Surg 1992;118:978–982.

119. Tan O, Atik B, Ergen D. A new method in the treatment of postburn scar contractures: double opposing V-Y-Z plasty. Burns 2006;32:499–503.

120. Taylor GI, Corlett RJ, Caddy CM, et al. An anatomic review of the delay phenomenon: II. Clinical applications. Plast Reconstr Surg 1992;89:408–416.

121. Taylor GI, Palmer JH, McManamny D. The vascular territories of the body (angiosomes) and their clinical applications. In: McCarthy M, ed. Plastic surgery general principles. Philadelphia: Saunders, 1990:329–378.

122. Thordarson DB. Congenital crossover fifth toe correction with soft tissue release and cutaneous Z-plasty. Foot Ankle Int 2001;22:511–512.

123. Tintle SM, Kovach SJ, Levin LS. Free tissue transfer to the foot and ankle: perforator flaps. Tech Foot Ankle Surg 2013;12:79–86.

124. Topp SG, Lovald S, Khraishi T, et al. Biomechanics of the rhombic transposition flap. Otolaryngol Head Neck Surg 2014;151:952–959.

125. Walike JW, Larrabee WF Jr. The "note flap." Arch Otolaryngol 1985;111:430–433.

126. Webster RC, Davidson TM, Smith RC. The thirty degree transposition flap. Laryngoscope 1978;88:85–94.

127. Yeh JT, Lin CH, Lin YT. Skin grafting as a salvage procedure in diabetic foot reconstruction to avoid major limb amputation. Chang Gung Med J 2010;33:389–396.

128. Zgonis T, Jolly GP, Blume P. A guide to closure techniques for open wounds. Podiatry Today 2003;16:40–48.

129. Zgonis T, Stapleton JJ, Roukis TS. Advanced plastic surgery techniques for soft tissue coverage of the diabetic foot. Clin Podiatr Med Surg 2007;24:547–568.

130. Zheng Y, Yi C, Xia W, et al. Mesenchymal stem cells transduced by vascular endothelial growth factor gene for ischemic random skin flaps. Plast Reconstr Surg 2008;121:59–69.

CHAPTER 13

Local Intrinsic Muscle Flap Reconstruction for Soft Tissue Coverage of the Diabetic Foot

Daniel J. Short • Thomas Zgonis

INTRODUCTION

Diabetic foot wounds impose a significant burden to the health care system with a constantly increasing cost to treat. Wounds themselves present with serious complications in the diabetic population that may lead to osteomyelitis and lower extremity amputation. Diabetic patients are commonly encountered with multiple medical comorbidities that can have a detrimental effect in the overall wound healing process which in turn can involve a complicated and prolonged course of treatment. Diabetic foot wounds differ from other areas in the body due to the amount of motion and biomechanical forces acting on the lower extremity. Diabetic foot wounds are mostly caused by repetitive stress injury to the affected region, which as a function of the peripheral neuropathy is often overlooked by the patients in the early development of the wound.

The utilization of local intrinsic muscle flaps for soft tissue coverage in the diabetic foot are advantageous in certain clinical case scenarios complicated by osteomyelitis, foot deformity such as Charcot neuroarthropathy (CN), avascular necrosis, and large osseous and soft tissue defects after osseous resection and/or implanted hardware removal. The unique characteristics of the local intrinsic muscle flaps of the foot involve the ability of providing increased blood flow to the recipient area and therefore enhancing the deliverance of antibiotics and white blood cells facilitating the healing process while eradicating the localized infection.

The most common local intrinsic muscle flaps in the diabetic foot are the extensor digitorum brevis (EDB), flexor digitorum brevis (FDB), abductor hallucis (ABH), and abductor digiti minimi (ABDM). These muscle flaps are predominantly dependent on a dominant vascular pedicle and several more distal minor pedicles that allow for easy mobilization and rotation to achieve soft tissue coverage about the foot and ankle. In the diabetic foot, local intrinsic muscles are usually harvested in isolation and covered in the recipient area by an autogenous split-thickness skin graft (STSG) or bioengineered alternative tissue.

PREOPERATIVE PLANNING

Vascular Examination

In the diabetic population, peripheral arterial disease (PAD) is quite common and carefully needs to be assessed before the muscle flap reconstruction. Initial physical examination includes manual palpation of the lower extremity arteries followed by the use of an arterial Doppler ultrasound. In addition, arterial noninvasive testing including the ankle-brachial index (ABI), toe-brachial index, transcutaneous oxygen pressures, and skin perfusion pressures are performed when indicated. In certain clinical case scenarios, the ABI may be falsely elevated, underestimating the severity of PAD secondary to multiple calcified vessels common in the diabetic population. After a thorough clinical and arterial noninvasive studies are performed, a vascular surgery consultation may be warranted based on the findings for further invasive diagnostic or revascularization procedures. Understanding the vascular anatomy and dominant blood supply to the desired muscle flap reconstruction is paramount before the planned surgical procedure. The Doppler ultrasound is also used to identify the desired muscle flap's main blood supply and accompanying perforators during the preoperative planning.

Wound Assessment

Careful assessment of the recipient wound bed and surrounding soft tissues is based on the anatomic location, size, depth, edema, soft tissue infection, osteomyelitis, underlying deformity, perfusion, sensation, previous surgical scars or implanted hardware, and equinus and biomechanical alterations. In the presence of a soft tissue or osseous infection, multiple-staged surgical débridements might be necessary before the definitive muscle flap reconstruction. In clinical case scenarios, where previous surgical procedures were performed along the desired muscle flap harvesting, the proposed muscle flap may not be the suitable option for soft tissue coverage.

Finally, it is also important to remember that in diabetic patients with dense peripheral neuropathy, intrinsic muscle atrophy can be quite common, and, therefore, muscle flap coverage with known muscle atrophy may not be robust to provide soft tissue coverage.

Concomitant Osteomyelitis

Acute or chronic diabetic foot wounds may present with a concomitant underlying osteomyelitis which needs to be addressed before the final muscle flap reconstructive procedure. Medical imaging including plain radiographs, magnetic resonance imaging, computed tomography, and/or bone scintigraphy may need to be performed in order to verify or assess the extent of the soft tissue and osseous involvement. In the presence of diabetic CN with osteomyelitis, medical imaging can be quite challenging and difficult in determining the extent and severity of underlying infection in an abnormal foot architecture. Intraoperative bone biopsy and histopathologic analysis along with soft tissue and bone cultures might be the most reliable source of providing valuable information in determining the presence of concomitant osteomyelitis in diabetic patients with CN. Lastly, special attention is emphasized when using contrast dye in diagnostic medical imaging and diabetic patients with kidney or heart disease.

Resected osteomyelitic defects in the diabetic foot and/or ankle can initially be managed by the application of antibiotic-impregnated polymethylmethacrylate (PMMA) cemented beads and/or spacers prior to the definitive muscle flap procedure. Culture-specific long-term parenteral antibiotics are managed by the infectious disease specialists and their duration is based on the clinical, laboratory, and surgical findings. Upon surgical removal of the nonbiodegradable implanted antibiotic-impregnated PMMA cemented beads and/or spacers, it is recommended that new intraoperative cultures are obtained before the definitive muscle flap procedure. In most clinical case scenarios, bone grafting and osseous reconstruction is necessary along with the proposed muscle flap coverage. The utilization of local intrinsic muscle flap closure can increase the arterial perfusion as well as the deliverance of antibiotics in the recipient defect.

Lower Extremity Deformity

Lower extremity biomechanical assessment is a valuable tool and adjunct component in any flap reconstruction for the diabetic foot and ankle. Lower extremity equinus contractures are often associated with numerous pathologic entities in the diabetic population including CN. A thorough clinical and radiographic assessment is necessary to determine the level and severity of equinus contracture and before surgical correction with an isolated gastrocnemius recession or tendo-Achilles lengthening procedure. Equinus contractures are often seen in diabetic patients with CN, forefoot ulceration(s), cerebrovascular accident, acquired pes planovalgus or cavovarus deformities, traumatic injuries, prolonged immobilization, casting, and partial foot amputations.

When performing a local intrinsic muscle flap for soft tissue coverage of the diabetic foot, the underlying osseous deformity as well as soft tissue contracture such as the equinus deformity is addressed at the time of muscle flap surgery. In patients with diabetic CN, preoperative plain radiographs include the foot, calcaneal axial, ankle, and leg views in a standing position when feasible. In addition, computed tomography scanning is highly recommended to further assess the quality of the affected joints and better evaluate the deformity during the preoperative planning process. Surgical procedures for correcting the associated diabetic CN or underlying osseous deformity vary from simple exostectomies to major arthrodesis and are dependent based on the anatomic location and overall medical status of the diabetic patient.

Medical Optimization

Diabetic patients with acute or chronic wounds that are in need of an intrinsic muscle flap coverage usually present with multiple medical comorbidities including, but not limited to, PAD, coronary arterial disease, hypertension, hypercholesterolemia, chronic hyperglycemia, kidney disease, anemia, venous stasis disease, deep vein thrombosis and pulmonary embolism, peripheral edema and neuropathy, retinopathy, malnutrition, obesity, and/or smoking. Based on this clinical presentation, the proposed muscle flap coverage may be associated with an increased risk of flap necrosis, surgical wound infection, reulceration, osteomyelitis, and potential amputation. During the preoperative planning, it is essential that a multidisciplinary health care team is actively involved in all medical and surgical aspects of the diabetic patient. Medical optimization prior to the proposed muscle reconstructive procedure is paramount to the patient's successful outcome.

PREOPERATIVE CONSIDERATIONS

Local intrinsic muscle flaps can be harvested to include the cutaneous portion supplied by the musculocutaneous perforating vessels or in isolation from their insertion or origin followed by coverage of an autogenous STSG or allogenic skin graft. Local intrinsic muscle flaps of the foot depend on a dominant vascular pedicle that will have perforating branches which supply a surrounding area of overlying skin. These anatomic areas were described by Taylor et al. as angiosomes and are supplied by a vessel (3,6–8). Based on the Mathes and Nahai muscle classification, the local intrinsic muscle flaps of the foot are type II muscles with at least one dominant vascular pedicle accompanied by varying minor vascular networks (1).

The identification of local, distant, and/or free muscle flaps as a source of donor tissue offered tremendous versatility and more options for wound closure techniques. As the vascular anatomy became understood, it was possible to detach the muscle at the origin, insertion, or both and transfer it to a new site while maintaining perfusion inflow. In addition to the patient's vascular status, several factors must be considered when planning a muscle flap including, but not limited to, the size and location of the defect, the damage to surrounding regional tissues, and the presence of exposed vital structures.

In the diabetic foot, a local intrinsic muscle flap is used predominately for soft tissue closure over osseous defects as a result of lower extremity deformities associated with a CN and/or resected osteomyelitis (5). The main advantage of a local intrinsic muscle flap is that extensive soft tissue coverage with perfusion inflow about all aspects of the foot can be provided without the microvascular anastomosis that is required of a free tissue transfer. In many cases, diabetic patients present with severely calcified vessels making microvascular anastomosis discouraging or impossible.

In clinical case scenarios where subsequent implanted hardware removal or revisional surgery may be required and a large osseous defect may be the result before the definitive closure procedure, a free tissue transfer or pedicle flap may be a preferable alternative for soft tissue coverage in the diabetic foot and ankle. Free tissue transfers or pedicle flaps permit the necessary surgical exposure to perform hardware removal, bone grafting, and osseous reconstruction if needed. However, vascularized pedicle flaps might be limited to specific anatomic regions (2).

DETAILED DESCRIPTION AND SURGICAL TECHNIQUE

Extensor Digitorum Brevis Muscle Flap

The EDB muscle flap is usually harvested without the overlying skin as the muscle lies deep to the extensor tendons and is used for soft tissue coverage of dorsolateral diabetic foot and/or ankle wounds. The dorsalis pedis artery and its lateral tarsal artery branch are mapped preoperatively with a Doppler ultrasound to ensure safety while identifying the anatomic landmarks. The skin incision should lie just laterally to the dorsalis pedis artery and follow the course of the EDB muscle belly from its origin of the dorsolateral surface of the calcaneus to the base of the proximal phalanges of the second, third, and fourth toes. The second, third, and fourth muscle slips are harvested along with their tendinous attachments distally while usually sparing the extensor hallucis brevis muscle. The EDB muscle flap is then rotated proximally and laterally as it is skeletonized from its tendinous attachments based on the proximal dominant pedicle and inset to the prepared recipient site followed by coverage of either an autogenous STSG or allogenic skin graft. The distal stumps of the EDB tendons can be sutured to the extensor digitorum longus tendons with a 2-0 polydioxanone suture (PDS II) if desired, but this technique is not usually required. The distal aspect of the skin incision for harvesting the EDB muscle may then be closed primarily (Fig. 13.1).

Flexor Digitorum Brevis Muscle Flap

The FDB muscle flap dissection begins as a midline incision to the plantar aspect of the foot. Typically, a "Z"-style incision is undertaken to minimize postoperative skin contracture as well as maximize exposure. The muscle is supplied by the lateral plantar artery as well as the medial plantar artery, whereas the dominant pedicle is supplied by the lateral plantar artery at the proximal plantar aspect of the FDB muscle. The mooring ligaments are released often through blunt and sharp dissection in order to expose the plantar fascia which the FDB muscle belly lies deep to. The plantar fascia is incised longitudinally and retracted medially and laterally with care to allow for further closure if desired. All dissection is carried distally until the FDB tendon slips to the second, third, fourth, and/or fifth toes are identified, whereas further distal dissection is not required once the sufficient tendons are identified. The harvested FDB tendons are transected from their distal tendinous attachments, tagged with a 2-0 PDS suture or grasped with an Allis clamp/hemostat distally and freed as a unit from the underlying deep fascia. The minor pedicles may be sacrificed as encountered during the dissection as the dominant vascular pedicle lies near the muscle origin at the proximal calcaneus but, depending on the location of the recipient site, may be left undisturbed if mobility of the flap is not restricted. The FDB muscle flap is then rotated proximally and centrally as it is skeletonized from its tendinous attachments based on the proximal dominant vascular pedicle and inset to the prepared recipient site followed by coverage of either an autogenous STSG or allogenic skin graft. The distal stumps of the FDB tendons can be sutured to the flexor digitorum longus tendons if desired, but this technique is not usually required. Similarly, the incised plantar fascia may be repaired if desired. The distal aspect of the skin incision for harvesting the FDB muscle may then be closed primarily (Fig. 13.2).

Abductor Hallucis Muscle Flap

The ABH muscle flap dissection begins at the medial and slightly plantar aspect of the first metatarsophalangeal joint (MTPJ) and at the insertion of the base of the first proximal phalangeal level. Once the ABH tendinous slip is identified distally, the skin incision is extended proximally along the course of the tendon and is followed medially and proximally until identifying the muscle belly. There is often a superficial venous complex within the incision that is retracted superiorly or ligated as necessary. The inferior side of the muscle is often tethered through a thick fibrous septum to the flexor hallucis brevis (FHB) muscle. Depending on the size of the recipient defect, the FHB muscle may be also harvested along to provide additional soft tissue coverage and blood supply or separated to harvest only the ABH muscle.

Limited dissection superior and inferior to the ABH tendinous slip is performed, and its distal attachment at the insertion of the first proximal phalanx is transected with a tenotomy scissor or a no. 15 surgical blade. The harvested ABH tendon is then tagged with a 2-0 PDS suture or grasped with an Allis clamp/hemostat at its distal stump and is raised while avoiding trauma to the undersurface of the muscle flap. Elevation and rotation of the ABH muscle with its harvested tendinous portion is performed by applying gradual tension in a proximal and medial direction toward the recipient site.

The distal perforating arteries that arise from the medial plantar artery are identified and ligated while maintaining the

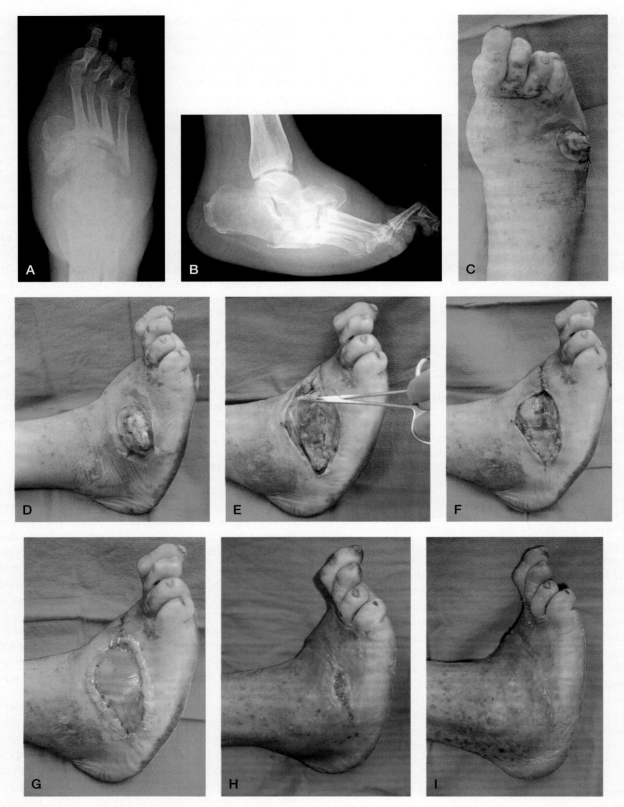

FIGURE 13.1 Preoperative radiographic **(A,B)** and intraoperative **(C,D)** pictures of a right foot severe dorsolateral soft tissue infection without osteomyelitis in a diabetic patient with a partial first ray (toe and metatarsal) amputation and Charcot neuroarthropathy. Patient underwent an initial surgical excisional débridement of all nonviable soft tissues followed by an extensor digitorum brevis (EDB) muscle flap covered with a dermoconductive acellular dermal replacement 2 days after the initial surgical procedure **(E–G)**. The patient was followed closely in an outpatient clinical setting for local wound care and lower extremity posterior splint changes. Clinical outcomes at 10 weeks **(H)** and 16 weeks **(I)** after the local intrinsic EDB muscle flap coverage.

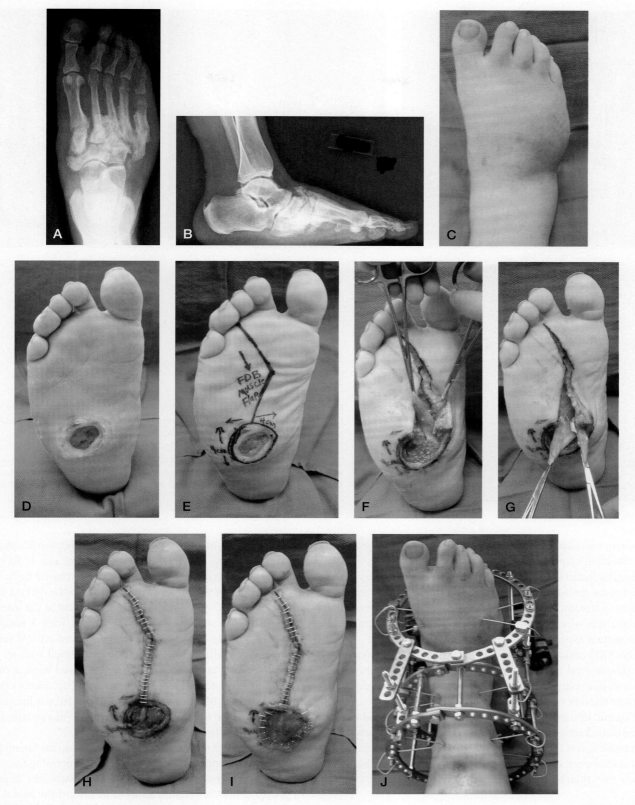

FIGURE 13.2 Preoperative radiographic **(A,B)** and intraoperative **(C,D)** pictures of a right foot chronic plantar central ulceration of a stable diabetic Charcot neuroarthropathy without osteomyelitis. Patient underwent an initial surgical excisional débridement of all nonviable soft tissues 2 days prior to the definitive reconstructive procedure. **E.** Picture shows the anatomic landmarks for harvesting the flexor digitorum brevis (FDB) muscle from its distal tendinous attachments. The harvested FDB muscle is then raised **(F)** and rotated proximally and centrally toward the recipient area **(G,H)**. Note the primary closure of the skin incision made for harvesting the FDB muscle followed by an application of a dermoconductive acellular dermal replacement at the superior surface of the inset FDB muscle's recipient site **(I)**. *(continued)*

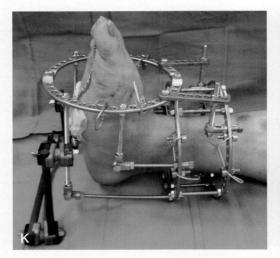
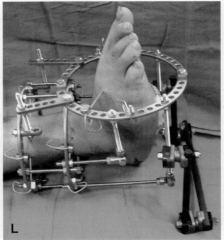
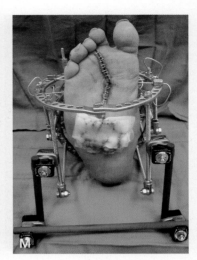

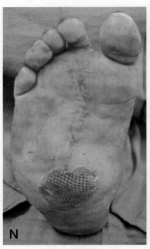
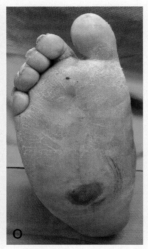

FIGURE 13.2 *(Continued)* **J–M.** The application of the circular external fixation device provided simultaneous surgical off-loading, stabilization of the foot to the lower extremity, and immobilization of the FDB muscle flap. **N.** The surgical off-loading circular external fixation device was removed at approximately 6 weeks postoperatively at which time an autogenous split-thickness skin graft was used for soft tissue coverage at the recipient area. **O.** Clinical outcome at approximately 19.5 weeks after the FDB muscle flap closure.

dominant vascular pedicle at the proximal aspect of the muscle. The direction of proximal muscle rotation tends to be toward the medial malleolus and is used to cover defects at the medial aspect of the diabetic foot and/or ankle. Rotation in this manner minimizes tension across the last perforating artery of the medial plantar artery which is commonly encountered 0.5 to 1 cm distal to the plantar aspect of the navicular tuberosity.

The ABH muscle flap is rotated proximally and medially as it is skeletonized from its tendinous attachment based on the proximal dominant vascular pedicle and is inset to the prepared recipient site followed by coverage of either an autogenous STSG or allogenic skin graft. The distal stump of the ABH tendon can be reattached with a 2-0 PDS suture to the retained severed tendinous portion at the insertion of the first MTPJ. The distal and/or proximal aspects of the skin incision for harvesting the ABH muscle may then be closed primarily (Fig. 13.3).

Abductor Digiti Minimi Muscle Flap

The ABDM muscle flap dissection begins at the lateral and slightly plantar aspect of the fifth MTPJ and at the insertion of the base of the fifth proximal phalangeal level. Once the ABDM

tendinous slip is identified distally, the skin incision is extended proximally along the course of the tendon and is followed laterally and proximally until identifying the muscle belly.

Limited dissection superior and inferior to the ABDM tendinous slip is performed, and its distal attachment at the insertion of the fifth proximal phalanx is transected with a tenotomy scissor or a no. 15 surgical blade. The harvested ABDM tendon is then tagged with a 2-0 PDS suture or grasped with an Allis clamp/hemostat at its distal stump and is raised while avoiding trauma to the undersurface of the muscle flap. Elevation and rotation of the ABDM muscle with its harvested tendinous portion is performed by applying gradual tension in a proximal and lateral direction toward the recipient site.

The distal perforating arteries that arise from the lateral plantar artery are identified and ligated while maintaining the dominant pedicle at the proximal aspect of the muscle. The direction of proximal muscle rotation tends to be toward the lateral malleolus and is used to cover defects at the lateral aspect of the diabetic foot and/or ankle. Rotation in this manner minimizes tension across the last perforating artery of the lateral plantar artery which is commonly encountered at the fifth metatarsal base or up to 1 cm proximal to the fifth metatarsal base.

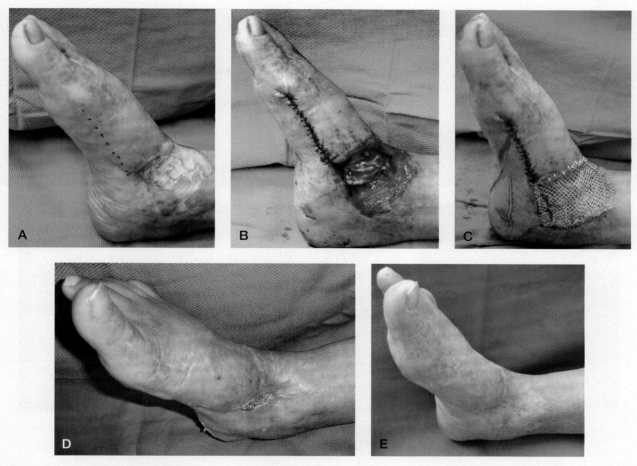

FIGURE 13.3 Intraoperative picture **(A)** of a large soft tissue defect at the proximal anteromedial aspect of the foot and ankle being covered by an abductor hallucis (ABH) muscle flap harvested from its distal attachment at the medial aspect of the first metatarso-phalangeal joint **(B)**. Note the primary closure of the skin incision made for harvesting the ABH muscle followed by an application of an autogenous split-thickness skin graft at the superior surface of the inset ABH muscle's recipient site **(C)**. **D,E.** Long-term clinical outcomes after minor débridements and local wound care.

The ABDM muscle flap is rotated proximally and laterally as it is skeletonized from its tendinous attachment based on the proximal dominant vascular pedicle and is inset to the prepared recipient site followed by coverage of either an autogenous STSG or allogenic skin graft. The distal stump of the ABDM tendon can be reattached with a 2-0 PDS suture to the retained severed tendinous portion at the insertion of the fifth MTPJ. The distal and/or proximal aspects of the skin incision for harvesting the ABDM muscle may then be closed primarily (Fig. 13.4).

INTRAOPERATIVE CONSIDERATIONS

One of the most common limiting factors with local intrinsic muscle flaps of the foot is the bulk and viability of the muscle, which is highly variable in the diabetic population. It is usually difficult to obtain a true estimation of viable and useable muscle bulk with preoperative imaging, and therefore, intraoperative findings of an atrophied muscle might result in further soft tissue coverage alternatives during or in staged reconstructive proce-

dures. Similarly, in large wounds with exposed deep structures, a local intrinsic muscle flap may be too small to completely close the entire defect, and therefore, adjunctive soft tissue reconstructive procedures may be needed to assist in wound closure.

In the local intrinsic muscle flaps of the foot, the dominant vascular pedicle is also always located close to the muscle origin, which allows confident dissection and ligation of minor pedicles when performing muscle flaps that fall within the arc of rotation. In muscle flaps which approach the limit of the arc of rotation, care must be taken to avoid damage to the dominant pedicle which is rarely skeletonized when performing the dissection.

Muscle flaps must be handled with care and especially in diabetic patients with calcified vessels and vascular insufficiency. Pneumatic tourniquet utilization during the muscle harvesting process along with intraoperative use of a Doppler ultrasound and loupe magnification are highly recommended in order to better visualize, expedite, and minimize intraoperative complications associated with disruption of the dominant vascular pedicle. It is also recommended to harvest

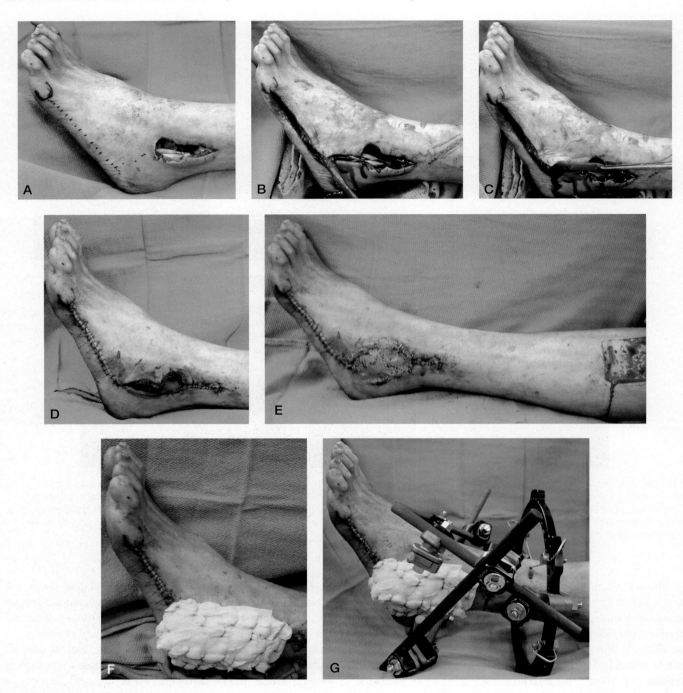

FIGURE 13.4 Intraoperative picture **(A)** of a large soft tissue defect at the proximal anterolateral aspect of the foot and ankle being covered by an abductor digiti minimi (ABDM) muscle flap harvested from its distal attachment at the lateral aspect of the fifth metatarsophalangeal joint **(B,C)**. Note the primary closure of the skin incision made for harvesting the ABDM muscle **(D)** followed by an application of an autogenous split-thickness skin graft at the superior surface of the inset ABDM muscle's recipient site **(E,F)**. **G.** The application of the hybrid external fixation device provided simultaneous surgical off-loading, stabilization of the foot to the lower extremity, and immobilization of the ABDM muscle flap.

the local intrinsic muscle with its tendinous attachment during the dissection process because it can be raised and inset as a unit without trauma to the muscle. Insetting of the skeletonized muscle from its tendinous attachment to the recipient site is performed without any excessive tension or torsion on the dominant vascular pedicle so that perfusion inflow and muscle viability is not compromised.

Frequent irrigation with warmed normal saline prevents desiccation and vasospasm from occurring. The harvested muscle is secured to the surrounding dermis and subdermal fascia at the perimeter of the recipient site with a 2-0, 3-0, or 4-0 monofilament absorbable suture such as PDS. The vascular inflow should be assessed intraoperatively with a Doppler ultrasound after insetting the muscle. If the vascular inflow is compromised, the muscle is repositioned in order to ensure adequate blood flow or might be resected and covered with a negative pressure wound therapy (NPWT) device. In certain cases, delayed muscle flap closure after it is raised may be indicated in order to improve the muscle vascularity and viability status.

Achieving adequate intraoperative hemostasis is essential in order to prevent hematoma formation and subsequent muscle flap failure. If a pneumatic tourniquet is utilized during the muscle harvesting, it should be released prior to insetting of the muscle flap to ensure muscle flap viability and perfusion inflow and to adequately achieve hemostasis. Topical thrombin and/or other hemostatic agents are commonly utilized throughout the surgical procedure along with manual compression or application of a compressive dressing while the tourniquet is released. Any active bleeding vessels are ligated as necessary making sure that the dominant vascular pedicle to the muscle flap is not compromised.

Local intrinsic muscle flaps of the foot are usually harvested without the overlying skin, and after they are inset in the recipient areas, they are covered with an autogenous STSG or allogenic skin graft. A bolster dressing composed from a non-adherent dressing and sterile sponge(s) soaked in normal saline solution or application of a non-adherent dressing with NPWT device on the superior surface of the muscle flap is recommended after the muscle flap insetting. If a NPWT device is applied as a bolster dressing on the muscle flap, it is usually left in a continuous low pressure mode for approximately 5 to 7 days postoperatively.

ADJUNCTIVE SURGICAL PROCEDURES

As discussed previously, local intrinsic muscle flaps of the foot are usually performed with an associated osseous and/or soft tissue reconstruction procedure(s). Such procedures may include, but are not limited to, osseous exostectomies, joint arthrodesis, management of osteomyelitis with antibiotic-impregnated PMMA cemented beads and/or spacers and subsequent bone grafting, soft tissue release(s), and/or equinus correction.

The utilization of a circular external fixation device as a primary method of underlying deformity correction or as a surgical off-loading tool for simultaneous lower extremity stabilization, muscle flap immobilization, and elevation while maintaining a non–weight-bearing status during the postoperative course is paramount in the patient's successful outcome (4).

In clinical case scenarios where implanted noninfected hardware are removed and a muscle flap is in need for soft tissue coverage of the osseous and soft tissue defect, autogenous or allogenic bone grafting might be necessary to fill the osseous defects of any intraosseous bleeding before the muscle insetting.

POSTOPERATIVE CONSIDERATIONS

The duration of the circular external fixation application is dependent on the type of adjunctive surgical procedures performed as well as the occurrence of any postoperative complications. During the postoperative course, a non–weight-bearing status is maintained with frequent visits for clinical and radiographic assessments. If a bolster dressing is applied without the NPWT device over the muscle flap, it is usually left undisrupted for approximately 2 to 6 weeks unless clinical signs of localized infection have occurred. If a NPWT device has been used as a bolster dressing, it is usually discontinued within 5 to 7 days after the muscle flap surgery. After removal of the circular external fixation device, further immobilization with frequent lower extremity posterior splint or below-the-knee casting changes is recommended until satisfactory closure of the wound has been achieved.

Throughout the postoperative course, the multidisciplinary team approach to the patient's medical optimization is maintained by the input of specialties in the management of medical comorbidities, deep vein thrombosis and pulmonary embolism prophylaxis, antibiotic dosage and administration, physical therapy, and rehabilitation. In the event of a postoperative infection, reulceration, or muscle necrosis, surgical débridement and staged reconstruction is established in an expedited manner (Fig. 13.5).

FIGURE 13.5 Intraoperative picture **(A)** of a right foot recurrent plantar central ulceration without osteomyelitis in a diabetic patient with Charcot neuroarthropathy, previous medial column arthrodesis, flexor digitorum brevis (FDB) muscle flap covered with a dermoconductive acellular dermal replacement and circular external fixation. Patient underwent an initial surgical excisional débridement of all nonviable soft tissues and partial cuboid resection **(B,C)** followed by a revisional soft tissue and osseous excisional débridement with a local random rhomboid advancement flap closure 2 days after the initial surgical procedure **(D,E)**. (continued)

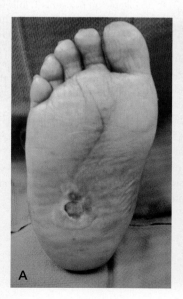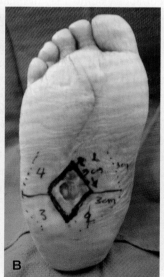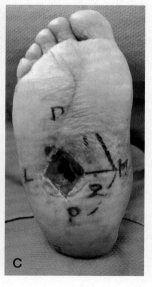

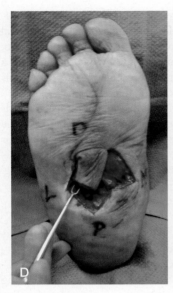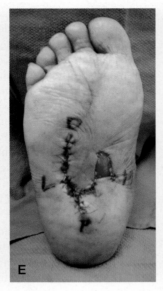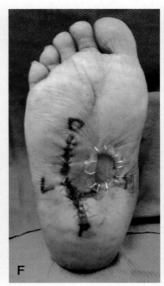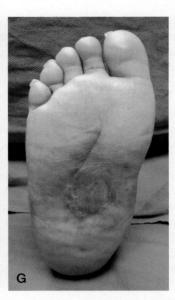

FIGURE 13.5 *(Continued)* Note the skin closure at the recipient site followed by the application of a dermoconductive acellular dermal replacement in the donor non–weight-bearing area of the foot **(F)**. **G.** Clinical outcome at approximately 28 weeks after a local random flap closure was utilized for a reulceration of a previous FDB muscle flap closure.

In cases where the muscle flap reconstruction is performed without the utilization of a circular external fixation device, the muscle flap is secured with a well-padded lower extremity posterior splint immediately after the muscle flap procedure. Continuous non–weight-bearing status is maintained throughout the postoperative period with frequent lower extremity posterior splint or below-the-knee casting applications. The patient is then progressed into a walking cast or fracture boot for an additional 4 to 6 weeks during which time custom-made diabetic shoes and/or bracing are prepared by a pedorthotist.

Conclusion

As our knowledge of diabetic foot wounds continues to increase, early recognition and timely referral to a specialized health care center is also mandated. Timely detection of complicated or at high-risk diabetic foot wounds may ultimately result in prompt intervention to direct and hopefully influence the ultimate result.

Local intrinsic muscle flaps of the foot provide an important tool in the closure of soft tissue defects in the diabetic foot and/or ankle. Although providing a bulk of soft tissue to cover vital structures and assisting in the management of localized infection, muscle flaps are also a viable option where other surgical procedures may not be durable enough for long-term success. The proximal location of the dominant vascular pedicles allows for rapid and confident dissection during the local intrinsic muscle flap harvesting. Lastly, the harvesting of intrinsic muscle flaps often exposes osseous prominences and joints

which are to be addressed surgically and therefore obviating the need for additional incisional approaches.

References

1. Mathes SJ, Nahai F. Classification of the vascular anatomy of muscles: experimental and clinical correlation. Plast Reconstr Surg 1981;67:177–187.
2. McGregor IA, Morgan G. Axial and random pattern flaps. Br J Plast Surg 1973;26:202–213.
3. Saint-Cyr M, Wong C, Schaverien M, et al. The perforasome theory: vascular anatomy and clinical implications. Plast Reconstr Surg 2009;124:1529–1544.
4. Short DJ, Zgonis T. Circular external fixation as a primary or adjunctive therapy for the podoplastic approach of the diabetic Charcot foot. Clin Podiatr Med Surg 2017;34:93–98.
5. Stapleton JJ, Zgonis T, Jolly GP, et al. Muscle flaps for soft tissue coverage of the diabetic foot. In: Zgonis T, ed. Surgical reconstruction of the diabetic foot and ankle. Philadelphia: Lippincott Williams & Wilkins, 2009:167–177.
6. Taylor GI, Corlett RJ, Dhar SC, et al. The anatomical (angiosome) and clinical territories of the cutaneous perforating arteries: development of the concept and designing safe flaps. Plast Reconstr Surg 2011;127:1447–1459.
7. Taylor GI, Gianoutsos MP, Morris SF. The neurovascular territories of the skin and muscles: anatomic study and clinical implications. Plast Reconstr Surg 1994;94:1–36.
8. Taylor GI, Palmer JH. The vascular territories (angiosomes) of the body: experimental study and clinical applications. Br J Plast Surg 1987;40:113–141.

CHAPTER 14

Pedicle Flap Reconstruction for Soft Tissue Coverage of the Diabetic Foot

Crystal L. Ramanujam • Hani M. Badahdah • Thomas Zgonis

INTRODUCTION

Complicated diabetic foot and ankle wounds with multidimensional defects call for restoration of not only the skin but also the underlying structural anatomy in order to provide the best functional outcomes. For cases of complex soft tissue and/or bone loss found in the diabetic foot and ankle, pedicle flaps are ideal for durable wound closure, are often used in combination with skeletal reconstruction, and in some cases can provide sensation to the recipient site. In navigating through the soft tissue reconstructive pyramid for the diabetic foot, local and/or distant pedicle flaps are found above local random and/or muscle flaps and just below free tissue transfers (6). Because local random and/or muscle flaps are limited by their extensibility and excursion potential of the surrounding tissue, pedicle flaps are favored because they avoid tension and can resemble the anatomy at the site of the original defect. Reported advantages supporting the use of a pedicle flap in comparison to free tissue transfer in diabetic patients include but are not limited to avoiding the need for microvascular anastomosis, reduced operating times, fewer perioperative complications, and better tissue durability. The most common local pedicle flaps used for the diabetic foot are the great toe artery (GTA) flap, medial plantar artery (MPA) flap, lateral plantar artery (LPA) flap, and lateral calcaneal artery (LCA) flap, whereas the most common distant pedicle flap is the distally based sural artery neurofasciocutaneous (SAN) flap. The versatility of pedicle flaps is evident in their ability to address a variety of diabetic foot and ankle defects on both weight bearing and non–weight-bearing areas and demonstrated in their success when properly performed in combination with other reconstructive surgical techniques such as osseous correction and autogenous or allogenic skin grafting.

ANATOMY, INDICATIONS, AND CONTRAINDICATIONS

A pedicle flap is composed of the skin, subcutaneous tissue, fascia, and neurovascular structures composed of the associated named artery, vein, and/or nerve that maintain its attachment to the donor site by a portion of tissue through which it receives its blood supply. The pedicle may also include the nerve when sensation is desired to the recipient site. Pedicle flaps are classified as either peninsular or island. Peninsular flaps maintain tissue continuity across the length of the donor area, whereas island pedicle flaps comprise an island of skin, subcutaneous tissue, and/or fascia maintained on a debulked or skeletonized pedicle. The unique anatomic structure and contours of the foot and ankle require careful consideration for long-term wound closure, durability, and function. The most common pedicle flaps in diabetic foot and ankle surgery each have characteristics making them ideal for application in certain regions. Table 14.1 includes these pedicle flaps with their specific vasculature, innervation, and location of their indicated recipient sites.

Indications for the use of pedicle flaps in the diabetic foot and ankle include but are not limited to soft tissue defects that have failed treatment with off-loading and are not candidates for primary wound closure using local random flaps or skin grafting, unstable scars resulting from prior surgery that are prone to ulceration, resected osteomyelitic areas with large defects, and surgical wounds that may require concomitant reconstruction of underlying osseous deformity. Contraindications for the use of pedicle flaps include but are not limited to active wound infection and/or osteomyelitis, compromised vascular status, hemodynamic instability, venous insufficiency, active smoking with potential wound healing complications, and soft tissue defects that can be addressed by other surgical techniques found lower on the reconstructive pyramid (6).

LITERATURE REVIEW AND CLINICAL OUTCOMES

Great Toe Artery Pedicle Flap

A pedicle flap based on the digital artery was initially described for use in hand reconstruction by Littler (21,22), whereas Moberg (26,27) first applied the technique for the foot in 1964. The highly specialized structure of the plantar soft tissues located at the forefoot often lends to difficult wound healing in diabetic patients. Simple primary wound closure and local

TABLE 14.1	Most Common Pedicle Flaps Utilized for Soft Tissue Coverage of the Diabetic Foot and Ankle		
Pedicle Flap	**Vasculature**	**Innervation**	**Recipient Sites**
Great Toe Artery Flap	• Great toe artery corresponding to donor site • Corresponding superficial digital vein(s)	Digital nerve corresponding to donor site	Plantar forefoot, central ray (toe and metatarsal) amputation, sesamoidectomy
Medial Plantar Artery Flap	• Collaterals from the dorsalis pedis artery and perforators of the medial plantar artery • Superficial venous system draining to the great saphenous vein	Cutaneous sensory nerve branches from the posterior tibial nerve	Heel, lateral plantar foot, dorsomedial foot, posterior and medial ankle
Lateral Plantar Artery Flap	• Lateral plantar artery • Superficial venous system draining to the great saphenous vein	Cutaneous sensory nerve branches from the posterior tibial nerve	Plantar forefoot, lateral plantar region
Lateral Calcaneal Artery Flap	• Lateral calcaneal artery • Lesser saphenous vein	Sural nerve	Posterior heel, plantar heel, and lateral malleolar regions
Sural Artery Neurofascio-cutaneous Flap	• Sural artery and peroneal perforator(s) • Lesser saphenous vein	Sural nerve (medial and/or lateral sural cutaneous nerves)	Distal lower extremity, ankle, heel, and proximal foot

random flaps are often of limited use due to lack of viable redundant skin at this region of the foot. The GTA flap offers surgeons the option to utilize soft tissue with similar characteristics as that of the plantar region of the foot without causing tension or further compromise to the area of skin adjacent to the recipient wound. Dutch et al. (11) reported on a series of 12 patients in which 15 GTA flaps were performed; however, 8 of these were for treatment of forefoot plantar wounds, whereas the remaining 7 were for dysfunctional scars. Two out of the 15 GTA flaps failed due to complete flap necrosis, whereas the others achieved complete healing. Demirtas et al. (8) utilized the same principle with the homodigital reverse flow island flap for coverage of diabetic neuropathic ulcerations of the great toe, showing satisfactory results in 3 out of a total 4 patients. Other successful case studies for the GTA flap in diabetic patients include those reported by Roukis and Zgonis (34) and Ramanujam and Zgonis (33).

Medial Plantar Artery Pedicle Flap

Building on the work of Shanahan and Gingrass (38) in their technique of an instep sensory skin flap for coverage of the heel, Harrison and Morgan (15) formally described the MPA pedicle island flap as a modification in 1981. The MPA flap has since become a popular option for extensive wound coverage at the plantar aspect of the diabetic foot given its ample blood supply and wide arc of rotation. The versatility of the MPA flap is evidenced by its use in several locations and types of soft tissue defects. Baker et al. (3) demonstrated successful outcomes for 11 patients who underwent the MPA flap for

coverage of mostly traumatic wounds at the plantar calcaneus, posterior ankle, lower leg, and plantar forefoot. Pallua et al. (30) studied 12 diabetic patients in which distally based dorsalis pedis artery flaps or MPA flaps were performed for coverage of defects at the plantar forefoot, demonstrating few complications consisting of temporary donor site pain and partial skin graft loss at the donor site. Acikel et al. (1) followed 20 patients with nondiabetic soft tissue defects who had the MPA flap performed via either proximally sensorial pedicle island flaps or reverse flow island flaps, showing only partial flap loss in 1 patient. Benito-Ruiz et al. (5) reported the successful healing of the MPA flap for 5 out of 6 patients with anterior heel defects secondary to chronic ulceration or trauma. Schwarz and Negrini (37) prospectively studied 51 MPA flaps in 48 patients with sensory impairment, resulting in a 98% overall flap survival rate. Zgonis et al. (40) further expanded the use of the MPA flap in combination with skeletal reconstruction via a lateral column arthrodesis for a diabetic Charcot neuroarthropathy midfoot deformity with chronic nonhealing ulceration.

Lateral Plantar Artery Pedicle Flap

The LPA flap is an instep island flap similar to the MPA flap for use at the weight bearing surface of the forefoot/midfoot; however, it is based on the LPA. The technique was first described by Martin et al. (24) in 1991. Sakai et al. (35) utilized the LPA flap to cover large soft tissue defects located at the lateral metatarsal head region of the foot. Luo et al. (23) found a 100% survival rate of 10 LPA flaps performed in 9 patients for coverage of soft tissue defects located at the anterior lateral plantar region of the foot. Oberlin et al. (28) also reported advantages of the LPA over the MPA flap including the potential for more distal advancement of the island flap with greater pedicle length.

Lateral Calcaneal Artery Pedicle Flap

Utilized for coverage of soft tissue defects about the heel and ankle, the LCA flap was initially reported by Grabb and Argenta (14) in 1981. The versatility of the LCA anatomy has led to modifications including the LCA island flap, LCA adipofascial flap, and the reverse LCA flap. In most cases, the sural nerve is retained in the dissection, therefore producing a sensate LCA flap. Holmes and Rayner (16) demonstrated successful healing of the LCA island flap for 9 out of 13 patients but cited the presence of infection and vascular disease as potential risk factors for flap failure. Favorable results using the LCA flap were shown by Gang (13) in 11 patients with medial malleolar wounds and Hovius et al. (17) for 7 patients with chronic ulcerations at the heel or lateral malleolus. Ağaoğlu et al. (2) successfully used the LCA flap in 3 patients, specifically mentioning 2 were diabetic wounds at the posterior calcaneal region with exposed Achilles tendon.

Through cadaveric study of the vascular network between the LCA and the lateral plantar and lateral tarsal arteries, Ishikawa et al. (19) detailed the possible reverse blood flow in the LCA artery and went on to perform the distally based LCA flap with complete healing in 2 patients. Lin et al. (20) modified the LCA flap as an adipofascial flap for coverage of defects at the posterior heel, lateral malleolus, and lateral supramalleolar regions. Likewise, Chung et al. (7) showed positive short-term results of the LCA adipofascial flap for 5 patients with wounds at the posterior heel described as either traumatic or chronic wounds. Lastly, Omokawa et al. (29) demonstrated successful long-term reconstruction in 4 patients using the LCA flap over defects with exposed bone or tendon at the lateral malleolus and posterior heel.

Sural Artery Neurofasciocutaneous Pedicle Flap

The inception of the SAN flap can be traced back to Pontén (31) in 1981 with his introduction of the fasciocutaneous flap based on the sural artery for reconstruction of lower leg defects. In that publication, along with the detailed description of the surgical technique, Pontén included a review of 23 fasciocutaneous flaps resulting in only 3 failures. In 1983, Donski and Fogdestam (10) described the distally based fasciocutaneous flap from the sural region with 3 successful cases involving defects at the middle and lower third of the leg. Then in 1992, while introducing the concept of the neurocutaneous island flap, Masquelet et al. (25) first described the sural neurocutaneous flap, which is now more frequently referred to as the reverse or retrograde SAN flap or simply the sural flap.

In contrast to the other pedicle flaps previously discussed, the literature contains several references that specifically applied the reverse flow SAN in diabetic reconstruction. In a large study by Dhamangaonkar and Patankar (9) of 109 cases, including 12 diabetic ulcerations that were addressed by using the SAN, the authors concluded that the risk of flap necrosis was higher in more distal soft tissue defects such as those on the plantar foot and anterior ankle, and in patients with diabetic and venous ulcers. Fraccalvieri et al. (12) analyzed 33 patients using the sural flap to cover defects of the foot, out of which 4 were diabetic and 1 of these had superficial skin necrosis following flap coverage but ultimately resolved with secondary healing. Baumeister et al. (4) provided an analysis of 70 sural flap cases to determine risk factors for complications, showing that the presence of diabetes mellitus, peripheral arterial disease or venous insufficiency, and/or patient age over 40 years increased risk of flap necrosis. A study of 37 patients by Tosun et al. (39) comprised the largest series of patients in which the sural flap was used for diabetic foot wounds located at the heel, dorsal foot, ankle, and plantar region; furthermore, the authors indicated that larger sural flaps especially in diabetic patients may avoid venous and arterial insufficiency by delay procedure.

Although most studies have shown use of the isolated SAN for the diabetic foot, the procedure has become increasingly popular in combination with corrective osseous techniques. Ignatiadis et al. (18) reported a case using the sural flap with partial calcanectomy for treatment of ulceration and osteomyelitis. Schannen et al. (36) presented a case report using both the SAN and rotational propeller flap based on the posterior tibial artery for revisional reconstruction of the medial and lateral ankle in an infected diabetic ankle fracture. Ramanujam and Zgonis (32) described a successful case utilizing the sural flap combined with subtalar joint arthrodesis for treatment of a nonhealing wound with osteomyelitis in a diabetic patient.

PREOPERATIVE CONSIDERATIONS

Proper diabetic patient selection and optimization is vital to successful outcomes in pedicle flap reconstruction. Detailed discussions with the patient including full disclosure of all possible risks and complications should be initiated early, and amputation should be reviewed as an alternative option in cases of a nonreconstructable lower extremity. Analysis of existing literature reveals several risk factors for pedicle complications, which are listed in Table 14.2.

Preoperative medical optimization of all comorbid conditions should be prioritized in the diabetic patient; therefore, a multidisciplinary team approach should be employed. The recipient wound should be free of infection, which is typically accomplished through staged surgical débridement and appropriate culture-based antibiotic therapy. Because successful outcomes are also dependent on intact vasculature, the inflow perfusion of the recipient wound should be thoroughly assessed via clinical examination and noninvasive vascular testing of the lower extremity including arterial Doppler ultrasound, ankle/toe brachial indices, and transcutaneous oxygen pressure measurements. If this initial vascular assessment reveals questionable inflow perfusion, a formal vascular surgery consultation is warranted to determine if further angiography and/or surgical revascularization procedure(s) are indicated.

<table>
<tr><td colspan="1">

TABLE 14.2

Most Commonly Reported Risk Factors in Pedicle Flap Complications

Risk Factors

Smoking
Older age
Hemodynamic instability
Diabetes mellitus
Cardiac disease
Peripheral arterial disease
Venous insufficiency
Renal disease
</td></tr>
</table>

Vascular testing and imaging through an arterial Doppler ultrasound or angiography may also be used to analyze the patency of the named artery to be included in the pedicle flap. Preoperative vein mapping is also helpful to evaluate the lesser saphenous vein for its location and diameter (usually >2 mm) prior to performing a SAN flap. Vein mapping of the lesser saphenous vein will help locate the donor site of the sural artery and sural nerve which accompany the lesser saphenous vein during the SAN flap dissection.

Thorough clinical examination of the affected lower extremity with corresponding appropriate medical imaging can determine other contributing factors such as underlying equinus contracture, osseous deformity, and/or osteomyelitis at the site of the recipient defect. This may prompt the surgeon to include additional surgical procedures for reconstruction at the time of the pedicle flap closure or in staged fashion. Surgical adjunctive procedures such as gastrocnemius recession or tendo-Achilles lengthening, exostectomy, arthrodesis, and/or soft tissue contracture release may also be utilized during the pedicle flap closure or in staged reconstruction. Furthermore, in certain cases where the pedicle flap donor site is compromised due to a previous musculoskeletal or vascular injury and is unavailable for harvesting, a cross-leg or cross-foot pedicle flap may be considered for harvesting the desired pedicle flap from the contralateral extremity.

Detailed surgical planning is of utmost importance to familiarize the surgeon with the anatomy of pedicle flaps. Because undue tension will initially impair venous return, many pedicle flaps are often designed of greater dimension than initially estimated to avoid tension. Another consideration is the "delay phenomenon." Delay procedure may increase flap survival by allowing more efficient functional blood flow to a segment of tissue via staged division of a portion of its vascular supply. This is performed in staged fashion in which the designed flap is partially dissected and inset at the donor site during the first stage and followed by a second stage in which pedicle transection and inset completion is executed after the flap has established ideal vascular connections at the recipient site. This delay maneuver allows the use of flaps with greater surface area than would otherwise be possible (39).

Delayed flap closure is usually performed within 5 to 14 days of the initial flap dissection and is dependent on the flap's characteristics and viability.

The donor sites of the pedicle flaps for the diabetic foot and ankle are usually covered by an autogenous or allogenic skin graft, plastic surgery closure techniques, and sometimes by primary closure. In addition, for major pedicle flaps that cover weight bearing surfaces of the foot, surgical off-loading of the lower extremity with the utilization of a circular external fixation device is recommended.

DETAILED SURGICAL TECHNIQUE

Great Toe Artery Pedicle Flap

The recipient wound is excised full-thickness in circular fashion. The digital vascular pedicle at the lateral aspect of the great toe is identified with a sterile handheld arterial Doppler probe, and the proposed flap at the donor site is marked with an identical size and shape as the recipient wound. With the tourniquet inflated, the full-thickness GTA flap is raised under loupe magnification and minimal direct handling of the pedicle flap. A skin incision is made to connect the recipient wound bed to the donor site and the GTA flap is carefully mobilized and inset at the recipient wound. The tourniquet is deflated, and the flap is secured using nonabsorbable sutures. The communicating incision is closed primarily, whereas the donor site can be closed with an autogenous split-thickness skin graft, allogenic skin graft, or primary closure. In certain cases, a lateral great toe phalangeal exostectomy may be performed to assist with primary closure of the donor site (Figs. 14.1 to 14.3).

Medial Plantar Artery and Lateral Plantar Artery Pedicle Flap

The recipient wound is excised in full-thickness triangular fashion with the base of the triangle oriented laterally. The MPA is identified for its course via a sterile handheld arterial Doppler probe, and the proposed flap is marked taking care to preserve the medial skin island while maintaining a large radius of elevation to prevent tension. With the tourniquet inflated, the proposed flap is incised in semicircular fashion extending from the base of the triangle and oriented in a distal medial direction. With minimal handling of the flap and under loupe magnification, dissection of the flap is carefully performed, beginning laterally at the apex of the flap and then medially toward the MPA. The surgeon can also access the underlying anatomy through this approach if further osseous reconstruction is indicated. The tourniquet is deflated, followed by insetting of the MPA flap at the recipient wound with minimal deep absorbable suture and skin approximated with nonabsorbable suture or skin staples. The donor site can be closed with an autogenous split-thickness skin graft, allogenic skin graft, or primary closure (Figs. 14.4 and 14.5). In certain cases, fasciocutaneous flaps can be raised as peninsular or island fashion and based on the MPA for closure in diabetic foot wounds (Fig. 14.6).

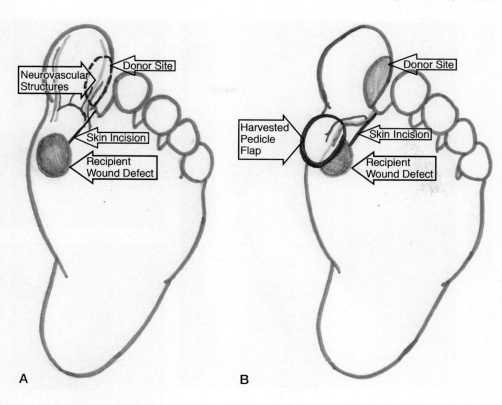

FIGURE 14.1 Schematic illustration showing a plantar forefoot ulceration **(A)** excised in full-thickness circular fashion and covered with a great toe artery (GTA) pedicle flap raised from the donor site at the lateral aspect of the great toe **(B)**. A skin incision is made to connect the recipient wound defect to the donor site while the GTA flap is carefully mobilized and inset at the recipient wound defect **(B)**. The donor site can be closed with an autogenous split-thickness skin graft, allogenic skin graft, or primary closure. In certain cases, a lateral great toe phalangeal exostectomy may be performed to assist with primary closure of the donor site.

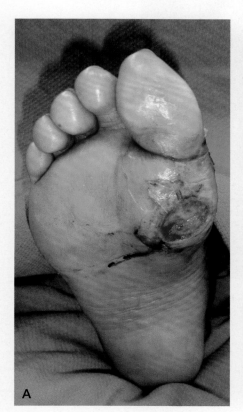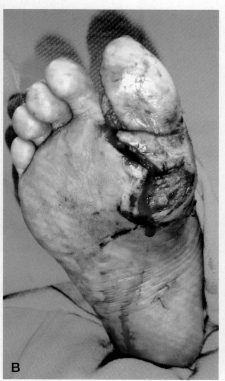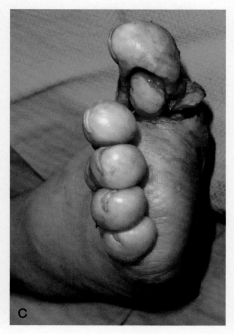

FIGURE 14.2 Intraoperative picture **(A)** of a right forefoot plantar ulceration covered with a great toe artery (GTA) pedicle flap harvested from the lateral aspect of the great toe **(B,C)**. *(continued)*

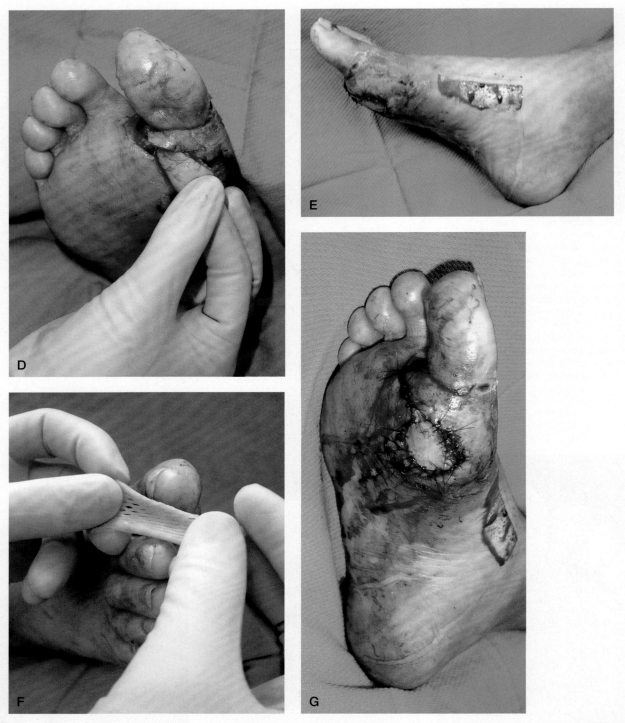

FIGURE 14.2 *(Continued)* **D.** A communicating skin incision is made to connect the recipient wound defect to the donor site, and the GTA flap is carefully mobilized and inset at the recipient wound defect. **E,F.** An autogenous split-thickness skin graft can be harvested from the medial aspect of the ipsilateral foot to cover the donor site. The GTA flap is inset and secured at the recipient wound defect using nonabsorbable sutures **(G)**. *(continued)*

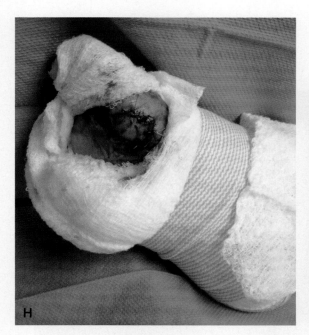
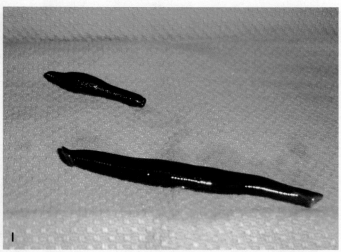

FIGURE 14.2 *(Continued)* Postoperative appearance of the GTA flap with signs of venous congestion **(H)** can be managed readily by the application of medicinal leeches and after the pedicle flap has been prepared by a "pie-crusting" technique to allow for bleeding and attachment of the medicinal leeches **(I)**.

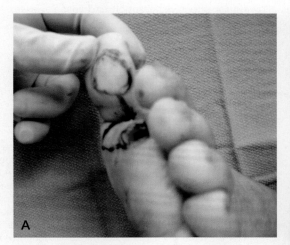
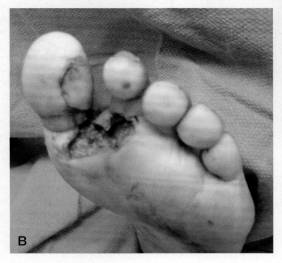
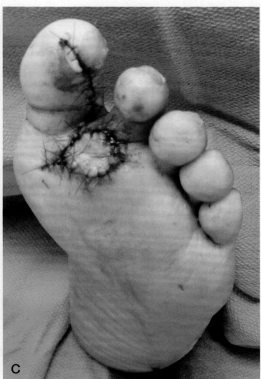

FIGURE 14.3 Intraoperative picture showing the marking of the great toe artery (GTA) pedicle flap from the donor site at the lateral aspect of the great toe **(A)**, followed by careful pedicle dissection **(B)** and insetting to the first web space at the plantar aspect of the foot **(C)**. Note that primary wound closure was performed at the donor site of the GTA flap **(C)**. *(continued)*

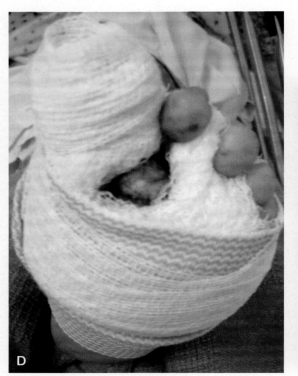
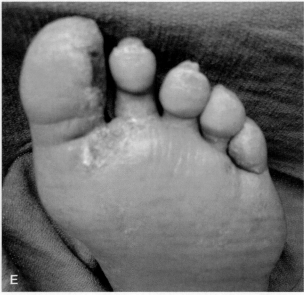

FIGURE 14.3 *(Continued)* **D.** Immediate postoperative dressings allowing for direct visualization and vascular assessment of the GTA flap. **E.** Final postoperative clinical outcome at 7 weeks.

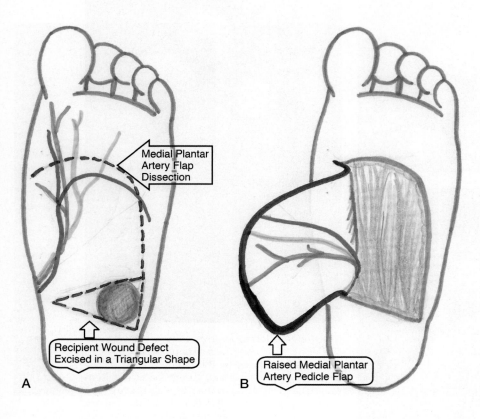

FIGURE 14.4 Schematic illustration showing a plantar midfoot/hindfoot ulceration **(A)** excised in full-thickness triangular fashion and covered with a medial plantar artery (MPA) pedicle flap **(B)**. The MPA flap is incised in a semicircular fashion extending from the base of the triangle and oriented in a distal medial direction **(A)**. With minimal handling of the pedicle flap and under loupe magnification, dissection of the pedicle flap is carefully performed, beginning laterally at the apex of the flap and then medially toward the MPA **(B)**. The raised MPA flap is then inset at the recipient wound defect with minimal deep absorbable sutures and the skin is approximated with nonabsorbable sutures or skin staples **(B)**. The donor site can be closed with an autogenous split-thickness skin graft, allogenic skin graft, or primary closure. A hybrid or circular external fixation device application is also highly recommended for simultaneous lower extremity stabilization, surgical off-loading, and direct access of the pedicle flap.

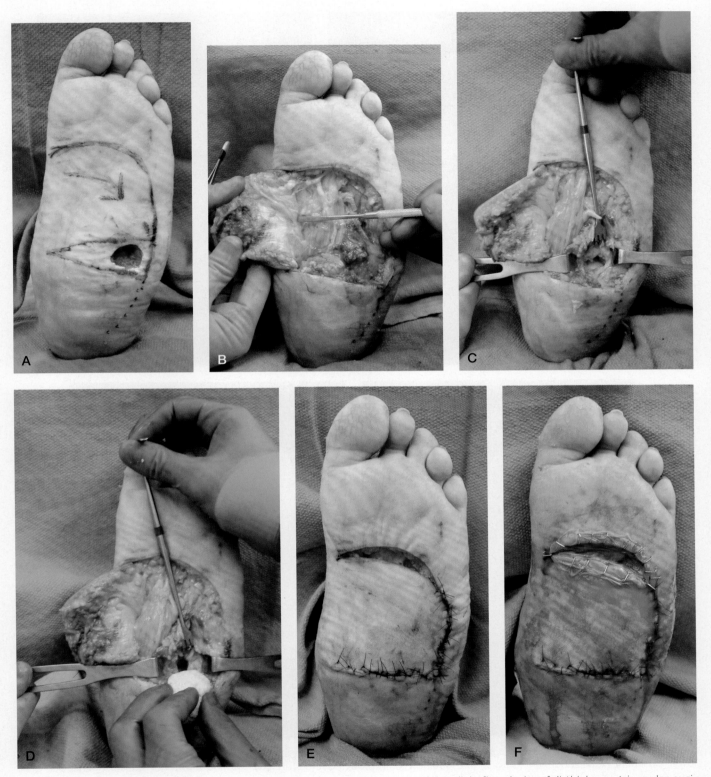

FIGURE 14.5 A. Intraoperative picture showing the medial plantar artery (MPA) pedicle flap design, full-thickness triangular excision of the plantar ulceration, and direct approach to the lateral column arthrodesis for a left foot diabetic Charcot neuroarthropathy. Intraoperative picture showing the MPA flap dissection **(B)**, followed by joint preparation **(C)** and application of allogenic bone graft at the lateral column arthrodesis site **(D)**. Closure of the MPA flap at the recipient wound defect **(E)** is followed by application of an allogenic skin graft at the non–weight-bearing donor site **(F)**. *(continued)*

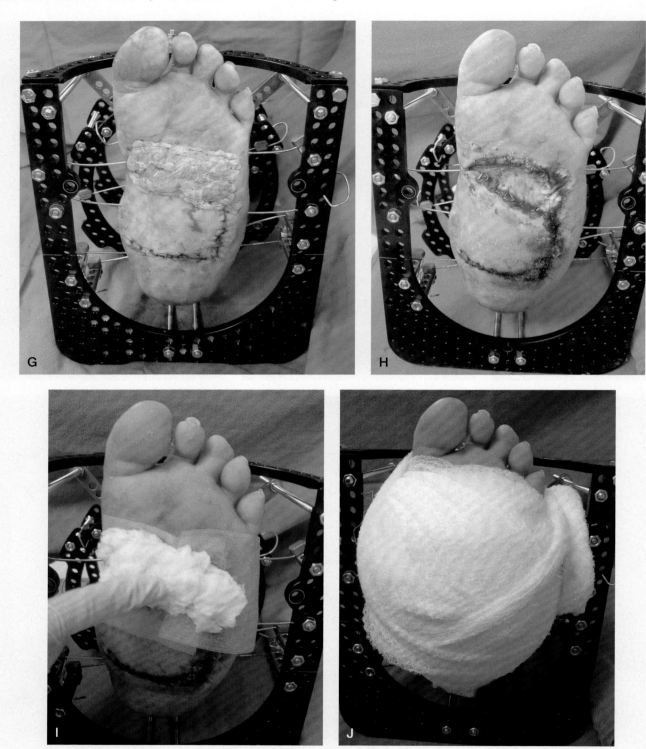

FIGURE 14.5 *(Continued)* A circular external fixation device is then applied for a simultaneous deformity correction and arthrodesis, lower extremity stabilization, and surgical off-loading **(G)**. Intraoperative picture **(G)** showing the donor site's allogenic skin graft covered by a bolster dressing composed of a nonadherent material and sterile sponges soaked in saline. Four weeks postoperative picture of the bolter dressing removal **(H)** followed by wet-to-dry sterile saline dressings at the donor site **(I)** and postoperative circular external fixation dressings **(J)**. *(continued)*

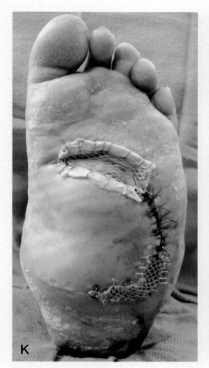
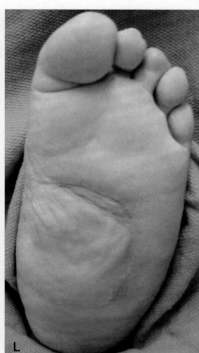

FIGURE 14.5 *(Continued)* **K.** Intraoperative picture 10 weeks postoperatively after the circular external fixation removal and application of autogenous split-thickness skin graft at the donor and recipient wound defects. **L.** Final postoperative clinical outcome at 14 weeks since the initial surgery.

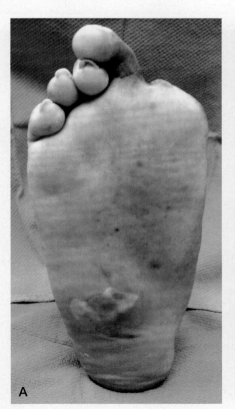
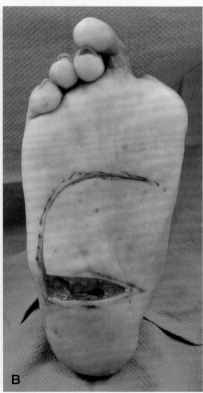
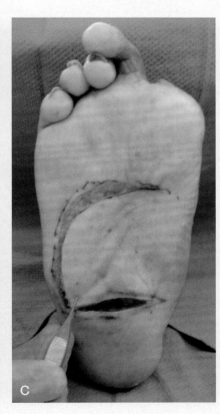

FIGURE 14.6 **A.** Intraoperative picture of a right foot plantar cuboid infected ulceration in a diabetic patient with Charcot neuroarthropathy and previous reconstruction with medial column arthrodesis, plantar cuboid exostectomy, excisional débridement, percutaneous tendo-Achilles lengthening, and utilization of internal and circular external fixation devices. Patient underwent an initial surgical excisional débridement of all nonviable soft tissues followed by a revisional excisional débridement, cuboid partial resection, removal of prominent internal screw from the previous medial column arthrodesis, and fasciocutaneous peninsular flap based on the medial plantar artery (MPA). Note that the recipient wound defect was excised in full-thickness triangular fashion with the base of the triangle laterally **(B)** and that the raised fasciocutaneous flap based on the MPA was rotated toward the base of the triangle **(C)**. *(continued)*

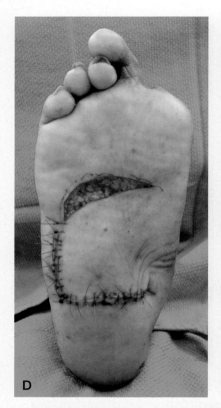
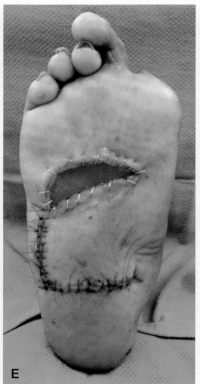
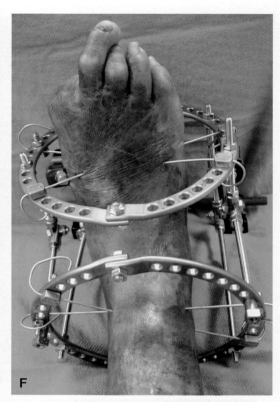
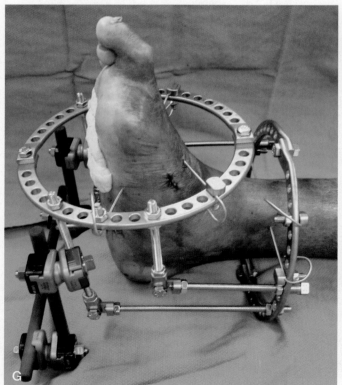
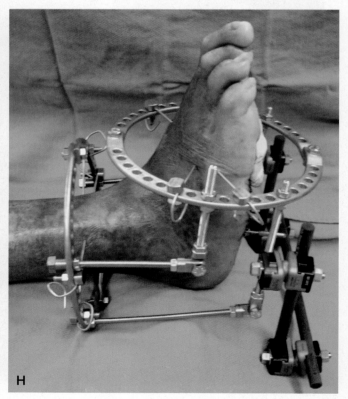

FIGURE 14.6 *(Continued)* The flap was then secured to the recipient wound defect with nonabsorbable sutures **(D)** while the donor site was covered with a dermoconductive acellular dermal replacement **(E)**. A circular external fixation device and Steinmann pin fixation were then applied for simultaneous lower extremity stabilization and surgical off-loading **(F–I)** while a bolster dressing composed of a nonadherent material and sterile sponges soaked in saline was applied over the dorsal surface of the dermoconductive acellular dermal replacement at the donor site **(I)**. *(continued)*

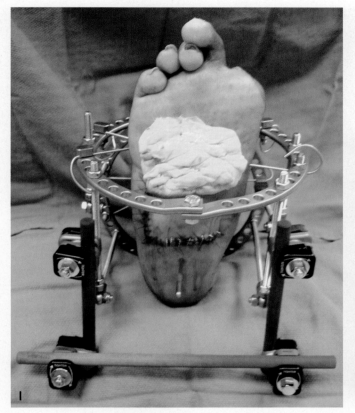

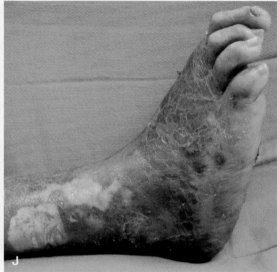

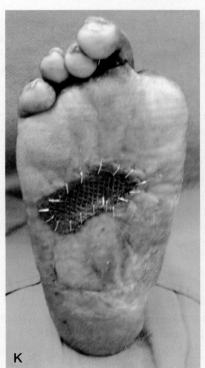

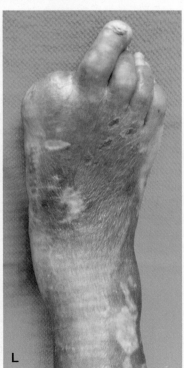

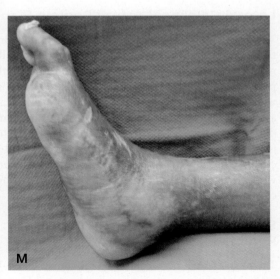

FIGURE 14.6 *(Continued)* The circular external fixation device and Steinmann pin fixation were removed at approximately 5 weeks postoperatively followed by an autogenous split-thickness skin graft harvested from the ipsilateral lateral aspect of the lower leg **(J)** to the donor site of the previously raised fasciocutaneous flap **(K)** 3 weeks after the circular external fixation and Steinmann pin fixation removal. **L–O**. Final postoperative clinical outcomes at 5 months since the initial surgery. *(continued)*

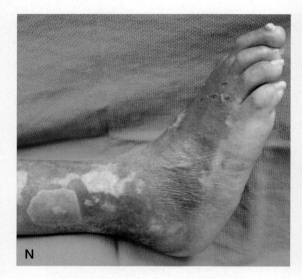

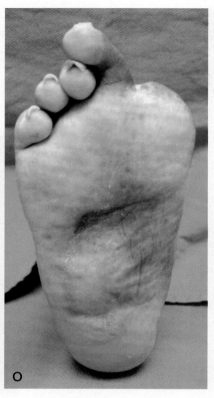

FIGURE 14.6 *(Continued)*

The LPA flap is generally performed in similar fashion; however, the LPA is identified and maintained in the neurovascular pedicle. When compared to the MPA flap, the LPA flap may also be elevated for more distal advancement of the flap to the recipient site.

Lateral Calcaneal Artery Pedicle Flap

The recipient wound is excised full-thickness in circular fashion. The LCA is identified with a sterile handheld arterial Doppler probe and its course marked along with the proposed flap. With the tourniquet inflated, the flap is elevated with minimal handling and under loupe magnification. This approach may also facilitate access to any underlying osseous deformity if correction is clinically indicated. The tourniquet is deflated, and the LCA flap is inset and secured to the recipient wound with minimal deep absorbable suture and skin with nonabsorbable suture or skin staples. The donor site is closed with an autogenous or allogenic skin graft.

Sural Artery Neurofasciocutaneous Pedicle Flap

The recipient wound is excised full thickness in oval or circular fashion. Using a sterile handheld arterial Doppler probe, the most distal perforator of the peroneal artery is identified and located generally 5 to 7 cm proximal to the distal tip of the lateral malleolus between the fibula and Achilles tendon. The surgeon can use the sterile wrapper from the sterile gloves to cut out a template of the recipient wound. That template is

then used to trace the proposed flap onto the posterior central aspect of the proximal lower leg. It may also be helpful to consider the following in the procedure: (a) inclusion of a cutaneous tail over the SAN pedicle to decrease tension at the pedicle components and (b) design the flap further distally from the popliteal crease to ensure the pedicle components are included throughout the entirety of the flap while allowing harvest of autogenous split-thickness skin graft just proximal to the donor site if needed for donor site closure. A "Z"-shaped incision is marked from the flap over the perforating peroneal artery to the recipient wound. Careful dissection under loupe magnification is carried out beginning midline at the most superior aspect of the outlined flap. This technique allows for continuous visualization of the pedicle (sural artery, sural nerve, and lesser saphenous vein) components to ensure proper width of the flap with the neurovascular structures maintained at the mid-axis of the dissected flap. Blunt dissection with minimal handling of the flap and without undermining is performed to the level of fascia overlying the gastrocnemius muscle belly. The flap is elevated from proximal to distal until the pivot point is reached, and then the flap is transposed onto the recipient wound, with the pedicle either tunneled or exteriorized. The tourniquet is deflated, and inflow perfusion is assessed for the next 5 to 10 minutes. If inflow perfusion is inadequate, delay procedure is performed over the next 5 to 14 days. The SAN flap is inset and secured with nonabsorbable suture.

Primary closure may be performed at the "Z" incision and donor site if <5 cm; however, if the donor site is >5 cm, an autogenous split-thickness skin graft or allogenic skin graft can be used to cover the donor site. Inflow perfusion at the pedicle can be assessed using the sterile handheld arterial Doppler probe but is best observed based on the color of the flap (Figs. 14.7 and 14.8). If the pedicle flap is harvested in an island fashion, an autogenous split-thickness skin graft is applied over the skeletonized pedicle at the pivot point approximately 5 to 7 cm proximal to the distal tip of the lateral malleolus. In certain cases, fasciocutaneous flaps can be raised as peninsular or island fashion and based on the peroneal perforator similar to SAN flap for closure in diabetic foot wounds (Fig. 14.9).

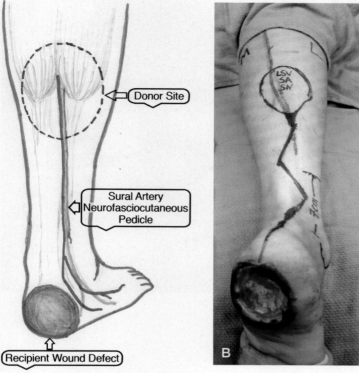

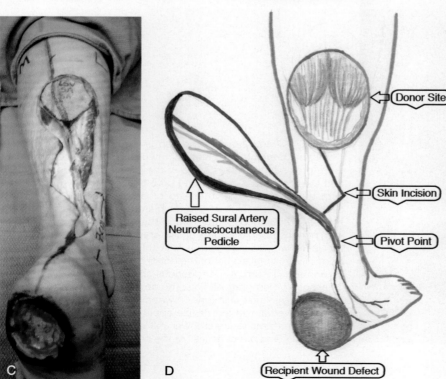

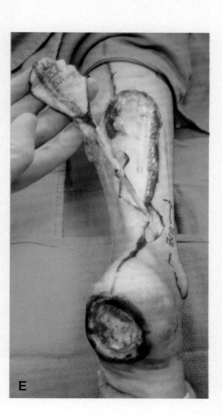

FIGURE 14.7 Schematic **(A)** and clinical **(B)** illustration showing a posterior hindfoot ulceration excised in full-thickness circular fashion and covered with a sural artery neurofasciocutaneous (SAN) pedicle flap. With minimal handling of the pedicle flap and under loupe magnification, dissection of the pedicle flap is carefully performed, beginning midline at the most superior and proximal aspect of the outlined flap **(C)**. This technique allows for continuous visualization of the pedicle (sural artery, sural nerve, and lesser saphenous vein) components to ensure proper width of the flap while the neurovascular structures are maintained at the mid-axis of the dissected flap **(D,E)**. *(continued)*

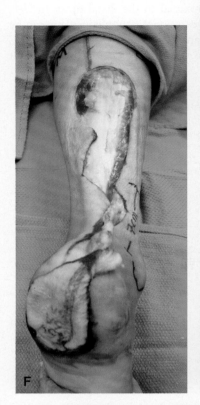

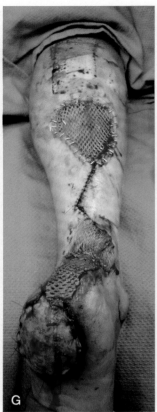

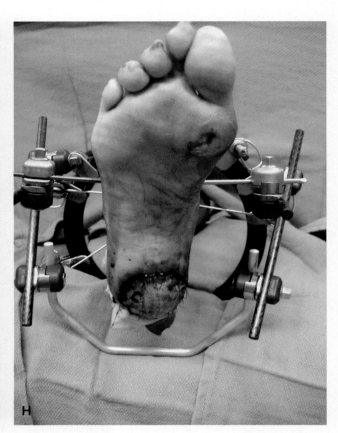

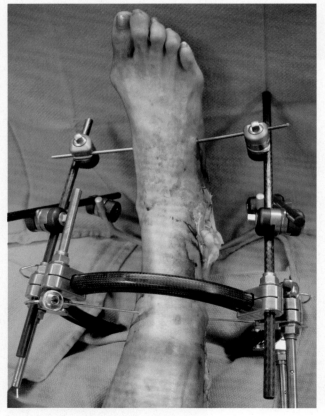

FIGURE 14.7 *(Continued)* The flap is elevated from proximal to distal direction until the pivot point which is located generally 5 to 7 cm proximal to the distal tip of the lateral malleolus is reached and then the flap is transposed onto the recipient wound defect, with the pedicle either tunneled or exteriorized **(F)**. The raised SAN flap is then inset at the recipient wound defect with minimal deep absorbable sutures, and the skin is then approximated with nonabsorbable sutures or skin staples **(G)**. The donor site can be closed with an autogenous split-thickness skin graft harvested from the proximal aspect of the donor site **(G)**, allogenic skin graft, or primary closure. An autogenous split-thickness skin graft **(G)** or allogenic skin graft can also be applied for coverage over the pedicle to minimize skin tension when necessary. A hybrid **(H,I)** or circular external fixation device application is also highly recommended for simultaneous lower extremity stabilization, surgical off-loading, and direct access of the pedicle flap.

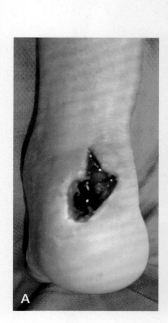
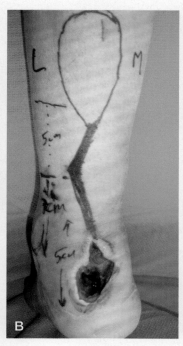
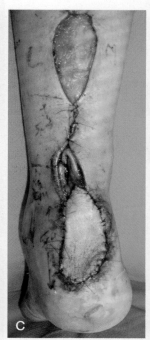
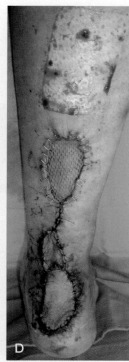

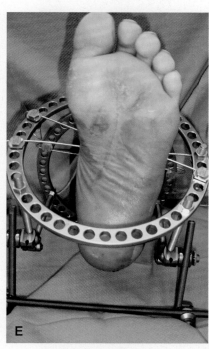
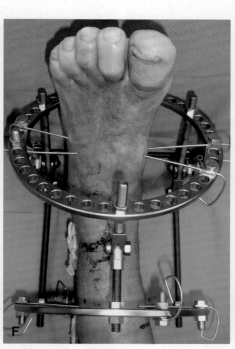
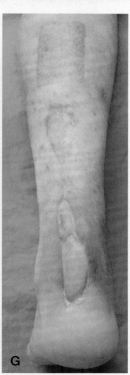

FIGURE 14.8 A. Intraoperative picture showing a posterior hindfoot ulceration with a history of previous recurrent infections that was surgically debrided with a minimal partial calcaneal resection. **B.** Picture shows harvesting of the sural artery neurofasciocutaneous (SAN) pedicle flap from the posterior aspect of the lower extremity. A modified "Z"-shaped incision from the pedicle flap to the level of the recipient wound defect is aiming at the most distal perforator from the peroneal artery with each arm of the skin incision designed in equal lengths **(B)**. The SAN flap is then inset to the recipient wound defect **(C)** while the donor site and part of the pedicle are closed with an autogenous split-thickness skin graft harvested just superior to the proximal aspect of the donor site **(D)**. **E,F.** Intraoperative pictures of the circular external fixation device application for simultaneous lower extremity stabilization, surgical off-loading, and direct access of the pedicle flap. The circular external fixation device was removed at approximately 6 weeks postoperatively. **G.** Final postoperative clinical outcome at approximately 6 months. (With permission from Ramanujam CL, Facaros Z, Zgonis T. Surgical off-loading external fixation and plastic reconstruction of the foot and ankle. In: Cooper PS, Polyzois VD, Zgonis T, eds. External fixators of the foot and ankle. Philadelphia: Lippincott Williams & Wilkins, 2013:375.)

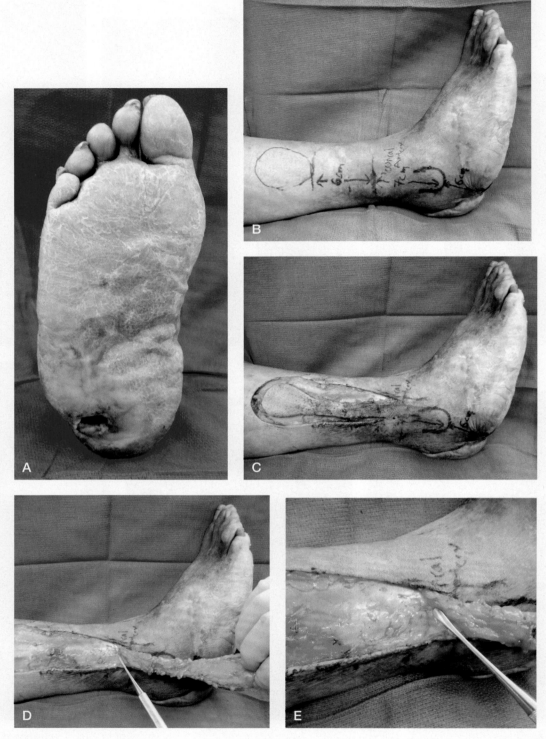

FIGURE 14.9 A. Intraoperative picture showing a plantar hindfoot ulceration in a diabetic patient with a right foot calcaneal osteomyelitis and Charcot neuroarthropathy with a history of multiple previous excisional surgical soft tissue and osseous débridements, application and removal of antibiotic-impregnated polymethylmethacrylate cemented beads, and negative pressure wound therapy. Patient underwent an initial surgical excisional débridement of all nonviable soft tissues followed by a revisional excisional débridement and soft tissue coverage with a fasciocutaneous peninsular flap based on the peroneal artery. Note the marking of the proposed fasciocutaneous flap based on the most distal perforator of the peroneal artery harvested in a peninsular fashion from the lateral aspect of the lower extremity **(B)**. With minimal handling of the flap and under loupe magnification, dissection of the flap was carefully performed, beginning midline at the most superior and proximal aspect of the outlined flap **(C)**. *(continued)*

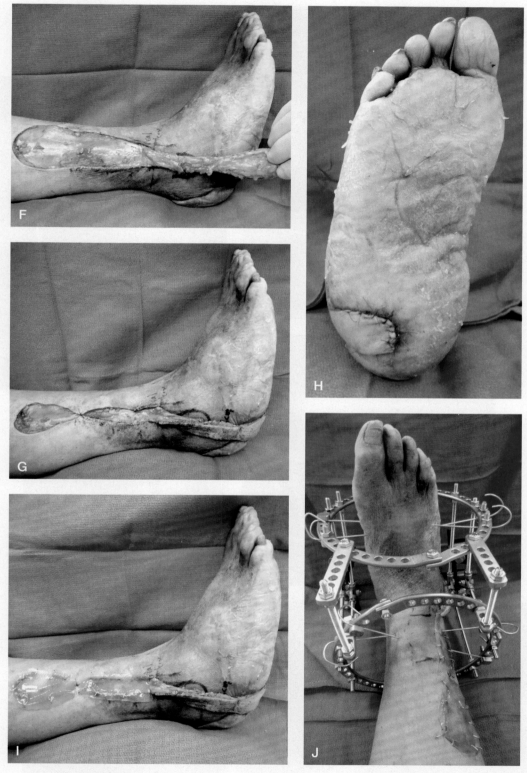

FIGURE 14.9 *(Continued)* The flap was elevated in a peninsular fashion from proximal to distal direction until the pivot point which is located generally 5 to 7 cm proximal to the distal tip of the lateral malleolus was reached **(D,E)** and secured to the recipient wound defect with nonabsorbable sutures **(F–H)**. The donor site can be closed with an autogenous split-thickness skin graft, allogenic skin graft **(I)**, or primary closure. A circular external fixation device was then applied for simultaneous lower extremity stabilization and surgical off-loading **(J–M)**, while a bolster dressing composed of a nonadherent material and sterile sponges soaked in saline was applied over the dorsal surface of the dermoconductive acellular dermal replacement at the donor site. *(continued)*

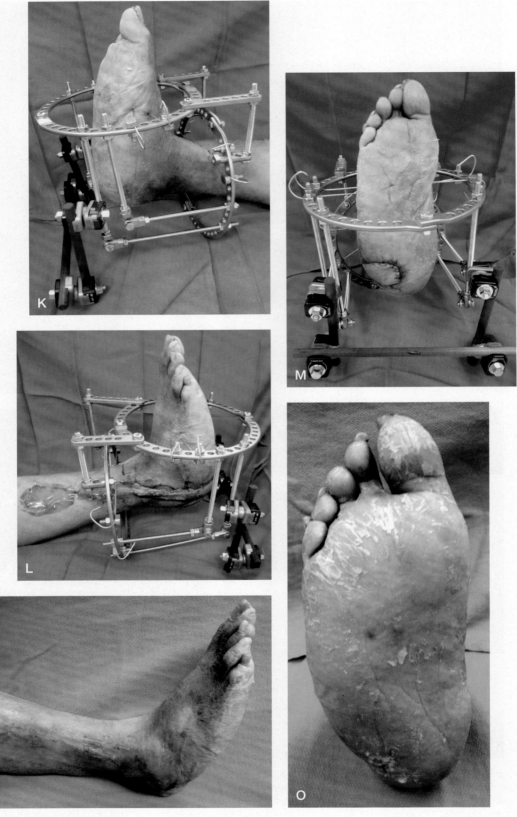

FIGURE 14.9 *(Continued)* The circular external fixation device was removed at 6 weeks postoperatively followed by an application of a dermoconductive acellular dermal replacement at the donor and recipient wound defects. The patient was followed closely in an outpatient clinic for lower extremity off-loading and local wound care. **N,O.** Final postoperative clinical outcomes at approximately 6 months since the flap surgery.

Overall, the pedicle flaps discussed in this chapter are covered minimally to allow easy access for frequent monitoring postoperatively. The donor site, whether covered by autogenous split-thickness or allogenic skin graft, can be dressed with sterile nonadherent gauze and mild compressive dressing. Depending on adjunctive surgical procedures such as equinus correction, osteotomies, and/or arthrodeses, further postoperative management may include a well-padded posterior splint or a surgical off-loading circular external fixation device with appropriate pin/wire site and incision site dressings.

POSTOPERATIVE CARE AND COMPLICATIONS

Most patients are admitted postoperatively on average 3 to 7 days for observation of the pedicle flap, pain management, and rehabilitation. Strict bed rest is typically imposed for the first 24 to 48 hours, with flap inspection and vascular checks every 2 to 4 hours for the first day and then every 4 to 6 hours for the second day. Prophylaxis for deep vein thrombosis may be administered during this period of immobility and is often based on hospital protocol. Weight bearing status and physical therapy thereafter often depends on other concomitant surgical procedures performed at the time of the pedicle flap reconstruction. Antibiotics should be administered postoperatively to prevent infection and are based on intraoperative soft tissue cultures, bone cultures, and/or bone biopsies.

Complications following pedicle flap reconstruction may be due to any or a combination of the following: flap choice, reconstructive timing, wound characteristics, and surgical and patient-related features. The most common complications for pedicle flaps are included in Table 14.3.

Early observation and prompt treatment of potential complications may improve clinical outcomes. Pallor of the flap often reflects inadequate arterial supply, whereas cyanosis indicates venous congestion. Surgical drains may be employed intraoperatively to facilitate removal of excess drainage and are typically removed within the first 24 to 48 hours. Hematoma or seroma at the recipient wound and flap interface can impede healing, cause infection, and/or eventual flap necrosis. If full-thickness necrosis is visualized, adequate surgical débridement is warranted to prevent further tissue loss and infection. Hydrosurgical or ultrasonic instrumentation can be very helpful in this regard to selectively remove necrotic or infected tissue at the site.

Venous congestion is mainly encountered with the SAN flap and is most often attributed to impaired venous drainage due to the presence of valves in the deep venous system that prevent uninterrupted retrograde venous flow. Modifications over the years in the operative technique for the SAN flap have attempted to decrease the occurrence of venous congestion. However, when venous congestion is present, medicinal leeches need to be available for treatment (see Fig. 14.2I). If mild pedicle flap dehiscence is encountered, further surgical wound closure may be facilitated with revisional surgical débridement and primary wound closure, autogenous or allogenic skin grafting, and/or local random flap closure. In complications resulting in significantly larger tissue loss, negative pressure wound therapy may be employed to facilitate wound healing prior to more definitive wound closure techniques.

Conclusion

The sheer diversity of the proposed surgical techniques available for soft tissue reconstruction of diabetic foot and ankle wounds reflects the potential complexity of these cases. The aforementioned local and distant pedicle flaps can offer surgeons the ability to restore the diabetic foot or ankle defects with soft tissue that resembles its original surface, but can also be utilized in combination with other reconstructive procedures to produce the optimal underlying structure and function.

References

1. Acikel C, Celikoz B, Yuksel F, et al. Various applications of the medial plantar flap to cover the defects of the plantar foot, posterior heel, and ankle. Ann Plast Surg 2003;50:498–503.

2. Ağaoğlu G, Kayikçiolu A, Safak T, et al. Lateral calcaneal artery skin flap. Ann Plast Surg 2001;46:572–573.

3. Baker GL, Newton ED, Franklin JD. Fasciocutaneous island flap based on the medial plantar artery: clinical applications for leg, ankle, and forefoot. Plast Reconstr Surg 1990;85:47–60.

4. Baumeister SP, Spierer R, Erdmann D, et al. A realistic complication analysis of 70 sural artery flaps in a multimorbid patient group. Plast Reconstr Surg 2003;112:129–142.

5. Benito-Ruiz J, Yoon T, Guisantes-Pintos E, et al. Reconstruction of soft-tissue defects of the heel with local fasciocutaneous flaps. Ann Plast Surg 2004;52:380–384.

6. Capobianco CM, Stapleton JJ, Zgonis T. Soft tissue reconstruction pyramid in the diabetic foot. Foot Ankle Spec 2010;3:241–248.

7. Chung MS, Baek GH, Gong HS, et al. Lateral calcaneal artery adipofascial flap for reconstruction of the posterior heel of the foot. Clin Orthop Surg 2009;1:1–5.

8. Demirtas Y, Ayhan S, Latifoglu O, et al. Homodigital reverse flow island flap for reconstruction of neuropathic great toe ulcers in diabetic patients. Br J Plast Surg 2005;58:717–719.

9. Dhamangaonkar AC, Patankar HS. Reverse sural fasciocutaneous flap with a cutaneous pedicle to cover distal lower limb soft tissue defects: experience of 109 clinical cases. J Orthop Traumatol 2014;15:225–229.

TABLE 14.3
Most Common Complications of Pedicle Flaps in Diabetic Foot and Ankle Surgery
Complications
Flap necrosis (partial or complete)
Incomplete and/or delayed flap take
Dehiscence
Venous congestion
Hematoma or seroma
Infection

10. Donski PK, Fogdestam I. Distally based fasciocutaneous flap from the sural region. A preliminary report. Scand J Plast Reconstr Surg 1983;17:191–196.

11. Dutch WM, Arnz M, Jolly GP. Digital artery flaps for closure of soft tissue defects of the forefoot. J Foot Ankle Surg 2003;42:208–214.

12. Fraccalvieri M, Bogetti P, Verna G, et al. Distally based fasciocutaneous sural flap for foot reconstruction: a retrospective review of 10 years experience. Foot Ankle Int 2008;29:191–198.

13. Gang RK. Reconstruction of soft-tissue defect of the posterior heel with a lateral calcaneal artery island flap. Plast Reconstr Surg 1987;79:415–421.

14. Grabb WC, Argenta LC. The lateral calcaneal artery skin flap (the lateral calcaneal artery, lesser saphenous vein, and sural nerve skin flap). Plast Reconstr Surg 1981;68:723–730.

15. Harrison DH, Morgan BD. The instep island flap to resurface plantar defects. Br J Plast Surg 1981;34:315–318.

16. Holmes J, Rayner CR. Lateral calcaneal artery island flaps. Br J Plast Surg 1984;37:402–405.

17. Hovius SE, Hofman A, van der Meulen JC. Experiences with the lateral calcaneal artery flap. Ann Plast Surg 1988;21:532–535.

18. Ignatiadis IA, Tsiampa VA, Arapoglou DK, et al. Surgical management of a diabetic calcaneal ulceration and osteomyelitis with a partial calcanectomy and a sural neurofasciocutaneous flap. Diabet Foot Ankle 2010;1.

19. Ishikawa K, Isshiki N, Hoshino K, et al. Distally based lateral calcaneal flap. Ann Plast Surg 1990;24:10–16.

20. Lin SD, Lai CS, Chiu YT, et al. The lateral calcaneal artery adipofascial flap. Br J Plast Surg 1996;49:52–57.

21. Littler JW. Neurovascular pedicle transfer of tissue in reconstructive surgery of the hand. J Bone Joint Surg 1956;38:917.

22. Littler JW. The neurovascular pedicle method of digital transposition for reconstruction of the thumb. Plast Reconstr Surg 1953;12:303–319.

23. Luo Y, Wang T, Fang H. Clinical application of retrograde island flap pedicled with lateral plantar artery. J Tongji Med Univ 1997;17:247–249.

24. Martin D, Gorowitz B, Peres JM, et al. Le lambeau plantaire interne sur pédicule plantaire externe: un moyen de couverture utilisable sur toute la surface du pied. Ann Chir Plast Esthet 1991;36:544–548.

25. Masquelet AC, Romana MC, Wolf G. Skin island flaps supplied by the vascular axis of the sensitive superficial nerves: anatomic study and clinical experience in the leg. Plast Reconstr Surg 1992;89:1115–1121.

26. Moberg E. Aspects of sensation in reconstructive surgery of the extremity. J Bone Joint Surg Am 1964;46:817–825.

27. Moberg E. Evaluation and management of nerve injuries in the hand. Surg Clin North Am 1964;44:1019–1029.

28. Oberlin C, Accioli de Vasconcellos Z, Touam C. Medial plantar flap based distally on the lateral plantar artery to cover a forefoot skin defect. Plast Reconstr Surg 2000;106:874–877.

29. Omokawa S, Yajima H, Tanaka Y, et al. Long-term results of lateral calcaneal artery flap for hindfoot reconstruction. J Reconstr Microsurg 2008;24:239–245.

30. Pallua N, Di Benedetto G, Berger A. Forefoot reconstruction by reversed island flaps in diabetic patients. Plast Reconstr Surg 2000;106:823–827.

31. Pontén B. The fasciocutaneous flap: its use in soft tissue defects of the lower leg. Br J Plast Surg 1981;34:215–220.

32. Ramanujam CL, Zgonis T. Primary arthrodesis and sural artery flap coverage for subtalar joint osteomyelitis in a diabetic patient. Clin Podiatr Med Surg 2011;28:421–427.

33. Ramanujam CL, Zgonis T. Reverse flow digital artery pedicle flap for closure of diabetic forefoot ulceration. Diabet Foot Ankle 2010;1.

34. Roukis TS, Zgonis T. Modifications of the great toe fibular flap for diabetic forefoot and toe reconstruction. Ostomy Wound Manage 2005;51:30–32.

35. Sakai S, Soeda S, Kanou T. Distally based lateral plantar artery island flap. Ann Plast Surg 1988;21:165–169.

36. Schannen AP, Goshima K, Latt LD, et al. Simultaneous soft tissue coverage of both medial and lateral ankle wounds: sural and rotational flap coverage after revision fixation in an infected diabetic ankle fracture. J Orthop 2014;11:19–22.

37. Schwarz RJ, Negrini JF. Medial plantar artery island flap for heel reconstruction. Ann Plast Surg 2006;57:658–661.

38. Shanahan RE, Gingrass RP. Medial plantar sensory flap for coverage of heel defects. Plast Reconstr Surg 1979;64:295–298.

39. Tosun Z, Ozkan A, Karaçor Z, et al. Delaying the reverse sural flap provides predictable results for complicated wounds in diabetic foot. Ann Plast Surg 2005;55:169–173.

40. Zgonis T, Roukis TS, Stapleton JJ, et al. Combined lateral column arthrodesis, medial plantar artery flap, and circular external fixation for Charcot midfoot collapse with chronic plantar ulceration. Adv Skin Wound Care 2008;21:521–525.

CHAPTER 15

Distant Leg Pedicle and Perforator Flap Reconstruction for Soft Tissue Coverage of the Diabetic Foot and Ankle

Alexandru V. Georgescu • Ileana R. Matei

INTRODUCTION

Based on the anatomic and functional characteristics of the distal lower leg, ankle, and foot, the reconstruction of soft tissue and osseous defects with exposed tendons, bones, and/or joints continues to be very challenging for the treating surgeon. This clinical case challenge becomes more than true in acute or chronic wounds as a result of minor trauma in patients with medical comorbidities such as diabetes mellitus, peripheral arterial, or venous disease which are often accompanied by infection, ischemia, neuropathy, and/or coagulopathy (155,180).

According to some epidemiologic studies conducted in the last years (169,181), a dramatic increase in the number of diabetic patients has been documented from 30 million cases in 1985, 177 million cases in 2000, 285 million cases in 2010, and with the estimation of more than 360 million cases for 2030. Over 12% to 25% (1,16,26,118) from those diabetic patients will develop foot ulcers during their lifetimes. As shown in a European study done in 2007, 49% of diabetic foot ulcers are associated with ischemia, 58% with infection, and 31% with combined ischemia and infection which further increases the amputation and mortality rates (166). Moreover, 10% to 20% of the mild diabetic foot infections and 50% to 60% of the moderate or severe soft tissue infections will develop osteomyelitis (68). These findings can explain why 7% to 20% of the expenditure on diabetes mellitus in North America and Europe is dedicated to the treatment of diabetic foot ulcers (20) which motivates the necessity of a selective surgery to improve outcomes on persistent nonhealing diabetic foot ulcers (82).

The first step in acute and not complicated cases with diabetic foot ulcers is the initiative to treat the diabetic foot ulcer by appropriate débridement, off-loading of pressure, control of infection, and local wound care strategy (154). After the relative aggressive débridement, a large variety of nonsurgical methods can be used, such as vacuum drainage systems (19,92), blood bank platelet concentrate as a source of growth factors (97), hyperbaric oxygen therapy (89,147,154), pulsed electromagnetic fields (154), gene therapy using synthetic growth factors (7), stem cell therapy (32), and skin graft substitutes (106). However, in the large majority of cases, reconstructive surgery may be necessary for closure of recalcitrant diabetic foot wounds (154).

Split- or full-thickness skin grafts can be successfully used in few cases involving only the skin and without deep structures exposure or, if deep structures are exposed, with preservation of the paratenon and periosteum and with the exposed bones being drilled with a burr to bleed (211). However, there is a high risk of ulcer recurrence after skin grafting (62,211). One of the most reasonable methods to cover a nonhealing diabetic foot ulcer is the use of flaps, the only procedure able to provide well-vascularized tissue to control infection, adequate contour, durability, and increased mechanical support to shearing pressure forces during ambulation (154).

The advances in microsurgery allowed the extension of the indication for free flaps also in patients with diabetic foot ulcers. Before the year of 2000, it was considered that microsurgery has an only low applicability in the treatment of the diabetic foot (104) due to some concerns related to systemic conditions and patient's compliance, flap's efficacy and viability, vascular disease, and economic burden (87). However, despite the higher incidence of involvement of the lower leg main arteries in diabetic patients, this does not result in occlusion very frequent and the degree of vascular involvement does not necessarily preclude arterial reconstruction (13). That means that in very well selected cases, the arterial reconstruction can be performed before the utilization of a free flap which can increase the chance of survival of such a procedure (11,201). Nowadays, it is considered that in the absence of some risk factors (i.e., peripheral arterial disease, history of angioplasties, and immunosuppressive therapy after surgery), the microsurgical procedures have a high chance to be successful and increase the 5-year survival rate (87,152,201). A large variety of free flaps have been used for soft tissue coverage in diabetic patients, such as the latissimus dorsi, gracilis, radial forearm, parascapular, tensor fascia lata, upper medial thigh, anterolateral thigh perforator, anteromedial thigh perforator, superficial circumflex iliac artery perforator, and deep inferior epigastric artery perforator (11,49,88,149,150,152). However, indifferent of these considerations, a main concern regarding the use of free flaps remains with the fact that when such a free flap has failed, the clinical case scenario may end up being even worse than the patient's preoperative status (62).

Taking into account all of these considerations and the advances in knowledge of the vascular anatomy of the lower leg, it may be more reasonable to use the local/regional flaps for soft tissue reconstruction of the diabetic foot and ankle. However, the question still remains of which kind of a flap can be used to cover a defect in a leg with an uncertain vascular supply. In addition, there are some concerns in using local flaps related to the possible involvement of the neighboring skin (10) and the close vicinity of the grafted donor site to the original defect (67). In contrary, the use of regional flaps can avoid these potential problems.

As a result of the small dimensions and restrictions in mobility, the use of local random pattern flaps is generally unreliable in the lower leg (168), with a possible necrosis rate up to 25% (4). However, local random flaps such as V-Y advancement flaps based on a subcutaneous pedicle (200), rotational flaps (79), bilobed flaps (132), and/or pedicled superior-based transposition flaps (71) can be used for smaller defects. Essentially, in order to avoid complications and to increase their mobility, all of these local random flaps can be harvested in a fasciocutaneous manner (200). In addition, these flaps offer a great advantage of primary closing the donor site (79,132,200) or of a minimally skin grafted donor site (71).

McGregor and Jackson (137) described in 1972 that the axial pattern flap blood supply was from an axial vascular pedicle. Unfortunately, because such a flap needs the sacrifice of a main artery (124,136,194,204) in a leg that may be already vascularly compromised, this procedure has only very limited indications in a diabetic patient. Flaps like the dorsalis pedis flap (110,136), distally based peroneal artery flap (194), distally based posterior tibial artery flap (124), or distally based anterior tibial artery flap (204) can be used but only in cases without vascular involvement of the main arteries.

The introduction of pedicled muscle and musculocutaneous flaps (63,64,151) proved to be a reliable alternative in covering small to medium defects, especially in the midfoot, hindfoot, or ankle (49). Unfortunately, because of inadequate reach, these flaps have only a very few indications in the distal third of the lower leg (73,167).

A real revolution in lower leg coverage was the inclusion by Pontén (164) of the deep fascia in the skin flaps harvested in this region which eliminated any restriction regarding the length-to-width ratio. The anatomic basis of these fasciocutaneous flaps was established later by other studies (12,40,69). However, a high necrosis rate of 25% of these flaps was reported as well (96). A very popular variant of the fasciocutaneous flaps used in the lower leg is the reverse sural fasciocutaneous flap, a neurocutaneous flap first described by Donski and Fogdestam (46) and later described in details from anatomic point of view by Masquelet et al. (135).

The contribution of Manchot (130), Salmon et al. (174), and Taylor and Palmer (189) in vascular anatomy of the skin was later fully fructified by Koshima and Soeda (109) and Kroll and Rosenfield (111), who performed the first perforator flaps, opening a new era in soft tissue coverage. A large contribution in vascular anatomy of the lower leg was brought by Taylor and Pan (190) which described the distribution of the branches of the cutaneous vessels. The use of local and regional perforator flaps in the lower leg and foot has proven to be very reliable (50,61,62,73,96,98,100,107,114,115,134,157,163,167,173,178,191,196) and with a high potential to find new or modified such flaps (60). These flaps can be used as advancement flaps and transposition flaps with the most reliable modality being the propeller flaps. Hyakusoku et al. (91) first described in 1991 the concept of propeller flap for an adipocutaneous flap rotated for 90 degrees, but the blood supply of the flap was through a random pedicle. Later on, Hallock (74) used the term of propeller perforator flap for a flap vascularized through a skeletonized perforator pedicle and rotated for 180 degrees. According to the first Tokyo meeting on perforator and propeller flaps, a propeller perforator flap is a skin island vascularized through a single perforator pedicle that has to rotate around the pedicle for at least 90 to 180 degrees (162). The main advantages of local and regional perforator flaps can be summarized as (a) the source artery and the underlying muscle are spared, (b) donor site morbidity is reduced, (c) replace "like with like" tissue for the defect area, (d) donor and recipient sites are in the same area, (e) possibility of complete or partial primary closure of the donor site, (f) technically less demanding than a free flap, and (g) shorter operating time (50,61,96,107,114,115,155,167,178).

CLINICAL PATIENT OUTCOMES

Nonhealing wounds and/or skin defects in diabetic patients may be the result of an acute injury or of wearing improper fitting shoes. However, independent to the etiologic factors, diabetic patients are exposed to a high predisposition of complications (i.e., infections, equinus deformities, peripheral neuropathy, peripheral arterial disease, ulcerations, and/or Charcot neuroarthropathy) which may affect in a high degree their quality of life (83). The quality of life is mostly affected in diabetic patients presenting with foot ulcers that did not heal or in those patients with recurrent foot ulcers (206). It is considered that in diabetic patients experiencing a first-time foot ulcer that does not heal after 18 months or is reulcerated, the quality of life deteriorates significantly (206). Because of the patient's limited mobility, uncontrolled medical comorbidities, and frequent hospitalizations, the lifespan for diabetic patients with foot ulcers or Charcot neuroarthropathy seems to be 14 years shorter than in nondiabetic patients as it was calculated in 1 study (199).

There is a multitude of risk factors that can aggravate the development of a diabetic foot ulcer that may be related to the patient's characteristics, systemic, and/or local causes (19,31, 57,142,202). General patient characteristics may include the following: (a) Males are more predisposed to develop a diabetic foot ulcer, (b) duration of diabetes mellitus for more than 10 years, (c) older age, and (d) diabetic patients have generally a higher body mass index. The systemic factors may include, but are not limited to, (a) peripheral arterial disease, (b) uncontrolled hyperglycemia, (c) high glycated hemoglobin level, (d) retinopathy, and/or (e) chronic renal disease. The local factors of major importance may include the following: (a) previous diabetic foot ulceration, (b) peripheral neuropathy (with a loss of protective sensation to 5.07/10 g monofilament), (c) poor foot care, (d) existence of structural deformities of the foot, (e) trauma, (f) improper fitted shoes, (g) presence of callus, (h) limited joint mobility, and/or (i) equinus deformities.

According to the risk chart developed by the International Working Group on the Diabetic Foot, there are 4 categories of risk (160):

- Group 0: patients without neuropathy, having an ulceration risk of 5% and no amputation risk
- Group 1: patients with neuropathy but without deformity or vascular disease, having a 14% ulceration risk and no amputation risk
- Group 2: patients with neuropathy and deformity or vascular disease, having a 19% ulceration risk and 3% amputation risk
- Group 3: patients with previous ulcer or amputation, having a 55% reulceration risk and 21% amputation risk.

Because the presence of vascular disease represents an independent higher risk, Lavery et al. (113) modified this risk chart into the following:

- Group 0: no neuropathy or vascular disease
- Group 1: neuropathy but no vascular disease or deformity
- Group 2A: neuropathy and deformity but no vascular disease
- Group 2B: vascular disease
- Group 3A: previous ulcer
- Group 3B: previous amputation

It is very clear that obtaining successful outcomes in a diabetic patient requires the work of a multidisciplinary team, including, but not limited to, a diabetologist, podiatrist, orthotist, orthopedic surgeon, vascular surgeon, wound care specialist, and plastic surgeon. Only such a multidisciplinary team approach will be able to reduce the burden of the diabetic foot by accurate prevention, early treatment, and good aftercare.

This approach allows a reduction with 40% to 80% of the amputation rate for the diabetic foot (47,176,177). Some recent studies consider that the prevention of the mortality rate in patients with diabetic foot complications can be achieved mainly by paying attention to cardiovascular risk factors (21).

A crucial element in avoiding or reducing the amputation and mortality rates in a diabetic patient is the prevention of foot ulceration (9,55,56), or the obtaining of the primary ulcer healing (42,86). Diabetic patient education on foot hygiene, daily inspection, and proper footwear has a very important preventive role (9,55,56). Diabetic patients should be encouraged to consult a surgeon in the attempt to correct the deformities that cannot be accommodated by therapeutic footwear, that is, tight Achilles tendon, hammertoe, plantar exostoses (26,28,55), or to ameliorate the signs of neuropathy by surgical decompression of peripheral nerves (44,45). Of same importance is the detection of a possible peripheral arterial disease which can benefit from revascularization without the need to surgically treat the diabetic foot ulcer (26).

In the presence of a diabetic foot ulcer, a successful clinical outcome can be obtained by the following:

- Obtaining an extensive past medical history (type of diabetes, how is it being treated, how well is it controlled, which general complications the patient already had or has, existence of a previous ulcer or Charcot neuroarthropathy, presence of neuropathy, venous insufficiency, and/or peripheral arterial occlusive disease) (9,66)
- Preventing the development of reulceration in a diabetic patient with a previously healed one by using off-loading modalities, education, and footwear advice (154)
- Performing the appropriate ulcer débridement in an expedited manner which improves the outcome (154,183) by favoring the wound healing process in absence of further surgery (154,159)
- Preventing the local infection by careful local and systemic management
- Managing the local treatment of the ulcer (appropriate débridement, off-loading of pressure, control of infection and local wound care strategy) (154) by utilizing nonsurgical methods first, that is, vacuum drainage systems (19,92), blood bank platelet concentrate as a source of growth factors (97), hyperbaric oxygen therapy (89,147,154), pulsed electromagnetic fields (154), gene therapy using synthetic growth factors (7), stem cells therapy (32), or skin graft substitutes (106)
- Recommending reconstructive surgery if the area of a diabetic foot ulcer does not heal or does not decrease by more than 10% (154)

The use of local or regional flaps can have satisfactory results in diabetic patients with well-controlled diabetes mellitus, have adequate vasculature, are free of infection, and willing to comply with the overall medical and surgical management. These reconstructive procedures can prevent and/or delay the development of a new ulceration and also decrease the amputation and/or mortality rates in the diabetic population.

PREOPERATIVE ASSESSMENT

A thorough lower extremity examination in the diabetic patient that will undergo a soft tissue reconstruction procedure may include the following:

1. Overall clinical appearance of the diabetic foot examining the color, temperature, and presence of edema: If there is no associated peripheral arterial disease, the foot can be warm and/or dry, and with bounding pedal pulses. If the diabetic foot ulcer is infected, the foot can present with edema, but the edema can also be associated in the presence of venous insufficiency.

2. Evaluating the diabetic foot ulcer characteristics, that is, location, size, depth, and presence of surrounding hyperkeratotic tissue: Exposed bone at the base of the ulcer may indicate the association of concomitant osteomyelitis. If hyperkeratotic tissues are present, they should be thoroughly débrided for being able to better assess the ulcer.

3. Determining the presence of peripheral neuropathy which is considered to be 1 of the main etiologic factors for the development of diabetic foot ulceration: The suspicion of peripheral neuropathy is usually raised by the presence of burning, tingling, and/or numbness of the feet. The diabetic foot ulcer is located mainly on the plantar aspect of the foot, usually at the level of the first metatarsal head, and often presents with hyperkeratotic tissue around it. Foot deformity is often associated with the presence of a diabetic foot ulcer. The light touch, pain, vibration, and proprioception signs should be tested on both lower extremities. Tests such as the Semmes-Weinstein neurofilament, 2-point discrimination, and Ipswich touch test can also be successfully used to assess for protective sensation on both feet (101,127,172,175).

4. Examining for the presence of peripheral arterial disease. Diabetic patients with peripheral arterial disease complain about intermittent claudication and pain in the extremities even during the night. Vascular examination reveals diminished or absent pulses, decreased hair growth, nail dystrophy, and shiny, cool, and pale skin. The diabetic foot ulcer is generally well demarcated, has a dry and dark base, and is usually located on the lateral aspect of the lower leg, posterior aspect of the heel, medial aspect of the first metatarsal head, lateral aspect of the fifth metatarsal head, and distal aspect of the toes. The Doppler probe can be used, but due to the sclerotic or calcified arteries, the test could not be relevant enough in diabetic patients. In these conditions, an arteriography can be more useful. In addition, the ankle-brachial index (ABI) and toe-brachial index (TBI) can be more relevant in predicting a peripheral arterial disease. It is considered that an ABI <0.9 or TBI <0.7 is predictive of peripheral arterial disease; if the ABI is <0.6, a poor wound healing will occur (177). Both venous and arterial Doppler tests can provide important information regarding the vascular status of the lower extremities; however, arteriography is the single one providing more reliable data.

5. Examining for the presence of venous insufficiency which plays a dominant role in the development of ulceration in a relatively important number of cases: Diabetic patients complaining about tired, swollen, or aching legs and presenting with edema and hyperpigmentation of the lower legs raise the suspicion of venous insufficiency. The ulcer is located usually in the distal medial leg, more frequent near the medial malleoli, has irregular margins, and presents with a shallow base. Pain can be present but is less than in the cases of an ischemic ulcer.

6. Determining the presence of infection which frequently accompanies any kind of diabetic foot ulcer. According to the Infectious Diseases Society of America, there are 4 categories of diabetic foot infections: (a) uninfected, (b) mild (only skin/subcutaneous infection and with less than 2 cm of erythema around the ulcer), (c) moderate (the infection involves muscles, joint, bone, and cellulitis for more than 2 cm around the ulcer; gangrene can also be present), and (d) severe (infected ulcer in a patient with compromised general status) (123). It is very important to appreciate from the beginning the existence and gravity of the infection because the presence of wet gangrene, necrotizing fasciitis, or abscess can be limb- or life-threatening (25).

7. Evaluating for the presence of foot deformities that are common in diabetic patients and generate focal areas of high pressure: Adding this fact to the presence of neuropathy explains the large number of ulcerations in diabetic patients (9).

If a surgical procedure is needed to be performed, the clinical examination should be completed with a series of studies to assess the local and overall medical status of the diabetic patient. The levels of blood glucose and glycosylated hemoglobin (HbA_{1c}) should be performed in the attempt to assess the management of diabetes mellitus and its metabolic effects. Of higher risk are the diabetic patients with HbA_{1c} above 8.5%. The cardiac and renal function should also be evaluated and appropriate consults can be initiated when necessary.

Special attention must be paid to the associated foot deformities which play an important role in the development of diabetic foot ulcerations. Plain foot and lower extremity radiographs are essential to differentiate simple deformities from Charcot neuroarthropathy. In some cases, computed tomography angiography (CTA) may be the only test that can provide important information in complex diabetic foot deformities with associated peripheral arterial disease. Plain foot and lower extremity radiographs, magnetic resonance imaging, bone scintigraphy, computed tomography, and/or positron emission tomography can also be used to diagnose bone infection versus Charcot neuroarthropathy (131,161).

INDICATIONS/CONTRAINDICATIONS FOR DISTANT LEG PEDICLE AND PERFORATOR FLAPS

Some studies have found a satisfactory remission rate for diabetic foot ulcerations nonsurgically treated, even in those with concomitant osteomyelitis, as demonstrated by the very recent work of Zeun et al. (214) which achieved a remission in 65.9% cases. However, other studies consider that reconstructive surgery may allow for an earlier functional rehabilitation and also reduce the incidence of long-term complications and amputations (99).

The indications for reconstructive surgery should be very carefully assessed emphasizing the overall medical status of the patient and his/her voluntary motivation (154). Of paramount importance is also the approach by a multidisciplinary diabetic team and the existence of an algorithm in managing and salvaging the diabetic foot from amputation (88).

Complex diabetic foot ulcerations and especially those with exposed tendons, bones, or other deeper anatomic structures represent an indication for flap surgery. In addition, the use of flaps will provide durable soft tissue coverage for weight bearing surfaces at the plantar aspect of the diabetic foot. The indication for using flaps to reconstruct the diabetic foot is related to the need to bring well-vascularized tissues able to control the infection and to provide durability, contour, and resistance to shearing forces (154). The choice of the flap depends on the location, dimensions, and depth of the diabetic foot ulceration.

One of the most essential circumstances for using flaps is to have a diabetic patient without a compromised vascular status. In a patient with complete arterial obstruction, the use of flap reconstruction is possible only after revascularization. Fortunately, diabetic patients with concomitant peripheral arterial disease usually still have a patent major vascular axis, most commonly being the peroneal artery (PA), with viable perforators to support a perforator flap (38,62,76). Moreover, sometimes even in diabetic patients with almost complete arterial obstruction, it is still possible to perform flap reconstruction because there are very well represented collateral vascular networks from which patent perforators emerge. In addition, despite the fact that the vascular involvement is more extensive in diabetic patients than in nondiabetic patients, it does not frequently generate occlusion on the small vessels (13,38). That means that arterial reconstruction should not be contraindicated in cases with suspected or apparent small vessel disease (13). Surgical nerve decompression surgery may also improve and compliment the results of soft tissue reconstruction (44,45).

Definitive contraindications to reconstructive flap surgery may include an overall compromised medical status and the absence of voluntary patient motivation. Some authors consider as obvious contraindication the association of peripheral arterial disease and/or the insulin dependence for management of diabetes mellitus (96,167). Additional contraindications include a severely compromised vascularization with complete arterial obstruction and the presence of uncontrollable infection/osteomyelitis and/or gangrene.

ANATOMIC CONSIDERATIONS

After the description of the angiosome concept which focuses on the source vessel (189), most recent studies focused only on the perforator vessels and thus initiating the new perforasome concept (173,178). According to this concept, the perforator vessels emerging from the source arteries anastomose by the mean of direct and indirect linking vessels with the above and below perforator vessels to form a longitudinal orientation of circulation; the direct linking vessels are macroscopic vessels that apprehend anastomoses between 2 branches of adjacent perforators (173), whereas the indirect linking vessels correspond to the "choke vessels" described by Taylor and Palmer (189) and represent the subdermal network. This longitudinal orientation of linking vessels sustains the necessity to design the flaps in a vertical direction (41,72,173,178,189). At the same time, the perforators from 1 source vessel anastomose also transversally with perforators from the neighboring source vessels.

Main Source Arteries in the Leg

The major arteries in the lower leg, that is, anterior tibial artery (ATA), posterior tibial artery (PTA), and PA, represent the main sources of musculocutaneous perforator (MCP) and septocutaneous perforator (SCP) vessels, which blood supply the skin of the lower leg (60,61,178). There are 3 vascular territories with a series of 4 longitudinal rows within the intermuscular septa (60,61,178) (Fig. 15.1). The perforators are located in 3 main clusters from the intermalleolar line to proximal: the first between 4 and 9 cm, the second between 13 and 18 cm, and the third between 21 and 26 cm (178). In the first cluster, there are perforators from all 3 source arteries, in the second from PTA and PA, and in the third from ATA and PTA. All these 3 arteries can represent the vascular source for *axial pedicled flaps* and *pedicled perforator flaps*.

The ATA gives about 6 ± 3 MCP and SCP of 0.6 ± 0.2 mm, and with a superficial length of 29 ± 13 mm (60). The largest perforators are distributed proximal in the third area. The distal perforators, distributed in the first area, are smaller

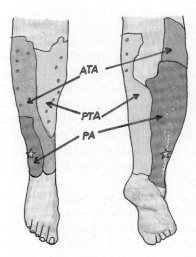

FIGURE 15.1 Distribution of perforators in the lower leg. *ATA,* anterior tibial artery; *PTA,* posterior tibial artery; *PA,* peroneal artery; *bullets,* main perforators; *stars,* main distal perforator of the PA.

and emerge between the tendons in the anterior compartment of the lower leg (178). From these, 1 to 2 perforators emerge above the extensor retinaculum and give branches to supply the skin over both malleoli, and anastomose with branches from the PTA and PA at the ankle level (107).

The PTA gives between 3 to 5 (50,107) and 10 ± 4 (60) cutaneous perforators with a diameter of 1 to 1.5 mm, the largest being found in the middle third of the lower leg (50,60,107,178). In some studies, the great amount of perforators was found in the area between 5 and 14 cm from the intermalleolar line (50,107,167), but other studies found that in all aforementioned clusters, there is an equal distribution of about 23% of the total number of perforators (178). At 5 cm above the medial malleolus can be found a very constant SCP (107). At the ankle region, the terminal branches of the PTA, ATA, and PA anastomose with each other forming a rich collateral vascular network (107).

From the PA emerge 5 ± 2 MCP and SCP of 0.8 ± 0.2 mm (17,60,205,213), with a predominant distribution in the second cluster (178). Similar to the PTA, the PA gives a very constant and large perforator at about 5 cm above the lateral malleolus which divides into an ascending and descending branch (60,107). The ascending branch anastomoses with the superficial peroneal artery, whereas the descending branch contributes to the collateral vascular network around the ankle.

Alternative Arterial Sources in the Leg

These alternative arterial sources are represented by some of the very distal branches of the main arteries, the networks apprehended by the anastomoses of these branches, and the perineural vascular networks of the sensory nerves.

The ATA continues beneath the extensor retinaculum with the dorsalis pedis artery. Along its route on the dorsal aspect of the foot, it gives tiny branches that supply the skin and represent the vascular basis of the *dorsalis pedis flap* (129). After giving its 1 to 2 main distal perforators above the extensor retinaculum, the ATA supplies an anterolateral and an anteromedial branch which vascularize the skin over the anterior aspect of the lateral and medial malleolus; the anterolateral branch, after passing deep to the extensor tendons to reach the anterior aspect of the lateral malleolus, divides into 1 deep and 1 to 2 superficial branches, the latest following an ascending direction and ensuring the vascular supply of the *anterolateral malleolar flap* (107). The anteromedial branch gives 2 to 3 small cutaneous branches for the skin over the anterior aspect of the medial malleolus which also go in an ascending direction and blood supplies the *anteromedial malleolar flap* (107).

The most distal perforator originating from the PTA is within the calcaneal canal after perforating the fascia posterior to the medial malleolus goes anteriorly and ascendant and represents the vascular basis of the *posteromedial malleolar flap* (107)

The PA gives a branch posterior to the lateral malleolus which represents the vascular basis of the *posterolateral malleolar flap* (107). The lateral calcaneal artery which ensures the blood supply for the *lateral calcaneal flap* (8,23,107) is an almost constant terminal branch of the PA, from which originates in between 87% (54) and 94.12% (23) of cases. In the remaining cases, it originates from the PTA. The most distal main perforator from the PA, located 5 cm above the lateral malleolus, terminates in 2 branches: the deep descending branch and the superficial ascendant branch, the last 1 representing the vascular basis of the *lateral supramalleolar flap* (107).

Just above the knee, from the popliteal artery emerge 4 to 5 branches named sural arteries, which contribute to the blood supply of the muscles and skin over the posterior aspect of the lower leg, especially in the distal two-thirds. One of them (i.e., the median superficial sural artery) accompanies the sural nerve (known also as the medial sural nerve) between the heads of the gastrocnemius muscle and then parallels it laterally to the Achilles tendon (77,135,139). Another one (i.e., the lateral superficial sural artery) parallels the lateral sural nerve.

The sural nerve results from the union of the medial sural (branch of the tibial nerve) and lateral sural (branch of the common peroneal nerve) nerves, usually at the distal third of the lower leg. However, in 33% of cases, the sural nerve is a direct prolongation of the medial sural nerve (144). Similarly, the lesser saphenous vein is accompanied by 1 to 2 arteries: Nakajima et al. (145) described 2 arteries, whereas Mojallal et al. (139) found only 1 artery in 73% of cases. Regarding the vascularization of the sural nerve, it is provided by the sural artery in its proximal third (135) and by SCPs from the PA (139). These perforators apprehend in fact 2 parallel networks: 1 for the sural nerve and another for the lesser saphenous vein.

The lesser saphenous vein arterial network contributes to the vascularization of the skin over the posterolateral aspect of the lower leg; it seems that this one is more important than the arterial contribution of the sural nerve because the arterial extrinsic network of the nerve anastomoses is mainly with the vein arterial network, and only few perforators from the nerve arterial extrinsic network are going to the skin (143,207).

The blood supply of the skin over the medial aspect of the lower leg is provided by perforators from the saphenous artery in the proximal third (usually, 12 cm below the knee joint), whereas in the middle and distal third by a rich arterial network around the saphenous nerve and perforators from the arteries which accompany the greater saphenous vein; these networks anastomose with the lowermost perforators from the PTA (36,146).

Regarding the venous drainage, in the proximally based pedicled and perforator flaps, it is apprehended in a normal direction, either through 1 of the subcutaneous veins when they are included in the flaps or from the suprafascial venous network through the perforator veins. Regarding the venous drainage in distally based pedicled flaps despite the presence of valves in the venae comitantes which can allow some reflux (194), it seems that the anastomoses apprehended between their branches form communicating channels able to bypass the valves (77,194). A contribution to the venous drainage in the distally based pedicled flaps can also have the incompetence of the valves secondary to the denervation of the veins and the increase of venous pressure secondary to the proximal tightening of the veins (165,195).

TYPES OF LOCAL/REGIONAL FLAPS IN THE LEG

The following types of local/regional flaps harvested from the lower leg can be used to cover defects in the foot, ankle, and distal lower leg: random flaps, axial flaps, perforator flaps, neurofasciocutaneous flaps, venofasciocutaneous flaps, and adipofascial flaps. Nowadays, it is considered that independent of the flap type, the inclusion of the deep fascia enhances the flap's survivability (164). It is proven that by including the deep fascia in local flaps harvested from the lower leg, the previously 1:1 length-to-width flap ratio can be changed to a 3:1 ratio or more (164,193). Therefore, by including the deep fascia, all of the flaps harvested from the lower leg are fasciocutaneous or adipofascial flaps.

Random Flaps

Although initially a random flap was defined as a flap with unknown vascularization (41), nowadays, such a flap should be considered as random only because it is harvested without the identification of any named artery (71). In this sense, a random flap is a *type A* fasciocutaneous flap because its blood supply is provided through multiple suprafascial vessels from well-known vascular sources (39). Therefore, any kind of pedicled fasciocutaneous flap, adipofascial pedicled flap, or advancement flap without identification of a distinct vascular source can be considered as a random flap.

Particular Types of Random Flaps

Proximally Based Fasciocutaneous Pedicled Flaps
Even if these proximally based fasciocutaneous flaps (Fig. 15.2) are considered more reliable than the distally based pedicled flaps, they have only few indications for the coverage of distal lower leg and ankle defects (72). The maximum reach for a safe flap is the upper part of the distal third of the lower leg. It is imperative to design the flap vertically and to include the deep fascia. The length-to-width ratio can be up to 3:1. A main advantage of these flaps is the possibility to include a major superficial vein which enhances the venous drainage. To compensate the length loss through rotation, a few centimeters should be added to the length of the flap. A drawback of these flaps is the necessity to skin graft the donor site.

Distally Based Fasciocutaneous Pedicled Flaps
The existence of the well-known reach anastomotic vascular networks in the distal lower leg explains the possibility to use distally pedicled fasciocutaneous random flaps (Fig. 15.3A) harvested from the lower leg to cover small

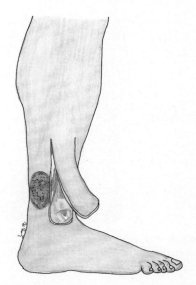

FIGURE 15.2 Schematic representation of a proximally based random fasciocutaneous pedicled flap.

and medium defects in the foot, ankle, and distal leg. The condition for having a safe flap is to appreciate the length-to-width ratio of maximum 3:1 and to include the deep fascia. To offer more safety and especially for very long flaps which can extend up to the knee joint, it is possible to perform a 3-stage procedure: (a) flap's incision including the deep fascia and suture of the wound, (b) transfer of the flap 1 week later, and (c) sectioning of the pedicle at 3 weeks (112). A very important point in performing these flaps is to plan their base not distally to the union of the middle and lower third of the leg. Besides the disadvantage of a long surgical procedure, other disadvantages are related to the slight kinking when the flap is rotated along the long axis and the necessity to skin graft the donor site (112). In cases of a smaller defect, the flap can be performed as a 1-stage procedure, and more distally, the donor site can be closed by using a second advancement V-Y flap (24) (see Fig. 15.3B,C).

Occasionally and especially in cases with scarred skin around the ulceration or in those with previously performed flaps, the distally pedicled flaps can be used as de-epithelialized "turnover" skin flaps (153,192). Such a flap needs to be de-epithelialized and turned over on itself. The base of the pedicle should define a gentle curve to not affect the blood supply. The main disadvantage of this flap is represented by the necessity of skin grafting both the flap and its donor site. The distally pedicled fasciocutaneous flaps can also be used as island fasciocutaneous flaps based on an adipofascial pedicle and with the skin island completely or partially de-epithelialized to fill some deep defects (Fig. 15.4).

To avoid the donor site skin grafting and improve its aspect, it is possible to use only distally pedicled random adipofascial flaps (81,119–121) or fascia flaps (53,75). These flaps are in fact

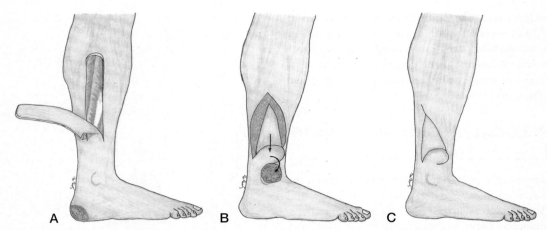

FIGURE 15.3 Schematic representation of a distally based random fasciocutaneous pedicled flap. **A.** Design of a larger flap. **B.** More distally possible design of a smaller flap and closure of the donor site by using a V-Y advancement flap. **C.** Final closure.

either distally pedicled adipofascial perforator flaps or distally based neuro- or venoadipofascial flaps (53,81,119,120,122). Such flaps harvested either on the posterior (53), anteromedial (81,120,122), or lateral aspect (119) of the lower leg can be successfully used to cover defects in the distal lower leg and ankle. They are mainly blood supplied through perforators from the PTA, PA, or from the rich vascular network around the ankle. To include as much as possible blood supply, the pivot point should be at 8 to 10 cm above the intermalleolar line. These flaps can not only cover superficial defects but can also fill deeper defects over or inside the bones (Fig. 15.5). Because of the vascular connections between the fascia and gastrocnemius muscle, sometimes, the flap can be harvested as a muscle-adipofascial flap by including a small segment of the muscle, which proves to be very useful in cases of resected osteomyelitis. To avoid the possible endurance of the skin flaps at the donor site in the adipofascial variant, care should be taken to leave enough adipose tissue on them. The coverage of the flaps with split-thickness skin grafts can be performed in the same operative procedure or after 3 to 5 days.

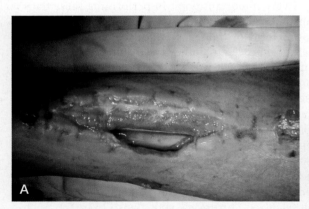

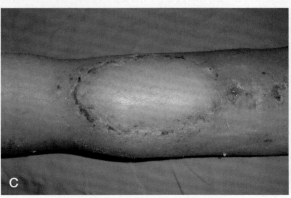

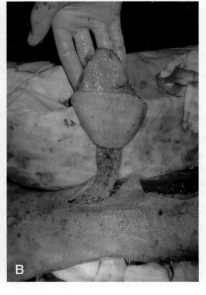

FIGURE 15.4 Dehiscence and infection after a sutured post-traumatic wound in a diabetic patient. **A.** Preoperative picture showing the wound dehiscence. **B.** After surgical débridement and superficial bone resection, the remaining defect was covered with an island fasciocutaneous flap based on an adipofascial pedicle with the skin island being partially de-epithelialized and filling the defect. **C.** Postoperative picture at 1-month follow-up.

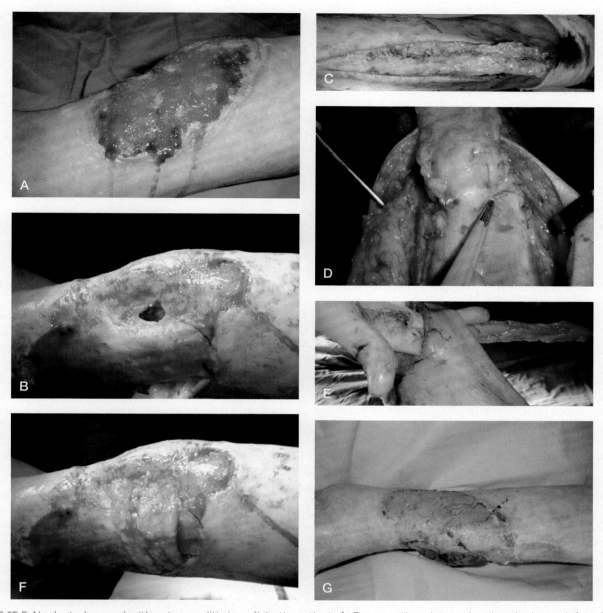

FIGURE 15.5 Neglected wound with osteomyelitis in a diabetic patient. **A.** Preoperative picture showing the large defect. **B.** After surgical soft tissue and osseous débridement. **C.** Harvesting of a distally pedicled adipofascial flap. **D.** A peroneal perforator is identified but is not skeletonized. **E.** The flap is passed to the recipient defect area through a large tunnel. **F.** Flap insetting at the recipient defect. **G.** Final postoperative outcome.

A bipedicled fasciocutaneous flap combines the advantages of both proximally and distally based pedicled fasciocutaneous flaps. Moreover, by adding a secondary source of vascularization, it allows the survival of longer and larger flaps (51,70). The flap can be designed either vertically (Fig. 15.6A) or horizontally (see Fig. 15.6B). It is generally accepted that the length of the flap should be twice that of the defect and that its width should be at least half the length (51). Other obvious advantages of the vertical variant are the possibility of performing small "V" cutback incisions at the level of the upper and lower ends of the lateral incisions which facilitate the mobilization of the flap (51) and the avoidance of bone or tendon exposure at the donor site, which are frequent with an unipedicled flap (70).

V-Y ADVANCEMENT SUBCUTANEOUS PEDICLE FLAPS

The V-Y advancement flap can be used as random flap based on a subcutaneous pedicle (Fig. 15.7), but its mobility is very limited in regions with small amount of subcutaneous tissue (i.e., the distal lower leg) (200). The flap can be successfully used to cover small defects up to 3 to 4 cm in diameter over the heel and ankle. The design of such a flap should respect the following rules: (a) The length of the flap should be 1.5 to 2 times as long as the diameter of the defect and (b) the base of the triangle should be equal to the width of the defect (133). The base of the flap should be undermined as little as possible, but the opposite part of the flap should be extensively undermined subfascially. Care should

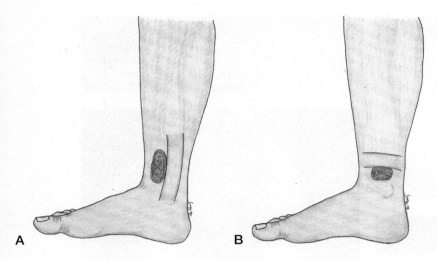

FIGURE 15.6 Schematic representation of a bipedicled random fasciocutaneous flap. **A.** Vertical variant. **B.** Horizontal variant.

be taken to preserve a broad and deep as possible subcutaneous pedicle (133).

The V-Y advancement flap can also be used to help the closure of the donor site of a pedicled transposition fasciocutaneous flap and especially for a distally based pedicled one (see Fig. 15.3B,C). Calderon et al. (24) described the fasciocutaneous cone flap which is a combination of a rotation transposition flap with a V-Y advancement flap. The original technique uses a rotation transposition distally pedicled flap with a 1:1 length-to-width ratio to close a defect up to 3.5 cm^2 and a V-Y advancement flap with a 3:1 height-to-base ratio to cover its donor site (24).

KEYSTONE ISLAND FLAPS

Even if these flaps are based on perforator vessels, they can be considered island random flaps because, as first described by Behan (15), they are harvested without identification of perforator vessels. This procedure can be performed in areas with

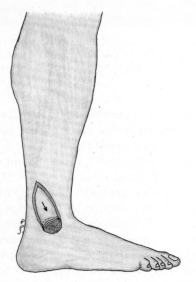

FIGURE 15.7 Schematic representation of the V-Y advancement flap.

enough skin laxity, that is, for the lower leg is better to harvest the flaps over the posterior aspect.

If a keystone flap (Fig. 15.8) is planned, the ulcer should be excised elliptically in the long axis of the lower leg. It is better to include in the flap the cutaneous nerves and superficial veins (15,105,158). The width of the flap should be equal with the width of the defect. From both ends of the defect, an incision at 90 degrees is performed until reaching the curvilinear further flaps' outer edge. Then, the incision is completed and deepened until the fascia, but the flap is not undermined. According with the original described technique (15), after incising the entire flap, the procedure can be continued in 5 different ways:

- Type I keystone flap: For defects with the width less than 2 cm, the deep fascia is not incised (see Fig. 15.8A–C).
- Type IIA keystone flap: For larger defects, when an increased mobility is necessary, the fascia on the outer edge of the flap is also incised (see Fig. 15.8D).
- Type IIB keystone flap: In cases of excessive tension, the donor site of the flap can be skin grafted (see Fig. 15.8E).
- Type III keystone flap: refers to the situations of larger defects, up to 5 to 10 cm in width, in which it is possible to use two opposite keystone flaps (see Fig. 15.8F,G)
- Type IV keystone flap: This flap is undermined subfascially up to 50% of its surface which enables the rotation of the undermined part (see Fig.15.8H).

Except of the type IIB keystone flap, in all other types, the donor site can be closed primarily by performing on each end of the remaining defect a V-Y advancement closure. One small triangle on each right angle of the flap should be generally excised which contributes to the narrowing of the defect. Sometimes, in types I and IIA, the excessive tension can be diminished by adding a third V-Y advancement flap in the central part of the defect, as described by Haydon and Caminer (78). In cases with enough skin laxity, the design of the flap can be modified by leaving a skin bridge along the outer edge of the flap which can prevent the venous and lymphatic congestion (141).

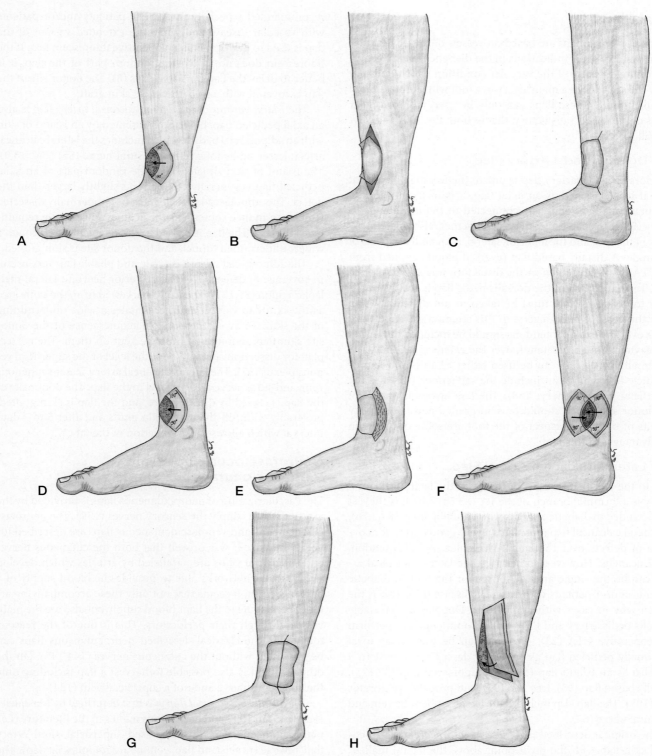

FIGURE 15.8 Schematic representation of the keystone flap. **A.** Design. **B.** Type I, without incision of the deep fascia. **C.** Final closure. **D.** Type II A, with incision of the deep fascia. **E.** Type II B, with skin grafting of the flap donor site. **F.** Type III, with two opposite keystone flaps and final closure after transposition **(G)**. **H.** Type IV, subfascial undermining up to 50% of a keystone flap.

Axial Flaps

The axial pattern flaps are based on vessels of the direct cutaneous system. Their indications in the diabetic foot are generally limited because of the vascular condition which does not allow the sacrifice of a main artery in a foot with compromised vascular status. These flaps can only be used if the vascular status of the foot is satisfactory, that is, both the ATA and PTA are still patent.

The Dorsalis Pedis Artery Flap

The dorsalis pedis artery flap is one of the few axial flaps that even if it is classified as an axial flap, it is in fact a random subcutaneous flap tenuously connected to the dorsalis pedis artery (58). This flap can easily reach the medial and lateral aspects of the foot and the anterior, lateral, and medial aspects of the ankle. A distally based flap reversed blood supplied from the PTA that is able to cover the distal foot was also described (94). The harvesting of the dorsalis pedis flap is relatively difficult to perform. Care must be taken to not dissect the flap from the dorsalis pedis artery. In this attempt, the superficial fascia over the extensor tendons should be included in the flap but leaving enough paratenon over the extensor tendons. The proximally based flap can be used either as an island flap or a pedicle flap which can include the saphenous vein and the superficial peroneal nerve (58). The less favorable aspect of the donor site which should be skin grafted and the sensory deficits of the dorsal aspect of the foot are some of the main disadvantages of this flap.

The Lateral Calcaneal Artery Flap

Due to the fact that in most of the cases the lateral calcaneal artery is a terminal branch of the PA (23,54) which is the last one occluded in diabetic patients with vasculopathy (38,62,76), the lateral calcaneal flap represents a very good option for coverage of defects over the lateral malleolus, Achilles tendon, and calcaneus. However, sometimes, the lateral calcaneal artery can be the single arterial source for the foot in diabetic patients and/or patients with vascular disease (67). This is the reason why in cases with clinical and Doppler undetectable dorsalis pedis artery and PTA, it is recommended to perform a preoperative CTA (23). This flap can be used as an axial proximally pedicled flap as originally described in 1981 (67) but also as an island flap (59,85), adipofascial flap (37,121), distally based flap (93), free flap (95), and propeller perforator flap (107). The flap also includes the lesser saphenous vein and the sural nerve (67).

The original described *axial lateral calcaneal flap* is a pedicled skin flap with the pivot point above the lateral malleolus and extending distally for 8 cm until at least 1 cm to the plantar aspect of the heel (8,67). An extended variant of the flap can also be used by adding a 6 cm distally skin random portion gently curved until the base of the fifth metatarsal bone (8). The lateral calcaneal artery which passes at a vertical distance from the most prominent point of the lateral malleolus of about 3 to 3.5 cm must be as close to the center of the flap (8). The width of the flap at the level of its base is at least 4 cm, but being an axial flap, its distal part can be larger. It is recommended especially in diabetic patients and/or patients with vascular disease and when the extended variant of the flap is used to perform an intraoperative fluorescein test: If the fluorescein does not reach the random part of the flap, it is better to delay the flap for 5 to 7 days (8). The donor site of the flap is covered with a split-thickness skin graft.

The *island variant of the lateral calcaneal artery flap* is also an axial pedicled flap, but it is represented by an island of skin with an adipofascial pedicle which includes the lateral calcaneal artery, lesser saphenous vein, and sural nerve (85) (Fig. 15.9). The island of skin situated over the random part of an axial pedicled flap is generally circular and slightly larger than the defect. The adipofascial pedicle must be subdermally dissected which can induce sometimes the acquiescence of the remaining skin flaps. The flap is passed to the recipient site through a widely undermined tunnel, and the donor site is skin grafted.

The adipofascial variant is a thin and pliable flap very useful in coverage of defects over the posterior heel and lateral malleolar region (37,121). The flap is harvested from the same area as the skin flap variant and necessitates a wide undermining of the skin. To avoid the possible acquiescence of the donor site skin flaps, enough fat must be kept on them. The correct plan for dissection seems to be at the level of the superficial venous plexus (37). The lateral calcaneal artery, lesser saphenous vein, and sural nerve are included in the flap. The donor site of the flap is closed by direct suture, and the flap is skin grafted, preferably with full-thickness skin grafts and after 5 to 7 days interval which allows the granulation of the fat (37).

Neurofasciocutaneous and Venofasciocutaneous Flaps

The vascularization of neurocutaneous flaps is provided by the arteries which supply the sensory nerves (139). The neurofasciocutaneous and venofasciocutaneous flaps are described together because it was proven that both the cutaneous nerves and superficial veins are paralleled by arteries which develop rich vascular networks able to provide the blood supply of a flap. Moreover, it seems that not only these accompanying arteries contribute to the flaps blood supply but also are the main vessels through their perforators. This is one of the reasons today why the classical described neurocutaneous flaps can be harvested without the cutaneous nerves (144,145). On the other hand, it is also possible to harvest a flap including only the cutaneous nerve and not a superficial vein (184).

The distally based sural flap was first described by Masquelet et al. (135) in 1992 and has various names in the literature (i.e., neurocutaneous flap, distally based superficial sural artery flap, reverse sural island flap, venoneuroadipofascial flap). The flap can be either used as a fasciocutaneous flap or adipofascial flap (140,179). The main indication of this flap is the coverage of defects over the heel, Achilles tendon, anterior and lateral aspects of the ankle, dorsal foot, lateral aspect of the hindfoot, and lower third of the lower extremity (14,90,125,135,171).

In the original description, it was considered that the vascular supply of the sural flap is provided mainly by the median superficial sural artery and the vascular network of the sural nerve (135). Actually, according to some recent studies, the

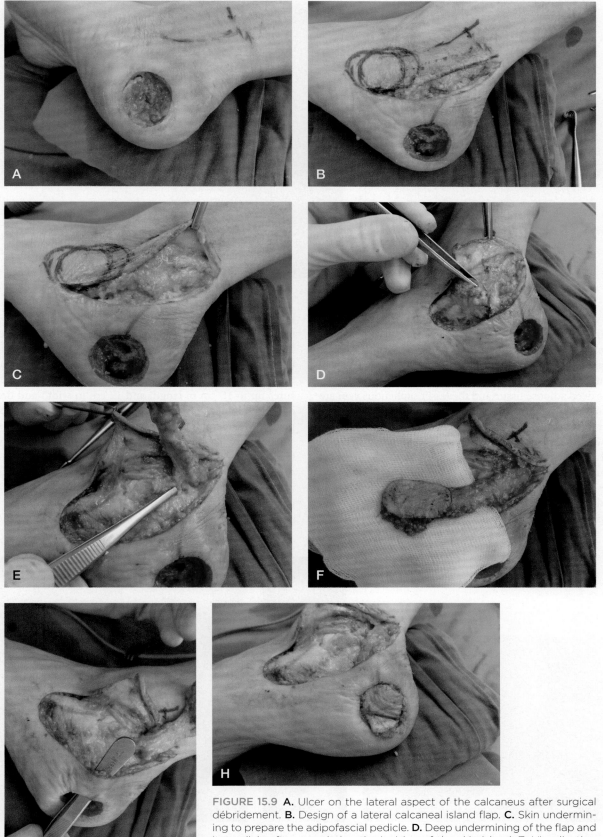

FIGURE 15.9 A. Ulcer on the lateral aspect of the calcaneus after surgical débridement. **B.** Design of a lateral calcaneal island flap. **C.** Skin undermining to prepare the adipofascial pedicle. **D.** Deep undermining of the flap and its pedicle after completing the incision of the skin island. **E.** Visualization of the vascular pedicle. **F.** The flap ready to be transferred to the recipient defect area. **G.** Preparing of a large tunnel for the pedicle. **H.** The flap being transferred into the defect. *(continued)*

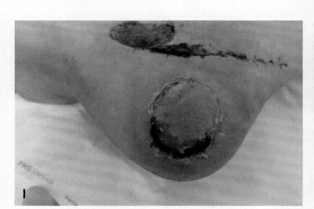

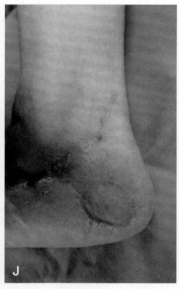

FIGURE 15.9 *(Continued)* **I.** Postoperative picture at 3 weeks follow-up. **J.** Postoperative picture at 2 years follow-up.

sural nerve does not have a very important contribution to the vascularization of the sural flap; it seems that the arterial extrinsic network of the sural nerve anastomoses with that of the lesser saphenous vein and does not send or sends only few perforators to the skin (139,143,208). According to Mojallal et al. (139), the deep adipose tissue and the lesser saphenous vein are the only mandatory anatomic elements for a good blood supply of the sural flap, whereas the deep fascia does not contribute to this. Nowadays, it is accepted that the main arterial supply of the sural flap is provided by distal perforators of the peroneal artery through 2 parallel networks, 1 for the sural nerve and 1 for the lesser saphenous vein (139). However, other authors harvested with the same success rate sural flaps based only on the intrinsic blood supply provided by the sural nerve, without

including subcutaneous tissue, superficial saphenous vein, and fascia (3,184). On the other hand, other studies report venocutaneous and venoadipofascial flaps by sparing the sural nerve but including the lesser saphenous vein (18,139,144,145).

As originally described, the skin island of the flap measures up to 15 cm in length and 12 cm in width and designed over the junction of the gastrocnemius heads, the adipofascial pedicle has a length to width ratio of 4:1, and the pivot point is situated lateral and 5 cm proximal to the lateral malleolus (135) (Fig. 15.10). According to some recent studies, the superior edge of the flap can be at 5 cm distal to the popliteal crease, and the mean length of the skin island can be up to 25 cm (139). Such flaps can be successfully used to cover the entire dorsal aspect of the foot (Fig. 15.11). In most of the studies about the sural

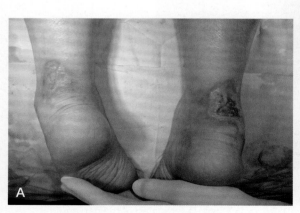

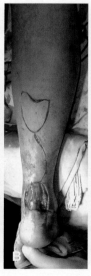

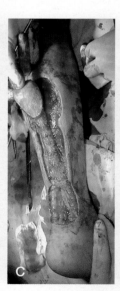

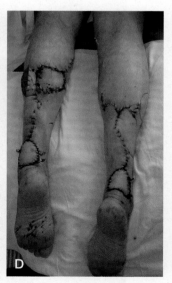

FIGURE 15.10 A. Preoperative picture of bilateral ulcers over both Achilles tendons. **B.** Design of the flap over the junction of the gastrocnemius heads on the right lower leg. **C.** The flap is harvested based on an adipofascial pedicle of 3.5 cm width and with the pivot point at about 5 cm above the lateral malleolus. **D.** Postoperative outcome of bilateral lower extremities.

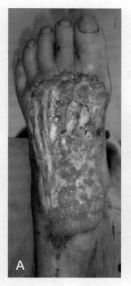
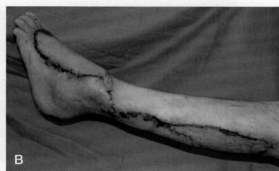

FIGURE 15.11 Distally based sural flap. **A.** Preoperative picture of a large defect on the dorsal aspect of the foot. **B.** Postoperative picture after using a flap of 20 × 9 cm.

flap, the width of the adipofascial pedicle is up to 3 to 4 cm, but being the relationship which seems to exist between the dimensions of the flap and the width of the pedicle, some other reports consider that as large the width of the pedicle, as large can be the flap's dimensions (124). Knowing that the most important distal perforator of the PA emerges at about 5 cm above the lateral malleolus, this point represents in some studies the pivot point of the flap (117,210). Other studies consider safer a pivot point located at 10 to 11 cm (18) or 7 to 8.5 cm (139) above the lateral malleolus. Moreover, some authors moved the pivot point more distally, considering that both the lateral malleolar artery and the lateral calcaneal artery can represent the main perforator of the sural flap (34,216).

One of the most important concerns in using the sural flap is how to manipulate its pedicle. Originally, the flap was passed to the donor site by tunneling its pedicle which could induce venous congestion (30,77,135). To minimize such a complication, the pedicle can be passed through a wider tunnel with about more than 3 cm of the pedicle width (198) (see Fig. 15.5E), or the tunnel can be enlarged by using an acute expansion (22). Other authors consider more safe to incise the skin bridge between the pedicle and recipient site (77,165,182) (see Fig. 15.10B), add a triangular skin limb extension in continuity with the flap and incise the skin bridge (91,124,165,212), or to transfer the flap in 2 steps as an interpolation flap by leaving the pedicle exposed and skin grafted and cutting it secondary after 2 weeks (126,128) (Fig. 15.12).

In an attempt to avoid the high rate of complications in using the sural flap reported in the literature which can be up 5% to 36% (2,4,14,84,148,171) or even up to 83% in some series (5), multiple modifications of the original design and use of the flap were described as follows:

- *Peninsular flap*, by keeping the skin over the pedicle
- *Sural artery fasciocutaneous flap*, which increases the flap survivability but has the disadvantage of a lesser arc of rotation (165)

- *Sural fasciomusculocutaneous flap*, which includes a small cuff of the gastrocnemius muscle allowing the filling of deeper defects (5,6,116). This flap seems to preserve the retrograde blood supply from the median sural artery to the MCPs and allows the filling of deep soft tissue or osseous defects (35). Sometimes, it is possible to use a part of one of the gastrocnemius muscles which is reversely vascularized through a MCP.
- *Supercharged reverse sural flap*, by anastomosing the lesser saphenous vein to a subcutaneous vein or to the great saphenous vein to increase the venous drainage (48,186)
- *Delayed sural flap*, which is very useful when using larger flaps and in patients with vascular risk factors (14,52, 65,103,156,188,197). Because the secondary dilatation of the arterial network and increasing of the perfusion pressure, flap delay contributes to the increasing of perfusion (52,65,103,188). Secondary to these effects, the length-to-width ratio of the flaps and the overall flap survival can be increased (52,65,103,188). Another advantage of the flap delay consists in the possibility of performing it during the débridement procedure (197).

The distally based saphenous flap, also well-known as distally based saphenous nerve-greater saphenous venofasciocutaneous flap (36,217), reverse pedicle-based greater saphenous neurovenofasciocutaneous flap (102), or reverse saphenous neurocutaneous flap (29), is the counterpart of the distally based sural flap. It has almost the same structure, type of blood supply, indications, and possible variants and designs with the sural flap. Similar with the sural flap, the blood supply is provided by the rich vascular networks which parallel the saphenous nerve (36) and great saphenous vein (146) which anastomose with the lower perforators of the PTA and especially with the lowermost one located at approximately 5 cm above the tip of the medial malleolus. The flap can be used as a fasciocutaneous island flap based on adipofascial pedicle, or as an adipofascial flap. In this flap, the structures included are

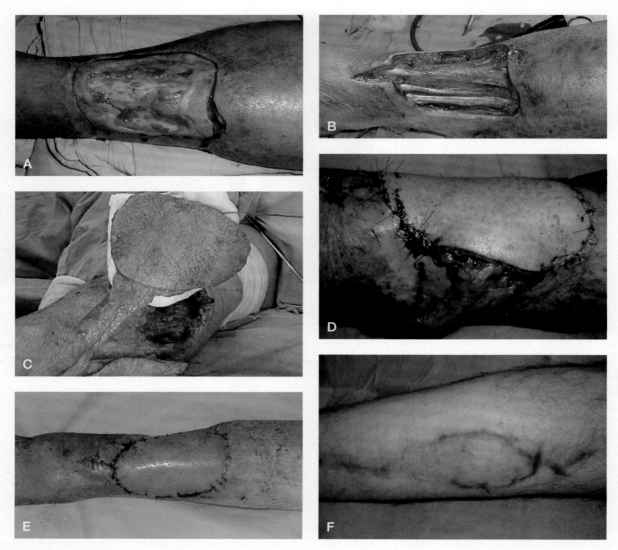

FIGURE 15.12 **A.** Preoperative picture of a chronic ulceration over the anterior aspect of the distal lower leg. **B.** Remaining defect after surgical débridement. **C.** Reverse island sural flap based on a very thin adipofascial pedicle including the sural nerve and lesser saphenous vein. **D.** The flap covering the recipient defect area with the adipofascial pedicle exteriorized. **E.** Postoperative picture at 2 weeks and after excising the pedicle. **F.** Skin-grafted donor site appearance; its dimensions were reduced by a purse-string suture technique.

the deep fascia, the saphenous nerve, and the great saphenous vein. Same with the sural flap, in a saphenous flap, either the saphenous nerve or the great saphenous vein can be spared (29,33). The long axis of the flap corresponds to a line between the medial condyle of the tibia and a point situated at 1 cm anterior to the tip of the medial malleolus, and the pivot point is considered at about 5 cm above the medial malleolus (36). The transversal extension of the flap is between the midline of the posterior calf and 1 to 1.5 cm medial to the tibial crest (36).

Perforator Flaps

The local perforator flaps gained a large popularity in the last years due to the recent advances in the vascular anatomy of the lower leg (27,60,61,80,107,108,167,178,187,205,209).

As mentioned earlier, all 3 main arteries of the lower leg (i.e., ATA, PTA, and PA) give perforator arteries able to blood supply a perforator flap (see Fig. 15.1). Of great importance in performing local perforator flaps able to cover defects in the foot and distal lower leg are the most distal perforators (Fig. 15.13). Both the PTA and the PA give a constant perforator of good caliber approximately 5 cm above the medial malleolus and the lateral malleolus, respectively, whereas the ATA gives more perforators of smaller caliber at 4 to 9 cm proximal to the intermalleolar line (60,107,178). The flaps harvested on these perforators are named according with the name of the main arteries from which they emerge (i.e., ATA, PTA, and PA perforator flaps). Koshima et al. (107) identified also distinct perforators emerging from the terminal part of the main arteries and described some specific perforator flaps, that is,

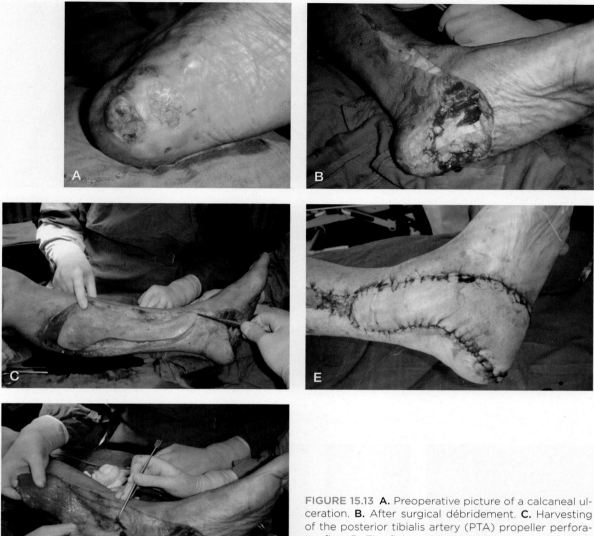

FIGURE 15.13 A. Preoperative picture of a calcaneal ulceration. **B.** After surgical débridement. **C.** Harvesting of the posterior tibialis artery (PTA) propeller perforator flap. **D.** The flap was harvested on the most distal perforator of PTA located at 5 cm above the medial malleolus. **E.** Final postoperative outcome.

anterolateral malleolar flap, anteromedial malleolar flap, posteromedial malleolar flap, posterolateral malleolar flap, and *lateral supramalleolar flap.*

The local perforator flaps harvested from the distal lower leg are very useful in covering defects over the distal lower leg, ankle, and foot. Among their advantages include replacement of soft tissue defects with "like-with-like" tissue, relatively simple to perform with shorter surgical times, do not require microsurgical anastomosis, and provide the possibility of direct closure of donor sites less than 6 cm wide, or reducing the surface of larger donor sites by using purse-string sutures (61,96,165,185).

The local perforator flaps can be used as V-Y advancement flaps, transposition flaps which rotate around the pivot point less than 90 degrees, and propeller flaps when the rotation around the pivot point is between 90 and 180 degrees. The V-Y advancement perforator flap (200) is a fasciocutaneous

flap that should be designed over a preoperatively detected perforator. It allows the coverage of small defects and the direct closure of the donor site. Sometimes, in order to increase the mobility of the flap, the perforator can be dissected until its origin from the main artery is identified.

The propeller perforator flaps can close medium defects and in many cases even much larger defects. Of very significant importance is the fact that they do not have to appreciate the length to width ratio of 2:1 to 3:1, sometimes being possible to harvest flaps up to a length-to-width ratio of 5:1 to 6:1 (Fig. 15.14). To increase the vasculature of larger flaps as well as increase their viability, these flaps can be designed as propeller perforator plus flaps which means to transform an island propeller perforator flap into a pedicled propeller perforator flap (61,115,138) (Fig. 15.15). The flaps can be harvested as cutaneous, fasciocutaneous, or adipofascial flaps. The preoperative detection of perforators is not mandatory, but it can

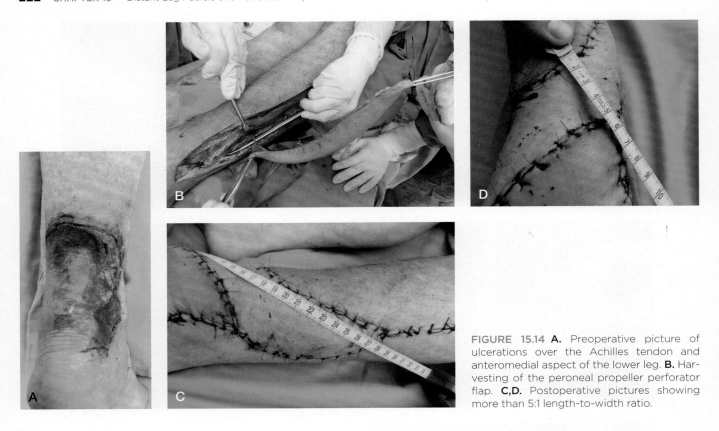

FIGURE 15.14 A. Preoperative picture of ulcerations over the Achilles tendon and anteromedial aspect of the lower leg. **B.** Harvesting of the peroneal propeller perforator flap. **C,D.** Postoperative pictures showing more than 5:1 length-to-width ratio.

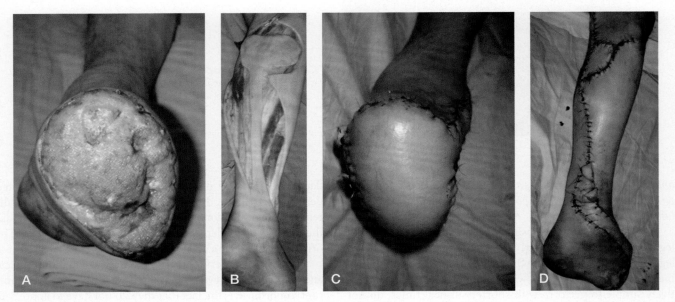

FIGURE 15.15 A. Preoperative picture of an infected midfoot amputation. **B.** Harvesting of the propeller plus flap based on a perforator of the peroneal artery located at 5 cm above the lateral malleolus. **C.** Postoperative picture showing the coverage at the recipient defect area. **D.** Picture of the donor site appearance. (In Georgescu AV. Propeller perforator flaps in distal lower leg: evolution and clinical applications. Arch Plast Surg 2012;39:94–105.)

assist especially when the skin is modified around the defect. It is also better to base the flap on a close as possible perforator to avoid the harvest of an unnecessarily long flap and attention should be emphasized to not use a perforator located close to the defect and surrounded by fibrotic tissue (185).

There are some very important steps in designing and harvesting a propeller perforator flap which are described as follows:

1. The flap has 2 unequal blades.
2. The dimensions of such a flap can be larger than the conventional flaps due to the interconnections of adjacent perforasomes through direct linking vessels (173,185).
3. Because the linking vessels are parallel to the long axis of the leg, these flaps should be designed longitudinally (173,185).
4. Because the direction of vascularity of the perforators located close to a joint is away from the joint as distally, the perforator as marginal will be located in the flap (173,185). In cases of a very marginal located perforator, less linking vessels will be included which can diminish drastically the vascularization of the flap. Therefore, it is better to harvest flaps based on perforators located few centimeters away from the edge of the flap. Also, this direction of the vascularity can explain some small acquiescence that appears on the distal end of the flap (Fig. 15.16).
5. The long blade of the flap should be directed away from the perforator (173,185).
6. The length of the long blade from the perforator should be 1 to 2 cm more than the distance from the perforator to the most distal point of the defect (191).
7. The width of the flap should be 0.5 to 1 cm more than the width of the defect (191).
8. Even if a preoperative identification of perforators is performed, only 1 edge of the planned flap is first incised, either up to or deep to the deep fascia (43,61,185,203) (see Fig. 15.16A).
9. Dissection under magnification with identification and preservation of all the perforators is mandated.
10. After choosing the most suitable perforator, it should be carefully dissected long enough under magnification to allow the rotation without kinking (61,185). The complete skeletonization of the pedicle is not recommended, but there are authors considering that for a perforator of 1 cm diameter, the pedicle should be cleared for a 3 cm length (208). Following this, the definitive design of the flap is accomplished, and the incision around the flap is completed (61).
11. If a tourniquet is used, it is released and time should be given for the perforator's spasm disappearance and apparition of perforator's pulsation and marginal flap's bleeding. Only after these steps, the flap can be rotated into the defect (61).

COMPLICATIONS

One of the most frequent complications after flap surgery for soft tissue reconstruction of the diabetic foot is the venous congestion of the tip or of the entire flap (61,62). Some of the

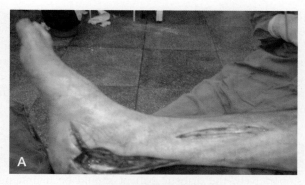

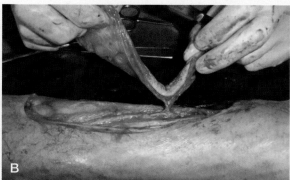

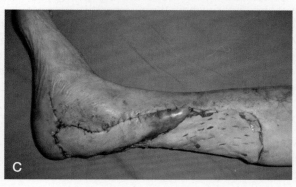

FIGURE 15.16 A. Surgically débrided wounds on the medial aspect of the calcaneus and lower leg showing the exploratory incision marking on of the edges of the designed flap. **B.** Harvested posterior tibialis artery propeller perforator flap. **C.** Superficial skin necrosis of the former distal part of the flap which is opposite to the normal direction of the blood flow.

causes of this complication can be due to underlying vascular disease, inadequate selection of the flap, kinking of the pedicle, and excessive pressure on the flap or its pedicle. Any complications of the flap should be addressed as soon as possible by releasing some sutures when there is skin tension, performing small incisions or punctures of the flap, or by utilizing medicinal leeches. Sometimes, if the venous congestion is observed very early, the flap can be reapplied in the original position and delay its reapplication. In local flaps and especially in local perforator flaps, even if the venous congestion is followed by necrosis, in more than 90% of the cases, it is only superficial. In these cases, the superficial débridement and skin grafting after granulation will lead to a successful outcome (61,62).

Other possible complications are wound dehiscence, either at the donor or recipient site, infection, or osteomyelitis.

In some cases, the persistence of peripheral neuropathy, peripheral arterial disease, and some of the soft tissue and osseous deformities predispose to the apparition of new ulcerations or septic complications which can lead to further amputation.

POSTOPERATIVE CARE

Postoperatively, the diabetic patient should be maintaining adequate control of blood glucose levels, with a well surveillance of all other medical comorbidities. In this attempt, the multidisciplinary team approach should be continued throughout the postoperative period to ensure a successful outcome.

Early postoperative course of mobilization, kinesiotherapy, occupational therapy, and in many cases, psychological therapy consultation are essential for the patient's overall postoperative recovery. In all the cases with local or regional flaps, but especially in those with perforator flaps, local wound care treatments should be very carefully pursued. It is important to not apply excessive pressure on the flap and its pedicle must be free of tension throughout the postoperative course.

Off-loading techniques are also very important by avoiding any contact of the flap and allowing simple dressing changes while monitoring the flap viability. Generally, surgical off-loading can be obtained by utilizing various types of external fixation (14,170,215).

Conclusion

Distant leg pedicle and perforator flap reconstruction in the diabetic population can provide a great source of surgical options when dealing with difficult-to-close diabetic foot soft tissue and osseous defects.

References

1. Abbott CA, Garrow AP, Carrington AL, et al. Foot ulcer risk is lower in South-Asian and African-Caribbean compared with European diabetic patients in the U.K.: the north-west diabetes foot care study. Diabetes Care 2005;28:1869–1875.

2. Akhtar S, Hameed A. Versatility of the sural fasciocutaneous flap in the coverage of lower third leg and hind foot defects. J Plast Reconstr Aesthet Surg 2006;59:839–845.

3. Akyürek M, Safak T, Sönmez E, et al. A new flap design: neural-island flap. Plast Reconstr Surg 2004;114:1467–1477.

4. Almeida MF, da Costa PR, Okawa RY. Reverse-flow island sural flap. Plast Reconstr Surg 2002;109:583–591.

5. Al-Qattan MM. A modified technique for harvesting the reverse sural artery flap from the upper part of the leg: inclusion of a gastrocnemius muscle "cuff" around the sural pedicle. Ann Plast Surg 2001;47:269–274.

6. Al-Qattan MM. Lower-limb reconstruction utilizing the reverse sural artery flap-gastrocnemius muscle cuff technique. Ann Plast Surg 2005;55:174–178.

7. Al-Zube L, Breitbart EA, O'Connor JP, et al. Recombinant human platelet-derived growth factor BB (rhPDGF-BB) and beta-tricalcium phosphate/collagen matrix enhance fracture healing in a diabetic rat model. J Orthop Res 2009;27:1074–1081.

8. Argenta LC. Lateral calcaneal artery skin flap. In: Strauch B, Vasconez LO, Herman CK, et al, eds. Grabb's encyclopedia of flaps: upper extremities, torso, pelvis, and lower extremities. 4th ed. Philadelphia: Wolters Kluwer, 2016:1472–1475.

9. Armstrong DG, Lavery LA. Diabetic foot ulcers: prevention, diagnosis and classification. Am Fam Physician 1998;57:1325–1332.

10. Attinger CE, Ducic I, Hess CL, et al. Outcome of skin graft versus flap surgery in the salvage of the exposed Achilles tendon in diabetics versus nondiabetics. Plast Reconstr Surg 2006;117:2460–2467.

11. Balakrishnan TM, Alalasundaram KV. Reconstruction in the revascularized diabetic foot. J Diab Foot Comp 2012;4:46–56.

12. Barclay TL, Cardoso E, Sharpe DT, et al. Repair of lower leg injuries with fascio-cutaneous flaps. Br J Plast Surg 1982;35:127–132.

13. Barner HB, Kaiser GC, Willman VL. Blood flow in the diabetic leg. Circulation 1971;43:391–394.

14. Baumeister SP, Spierer R, Erdmann D, et al. A realistic complication analysis of 70 sural artery flaps in a multimorbid patient group. Plast Reconstr Surg 2003;112:129–140.

15. Behan FC. The keystone design perforator island flap in reconstructive surgery. ANZ J Surg 2003;73:112–120.

16. Bennett MS. Lower extremity management in patients with diabetes. J Am Pharm Assoc (Wash) 2000;40(5 suppl 1):S40–S41.

17. Beppu M, Hanel DP, Johnston GH, et al. The osteocutaneous fibula flap: an anatomic study. J Reconstr Microsurg 1992;8:215–223.

18. Bocchi A, Merelli S, Morellini A, et al. Reverse fasciocutaneous flap versus distally pedicled sural island flap: two elective methods for distal-third leg reconstruction. Ann Plast Surg 2000;45:284–291.

19. Bortoletto MS, de Andrade SM, Matsuo T, et al. Risk factors for foot ulcers—a cross sectional survey from a primary care setting in Brazil. Prim Care Diabetes 2014;8:71–76.

20. Boulton AJ, Vileikyte L, Ragnarson-Tennvall G, et al. The global burden of diabetic foot disease. Lancet 2005;366:1719–1724.

21. Brownrigg JR, Davey J, Holt PJ, et al. The association of ulceration of the foot with cardiovascular and all-cause mortality in patients with diabetes: a meta-analysis. Diabetologia 2012;55:2906–2912.

22. Buluç L, Tosun B, Sen C, et al. A modified technique for transposition of the reverse sural artery flap. Plast Reconstr Surg 2006;117:2488–2492.

23. Burusapat C, Tanthanatip P, Kuhaphensaeng P, et al. Lateral calcaneal artery flaps in atherosclerosis: cadaveric study, vascular assessment and clinical applications. Plast Reconstr Surg Glob Open 2015;3(9):e517.

24. Calderón W, Andrades P, Leniz P, et al. Fasciocutaneous cone flap. In: Strauch B, Vasconez LO, Herman CK, et al, eds. Grabb's encyclopedia of flaps: upper extremities, torso, pelvis, and lower extremities. 4th ed. Philadelphia: Wolters Kluwer, 2016:1448–1450.

25. Capobianco CM, Stapleton JJ. Diabetic foot infections: a team-oriented review of medical and surgical management. Diabetic Foot Ankle 2010;1.

26. Caputo GM, Cavanagh PR, Ulbrecht JS, et al. Assessment and management of foot disease in patients with diabetes. N Engl J Med 1994;331:854–860.

27. Carriquiry C, Aparecida Costa MA, Vasconez LO. An anatomic study of the septocutaneous vessels of the leg. Plast Reconstr Surg 1985;76:354–363.

28. Catanzariti AR, Blitch EL, Karlock LG. Elective foot and ankle surgery in the diabetic patient. J Foot Ankle Surg 1995;34:23–41.

29. Cavadas PC. Reversed saphenous neurocutaneous island flap: clinical experience and evolution to the posterior tibial perforator-saphenous subcutaneous flap. Plast Reconstr Surg 2003;111:837–839.

30. Cavadas PC, Bonanad B. Reverse-flow sural island flap in the varicose leg. Plast Reconstr Surg 1996;98:901–902.

31. Cavanagh PR, Lipsky BA, Bradbury AW, et al. Treatment for diabetic foot ulcers. Lancet 2005;366:1725–1735.

32. Chan RK, Garfein E, Gigante PR, et al. Side population hematopoietic stem cells promote wound healing in diabetic mice. Plast Reconstr Surg 2007;120:407–411.

33. Chang SM, Hou CL. Role of large superficial veins in distally based flaps of the extremities. Plast Reconstr Surg 2000;106:230–231.

34. Chang SM, Zhang F, Xu DC, et al. Lateral retromalleolar perforator-based flap: anatomical study and preliminary clinical report for heel coverage. Plast Reconstr Surg 2007;120:697–704.

35. Chen SL, Chen TM, Wang HJ. The distally based sural fasciomusculocutaneous flap for foot reconstruction. J Plast Reconstr Aesthet Surg 2006;59:846–855.

36. Cheng Z, Wu W, Hu P, et al. Distally based saphenous nerve-greater saphenous venofasciocutaneous flap for reconstruction of soft tissue defects in distal lower leg. Ann Plast Surg 2016;77:102–105.

37. Chung MS, Baek GH, Gong HS, et al. Lateral calcaneal artery adipofascial flap for reconstruction of the posterior heel of the foot. Clin Orthop Surg 2009;1:1–5.

38. Conrad MC. Large and small artery occlusion in diabetics and nondiabetics with severe vascular disease. Circulation 1967;36:83–91.

39. Cormack GC, Lamberty BGH. A classification of fasciocutaneous flaps according to their patterns of vascularisation. Br J Plast Surg 1984;37:80–87.

40. Cormack GC, Lamberty BGH. Fasciocutaneous vessels. Their distribution on the trunk and limbs, and their clinical application in tissue transfer. Anat Clin 1984;6:121–131.

41. Cormack GC, Lamberty BGH. The arterial anatomy of skin flaps. Edinburgh, Scotland: Churchill-Livingstone, 1986.

42. Dargis V, Pantelejeva O, Jonushaite A, et al. Benefits of a multidisciplinary approach in the management of recurrent diabetic foot ulceration in Lithuania: a prospective study. Diabetes Care 1999;22:1428–1431.

43. D'Arpa S, Cordova A, Pignatti M, et al. Freestyle pedicled perforator flaps: safety, prevention of complications, and management based on 85 consecutive cases. Plast Reconstr Surg 2011;128:892–906.

44. Dellon AL. Treatment of symptomatic diabetic neuropathy by surgical decompression of multiple peripheral nerves. Plast Reconstr Surg 1992;89:689–697.

45. Dellon AL, Muse VL, Nickerson DS, et al. Prevention of ulceration, amputation, and reduction of hospitalization: outcomes of a prospective multicenter trial of tibial neurolysis in patients with diabetic neuropathy. J Reconstr Microsurg 2012;28:241–246.

46. Donski PK, Fogdestam I. Distally based fasciocutaneous flap from the sural region: a preliminary report. Scand J Plast Reconstr Surg 1983;17:191–196.

47. Dorresteijn JAN, Kriegsman DMW, Assendelft WJJ, et al. Patient education for preventing diabetic foot ulceration. Cochrane Database of Syst Rev 2010;(5):CD001488.

48. Dragu A, Bach AD, Kneser U, et al. Two easy and simple modifications when using a distally based sural flap to reduce the risk of venous congestion. Plast Reconstr Surg 2008;122:683–684.

49. Ducic I, Attinger CE. Foot and ankle reconstruction: pedicled muscle flaps versus free flaps and the role of diabetes. Plast Reconstr Surg 2011;128:173–180.

50. El-Sabbagh AH. Skin perforator flaps: an algorithm for leg reconstruction. J Reconstr Microsurg 2011;27:511–523.

51. Elsahy NI. Bipedicle skin flap to the heel. In: Strauch B, Vasconez LO, Herman CK, et al, eds. Grabb's encyclopedia of flaps: upper extremities, torso, pelvis, and lower extremities. 4th ed. Philadelphia: Wolters Kluwer, 2016:1450–1451.

52. Erdmann D, Gottlieb N, Humphrey JS, et al. Sural flap delay procedure: a preliminary report. Ann Plast Surg 2005;54:562–565.

53. Ferreira MC, Gabbianelli G, Alonso N, et al. The distal pedicle fascia flap of the leg. Scand J Plast Reconstr Surg 1986;20:133–136.

54. Freeman BJ, Duff S, Allen PE, et al. The extended lateral approach to the hindfoot. Anatomical basis and surgical implications. J Bone Joint Surg Br 1998;80:139–142.

55. Frykberg RG. Diabetic foot ulcers: pathogenesis and management. Am Fam Physician 2002;66:1655–1662.

56. Frykberg RG. Team approach toward lower extremity amputation prevention in diabetes. J Am Podiatr Med Assoc 1997;87:305–312.

57. Frykberg RG, Zgonis T, Armstrong DG, et al. Diabetic foot disorders. A clinical practice guideline (2006 revision). J Foot Ankle Surg 2006;45(5 suppl):S1–S66.

58. Furlow LT Jr. Dorsalis pedis flap. In: Strauch B, Vasconez LO, Herman CK, et al, eds. Grabb's encyclopedia of flaps: upper extremities, torso, pelvis, and lower extremities. 4th ed. Philadelphia: Wolters Kluwer, 2016:1495–1499.

59. Gang RK. Reconstruction of soft-tissue defect of the posterior heel with a lateral calcaneal artery island flap. Plast Reconstr Surg 1987;79:415–421.

60. Geddes CR, Tang M, Yang D, et al. Anatomy of the integument of the lower extremity. In: Blondeel PN, Morris SF, Hallock GG, et al, eds. Perforator flaps: anatomy, technique & clinical applications. St. Louis: Quality Medical, 2006:541–578.

61. Georgescu AV. Propeller perforator flaps in distal lower leg: evolution and clinical applications. Arch Plast Surg 2012;39:94–105.

62. Georgescu AV, Matei IR, Capota IM. The use of propeller perforator flaps for diabetic limb salvage: a retrospective review of 25 cases. Diabet Foot Ankle 2012;3.

63. Ger R. The operative treatment of the advanced stasis ulcer. A preliminary communication. Am J Surg 1966;111:659–663.

64. Ger R. The technique of muscle transposition in the operative treatment of traumatic and ulcerative lesions of the leg. J Trauma 1971;11:502–510.

65. Ghali S, Butler PE, Tepper OM, et al. Vascular delay revisited. Plast Reconstr Surg 2007;119:1735–1744.

66. Ghanassia E, Villon L, Thuan Dit Dieudonné JF, et al. Long-term outcome and disability of diabetic patients hospitalized for diabetic foot ulcers: a 6.5-year follow-up study. Diabetes Care 2008;31:1288–1292.

67. Grabb WC, Argenta LC. The lateral calcaneal artery skin flap (the lateral calcaneal artery, lesser saphenous vein, and sural nerve skin flap). Plast Reconstr Surg 1981;68:723–730.

68. Grayson ML, Gibbons GW, Balogh K, et al. Probing to bone in infected pedal ulcers. A clinical sign of underlying osteomyelitis in diabetic patients. JAMA 1995;273:721–723.

69. Haertsch P. The surgical plane in the leg. Br J Plast Surg 1981;34:464–469.

70. Hallock GG. Bipedicled fasciocutaneous flaps in the lower extremity. Ann Plast Surg 1992;29:397–401.

71. Hallock GG. Distal lower leg local random fasciocutaneous flaps. Plast Reconstr Surg 1990;86:304–311.

72. Hallock GG. Local fasciocutaneous flaps for cutaneous coverage of lower extremity wounds. J Trauma 1989;29:1240–1244.

73. Hallock GG. Lower extremity muscle perforator flaps for lower extremity reconstruction. Plast Reconstr Surg 2004;114:1123–1130.

74. Hallock GG. The propeller flap version of the adductor muscle perforator flap for coverage of ischial or trochanteric pressure sores. Ann Plast Surg 2006;56:540–542.

75. Hallock GG. Utility of both muscle and fascia flaps in severe lower extremity trauma. J Trauma 2000;48:913–917.

76. Hansen T, Wikström J, Johansson LO, et al. The prevalence and quantification of atherosclerosis in an elderly population assessed by whole-body magnetic resonance angiography. Arterioscler Thromb Vasc Biol 2007;27:649–654.

77. Hasegawa M, Torii S, Katoh H, et al. The distally based superficial sural artery flap. Plast Reconstr Surg 1994;93:1012–1020.

78. Haydon NB, Caminer D. 'The Crown flap': a modification to the keystone flap types I and IIA. European J Plast Surg 2014;37:347–348.

79. Healy C, Tiernan E, Lamberty BGH, et al. Rotation fasciocutaneous flap repair of lower limb defects. Plast Reconstr Surg 1995;95:243–251.

80. Heitmann C, Khan FN, Levin LS. Vasculature of the peroneal artery: an anatomic study focused on the perforator vessels. J Reconstr Microsurg 2003;19:157–162.

81. Heymans O, Verhelle N, Peters S. The medial adipofascial flap of the leg: anatomical basis and clinical applications. Plast Reconstr Surg 2005;115:793–801.

82. Hinchliffe RJ, Valk GD, Apelqvist J, et al. A systematic review of the effectiveness of interventions to enhance the healing of chronic ulcers of the foot in diabetes. Diabetes Metab Res Rev 2008;24(suppl 1):S119–S144.

83. Hogg FR, Peach G, Price P, et al. Measures of health-related quality of life in diabetes-related foot disease: a systematic review. Diabetologia 2012;55:552–565.

84. Hollier L, Sharma S, Babigumira E, et al. Versatility of the sural fasciocutaneous flap in the coverage of lower extremity wounds. Plast Reconstr Surg 2002;110:1673–1679.

85. Holmes J, Rayner CR. Lateral calcaneal artery island flap. Br J Plast Surg 1984;37:402–405.

86. Holstein PE, Sørensen S. Limb salvage experience in a multidisciplinary diabetic foot unit. Diabetes Care 1999;22(suppl 2):B97–B103.

87. Hong JP. Reconstruction of the diabetic foot using the anterolateral thigh perforator flap. Plast Reconstr Surg 2006;117:1599–1608.

88. Hong JP, Oh TS. An algorithm for limb salvage for diabetic foot ulcers. Clin Plast Surg 2012;39:341–352.

89. Hunter S, Langemo DK, Anderson J, et al. Hyperbaric oxygen therapy for chronic wounds. Adv Skin Wound Care 2010;23:116–119.

90. Hyakusoku H, Tonegawa H, Fumiiri M. Heel coverage with a T-shaped distally based sural island fasciocutaneous flap. Plast Reconstr Surg 1994;93:872–876.

91. Hyakusoku H, Yamamoto T, Fumiiri M. The propeller flap method. Br J Plast Surg 1991;44:53–54.

92. Iraj B, Khorvash F, Ebneshahidi A, et al. Prevention of diabetic foot ulcer. Int J Prev Med 2013;4:373–376.

93. Ishikawa K, Isshiki N, Hoshino K, et al. Distally based lateral calcaneal flap. Ann Plast Surg 1990;24:10–16.

94. Ishikawa K, Isshiki N, Suzuki S, et al. Distally based dorsalis pedis island flap for coverage of the distal portion of the foot. Br J Plast Surg 1987;40:521–525.

95. Ishikawa K, Kyutoku S, Takeuchi E. Free lateral calcaneal flap. Ann Plast Surg 1993;30:167–170.

96. Jakubietz RG, Jakubietz MG, Gruenert JG, et al. The 180-degree perforator-based propeller flap for soft tissue coverage of the distal, lower extremity: a new method to achieve reliable coverage of the distal lower extremity with a local, fasciocutaneous perforator flap. Ann Plast Surg 2007;59:667–671.

97. Jeong SH, Han SK, Kim WK. Treatment of diabetic foot ulcers using a blood bank platelet concentrate. Plast Reconstr Surg 2010;125:944–952.

98. Jiga LP, Barac S, Taranu G, et al. The versatility of propeller flaps for lower limb reconstruction in patients with peripheral arterial obstructive disease: initial experience. Ann Plast Surg 2010;64:193–197.

99. Kamalov T, Ismailov S, Dosova Z, et al. Surgical reconstruction in diabetic foot syndrome. Med Health Sci J (On-line) 2011;6:55–59.

100. Kamath BJ, Joshua TV, Pramod S. Perforator based flap coverage from the anterior and lateral compartment of the leg for medium sized traumatic pretibial soft tissue defects—a simple solution for a complex problem. J Plast Reconstr Aesthet Surg 2006;59:515–520.

101. Kamei N, Yamane K, Nakanishi S, et al. Effectiveness of Semmes-Weinstein monofilament examination for diabetic peripheral neuropathy screening. J Diabetes Complications 2005;19:47–53.

102. Kansal S, Goil P, Agarwal V, et al. Reverse pedicle-based greater saphenous neuro-veno-fasciocutaneous flap for reconstruction of lower leg and foot. Eur J Orthop Surg Traumatol 2014;24:62–72.

103. Karacalar A, Idil O, Demir A, et al. Delay in neurovenous flaps: experimental and clinical experience. Ann Plast Surg 2004;53:481–487.

104. Karp NS, Kasabian AK, Siebert JW, et al. Microvascular free-flap salvage of the diabetic foot: a 5-year experience. Plast Reconstr Surg 1994;94:834–840.

105. Khouri JS, Egeland BM, Daily SD, et al. The keystone island flap: use in large defects of the trunk and extremities in soft-tissue reconstruction. Plast Reconstr Surg 2011;127:1212–1221.

106. Koob TJ, Rennert R, Zabek N, et al. Biological properties of dehydrated human amnion/chorion composite graft: implications for chronic wound healing. Int Wound J 2013;10:493–500.

107. Koshima I, Itoh S, Nanba Y, et al. Medial and lateral malleolar perforator flaps for repair of defects around the ankle. Ann Plast Surg 2003;51:579–583.

108. Koshima I, Moriguchi T, Ohta S, et al. The vasculature and clinical application of the posterior tibial perforator-based flap. Plast Reconstr Surg 1992;90:643–649.

109. Koshima I, Soeda S. Inferior epigastric artery skin flaps without rectus abdominis muscle. Br J Plast Surg 1989;42:645–648.

110. Krag C, Riegels-Nielsen P. The dorsalis pedis flap for lower leg reconstruction. Acta Orthop Scand 1982;53:487–493.

111. Kroll SS, Rosenfield L. Perforator-based flaps for low posterior midline defects. Plast Reconstr Surg 1988;81:561–566.

112. Lagvankar SP. Distally-based random fasciocutaneous flaps for multi-staged reconstruction of defects in the lower third of the leg, ankle and heel. Br J Plast Surg 1990;43:541–545.

113. Lavery LA, Peters EJ, Armstrong DG. What are the most effective interventions in preventing diabetic foot ulcers? Int Wound J 2008;5:425–433.

114. Lecours C, Saint-Cyr M, Wong C, et al. Freestyle pedicle perforator flaps: clinical results and vascular anatomy. Plast Reconstr Surg 2010;126:1589–1603.

115. Lee BT, Lin SJ, Bar-Meir ED, et al. Pedicled perforator flaps: a new principle in reconstructive surgery. Plast Reconstr Surg 2010;125:201–208.

116. Le Fourn B, Caye N, Pannier M. Distally based sural fascimuscular flap: anatomic study and application for filling leg or foot defects. Plast Reconstr Surg 2001;107:67–72.

117. Le Huec JC, Midy D, Chauveaux D, et al. Anatomic basis of the sural fascio-cutaneous flap: surgical applications. Surg Radiol Anat 1988;10:5–13.

118. Leone S, Pascale R, Vitale M, et al. Epidemiology of diabetic foot [in Italian]. Infez Med 2012;20(suppl 1):8–13.

119. Lin SD, Chou CK, Lin TM, et al. The distally based lateral adipofascial flap. Br J Plast Surg 1998;51:96–102.

120. Lin SD, Lai CS, Chiu YT, et al. Adipofascial flap of the lower leg based on the saphenous artery. Br J Plast Surg 1996;49:390–395.

121. Lin SD, Lai CS, Chiu YT, et al. The lateral calcaneal artery adipofascial flap. Br J Plast Surg 1996;49:52–57.

122. Lin SD, Lai CS, Tsai CC, et al. Clinical application of the distally based medial adipofascial flap for soft tissue defects on the lower half of the leg. J Trauma 1995;38:623–629.

123. Lipski BA, Berendt AR, Deery HG, et al. Diagnosis and treatment of diabetic foot infection. Clin Infect Dis 2004;39:885–910.

124. Liu K, Li Z, Lin Y, et al. The reverse-flow posterior tibial artery island flap: anatomic study and 72 clinical cases. Plast Reconstr Surg 1990;86:312–316.

125. Liu L, Zou L, Li Z, et al. The extended distally based sural neurocutaneous flap for foot and ankle reconstruction: a retrospective review of 10 years of experience. Ann Plast Surg 2014;72:689–694.

126. Lo JC, Chen HC, Chen HH, et al. Modified reverse sural artery flap. Changgeng Yi Xue Za Hi 1997;20:293–298.

127. Madanat A, Sheshah E, Badawy El-B, et al. Response to the comment by Vas P.R. et al.: "P.R. Vas, S. Sharma, G. Rayman, Utilizing the Ipswich Touch Test to simplify screening methods for identifying the risk of foot ulceration among diabetics: comment on the Saudi experience. Prim. Care Diabetes (2015) http://dx.doi.org/10.1016/j.pcd.2015.01.003." Prim Care Diabetes 2015;9:401–402.

128. Maffi TR, Knoetgen J III, Turner NS, et al. Enhanced survival using the distally based sural artery interpolation flap. Ann Plast Surg 2005;54:302–305.

129. Man D, Acland R. The microarterial anatomy of the dorsalis pedis flap and its clinical applications. Plast Reconstr Surg 1980;65:419–423.

130. Manchot C. The cutaneous arteries of the human body. New York: Springer Publishing, 1983.

131. Markanday A. Diagnosing diabetic foot osteomyelitis: narrative review and a suggested 2-step score-based diagnostic pathway for clinicians. Open Forum Infect Dis 2014;1(2):ofu060.

132. Maruyama Y. Bilobed fasciocutaneous flap. Br J Plast Surg 1985;38:515–517.

133. Maruyama Y, Iwahira Y. V-Y advancement flaps to the heel and ankle. In: Strauch B, Vasconez LO, Herman CK, et al, eds. Grabb's encyclopedia of flaps: upper extremities, torso, pelvis, and lower extremities. 4th ed. Philadelphia: Wolters Kluwer, 2016:1452–1453.

134. Masia J, Moscatiello F, Pons G, et al. Our experience in lower limb reconstruction with perforator flaps. Ann Plast Surg 2007;58:507–512.

135. Masquelet AC, Romana MC, Wolf G. Skin island flaps supplied by the vascular axis of the sensitive superficial nerve: anatomic study and clinical experience in the leg. Plast Reconstr Surg 1992;89:1115–1121.

136. McCraw JB, Furlow LT Jr. The dorsalis pedis arterialized flap. A clinical study. Plast Reconstr Surg 1975;55:177–185.

137. McGregor IA, Jackson IT. The groin flap. Br J Plast Surg 1972; 25:3–16.

138. Mehrotra S. Perforator-plus flaps: a new concept in traditional flap design. Plast Reconstr Surg 2007;119:590–598.

139. Mojallal A, Wong C, Shipkov C, et al. Vascular supply of the distally based superficial sural artery flap: surgical safe zones based on component analysis using three-dimensional computed tomographic angiography. Plast Reconstr Surg 2010;126:1240–1252.

140. Mok WL, Por YC, Tan BK. Distally based sural artery adipofascial flap based on a single sural nerve branch: anatomy and clinical applications. Arch Plast Surg 2014;41:709–715.

141. Moncrieff MD, Thompson JF, Stretch JR. Extended experience and modifications in the design and concepts of the keystone design island flap. J Plast Reconstr Aesthet Surg 2010;63: 1359–1363.

142. Monteiro-Soares M, Boyko EJ, Ribeiro J, et al. Predictive factors for diabetic foot ulceration: a systematic review. Diabetes Metab Res Rev 2012;28:574–600.

143. Moutran M, Mojallal A, Chekaroua K, et al. Foot defect with vascular and neural injury due to freshwater stingray sting: reconstruction with a lesser saphenous vein adipo-fascial flap [in French]. Ann Chir Plast Esthet 2009;54:156–160.

144. Nakajima H, Imanishi N, Fukuzumi S, et al. Accompanying arteries of the cutaneous veins and cutaneous nerves in the extremities: anatomical study and a concept of the venoadipofascial and/or neuroadipofascial pedicled fasciocutaneous flap. Plast Reconstr Surg 1998;102:779–791.

145. Nakajima H, Imanishi N, Fukuzumi S, et al. Accompanying arteries of the lesser saphenous vein and sural nerve: anatomic study and its clinical applications. Plast Reconstr Surg 1999;103:104–120.

146. Nayak BB, Thatte RL, Thatte MR, et al. A microneurovascular study of the great saphenous vein in man and the possible implications for survival of venous flaps. Br J Plast Surg 2000;53:230–233.

147. Niinikoski J. Hyperbaric oxygen therapy of diabetic foot ulcers, transcutaneous oxymetry in clinical decision making. Wound Repair Regen 2003;11:458–461.

148. Noack N, Hartmann B, Küntscher M. Measures to prevent complications of distally based neurovascular sural flap. Ann Plast Surg 2006;57:37–40.

149. Oh TS, Lee HS, Hong JP. Diabetic foot reconstruction using free flaps increases 5-year-survival rate. J Plast Reconstr Aesthet Surg 2013;66:243–250.

150. Oishi SN, Levin LS, Pederson W. Microsurgical management of extremity wounds in diabetics with peripheral vascular disease. Plast Reconstr Surg 1993;92:485–492.

151. Orticochea M. The musculo-cutaneous flap method: an immediate and heroic substitute for the method of delay. Br J Plast Surg 1972;25:106–110.

152. Ozkan O, Coskunfirat OK, Ozgentas HE. Reliability of free-flap coverage in diabetic foot ulcers. Microsurgery 2005;25:107–112.

153. Pakiam AI. Reversed dermis flap. In: Strauch B, Vasconez LO, Herman CK, et al, eds. Grabb's encyclopedia of flaps: upper extremities, torso, pelvis, and lower extremity. 4th ed. Philadelphia: Wolters Kluwer, 2016:1459–1460.

154. Park TH, Anand A. Management of diabetic foot: brief synopsis for busy orthopedist. J Clin Orthop Trauma 2015;6:24–29.

155. Parrett BM, Pribaz JJ. Lower extremity reconstruction. Rev Med Clin Condes 2010;21:66–75.

156. Parrett BM, Pribaz JJ, Matros E, et al. Risk analysis for the reverse sural fasciocutaneous flap in distal leg reconstruction. Plast Reconstr Surg 2009;123:1499–1504.

157. Parrett BM, Talbot SG, Pribaz JJ, et al. A review of local and regional flaps for distal leg reconstruction. J Reconstr Microsurg 2009;25:445–455.

158. Pelissier P, Gardet H, Pinsolle V, et al. The keystone design perforator island flap. Part II: clinical applications. J Plast Reconstr Aesthet Surg 2007;60:888–891.

159. Pelle MT, Miller OF III. Debridement of necrotic eschar with 40% urea paste speeds healing of residual limbs and avoids further surgery. Arch Dermatol 2001;137:1288–1290.

160. Peters E, Lavery L. Effectiveness of the diabetic foot risk classification system of the International Working Group on the Diabetic Foot. Diabetes Care 2001;24:1442–1447.

161. Peters EJ, Lipsky BA. Diagnosis and management of infection in the diabetic foot. Med Clin North Am 2013;97:911–946.

162. Pignatti M, Ogawa R, Hallock GG, et al. The "Tokyo" consensus on propeller flaps. Plast Reconstr Surg 2011;127:716–722.

163. Pignatti M, Pasqualini M, Governa M, et al. Propeller flaps for leg reconstruction. J Plast Reconstr Aesthet Surg 2008;61:777–783.

164. Pontén B. The fasciocutaneous flap: its use in soft tissue defects of the lower leg. Br J Plast Surg 1981;34:215–220.

165. Price MF, Capizzi PJ, Watterson PA, et al. Reverse sural artery flap: caveats for success. Ann Plast Surg 2002;48:496–504.

166. Prompers L, Huijberts M, Apelqvist J, et al. High prevalence of ischemia, infection and serious comorbidity in patients with diabetic foot disease in Europe. Baseline results from the Eurodiale study. Diabetologia 2007;50:18–25.

167. Quaba O, Quaba AA. Pedicled perforator flaps for the lower limb. Semin Plast Surg 2006;20:103–111.

168. Rad AN, Singh NK, Rosson GD. Peroneal artery perforator-based propeller flap reconstruction of the lateral distal lower extremity after tumor extirpation: case report and literature review. Microsurgery 2008;28:663–670.

169. Ramachandran A, Snehalatha C, Shetty AS, et al. Trends in prevalence of diabetes in Asian countries. World J Diabetes 2012;3:110–117.

170. Ramanujam CL, Facaros Z, Zgonis T. External fixation for surgical off-loading of diabetic foot soft tissue reconstruction. Clin Podiatr Med Surg 2011;28:211–216.

171. Raveendran SS, Perera D, Happuharachchi T, et al. Superficial sural artery flap—a study in 40 cases. Br J Plast Surg 2004;57:266–269.

172. Rayman G, Vas PR, Baker N, et al. The Ipswich Touch Test: a simple and novel method to identify inpatients with diabetes at risk of foot ulceration. Diabetes Care 2011;34:1517–1518.

173. Saint-Cyr M, Wong C, Schaverien M, et al. The perforasome theory: vascular anatomy and clinical implications. Plast Reconstr Surg 2009;124:1529–1544.

174. Salmon M, Taylor GI, Tempest M. Arteries of the skin. London: Churchill Livingstone, 1988.

175. Saltzman CL, Rashid R, Hayes A, et al. 4.5-gram monofilament sensation beneath both first metatarsal heads indicates protective foot sensation in diabetic patients. J Bone Joint Surg Am 2004;86:717–723.

176. Sanders A. Impact of polyclinics on diabetes care. Pract Diab Int 2009;26:48–49.

177. Schaper NC, Apelqvist J, Bakker K. Reducing lower leg amputations in diabetes: a challenge for patients, healthcare providers and the healthcare system. Diabetologia 2012;55:1869–1872.

178. Schaverien M, Saint-Cyr M. Perforators of the lower leg: analysis of perforator locations and clinical application for pedicled perforator flaps. Plast Reconstr Surg 2008;122:161–170.

179. Schmidt K, Jakubietz M, Djalek S, et al. The distally based adipofascial sural artery flap: faster, safer, and easier? A long-term comparison of the fasciocutaneous and adipofascial method in a multimorbid patient population. Plast Reconstr Surg 2012;130:360–368.

180. Searles JM Jr, Colen LB. Foot reconstruction in diabetes mellitus and peripheral vascular insufficiency. Clin Plast Surg 1991;18:467–483.

181. Shahbazian H, Yazdanpanah L, Latifi SM. Risk assessment of patients with diabetes for foot ulcers according to risk classification consensus of International Working Group on Diabetic Foot (IWGDF). Pak J Med Sci 2013;29:730–734.

182. Singh S, Naasan A. Use of distally based superficial sural island artery flaps in acute open fractures of the lower leg. Ann Plast Surg 2001;47:505–510.

183. Smith J. Debridement of diabetic foot ulcers. Cochrane Database Syst Rev 2002;(4):CD003556.

184. Sönmez E, Silistireli ÖK, Safak T. Reconstruction of the soft-tissue defects of foot and ankle with neural-island flaps. In: Strauch B, Vasconez LO, Herman CK, et al, eds. Grabb's encyclopedia of flaps: upper extremities, torso, pelvis, and lower extremities. 4th ed. Philadelphia: Wolters Kluwer, 2016:1467–1469.

185. Sur YJ. Morsy M, Saint-Cyr M. The pedicled perforator (propeller) flap in lower extremity defects. In: Strauch B, Vasconez LO, Herman CK, et al, eds. Grabb's encyclopedia of flaps: upper extremities, torso, pelvis, and lower extremities. 4th ed. Philadelphia: Wolters Kluwer, 2016:1420–1426.

186. Tan O, Atik B, Bekerecioglu M. Supercharged reverse-flow sural flap: a new modification increasing the reliability of the flap. Microsurgery 2005;25:36–43.

187. Tang M, Mao Y, Almutairi K, et al. Three-dimensional analysis of perforators of the posterior leg. Plast Reconstr Surg 2009;123:1729–1738.

188. Taylor GI, Corlett RJ, Caddy CM, et al. An anatomic review of the delay phenomenon: II. Clinical applications. Plast Reconstr Surg 1992;89:408–416.

189. Taylor GI, Palmer JH. The vascular territories (angiosomes) of the body: experimental study and clinical applications. Br J Plast Surg 1987;40:113–141.

190. Taylor GI, Pan WR. Angiosomes of the leg: anatomic study and clinical implications. Plast Reconstr Surg 1998;102:599–616.

191. Teo TC. Perforator local flaps in lower limb reconstruction. Cir Plast Iberlatinamer 2006;32:15–16.

192. Thatte RL, Laud N. Deepithelialized "turnover" skin flap of the lower leg and foot. In: Strauch B, Vasconez LO, Herman CK, et al, eds. Grabb's encyclopedia of flaps: upper extremities, torso, pelvis, and lower extremities. 4th ed. Philadelphia: Wolters Kluwer, 2016:1454–1459.

193. Tolhurst DE, Haeseker B, Zeeman RJ. The development of the fasciocutaneous flap and its clinical application. Plast Reconstr Surg 1983;71:597–606.

194. Torii S, Namiki Y, Hayashi Y, et al. Reverse-flow peroneal island flap for the reconstruction of leg and foot. Eur J Plast Surg 1988;11:26–31.

195. Torii S, Namiki Y, Mori R. Reverse-flow island flap: clinical report and venous drainage. Plast Reconstr Surg 1987;79:600–609.

196. Tos P, Innocenti M, Artiaco S, et al. Perforator-based propeller flaps treating loss of substance in the lower limb. J Orthop Traumatol 2011;12:93–99.

197. Tosun Z, Ozkan A, Karaçor Z, et al. Delaying the reverse sural flap provides predictable results for complicated wounds in diabetic foot. Ann Plast Surg 2005;55:169–173.

198. Uygur F, Evinç R, Noyan N, et al. Should we hesitate to use subcutaneous tunneling for fear of damaging the sural flap pedicle? Ann Plast Surg 2009;63:89–93.

199. van Baal J, Hubbard R, Game F, et al. Mortality associated with acute Charcot foot and neuropathic foot ulceration. Diabetes Care 2010;33:1086–1089.

200. Venkataramakrishnan V, Mohan D, Villafane O. Perforator based V-Y advancement flaps in the leg. Br J Plast Surg 1998;51:431–435.

201. Verhelle NA, Lemaire V, Nelissen X, et al. Combined reconstruction of the diabetic foot including revascularization and free-tissue transfer. J Reconstr Microsurg 2004;20:511–517.

202. Waaijman R, de Haart M, Arts ML, et al. Risk factors for plantar foot ulcer recurrence in neuropathic diabetic patients. Diabetes Care 2014;37:1697–1705.

203. Wallace CG, Kao HK, Jeng SF, et al. Free-style flaps: a further step forward for perforator flap surgery. Plast Reconstr Surg 2009;124:419–426.

204. Wee JT. Reconstruction of the lower leg and foot with the reverse-pedicled anterior tibial flap: preliminary report of a new fasciocutaneous flap. Br J Plast Surg 1986;39:327–337.

205. Wei FC, Chen HC, Chuang CC, et al. Fibular osteoseptocutaneous flap: anatomic study and clinical application. Plast Reconstr Surg 1986;78:191–200.

206. Winkley K, Stahl D, Chalder T, et al. Quality of life in people with their first diabetic foot ulcer: a prospective cohort study. J Am Podiatr Med Assoc 2009;99:406–414.

207. Wong CH, Cui F, Tan BK, et al. Nonlinear finite element simulations to elucidate the determinants of perforator patency in propeller flaps. Ann Plast Surg 2007;59:672–678.

208. Wong CH, Tan BK. Maximizing the reliability and safety of the distally based sural artery flap. J Reconstr Microsurg 2008;24:589–594.

209. Wu WC, Chang YP, So YC, et al. The anatomic basis and clinical applications of flaps based on the posterior tibial vessels. Br J Plast Surg 1993;46:470–479.

210. Yang D, Morris SF. Reversed sural island flap supplied by the lower septocutaneous perforator of the peroneal artery. Ann Plast Surg 2002;49:375–378.

211. Yeh JT, Lin CH, Lin YT. Skin grafting as a salvage procedure in diabetic foot reconstruction to avoid major limb amputation. Chang Gung Med J 2010;33:389–396.

212. Yilmaz M, Karatas O, Barutcu A. The distally based superficial sural artery island flap: clinical experiences and modifications. Plast Reconstr Surg 1998;102:2358–2367.

213. Yoshimura M, Shimada T, Hosokawa M. The vasculature of the peroneal tissue transfer. Plast Reconstr Surg 1990;85:917–921.

214. Zeun P, Gooday C, Nunney I, et al. Predictors of outcomes in diabetic foot osteomyelitis treated initially with conservative (nonsurgical) medical management: a retrospective study. Int J Low Extrem Wounds 2016;15:19–25.

215. Zgonis T, Roukis TS. Off-loading large posterior heel defects after sural artery soft-tissue flap coverage with a stacked Taylor spatial frame foot plate system. Oper Tech Ortho 2006;16:32–37.

216. Zhang FH, Chang SM, Lin SQ, et al. Modified distally based sural neuro-veno-fasciocutaneous flap: anatomical study and clinical applications. Microsurgery 2005;25:543–550.

217. Zhang F, Zhang CC, Lin S, et al. Distally based saphenous nerve-great saphenous veno-fasciocutaneous compound flap with nutrient vessels: microdissection and clinical application. Ann Plast Surg 2009;63:81–88.

CHAPTER 16

Free Flap Reconstruction for Soft Tissue Coverage of the Diabetic Lower Extremity

Chrisovalantis Lakhiani • Karen K. Evans • Christopher E. Attinger

INTRODUCTION

Advances in microvascular surgery have redefined the way plastic surgeons approach lower extremity reconstruction today. Wounds that once would have destined a lower extremity for amputation are now salvageable and functional. Nevertheless, despite these advances, many patients with complex lower extremity wounds and ischemic lower extremities continue to undergo amputation. This is largely due to a misconception in the medical community that patients with multiple medical problems, such as diabetes mellitus, hypertension, peripheral arterial disease, and coronary artery disease, are poor candidates for major lower extremity reconstruction. Many subscribers to this misconception believe that amputation may afford a safer and more reliable option.

Lower extremity amputation carries significant postoperative morbidity, and societal costs associated with this procedure are not necessarily less when comparing amputation versus limb salvage (10,19). It is well known that soon after lower extremity amputation in diabetic patients, the contralateral limb may be threatened with the same fate (12,22). These patients are less likely to ambulate (36), and overall postamputation mortality is higher in this group of patients than in nondiabetic patients (30). As a group, diabetic patients with multiple comorbidities are ill equipped to tolerate the increased physical demands that come with one amputation and are even less able to tolerate bilateral amputations (9,18,34). The fundamental reason for emphasis on limb salvage and the preservation of limb length is that the increased energy of ambulation in amputees results in greater cardiopulmonary demands. In conjunction with often accompanied medical comorbidities and decreased physiologic reserve, this increased demand leads to higher morbidity and mortality rates among amputees following surgery.

The diabetic foot offers unique and challenging properties that preclude soft tissue reconstruction from being a straightforward task. Diabetic foot ulcerations (DFUs) are usually due to a myriad of factors including foot and ankle biomechanics,

peripheral neuropathy, arterial insufficiency, venous stasis, and hyperglycemia, which is an independent risk factor for poor healing or reconstruction complications. Often, what may present as a small ulceration reveals a much larger defect after serial débridements to healthy, noninfected, or nonischemic tissue. Management of DFUs therefore is best accomplished with a multidisciplinary care team involving podiatrists, vascular surgeons, plastic surgeons, orthopedists, physiatrists, internists, and many other health care providers who are able to manage the complex medical comorbidities. Prior to soft tissue reconstruction, the inciting factors which contributed to DFUs should be addressed. This may include correction of biomechanical abnormalities with off-loading shoe wear, tendon rebalancing, or osseous procedures. Revascularization may also be necessary in order to accomplish primary healing at the wound site or open occluded vessels to use as a source for microvascular free tissue transfer (4,6). Because of the size of some wounds, even with adequate arterial inflow, they may not heal without some type of soft tissue procedure, and the lower extremity may still be at risk for amputation. Free tissue transfer can cover vital structures, achieve wound closure of large defects, and bring in a reliable source of vascularized tissue that introduces antibiotic delivery and immune cells that can combat infection (20).

This chapter reviews the indications and contraindications for free tissue transfer, preoperative planning, anatomy, and surgical techniques for the most commonly utilized flaps as well as postoperative management in order to maximize the chance for a successful outcome.

PREOPERATIVE CONSIDERATIONS

Free tissue transfer is a commonly performed procedure that has been demonstrated to have a high rate of success for traumatic or oncologic procedures. However, in the past, consistent success for salvage of the diabetic foot has been more difficult to achieve (23,31). Due to host comorbidities, presence of ischemic lower extremities or calcified vessels, and a propensity for venous stasis or thrombosis in this population, a stepwise approach to preoperative planning should be employed for all patients in order to maximize a successful outcome. This includes assessment and optimization of the patient, the wound, arterial inflow, and venous outflow. Finally, a decision needs to be made if the defect requires microvascular free tissue transfer and of the selection of an appropriate flap.

Patient Assessment and Optimization

A thorough history and physical examination are crucial to determine if patients are candidates for microvascular reconstruction. This includes determining what comorbid conditions the patient possesses, including cardiac disease, renal disease (and if they are hemodialysis dependent), diabetes mellitus, history of cerebrovascular accident, heart attack, venous thromboembolism (VTE), bleeding disorders, and psychiatric history (Table 16.1).

The medical history alerts the reconstructive surgeon to the possible need for additional consultants and possibly eliminates patients who do not have the physiologic reserve to undergo an operative procedure that may lead to their demise. If necessary, an internist or cardiologist should be available to provide preoperative clearance and medically optimize the patient for surgery. This should include preoperatively ensuring that glucose levels are controlled (ideally <200 mg/dL perioperatively) (8). Hemoglobin A_{1c} level should be less than 8.0 prior to any elective reconstruction. It is also important to ask about nutritional status and consider obtaining nutritional labs because low preoperative serum albumin levels increase the risk of postoperative wound dehiscence. It is generally accepted that a patient with an American Society of Anesthesiologists (ASA) class IV or above is not a candidate for major reconstructive surgery. Additionally, the psychiatric history may exclude patients who are unable to adhere to strict postoperative instructions (7). Table 16.2 displays a list of absolute and relative contraindications for microvascular tissue transfer.

A history of VTE, such as deep vein thrombosis (DVT) or pulmonary embolus, should alert the surgeon to the possibility of an inherent or acquired hypercoagulable disorder. Patients should be asked the number of venous thromboembolic events they have had, the age at onset, and if they have family members who have had VTEs. If these are positive, referral to

TABLE 16.1
Relevant Questions to Ask in the Past Medical History

Have you ever had a heart attack or stroke?
Have you suffered a blood clot in your legs or lungs?
Have any family members suffered a blood clot?
Have you had any lower extremity vascular intervention?

TABLE 16.2
Absolute and Relative Contraindications to Microvascular Reconstruction

Absolute Contraindications

American Society of Anesthesiologists (ASA) class IV or greater
Unstable cardiac disease
Unstable psychiatric disorder
Ischemic lower extremity below-the-knee
Nonfunctional lower extremity

Relative Contraindications

Alcoholism
Intravenous drug use
Poor home care
Poor nutrition
End-stage renal disease

a hematologist may be beneficial for working up a hypercoagulable disorder. Furthermore, a history of DVT should alert the surgeon to assess the deep venous system for insufficiency preoperatively because this may affect the surgical plan. For patients in whom a hypercoagulable disorder is known or discovered, beginning a heparin drip intraoperatively may help prevent venous thrombosis of the free flap anastomosis (5).

Surgical history taking should include prior interventions for the wound, including reconstructive procedures and local or free flap that may have been attempted. In addition, patients should be asked about any prior vascular interventions such as a lower extremity bypass or endovascular stenting.

All patients should be asked regarding their social history and use of tobacco, alcohol, or illicit substances. Active tobacco smoking has repeatedly been shown to be a risk factor for total or partial flap loss, and cessation of smoking should be attempted for all patients prior to any microvascular reconstruction. Alcoholic patients or intravenous drug users should be monitored or encouraged to undergo detoxification prior to any microvascular procedure because both withdrawal symptoms and active use may lead to inadvertent flap damage. Finally, the patient's living situation should be assessed. For patients without societal support, or ability to enter a physical rehabilitation postoperatively, certain amputations provide a better alternative to free tissue transfer because they do not require the same level of postoperative care. It is also crucial to understand preoperative function, and it may be useful to use patient-reported preoperative functional scales such as the Short Form (SF)-12 or SF-36.

Assessment and Optimization of the Diabetic Wound and Lower Extremity

The patient's history should provide information on the etiology of the wound, its progression, and any interventions that have been performed up to the time of consultation.

Physical examination of the wound itself should include an analysis of the etiology, location, dimensions, depth, and assessment of which structures are exposed or missing. If bone or tendon is involved, it is more complex and will likely require local versus free tissue transfer. A patient's history should be taken which includes the origin (usually traumatic) and age of the wound. The trauma is usually related to biomechanical abnormalities and neuropathy causing excessive local pressure during gait, changes in shoe gear, penetrating trauma, or burn. It is important to ask what previous therapy has been used because topical agents can contribute to the wound's chronicity (e.g., caustic agents such as hydrogen peroxide, 10% iodine, alcohol, and others) (27).

Attention should be directed to the lower extremity itself, which should be examined for signs of arterial ischemia, venous insufficiency, or lymphedema. A thorough Doppler examination should be performed in all patients. The presence of arterial insufficiency should alert the physician to the need for further testing, beginning with noninvasive arterial studies, and, finally, interventional or computed tomography angiography after consultation with a vascular surgeon.

Biomechanical evaluation should also be performed in all patients when feasible. For those patients with soft tissue or osseous deformities of the foot, tendon rebalancing, equinus correction, and/or osseous reconstruction may need to be performed in order to mitigate the risk of reulceration. The presence of these issues may prompt consultation with an orthopedic or podiatric surgeon.

Lower extremity sensation must also be assessed. Lack of protective sensation can be established when the patient is unable to feel 10 g of pressure (5.07 Semmes-Weinstein monofilament). A more simple and equally effective assessment is the Ipswich Touch Test where one lightly touches the foot in 5 places to assess sensitivity to touch (26). Assessing sensation is critical to help understand the etiology of the DFU, determine off-loading regimens, and prevent ulceration with more vigilant follow-up (2).

Following the wound assessment, the wound should be appropriately prepared. This may require serial débridements of the wound and appropriate cultures if the wound is infected. Antibiotic therapy should be modified based on culture sensitivities and/or bone biopsies. The wound should be reassessed after the final débridement because the dimensions, depth, and missing or exposed anatomic structures have likely changed.

Addressing Ischemia Preoperatively

All patients should undergo a thorough Doppler examination to assess for arterial insufficiency. The posterior tibial, dorsalis pedis, and both branches of the peroneal artery should be assessed. Triphasic flow is normal, biphasic flow may be normal, and monophasic flow mandates an angiogram. Diminished flow to the angiosome on which the wound is located may require percutaneous transluminal angioplasty or stenting. The patient should then be referred to a vascular surgeon who specializes in distal lower extremity endovascular and bypass revascularizations. Noninvasive arterial testing should be obtained at the very least. Although ankle-brachial indices (ABIs) are often falsely

elevated due to arterial calcification in this patient population, pulse volume recordings and segmental limb pressures can help isolate the level of arterial occlusion. At this point, computed tomography or interventional angiography is useful both for identifying the site of any arterial lesion, assessing whether the affected artery is suitable for intervention and for recipient vessel flap planning. For this reason, angiography performed by an interventional physician is superior to computed tomography angiography because arterial lesions may be suitable to endovascular intervention at the time. When endovascular intervention is not possible, consultation with a vascular surgeon is warranted in order to determine if there is a role for vascular lower extremity bypass surgery. A bypass is useful not only for increasing angiosome-directed blood flow but also for serving as the vascular pedicle to any microvascular tissue transfer.

Angiography of the recipient extremity should generally be performed in order to identify which vessels will be suitable as a recipient for anastomosis. If no vessels are identified near the defect which could be reached by a flap with sufficiently long pedicle, then endovascular intervention or bypass surgery may be warranted. If endovascular intervention or bypass is unable to provide flow, then the leg may not be salvageable.

Venous Insufficiency

Patients should be asked if they have had a previous DVT and examined for signs of venous stasis and superficial phlebitis. These may indicate insufficiency of the deep or superficial venous systems and warrant exploration via Duplex ultrasonography. The presence of deep venous insufficiency should prompt the surgeon to consider performing 1 or both venous anastomoses to the superficial (saphenous) system, whereas the converse is true in the presence of insufficiency in the superficial system.

Flap Selection

Flap selection should begin with an assessment of the wound site and determining what flap characteristics would be ideal for a given location. Authors have attempted to classify the foot and ankle into distinct functional and aesthetic subunits (11); however, these are not widely used to date. Instead, the foot and ankle may be divided into 6 separate functional and aesthetic subunits based solely on anatomic landmarks. These include the distal forefoot, plantar forefoot, plantar midfoot, dorsal foot, calcaneus, and ankle. Table 16.3 showcases each subunit, the functional and aesthetic characteristics of each, ideal flap properties, and various flap options.

The choice of the flap may be altered by the contour of the recipient site; for wounds with irregular contours, muscle flaps may be easier to inset and occlude any dead space. Muscle flaps are able to provide thin, pliable, and well-contoured coverage. Although the original inset may appear bulky, muscular atrophy due to denervation will almost always lead to a thin and highly contoured flap, whereas debulking can be performed in the future if necessary. This is ideal for areas with low functional or weight bearing demands but have a requirement for covering an irregular surface area, such as the ankle.

TABLE 16.3	Subunits of the Foot and Ankle and Desired Flap Properties		
Subunits of the Foot and Ankle	Characteristics	Desired Flap Properties	Flap Options
Distal forefoot	Low functional Moderate aesthetic	Pliable Thin	Radial forearm free flap > lateral arm
Plantar forefoot	High functional Low aesthetic	Durable Thin	Radial forearm free flap > lateral arm > gracilis + split-thickness skin graft > anterolateral thigh
Plantar midfoot	Moderate functional Low aesthetic	Pliable Thin	Radial forearm free flap > anterolateral thigh > scapular > latissimus dorsi
Dorsal foot	Low functional High aesthetic	Pliable Very thin	Radial forearm free flap > anterolateral thigh > scapular > latissimus dorsi
Calcaneus	High functional Low aesthetic	Durable Moderate bulk	Anterolateral thigh > gracilis + split-thickness skin graft > latissimus dorsi
Ankle	Moderate functional Moderate aesthetic	Pliable Thin or bulky	Gracilis + split-thickness skin graft > latissimus dorsi > anterolateral thigh

When placing a flap around the area of the foot in contact with footwear, fasciocutaneous flaps are good choices because they provide durable coverage. However, depending on the patient's body mass index, some fasciocutaneous flaps may be very bulky due to subcutaneous fat. These flaps can undergo surgical debulking procedures or liposuction in the future in order to improve contour. As a general rule, weight bearing surfaces should be reconstructed using fasciocutaneous or adipocutaneous flaps. The reason for this is twofold: (a) muscle is more sensitive to pressure necrosis, and (b) reconstruction with a muscle flap and then a skin graft adds the possibility of a second site for shear during ambulation.

Neurotized flaps are able to provide protective sensation to the plantar foot via neural anastomosis to the tibial nerve. Various flaps may be harvested with cutaneous nerves in order to accomplish this. The anterolateral thigh (ALT) flap may be harvested with the lateral femoral cutaneous nerve or the free radial forearm flap with the lateral antebrachial cutaneous nerve.

Although microsurgeons are adept at working with vessels as small as 1 mm, microvascular surgery should be made as macrovascular as possible under the microscope. This means choosing flaps that have large-diameter vessels and a pedicle of sufficient length to reach outside the zone of injury. The longer the pedicle, the easier it will be to work out of the zone of inflammation at the recipient site, and the larger the diameter of the flap's vessels, the easier it will be to work with the vessels which may be calcified or diseased.

ANATOMY AND NOMENCLATURE OF FLAPS

A flap is unit of tissue that maintains its own blood supply when transferred from a donor to a recipient site. The spectrum of flaps ranges from simple local flaps containing skin and subcutaneous tissue to composite flaps which can contain combinations of skin, fat, fascia, muscle, or bone. Flaps are used to cover recipient sites with exposed neurovascular or devascularized structures.

Muscle flaps can provide a means of motor function to a defect. Importantly in lower extremity reconstruction, they are able to fill large soft tissue defects, cover irregular surface areas, and provide a robust blood supply for the delivery of antibiotics and increase oxygen tension to the wound area (20). Muscle flaps may include a cutaneous component (i.e., a musculocutaneous flap) or be skin grafted upon transfer to the recipient site. Mathes and Nahai (21) have classically divided muscle flaps into 5 distinct categories based on their blood supply. It is important to understand this classification and how it relates to preserving the vascular inflow pedicle during flap dissection. Table 16.4 lists the Mathes and Nahai (21) muscle flap classification.

Although muscle flaps provide reliable flap harvest, there are times when the added bulk of muscle is not wanted or a durable fasciocutaneous flap would be preferred. To this end, perforator flaps have revolutionized the field of reconstructive microsurgery. A perforator flap is composed of skin and subcutaneous

TABLE 16.4	
Mathes and Nahai (21) Muscle Flap Classification	
Type I	Single dominant vessel
Type II	Dominant and minor vessel
Type III	Two dominant vessels
Type IV	Segmental vascular supply
Type V	Dominant vessel and segmental supply

tissue supplied by a musculofascial perforating vessel. Perforating vessels (also known as perforators) pass from their vessel of origin to the flap through muscle or the fascial septum. In this way, the underlying muscle is entirely spared. Perforator flap may be taken with or without the underlying fascia. With regard to its ability to combat infection, research has demonstrated that fasciocutaneous flaps are as efficacious as muscle flaps for the clearance of infection (29). Three different perforator types are commonly recognized (1):

1. Indirect muscle perforators (also known as musculocutaneous perforators)
2. Indirect septal perforators (also known as septocutaneous perforators)
3. Direct cutaneous perforators

Perforators possess several advantages:

- Reduced donor site morbidity
- Ability to tailor flap size and thickness
- Improved postoperative recovery

Despite these advantages, perforator flaps do possess disadvantageous traits which should be kept in mind prior to flap selection (24,37):

- Greater variability in perforator size and location than musculocutaneous flaps
- Meticulous dissection of the pedicle
- Longer case duration
- Greater risk of fat necrosis than with musculocutaneous flaps

Taylor and Palmer (33) identified 374 distinct angiosomes of the human body which are able to supply a cutaneous vascular territory as flaps. Today, however, the most commonly used flap in lower extremity reconstruction is the ALT flap (37).

TECHNICAL ASPECTS OF MICROVASCULAR FREE TISSUE TRANSFER

Prior to the operative procedure, all aspects of the preoperative management should be addressed and plan for the surgery made. This includes which flap to be harvested, the recipient vessel, whether an end-to-side or end-to-end anastomosis will be performed, the recipient vein, if the flap will be neurotized, patient positioning, anticoagulation therapy, and health care team approach. Table 16.5 summarizes the operative considerations.

Before beginning the operative procedure, the anesthesiologist is also asked to avoid vasopressors if possible during the procedure because this could cause arterial constriction. If a vasopressor must be used, dobutamine or dopamine is preferred.

Unfortunately, diabetic patients frequently have peripheral arterial disease with poor arterial inflow. Thus, a team approach with a vascular surgeon may be required to provide arterial inflow into the leg. This conduit can serve as the arterial source for the free flap or it can revascularize the leg so

that another vessel can be used to provide arterial inflow to the flap. Technically, the former is easier to sew to in view of the fact that the graft is unlikely to be calcified because the patient's native leg arteries are likely to be. In addition, an end-to-side anastomosis is preferred in order to minimize risk of future ischemia. The exception to this is when there is an anterior tibial or posterior tibial vessel that ends just above the ankle; these may be safely anastomosed to in an end-to-end fashion without any risk for increasing ischemic complications to the native foot.

When performing free tissue transfer, a multiteam approach is ideal if feasible. This decreases operative times, costs, and surgeon fatigue. The patient should be appropriately positioned, and the donor and recipient sites should be prepped and draped. While the flap is being harvested by 1 team, the wound should be appropriately débrided a final time and the vessels are exposed.

Exposure of the native artery can be proximal or distal to the wound bed and outside the zone of tissue inflammation and injury. Any arterial branches that may serve as arterial inflow for the flap should be preserved; this may permit an end-to-end anastomosis for the flap's artery, which some surgeons may find easier; otherwise, an end-to-side anastomosis between the flap and the donor artery will be required. To facilitate vascular anastomosis, a noncalcified soft spot in the arterial recipient site should be chosen if possible. Once the recipient artery and vein are dissected out, an arteriotomy should be performed to ensure pulsatile flow. If there is no pulsatile flow, then efforts should be made to correct the cause for this or find an alternative inflow vessel with pulsatile flow.

If possible, the native saphenous veins can be mapped and marked prior to the operation for use during the surgery. Should preoperative duplex imaging have revealed insufficiency of the deep venous system, then the superficial saphenous system may be used for venous outflow and the flap should be inset in order to facilitate this. Generally, the deep venous system of paired venae comitantes can be used for

TABLE 16.5

Stepwise Approach to Free Flap Planning

1. History and physical examination
2. Wound assessment
3. Medical optimization of comorbidities
4. Recipient vessel angiography
5. Venous duplex imaging (if indicated)
6. Determine flap type based on wound location/dimensions
7. Assess anticoagulation therapy needs
8. Surgical planning for alternative procedures
9. Determine patient positioning; 1 or 2 team surgical approach
10. Determine perioperative flap monitoring (implantable Doppler, near-infrared spectroscopy, pen Doppler, nursing checks)

outflow when an end-to-end anastomosis can be performed. If the donor flap possesses 2 venae comitantes, then it is always safer to perform a second venous anastomosis when feasible.

The flap pedicle should only be ligated when the recipient vessels are fully exposed, and the surgical team is ready to move forward with microsurgical transfer. This includes bringing the microscope into the room, ensuring the microsurgical instruments and sutures are open, that there is pulsatile flow of the recipient vessel, and the patient is stable and not on any vasopressors. Some surgeons choose to give a single dose of 5000 units of heparin infusion prior to harvesting the flap. The flap pedicle is ligated to provide as much length as possible. The recipient veins are prepared under the microscope and cut distally. Any back bleeding is noted and should indicate a symptom of venous insufficiency. When this occurs, thought should be given to have at least 1 outflow vein to the superficial system. The flap is next transferred near the wound edge and either sutured or stapled in order to have it remain in place during the microvascular anastomosis. The flap may be irrigated with heparin–saline solution at this point through its artery until clear effluent is noted from the venae comitantes. If there is a history of VTE in the patient or a known hypercoagulable disorder, a fixed-dose or weight-based heparin drip can now be begun in order to decrease the risk of anastomotic thrombosis.

Venous anastomosis usually occurs first. This may be accomplished using either the venous coupler technique or suture. Large studies have shown the venous coupler to be comparable to suture anastomosis and may actually afford a slightly higher patency rate (13). After a vein anastomosis is completed, attention is directed to the recipient artery. This is then prepared under the microscope, and adventitia near the anastomotic site is stripped in order to prevent arterial vasoconstriction via sympathetic fibers. The same procedure is then performed on the flap pedicle.

To prepare the vessel for end-to-side anastomosis, an Acland clamp is placed proximally and distally on the recipient pedicle. A small arteriotomy is then made. Care should be taken to never damage or touch the intima. The Acland clamp is removed, and pulsatile flow is confirmed. To prepare a vessel for end-to-end anastomosis, it needs only to have an Acland clamp placed proximally and then be cut distally using the microsurgical scissors or other sharp scissors which will provide a smooth clean edge to suture to.

An arterial anastomosis is then performed in an end-to-side or end-to-end fashion using either 8-0 or 9-0 nylon suture. Various techniques that have been described in order to facilitate arterial anastomosis using sutures include interrupted, running, or Takahashi patterns. Regardless of the technique chosen, a double-opposing Acland or bulldog clamp to approximate the ends when performing an end-to-end anastomosis will facilitate an easier operation. It is generally easier to begin by placing the first suture at the point furthest away from the surgeon and the second at the point directly opposite to that. By leaving the suture tails long, this will allow repositioning of the arteries without repeated manipulation of the vessels themselves. The posterior wall formed by the arteries can then be addressed, followed by the anterior wall. The clamps can then be removed and pulsatile flow across the anastomosis confirmed via Doppler.

At this point, the venous anastomosis should also be checked for flow, and this too may be confirmed via Doppler. If the second venae comitantes were present during the flap harvest, these can now be unclamped or cut in order to observe if there is good drainage. If possible, a second venous anastomosis should be performed.

After all anastomotic connections are complete, the flap itself should be checked for a Doppler signal, and this site should be marked with a suture. If implantable Doppler monitoring is planned to be used, it should be placed along the venous anastomosis at this point. One advantage of the implantable Doppler is that venous outflow obstruction can be auscultated in real time during the flap inset. Flap inset should occur so that it covers the desired wound bed but does not cause undue tension on the arterial pedicle or venous outflow.

Following flap inset and donor site closure, the flap should be covered in a bulky soft dressing and gently elevated. A window is created in the dressing for flap monitoring and a Bair Hugger or warming blanket is used to warm the extremity to prevent venous constriction.

DONOR FLAP ANATOMY AND HARVEST TECHNIQUE

Anterolateral Thigh Flap

The ALT flap has seen an enormous growth in popularity since its introduction by Song in 1984 (37). This popularity is due largely to the fact that it possesses many of the characteristics which make it an "ideal soft tissue flap" (37). It can be harvested quickly and reliably; has limited donor site morbidity; can be designed as a large or small flap; and can be engineered as either myocutaneous, adipofascial, or as a super-thin suprafascially harvested adipocutaneous flap (15). Inclusion of the lateral femoral cutaneous nerve potentiates sensation after transfer (15). Clinical application of the ALT flap is broad, and it has been used for reconstruction of the head and neck, trunk, upper extremity, abdomen, and lower extremity (28). In complex reconstruction, the ALT flap benefits from a large pedicle length and diameter facilitating ease of transfer.

Use of the ALT flap in lower extremity and diabetic foot reconstruction is well described (25). The flap is best suited where durable coverage is needed. One of the most untoward aspects of the ALT flap in the diabetic population is flap thickness. Although it has been touted as a thin flap option in healthy individuals, in the diabetic limb salvage population, the flap may be as thick as 4 to 6 cm. This leads to a bulky flap at time of inset, but some lipoatrophy does occur with time, and the flap may be secondarily surgically debulked. In addition, liposuction of the flap either at the time of inset or in the future has been described as safe and effective way for thinning the flap.

The vascular supply to the ALT flap is derived from perforators originating from the descending branch of the lateral circumflex femoral artery (LCFA). Although there is some variability in perforator origin, this is now well described, and the perforator can routinely be traced to a source vessel (15). Perforators are either musculocutaneous and pierce the vastus lateralis muscle or are septocutaneous and travel through the fascial interval between the vastus lateralis and rectus femoris muscles. Importantly, in approximately 1% to 3% of patients, no suitable perforators are found. In these cases, it is generally possible to find a suitable perforator on the contralateral thigh. It is thus imperative to use the Doppler probe to identify if the thigh has any suitable perforators preoperatively. Table 16.6 further lists the characteristics of the various flap options.

Surgical Technique

The patient is placed supine on the operating table. A line is drawn from the anterior superior iliac spine (ASIS) to the superolateral border of the patella. The majority of the time perforators are located within a 3 to 5 cm radius around the midpoint of this line. More proximally located perforators tend to be septocutaneous and therefore have an easier dissection; however, they sacrifice pedicle length; more distally located perforators are commonly musculocutaneous but have a longer pedicle.

Doppler ultrasound is used to discover these perforators, and the skin paddle is designed around them. The anterior incision is first made, and dissection immediately is carried down to the investing fascia of the thigh. This is incised to expose the rectus femoris and vastus lateralis muscles. The rectus femoris muscle is then retracted to expose the descending branch of the LCFA. The pedicle is then traced proximally to expose its takeoff from the LCFA. If a septocutaneous perforator is present, it should be exposed at this point. If there is no obvious septocutaneous perforator, then the skin perforator is musculocutaneous and must be carefully traced through the vastus lateralis muscle to be exposed. This is best accomplished by first finding either its proximal or distal ends and then using bipolar electrocautery to dissect through the muscle. Following the perforator dissection, the posterior incision can be made, and the flap is raised from the thigh. Proximally, the branches to the rectus femoris or vastus lateralis can be ligated if extra pedicle length is needed; when possible, it is prudent to save these branches and ligate the pedicle just distal to them.

Closure of the donor site may be accomplished primarily if it is less than 8 cm in width. Larger donor sites may require split-thickness skin grafting, however (Case Study 1).

TABLE 16.6	Characteristics of Various Free Flap Types						
Free Flap	**Vascular Pedicle**	**Components**	**Maximum Size**	**Pedicle Length**	**Pedicle Size**	**Advantages**	**Disadvantages**
Anterolateral thigh	Perforators from the descending branch of the lateral circumflex femoral artery	Fasciocutaneous Adipofascial	35 × 10 cm	8 cm	1.0–2.5 mm	Thin Durable Long pedicle	Pedicle may be variable
Vastus lateralis	Muscular branch from the descending branch of the lateral circumflex femoral artery	Muscle Myocutaneous	30 × 10 cm	8 cm	1.0–2.5 mm	Pliable Bulky Possible muscle sparing	Bulk (if not harvested as muscle sparing)
Radial forearm	Radial artery	Fasciocutaneous	35 × 15 cm	15 cm	1.5–2.5 mm	Thin Pliable Durable Reliable Very long pedicle Ease of harvest	Sacrifice radial artery Not possible if palmar arch incomplete
Latissimus dorsi	Thoracodorsal artery	Muscle Musculocutaneous	40 × 20 cm	15 cm	2.0–3.0 mm	Reliable Large area	Positioning Donor site morbidity
Gracilis	Medial circumflex femoral artery	Muscle Musculocutaneous	20 × 6 cm	6 cm	1.0–2.0 mm	Thin Pliable Easy harvest	Small Skin paddle distally unreliable Short pedicle

CASE STUDY **1**

This is a 55-year-old male with a history of diabetes mellitus controlled by insulin and peripheral arterial disease who presented with a Charcot neuroarthropathy midfoot collapse. He was scheduled for midfoot reconstruction with orthopedic surgery, but it was postponed due to concern for infection. At clinical presentation, he had a draining sinus of his medial ankle with radiographic evidence of osteomyelitis of the midfoot, hindfoot, and medial ankle. The patient underwent serial wound débridements including partial resection of his talus, calcaneus, and distal tibia (Fig. 16.1). A multiplane circular external fixator was placed in order to maintain bony stabilization. A 10 × 5 cm soft tissue defect with exposed bone was left following osseous and soft tissue resection to healthy tissue (Fig. 16.2). Thus, free tissue transfer was indicated for reconstruction of the defect. Recipient-site angiography revealed that his only distal flow was the posterior tibial artery (Fig. 16.3). A free ALT flap with planned end-to-side anastomosis to the posterior tibial artery was used to cover his defect (Figs. 16.4 to 16.7). The patient had no recurrence of wound infection and was doing well at long-term follow-up (Figs. 16.8 and 16.9). Patient was ambulatory in a custom-made shoe (Fig. 16.10).

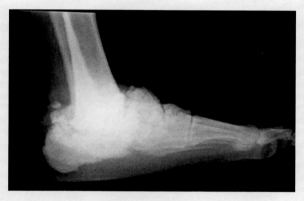

FIGURE 16.1 Preoperative ankle radiograph of a patient with an infected Charcot neuroarthropathy and severe collapse.

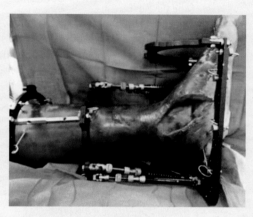

FIGURE 16.2 Following resection of the infected and nonviable osseous and soft tissue, the patient had a 10 × 5 cm defect with exposed bone.

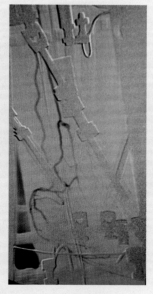

FIGURE 16.3 Recipient-site angiography revealed distal flow through the posterior tibial artery only.

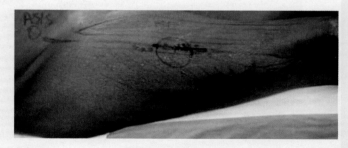

FIGURE 16.4 The anterolateral thigh flap is marked. A line is drawn from the anterior superior iliac spine to the superolateral border of the patella to mark the interval between the rectus femoris and vastus lateralis muscles. The majority of perforators can be found in a 3 cm circle located at the midpoint of this line.

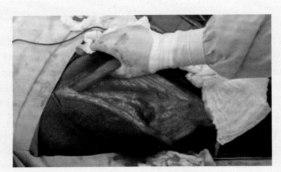

FIGURE 16.5 The anterior incision is made, and the rectus femoris muscle is retracted medially to expose the septum through which the descending branch of the lateral circumflex femoral artery passes. Perforators to the anterolateral thigh flap can be seen traveling in the septum or through the vastus lateralis muscle.

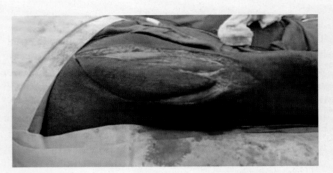

FIGURE 16.6 The posterior incision is made, and the antero-lateral thigh flap is raised based on 1 or more of its perforators.

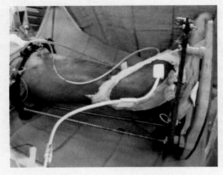

FIGURE 16.7 The flap is inset end-to-side to the posterior tibial artery. In this instance, a real-time tissue oximeter was used for flap monitoring and an external fixation device provided osseous stabilization as well as surgical off-loading of the an-terolateral thigh flap.

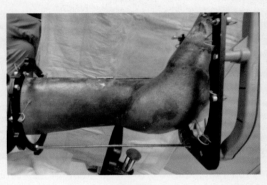

FIGURE 16.8 Short-term follow-up shows good flap contour and viability with an intact external fixation device.

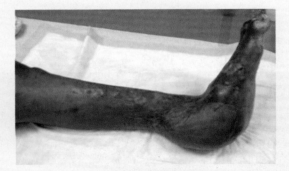

FIGURE 16.9 Long-term follow-up shows good flap contour and viability after removal of the external fixation device.

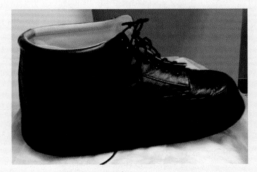

FIGURE 16.10 Example of a custom-made shoe which allowed the patient to ambulate comfortably with the anterolateral thigh flap.

Vastus Lateralis Muscle Flap

Like the ALT flap, the vastus lateralis muscle flap is based off the lateral circumflex femoral arterial system. It is a type II muscle flap; its dominant pedicle arises from a muscular branch via the descending branch of the LCFA, and minor pedicle arises from the transverse branch of the LCFA and small branches of the profunda femoris artery. Its origin is from the greater trochanter and lateral intermuscular septum, and it inserts onto the quadriceps tendon. The muscle functions as the largest of the quadriceps muscles; it is a knee stabilizer and leg extensor. Nevertheless, functional limitation following flap harvest has been reported to be minimal via dynamometric testing (14). It possesses 3 segments which each have an independent vascular supply: the superficial, intermediate, and deep segments (35).

The entire vastus lateralis muscle may be reliably harvested based solely off its muscular branches from the descending branch of the LCFA. However, it is unusual to need the entire muscle bulk. A muscle-sparing approach allows for harvest of the superficial segment of the vastus lateralis muscle while preserving the intermediate and deep segments of the muscle (35). The motor nerve to the vastus lateralis muscle from the femoral nerve can thus also be spared and its benefit as a knee stabilizer is maintained. Transfer of a vastus lateralis flap will require subsequent skin grafting over the muscle; however, the donor site can always be closed primarily when there is no cutaneous portion taken.

Surgical Technique

A line is drawn from the ASIS to the superolateral border of the patella. This delineates the septum between the vastus lateralis and rectus femoris muscles. The rectus femoris muscle is retracted medially to expose the descending branch of the LCFA. Dissection of the pedicle is then carried proximally to its origin off the LCFA proper. The muscular branch to the rectus femoris muscle is ligated if extra pedicle length is needed. At this stage, the entire vastus lateralis muscle may be safely disinserted and raised en bloc while protecting the pedicle superomedially. If less bulk is needed, the superficial segment of the vastus lateralis may be raised. This is approached by identifying the thin adipose layer between the segments distally and medially. Electrocautery is then used to carefully separate the superficial segment from the intermediate and deep segments. Careful dissection is needed here because the muscular branches may course in the deep part of the superficial segment, which is just above the plane of dissection. After the muscle has been sufficiently freed distally, it can be disoriginated from the greater trochanter and septum. The donor area is always able to close primarily when this is harvested as a muscle flap and without the cutaneous portion (Case Study 2).

CASE STUDY 2

This is a 45-year-old male with a history of diabetes mellitus and infected internal fixation hardware following a midfoot arthrodesis (Fig. 16.11). The patient was brought to the operating room for surgical débridement with hardware removal and placement of a polymethylmethacrylate antibiotic spacer (Fig. 16.12). Osseous stabilization was achieved through the application of a unilateral external fixation system (see Fig. 16.12). Following serial débridements to clean intraoperative cultures, a free vastus lateralis flap was used to cover the defect and a skin graft was placed over the muscle (Figs. 16.13 and 16.14). The flap had significant edema which resolved with compression. At long-term follow-up, the patient had excellent contour (Fig. 16.15).

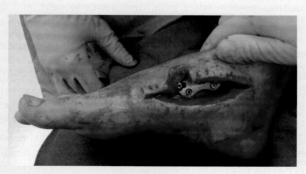

FIGURE 16.11 Clinical presentation of a diabetic patient with infected retained hardware following a midfoot arthrodesis.

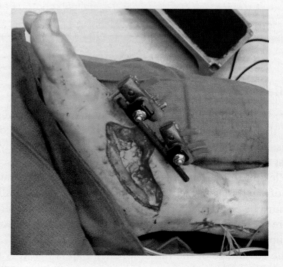

FIGURE 16.12 The hardware was removed, and a cemented antibiotic spacer with a unilateral external fixation device was used to achieve osseous stabilization.

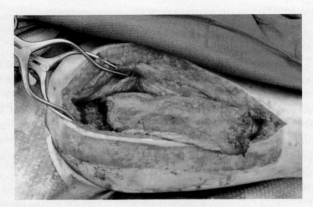

FIGURE 16.13 A vastus lateralis free flap was used to reconstruct the soft tissue defect at the medial aspect of the foot. An incision is made through a line drawn from the anterior superior iliac spine to the superolateral patella. The muscle is exposed and raised off the descending branch of the lateral circumflex femoral artery.

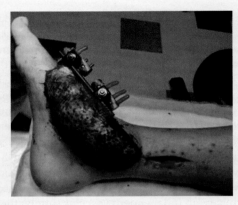

FIGURE 16.14 The vastus lateralis flap is inset with a split-thickness skin graft to cover it at the time of surgery. Note the significant edema that is present. At 6 to 12 weeks following surgery, gentle compression can be used to reduce edema and help contour the flap.

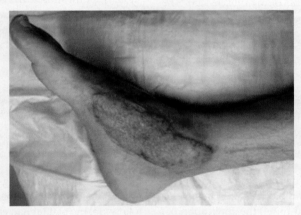

FIGURE 16.15 Long-term follow-up shows a good color match and excellent contour after removal of the external fixation device.

Radial Forearm Flap

The radial forearm flap is a thin fasciocutaneous flap harvested from the forearm with the radial artery and its venae comitantes. The radial forearm flap is a good option especially for dorsal foot wounds (32,38). It provides an excellent vascular pedicle up to 14 cm in length. The flap, if inset properly at the time of flap transfer, rarely needs tailoring. Preoperative Allen's test must be performed prior to harvesting the radial artery to ensure the hand has adequate flow via the ulnar artery through the superficial palmar arch.

The advantage of the radial forearm flap is that it is thin and pliable and can be harvested with a sensory nerve (lateral antebrachial cutaneous nerve) and the palmaris longus tendon can also be used to reconstruct missing tendons if necessary. The biggest disadvantage of the radial forearm flap is the donor site morbidity that includes need for a skin graft, scarring, postoperative pain, intolerance to cold, and difficulty healing (38).

Surgical Technique

The skin paddle of the radial forearm flap is designed on the distal volar forearm where the major perforators exist from the radial artery to the skin. A template of the size of the defect is made and placed distally along the distal volar forearm. This may be centered along the radial artery and extend onto the dorsal forearm or be volarly centered with the radial artery at the periphery. The radial artery follows a course from the antecubital fossa to the scaphoid tubercle and distally lies between the brachioradialis and flexor carpi radialis muscles. A Doppler is used to confirm and mark out the course of the radial artery because it takes off from the brachial artery. The flap can be harvested with or without the use of a tourniquet. The margins of the flap are incised down to the subcutaneous tissue and through the fascia. Flap elevation usually starts from the ulnar side of the flap where the fascia is thicker and the plane above paratenon is more obvious. It is important to preserve the paratenon on the tendons or consider harvesting in a suprafascial plane. Dissection then proceeds radially, where the radial artery and its septum can be found between the tendons of the flexor carpi radialis and brachioradialis. Dissection is continued from radial to ulnar toward the septum. A clamp is then placed on the distal radial artery and a Doppler exam is performed on the thumb to ensure that adequate ulnar flow exists.

The distal artery and venae comitantes are ligated distally, and proximal dissection takes place toward the brachial artery. The length of the pedicle dissection depends on the needs of the reconstruction; however, the dissection must stop prior to the brachial artery. The donor site can be closed primarily or skin grafted. If the tendons are exposed, acellular dermal replacement (Integra Dermal Regeneration Template, Integra LifeSciences, Plainsboro, NJ) can be used as a dermal substitute. A splint should be placed on the arm for immobilization for 2 to 3 weeks to facilitate autogenous skin graft or acellular dermal replacement take (Case Study 3).

CASE STUDY 3

This is a 59-year-old female with a history of diabetes mellitus who suffered skin necrosis of the anteromedial ankle following a total ankle arthroplasty (Figs. 16.16 and 16.17). After surgical débridement and exchange for a cemented antibiotic spacer, a radial forearm free flap was used to cover the anteromedial ankle (Fig. 16.18). The donor site was closed using a split-thickness skin graft (Fig. 16.19). The patient healed without any further complications.

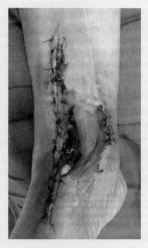

FIGURE 16.16 Clinical presentation of a diabetic patient with a failed total ankle arthroplasty. Subsequently, the patient developed skin necrosis between the 2 surgical incisions used for exposure.

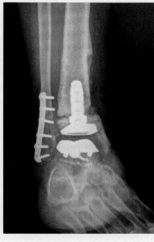

FIGURE 16.17 Preoperative ankle radiograph showing the failed total ankle implant.

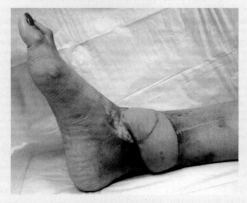

FIGURE 16.18 A radial forearm free flap was used to reconstruct the soft tissue defect.

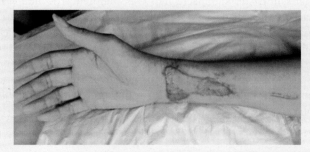

FIGURE 16.19 Clinical picture of the donor site radial forearm free flap which was closed using an autogenous split-thickness skin graft that was not meshed in order to improve cosmesis.

Latissimus Dorsi Flap

The latissimus dorsi muscle flap is one of the most commonly used donor flaps in reconstructive plastic surgery. As such, it has come to be known as a "workhorse" flap for its versatility, reliability, and ease of harvest. Since its inception, this flap has undergone rigorous study and evolution into muscle-sparing and even perforator flap variants. When not harvesting the latissimus dorsi as a muscle-sparing flap, it is important to remember that it does confer significant donor site morbidity. In the lower extremity patient, this flap muscle-sparing variant should always be used if ambulation with crutches, wheelchair, or a walker is expected because their shoulder adduction and stabilization will be significantly impaired (17).

The latissimus dorsi muscle is a type V muscle. Its dominant blood supply is via the thoracodorsal artery, and it derives minor segmental vascular inflow from branches of the intercostal and lumbar arteries. The thoracodorsal artery splits into a transverse and descending branch, either of which can be used as the basis for a muscle-sparing (or hemi-) latissimus dorsi flap. The thoracodorsal nerve follows the artery and splits into a transverse and descending branch approximately 1 to 2 cm proximal to where the artery splits. The thoracodorsal nerve can be included in a sensate or motor flap or spared during a muscle-sparing harvest (3,16).

The latissimus dorsi can be harvested as a muscle, myocutaneous, muscle-sparing, or perforator flap variant (3). The latter is commonly referred to as the thoracodorsal artery perforator flap. When harvesting a muscle-only flap, the flap will need to be skin grafted after transfer to the recipient site.

Surgical Technique

The patient is positioned laterally with the donor site upward and arm abducted. The entire arm is prepped and covered so that it can be manipulated during surgery. When harvesting the latissimus dorsi as a muscle-only flap, the dissection begins by marking along the posterior axillary line, 2 to 3 cm medial to the latissimus border. Anterior and posterior skin flaps are then raised to expose the lateral border of the muscle. Dissection then proceeds by raising the latissimus muscle off the chest wall from inferior and lateral to superior and medial. Care should be taken to identify the thoracodorsal artery as it enters the muscle's deep surface; this occurs approximately 9 cm inferior to the apex of the axilla and 2 to 3 cm medial to the lateral border of the muscle. The transverse and descending branch are preserved if harvesting the entire latissimus dorsi muscle. The pedicle is traced to its origin from the subscapular artery or simply to the circumflex scapular branch if such length is needed. Routinely, the branch to the serratus muscle is divided to obtain additional pedicle length as well. The muscle may then be disinserted from the humerus.

If performing the muscle-sparing variant, the descending branch is used as the flap pedicle, and this is traced to where it branches from the thoracodorsal artery proper. The descending branch is used in preference to the transverse branch because it supplies a large muscular area and affords an easier lateral approach (3).

The latissimus dorsi may also be harvested as a myocutaneous flap. In this case, an obliquely oriented skin paddle is marked over the latissimus dorsi muscle. The lateral border of the skin paddle is incised, and dissection then proceeds as normal to the lateral border of the latissimus muscle. Suturing the skin paddle to the muscle can avoid inadvertent avulsion and flap compromise. Although defects up to 10 cm may be closed primarily, the donor site may require skin grafting (Case Study 4).

CASE STUDY | **4**

This is a 65-year-old male with history of diabetes mellitus and radiation to his right foot for treatment of leiomyosarcoma. He presented with a full-thickness, exudative, medial ankle wound and extensive radiation damage (Fig. 16.20). In order to cover the extensive area of radiation damage, a latissimus dorsi muscle flap was planned. The flap was marked and raised with the patient in the lateral position (Figs. 16.21 and 16.22). The flap was inset, and the anastomosis was performed outside the zone of injury to the proximal posterior tibial artery and vein (Figs. 16.23 and 16.24). Skin grafting was performed over the muscle, and the patient had a good long-term outcome with acceptable contour (Figs. 16.25 and 16.26).

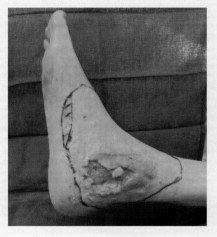

FIGURE 16.20 Clinical presentation of a diabetic patient with a history of radiation to the right foot for treatment of leiomyosarcoma who presented with an open wound and extensive radiation changes.

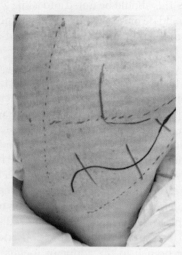

FIGURE 16.21 A latissimus dorsi free flap was used in order to provide a well-contoured coverage of the entire area of radiation damage. The scapular border is marked along with the anterior axillary fold and the borders of the latissimus dorsi. An oblique, sigmoidal incision is used to expose the muscle.

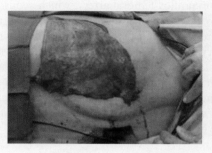

FIGURE 16.22 The patient is positioned laterally, and the latissimus dorsi flap is raised off the thoracodorsal artery and its venae comitantes.

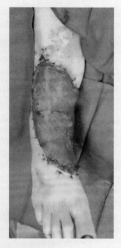

FIGURE 16.23 The latissimus dorsi flap is inset after anastomosis to the posterior tibial artery and vein.

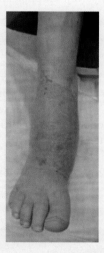

FIGURE 16.25 Clinical picture of the anterior ankle and lower extremity with a long-term follow-up of the latissimus dorsi flap shows good color match and excellent contour.

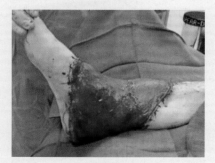

FIGURE 16.24 Note the latissimus dorsi flap's ability to contour and cover over the ankle. A split-thickness skin graft was placed over the flap.

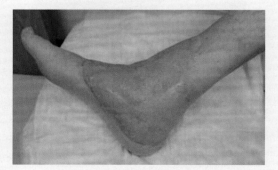

FIGURE 16.26 Clinical picture of the medial ankle and lower extremity with a long-term follow-up of the latissimus dorsi flap shows good color match and excellent contour.

Gracilis Flap

This gracilis is a flat thin muscle located superficially in the medial compartment of the thigh between the adductor longus and semimembranosus muscles. It is ideal for small wounds which require pliable flaps over an irregular surface area. The gracilis is a type II muscle deriving its dominant supply from the medial circumflex femoral artery, which sends a muscular branch to the gracilis. Minor branches supply to gracilis muscle via the obturator artery proximally, and the superficial femoral artery distally. If harvesting the gracilis for functional muscle transfer or to preserve sensation, the obturator nerve is taken with the flap. The muscle originates from the pubic symphysis and inserts onto the pes anserinus. Clinical and dynamometric studies have not revealed significant functional deficit following a gracilis flap harvest (14).

Surgical Technique

The patient is positioned either frog-leg or in stirrups so that the hips are abducted and the knees flexed. In this position, the adductor longus can be palpated in the medial thigh. It follows a trajectory roughly from the pubic tubercle to the medial tibial condyle. This should be noted and a line 2 to 3 posterior to this should be marked along the length of the thigh. The length of the marked line may now be incised down through the investing fascia of the thigh. Distally, the musculotendinous portion of the gracilis muscle is easily identified deep to the muscular fibers of the sartorius and superficial to the fascial expanse of the semimembranosus. The gracilis muscle may then be identified and traced proximally. There, the adductor longus should be retracted superiorly. The pedicle entering the gracilis muscle is reliably found between the adductor longus and gracilis muscles approximately 10 cm inferior to the pubic tubercle. At this point, the pedicle can be dissected proximally in order to free it from the surrounding tissue. Disinserting the gracilis inferiorly and ligating the minor pedicles at this time will aid dissection by allowing visualization of the superior and inferior aspects of the pedicle. If additional length is needed, the branch to the adductor longus can be ligated without risk of functional loss or necrosis. Following adequate pedicle exposure, the muscle may then be disoriginated and the pedicle ligated. As a muscle flap, it will require secondary skin grafting after transfer. The donor site is closed over drains primarily (Case Study 5).

This is a 66-year-old male with a history of diabetes mellitus and ankle arthrodesis with placement of a tibiocalcaneal intramedullary (IM) nail which subsequently became infected and developed osteomyelitis. Following serial surgical débridements, removal of the IM nail, and placement of a cemented antibiotic spacer, a 12 × 5 cm medial ankle wound was present (Fig. 16.27). Recipient vessel angiography revealed a widely patent peroneal and posterior tibial artery (Fig. 16.28). A gracilis muscle free flap with a split-thickness skin graft was used to cover the osseous and soft tissue defect (Figs. 16.29 to 16.31). Long-term results were good with excellent contour. Note the edema resolution over time of the muscle flap with appropriate compression (Fig. 16.32).

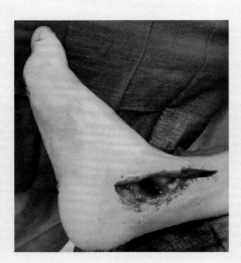

FIGURE 16.27 Clinical presentation of a diabetic patient with a history of an infected ankle fusion with a tibiocalcaneal intramedullary nail. A 12 × 5 cm medial ankle wound was present following hardware removal and serial surgical débridements.

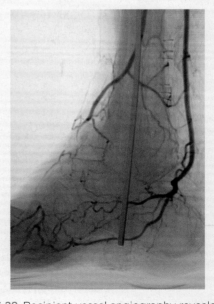

FIGURE 16.28 Recipient vessel angiography revealed a widely patent peroneal and posterior tibial artery.

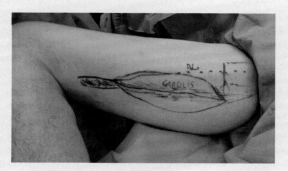

FIGURE 16.29 A gracilis muscle free flap was planned. The adductor longus muscle is marked, and the gracilis muscle is located below this. The pedicle is a muscular branch from the medial circumflex femoral artery.

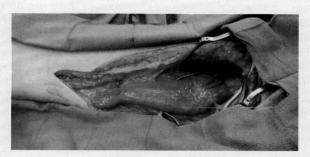

FIGURE 16.30 Intraoperative picture showing the harvesting of the gracilis muscle free flap.

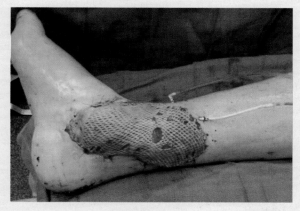

FIGURE 16.31 The gracilis muscle is raised and inset into the defect after anastomosis end-to-side to the posterior tibial artery. A meshed, autogenous split-thickness skin graft is used to cover the harvested gracilis muscle.

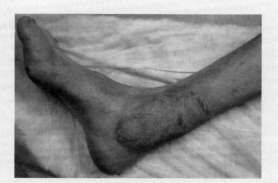

FIGURE 16.32 Clinical picture of the medial ankle and lower extremity with a long-term result of the gracilis muscle free flap shows good color match and excellent contour.

POSTOPERATIVE CARE

Postoperatively, the patient is transferred to the intensive care unit or a floor with nursing capable of performing frequent flap checks. The flap is generally checked at least once every hour for the first postoperative day, and the patient is kept on withhold from food or fluids by mouth should a complication arise, and need to return to the operating room. At our institution, flaps are checked once every 15 minutes for the first 4 hours, then every half hour for the next 4 hours, and every hour thereafter. If an implantable Doppler was placed during surgery, this should be checked immediately upon transfer and listened to with nursing. Similarly, a flap check to assess for color, turgor, and Doppler signals should be performed by the surgeon in conjunction with nursing with explicit instructions for when to call.

Aspirin is routinely given postoperatively and continued at least while the patient is admitted to the hospital. If a heparin drip has been ordered, then this should be appropriately titrated with a plan for when to discontinue it. In cases for which the patient has a known thromboembolic disorder, the hematologist may wish to continue an oral anticoagulant postoperatively as well (5). The flap should be protected with a bulky dressing, and dressing changes should only be performed by the team because simple dressing changes may lead to inadvertent flap compromise and tissue loss.

COMPLICATIONS AND REVISIONAL SURGERY

The most common complication of microsurgical tissue transfer is partial flap necrosis. In a muscle flap, this may manifest as areas of muscle (usually distally) with microvascular thrombosis and eventual sloughing. In perforator flaps, this generally manifests as fat necrosis or distal tip loss. In either event, the solution is to return to the operating room after the ischemic area has confirmed itself. The wound should be resected to healthy tissue, and the flap may then be advanced to close the defect.

The most serious complications of microsurgical tissue transfer are arterial or venous thrombosis. These are most likely to occur within the first 24 hours postoperatively. Arterial thrombosis presents as a cool, pale, and soft flap. When this is detected, it represents a surgical emergency, and the patient should immediately be made ready to go to the operating room for reexploration. Most commonly, a thrombosis at the anastomotic segment is detected. This is commonly resolved by flushing the flap with heparin–saline solution to ensure there is still flow and microvascular thrombosis has not occurred, followed by resecting the pedicle to healthy margins. The pedicle is now checked for pulsatile flow once again, and the anastomosis is performed. Generally, if this results in success, then a heparin drip is started and maintained while the patient is on the hospital unit. Consideration should also be given to performing a hypercoagulable workup and consulting with a hematologist.

In contrast, venous thrombosis presents as a cool, blue or mottled, tense flap. Rapid capillary refill or bleeding to pinprick can be observed. As with arterial thrombosis, this represents a surgical emergency, and the patient should be returned to the operating room for reexploration. The venous anastomosis should be resected and arterial flow allowed to progress while the distal vein is checked for appropriate bleeding. If there is good flow through the flap, then one can safely proceed with a revision venous anastomosis. Again, a heparin drip should be started and consideration given to a hypercoagulable workup.

Excessive tissue bulk leads to aesthetic and functional limitations of the microsurgical reconstruction. This can be addressed generally 3 to 6 months postoperatively. Myocutaneous or perforator flaps with a significant adipose component can safely undergo liposuction in order to contour the flap and minimize bulk. It is important to warn the patient that he or she may require further revisional operations with this technique. Alternatively, direct surgical lipectomy or flap re-inset can be safely performed. This can help contour the flap and improve aesthetics but more importantly to debulk the flap and allow for functional shoe gear.

Conclusion

Microsurgical free tissue transfer represents an important and powerful tool in the surgical armamentarium. As with any surgery, creating a thorough surgical plan, understanding how to manage complications and patient expectations remain the most important tools for performing a reconstruction that is satisfying to both patient and surgeon.

References

1. Blondeel PN, Van Landuyt KH, Monstrey SJ, et al. The "Gent" consensus on perforator flap terminology: preliminary definitions. Plast Reconstr Surg 2003;112:1378–1383.
2. Boulton AJ. What you can't feel can hurt you. J Vasc Surg 2010; 52(3 suppl):28–30.
3. Colohan S, Wong C, Lakhiani C, et al. The free descending branch muscle-sparing latissimus dorsi flap: vascular anatomy and clinical applications. Plast Reconstr Surg 2012;130:776e–787e.
4. DeFazio MV, Han KD, Akbari CM, et al. Free tissue transfer after targeted endovascular reperfusion for complex lower extremity reconstruction: setting the stage for success in the presence of mutlivessel disease. Ann Vasc Surg 2015;29:1316.e7–1316.e15.
5. DeFazio MV, Hung RW, Han KD, et al. Lower extremity flap salvage in thrombophilic patients: managing expectations in the setting of microvascular thrombosis. J Reconstr Microsurg 2016;32:431–444.
6. Ducic I, Rao SS, Attinger CE. Outcomes of microvascular reconstruction of single-vessel lower extremities: limb salvage versus amputation. J Reconstr Microsurg 2009;25:475–478.
7. Economides JM, Patel KM, Evans KK, et al. Systematic review of patient-centered outcomes following lower extremity flap reconstruction in comorbid patients. J Reconstr Microsurg 2013;29: 307–316.
8. Endara M, Masden D, Goldstein J, et al. The role of chronic and perioperative glucose management in high-risk surgical closures: a case for tighter glycemic control. Plast Reconstr Surg 2013;132:996–1004.
9. Evans KK, Attinger CE, Al-Attar A, et al. The importance of limb preservation in the diabetic population. J Diabetes Complications 2011;25:227–231.
10. Gupta SK, Veith FJ, Ascer E, et al. Cost factors in limb-threatening ischaemia due to infrainguinal arteriosclerosis. Eur J Vasc Surg 1988;2:151–154.
11. Hollenbeck ST, Woo S, Komatsu I, et al. Longitudinal outcomes and application of the subunit principle to 165 foot and ankle free tissue transfers. Plast Reconstr Surg 2010;125:924–934.
12. Kucan JO, Robson MC. Diabetic foot infections: fate of the contralateral foot. Plast Reconstr Surg 1986;77:439–441.
13. Kulkarni AR, Mehrara BJ, Pusic AL, et al. Venous thrombosis in handsewn versus coupled venous anastomoses in 857 consecutive breast free flaps. J Reconstr Microsurg 2016;32:178–182.
14. Lakhiani C, DeFazio MV, Han K, et al. Donor-site morbidity following free tissue harvest from the thigh: a systematic review and pooled analysis of complications. J Reconstr Microsurg 2016;32: 342–357.
15. Lakhiani C, Lee MR, Saint-Cyr M. Vascular anatomy of the anterolateral thigh flap: a systematic review. Plast Reconstr Surg 2012;130:1254–1268.
16. Lee KT, Kim A, Mun GH. Comprehensive analysis of donor-site morbidity following free thoracodorsal artery perforator flap harvest. Plast Reconstr Surg 2016;138:899–909.
17. Lee KT, Mun GH. A systematic review of functional donor-site morbidity after latissimus dorsi muscle transfer. Plast Reconstr Surg 2014;134:303–314.
18. Lin CW, Hsu BR, Tsai JS, et al. Effect of limb preservation status and body mass index on the survival of patients with limb-threatening diabetic foot ulcers. J Diabetes Complications 2017;31:180–185.
19. Mackey WC, McCullough JL, Conlon TP, et al. The costs of surgery for limb-threatening ischemia. Surgery 1986;99:26–35.
20. Mathes SJ, Feng LJ, Hunt TK. Coverage of the infected wound. Ann Surg 1983;198:420–429.
21. Mathes SJ, Nahai F. Classification of the vascular anatomy of muscles: experimental and clinical correlation. Plast Reconstr Surg 1981;67:177–187.
22. Moran SL, Illig KA, Green RM, et al. Free-tissue transfer in patients with peripheral vascular disease: a 10-year experience. Plast Reconstr Surg 2002;109:999–1006.

23. Moucharafieh RS, Saghieh S, Macari G, et al. Diabetic foot salvage with microsurgical free-tissue transfer. Microsurgery 2003;23: 257–261.

24. Nahabedian MY, Momen B, Galdino G, et al. Breast reconstruction with the free TRAM or DIEP flap: patient selection, choice of flap, and outcome. Plast Reconstr Surg 2002;110:466–475.

25. Oh TS, Lee HS, Hong JP. Diabetic foot reconstruction using free flaps increases 5-year-survival rate. J Plast Reconstr Aesthet Surg 2013;66:243–250.

26. Rayman G, Vas PR, Baker N, et al. The Ipswich Touch Test: a simple and novel method to identify inpatients with diabetes at risk of foot ulceration. Diabetes Care 2011;34:1517–1518.

27. Rodeheaver GT. Wound cleansing, wound irrigation, wound disinfection. In: Krasner D, Kane D, eds. Chronic wound care: a clinical source book for healthcare professionals. 2nd ed. Wayne, PA: Health Management, 1997:97–108.

28. Rozen WM, Ashton M-W, Pan WR, et al. Anatomical variations in the harvest of anterolateral thigh flap perforators: a cadaveric and clinical study. Microsurgery 2009;29:16–23.

29. Salgado CJ, Mardini S, Jamali AA, et al. Muscle versus nonmuscle flaps in the reconstruction of chronic osteomyelitis defects. Plast Reconstr Surg 2006;118:1401–1411.

30. Schofield CJ, Libby G, Brennan GM, et al. Mortality and hospitalization in patients after amputation: a comparison between patients with and without diabetes. Diabetes Care 2006;29:2252–2256.

31. Serletti JM, Deuber MA, Guidera PM, et al. Atherosclerosis of the lower extremity and free-tissue reconstruction for limb salvage. Plast Reconstr Surg 1995;96:1136–1144.

32. Soutar DS, McGregor IA. The radial forearm flap in intraoral reconstruction: the experience of 60 consecutive cases. Plast Reconstr Surg 1986;78:1–8.

33. Taylor GI, Palmer JH. The vascular territories (angiosomes) of the body: experimental study and clinical applications. Br J Plast Surg 1987;40:113–141.

34. Thorud JC, Plemmons B, Buckley CJ, et al. Mortality after non-traumatic major amputation among patients with diabetes and peripheral vascular disease: a systematic review. J Foot Ankle Surg 2016;55:591–599.

35. Toia F, D'Arpa S, Brenner E, et al. Segmental anatomy of the vastus lateralis: guidelines for muscle-sparing flap harvest. Plast Reconstr Surg 2015;135:185e–198e.

36. Toursarkissian B, Shireman PK, Harrison A, et al. Major lower-extremity amputation: contemporary experience in a single Veterans Affairs institution. Am Surg 2002;68:606–610.

37. Wei F, Jain V, Celik N, et al. Have we found an ideal soft-tissue flap? An experience with 672 anterolateral thigh flaps. Plast Reconstr Surg 2002;109:2219–2226.

38. Weinzweig N, Davies BW. Foot and ankle reconstruction using the radial forearm flap: a review of 25 cases. Plast Reconstr Surg 1998;102:1999–2005.

CHAPTER 17

Stepwise Surgical Approach to Acute Diabetic Charcot Foot and Ankle Neuroarthropathy

Bradley M. Lamm • Kyle R. Moore

INTRODUCTION

Charcot neuroarthropathy (CN) of the foot and/or ankle causes bone loss and joint subluxation/dislocation, which produces abnormal osseous prominences that are areas for potential ulceration. The resultant deformed pedal position alters the lower extremity muscle–tendon balance and weight bearing forces which increases the risk for ulceration. When ulcerations are present, osteomyelitis can develop; thus, the best treatment results are achieved when treatment is initiated early (5,16). Treatment of CN often is based on the stage at which the deformity presents. The Eichenholtz system is the most commonly used classification system that divides CN into 3 stages (developmental, coalescent, and reconstructive) (4).

The duration of acute CN is highly variable. Currently, there is no consensus on the average time from the acute CN onset to cessation, which can range from weeks to months. In a prospective magnetic resonance imaging (MRI) study of 40 diabetic patients with acute CN of the foot by Zampa et al. (18), the authors reported a mean time of 6.8 ± 2.3 months until clinical healing was noted. They reported that MRI findings such as bone marrow edema and fractures resolved at a mean time of 8.3 ± 2.9 months after off-loading treatment was initiated (18).

Normalizing skin temperature, swelling, and erythema remain the traditional clinical features of the resolving acute CN process. Skin temperature measurements between the involved and uninvolved foot is an effective and objective clinical tool. Skin temperature has been shown to correlate with the radiographic stages in CN, and it is conventional to use a 2°C or less difference between feet to indicate acute CN resolution (11). Gradual cooling of 2.1°C per 100 days has been reported in patients receiving off-loading treatment for acute CN (8). Recently, investigators have begun to develop a greater understanding of the role inflammatory markers contribute in monitoring the acute CN process. Previous studies have shown that common inflammatory markers including C-reactive protein,

white blood cell count, and erythrocyte sedimentation rate are frequently normal during the acute CN process (11,12). By assessing numerous markers for inflammation and bone turnover including interleukin-6 (IL-6), C-reactive protein, serum C-terminal telopeptide, tumor necrosis factor-alpha (TNF-α), and alkaline phosphatase, Petrova and colleagues (10) demonstrated that IL-6 and TNF-α are significantly elevated in patients with acute CN. Also, IL-6 and TNF-α decreased significantly after 3 months of off-loading therapy, but this was not the case for C-reactive protein, serum C-terminal telopeptide, or alkaline phosphatase. They concluded that IL-6 and TNF-α could be useful to monitor disease activity and could potentially be obtained in clinical practice (10).

In CN deformities of the foot and/or ankle, the ulcer location is a significant indicator of the overall prognosis and treatment plan. Plantar ulcerations correlate to the anatomic location of the CN and are associated with the degree of stability of the foot. Ulcerations along the medial column of the foot are generally associated with a Lisfranc fracture and/or dislocation and medial column collapse. CN deformities at the Lisfranc joint are typically stable due to the interlocking anatomy and are successfully treated conservatively or with a limited surgical approach (1,15). However, CN ulcerations that are located plantar central or plantar lateral are associated with a midfoot/hindfoot collapse and are typically unstable. Instability of the lateral column of the foot leads to recurrent ulcerations, whereby complex surgical reconstruction often becomes necessary (2,9). Similarly, CN deformities at the ankle level can present with ulcerations at the lateral or medial malleolus with a significant varus or valgus fracture and/or dislocation, respectively.

The goal of treatment for acute CN deformities of the foot and/or ankle (i.e., Eichenholtz stage 1) is to stabilize the osseous anatomy in order to avoid bone loss and joint subluxation/dislocation (6,14). Total contact casting for immobilization is one of the traditional treatment options in the initial stages of acute CN. Total contact casting or cast immobilization has been the treatment of choice to allow the acute CN process to stabilize and convert to stage 2. However, total contact casting has disadvantages due to the patient's inability to bear weight while in the cast, which produces osteopenia of the ipsilateral foot and an increase in the weight bearing forces on the contralateral foot. Disuse osteopenia and prolonged immobilization makes it difficult for sequent surgical reconstruction and further non–weight-bearing status throughout the postoperative period. In addition, overloading of the contralateral foot can result in ulceration and/or contralateral CN event. Maintaining continuous non–weight-bearing status is not easy for the diabetic patient with peripheral neuropathy for multiple reasons (e.g., muscle atrophy, diminished proprioception, and obesity), and therefore, early surgical intervention might be necessary in certain clinical scenarios with an acute CN of the foot and/or ankle.

Recently, a surgical technique was described for treating acute CN deformities of the foot and/or ankle by applying a static external fixation device, which acts like a cast by stabilizing the affected joints and bones (17). The advantage of the static external fixation is that it allows partial weight bearing when necessary by limiting osteopenia and maintaining the existing foot position. Applying a static external fixation device in the acute CN deformities of the foot and/or ankle is performed by avoiding the affected CN region. External fixation pins and/or transosseous wires are placed adjacent but not into the CN joint(s) and region. Additionally, olive wires and threaded rods or struts are strategically placed to afford dynamic gradual correction once the acute CN has subsided. After gradual realignment of the osseous segments is established, a second-stage reconstructive surgery with joint arthrodesis is performed to maintain the foot position. The external fixation device is maintained for at least 3 months thereafter. A third surgery is required for removal of the external fixation device. The ability to early detect a patient in the acute stage of CN is not common as most diabetic patients with CN typically present with an ulceration and foot collapse (Fig. 17.1).

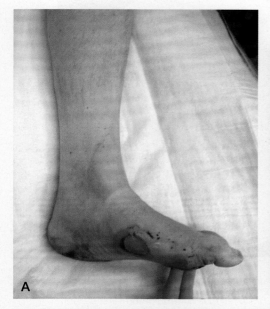
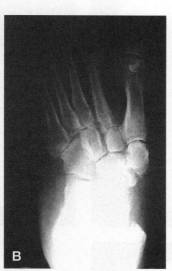
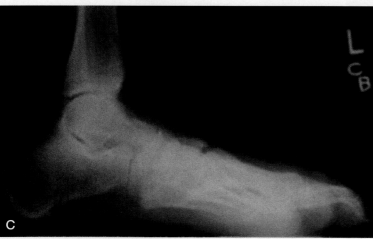

FIGURE 17.1 **A.** Clinical presentation of a Charcot neuroarthropathy (CN) midfoot deformity of a 60-year-old male who initially presented with a red, hot, and swollen left foot without an ulceration. The patient was placed in a non–weight-bearing cast for 2 weeks and developed a superficial ulcer at the medial aspect of the foot just prior to surgery. **B.** An anteroposterior radiographic view of the foot shows a shortened first ray with a collapsed navicular medially. **C.** A lateral radiographic view of the foot shows an elevated and shorted first ray with a break in the Meary's (lateral talo-first metatarsal) angle. *(continued)*

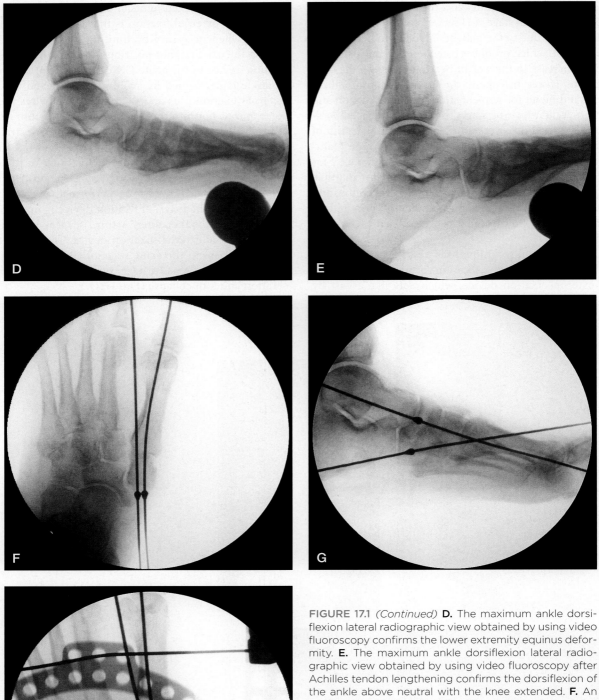

FIGURE 17.1 *(Continued)* **D.** The maximum ankle dorsiflexion lateral radiographic view obtained by using video fluoroscopy confirms the lower extremity equinus deformity. **E.** The maximum ankle dorsiflexion lateral radiographic view obtained by using video fluoroscopy after Achilles tendon lengthening confirms the dorsiflexion of the ankle above neutral with the knee extended. **F.** An anteroposterior radiographic view obtained by using video fluoroscopy shows insertion of the olive wires from proximal to distal capturing the medial cuneiform. **G.** A lateral radiographic view obtained by using video fluoroscopy shows insertion of the olive wires from proximal to distal capturing the medial cuneiform in 2 different directions. This allows the olive wires to have separate vectors of pull, thus increasing the strength and decreasing the risk of pullout. **H.** An anteroposterior radiographic view obtained by using video fluoroscopy shows a trail distraction of the medial cuneiform; note the 5 mm gap. The transverse metatarsal wire captures only the lesser metatarsals. *(continued)*

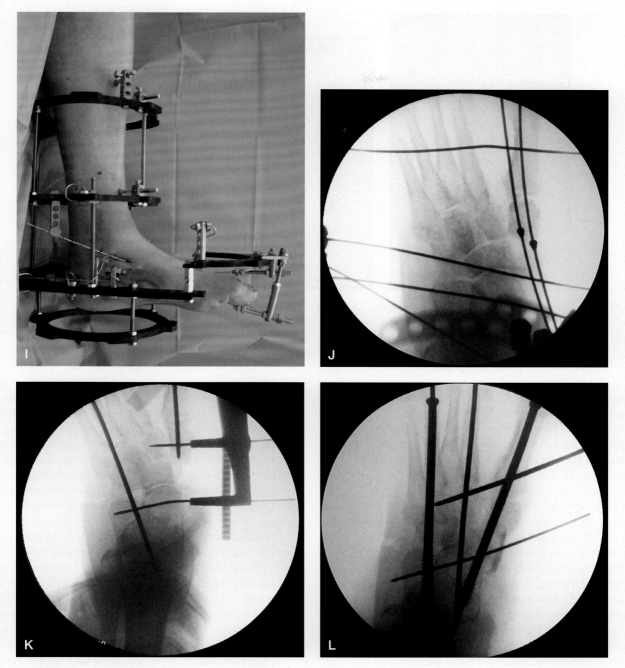

FIGURE 17.1 *(Continued)* **I.** A clinical picture of the stable external fixation device is shown. Note the 2 slotted threaded rods that hold the 2 olive wires at the tip of the great toe which are set up for distraction. **J.** An anteroposterior radiographic view obtained by using video fluoroscopy shows a distraction of the medial cuneiform adjacent to the intermediate cuneiform; note the 1.5 cm distraction gap. **K.** An anteroposterior radiographic view obtained by using video fluoroscopy shows a Hintermann distractor maintaining the distraction gap for placement of the bone graft. Note the guidewire placed in the medullary canal of the first metatarsal. **L.** An anteroposterior radiographic view obtained by using video fluoroscopy shows a fresh frozen fibula allograft with fixation in position. *(continued)*

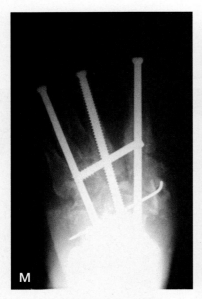
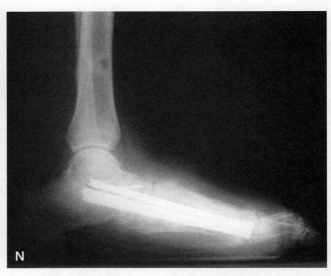

FIGURE 17.1 *(Continued)* **M.** A weight bearing anteroposterior radiographic view postdistraction and arthrodesis of the CN medial column of the foot shows a stable lengthened medial column, intact intramedullary metatarsal screws, and healed ulceration. **N.** A weight bearing lateral radiographic view postdistraction and arthrodesis of the CN medial column of the foot shows a normal or zero Meary's (lateral talo-first metatarsal) angle.

The chronic CN deformities of the foot and/or ankle (i.e., Eichenholtz stage 2 or 3) can be stable or unstable. The unstable chronic CN foot and/or ankle is difficult to shoe or brace and typically results in ulceration. The stable chronic CN foot and/or ankle is easier to shoe or brace and can be treated without surgery while it is still prone to ulceration. The goal of surgical treatment in cases of chronic CN is to establish a stable plantigrade foot. Achilles tendon lengthening, gastrocnemius recession, exostectomy, osteotomy, arthrodesis, and open reduction with internal fixation are well-known surgical reconstructive procedures aimed to re-establish the normal foot position. Acute deformity correction via open reduction with rigid internal fixation or plantar plating is frequently used for chronic CN reconstruction (13). Similarly, acute correction via open reduction with application of static external fixation (3,17) and minimally invasive techniques of gradual distraction with external fixation that provides both realignment and stabilization have also been reported in the literature (7).

MINIMALLY INVASIVE GRADUAL DIABETIC CHARCOT NEUROARTHROPATHY FOOT RECONSTRUCTION

The goals of surgical intervention for the acute and/or chronic CN of the foot and/or ankle are to restore alignment and stability, prevent amputation, and allow the patient to be ambulatory in custom-made diabetic shoes and/or bracing. Historically, open reduction with internal fixation was the mainstay for treatment of CN foot and/or ankle deformities.

Large open incisions were made to remove the excess bone, reduce the fragmented or dislocated bone, and fix the deformity with screw(s), intramedullary nailing, or plantar plating in an attempt to stabilize the CN joint. These invasive surgical procedures generally resulted in a nonanatomic correction (e.g., shortening of the foot or incomplete deformity correction) and occasionally resulted in neurovascular compromise, incision healing problems, infection, and the use of non–weight-bearing casts or boots.

Gradual deformity correction with external fixation is preferred for significant CN foot deformity reductions. Correction with external fixation is minimally invasive, allows for gradual, accurate anatomic realignment of the dislocated/subluxated CN joints without loss of foot length or bone mass, provides support for partial weight bearing if necessary, and limits neurovascular compromise as the correction occurs slowly during a certain period of time.

A stable or coalesced CN foot deformity requires an osteotomy for correction of the deformity. For an unstable or an incompletely coalesced CN foot, correction can be obtained through gradual distraction. Despite the radiographic appearance of coalescence, the majority of CN foot deformities can be distracted through the joints to realign the pedal anatomy without osteotomy. During the first stage, osseous realignment is achieved with a Taylor spatial frame (TSF) (Smith & Nephew, Inc., Memphis, TN) using the principle of ligamentotaxis. After realignment, the correction is maintained by joint arthrodesis (second stage) using percutaneously inserted intramedullary metatarsal screws. This minimally invasive 2-stage correction is a relatively new technique that has been shown to have excellent short-term follow-up results (7).

Surgical Technique

The first stage consists of osseous realignment achieved by performing ligamentotaxis. The TSF forefoot 6 × 6 butt frame construct is applied and provides gradual relocation of the forefoot on the hindfoot. The distal tibia, talus, and calcaneus are fixed with 2 U-plates joined and first mounted orthogonal to the tibia in both the anteroposterior and lateral planes. The U-plate is affixed to the tibia with one lateromedial 1.8 mm wire and 2 to 3 other points of fixation (combination of smooth transosseous wires or half-pins). For additional stability, a second distal tibial ring can be added to create a distal tibial fixation block. It is essential to fix the hindfoot in a neutral position; an Achilles tendon lengthening or gastrocnemius recession typically is required to achieve a neutral hindfoot position. With the hindfoot manually held in a neutral position, the U-plate is fixed to the calcaneus with 2 crossing 1.8 mm wires. A 1.8 mm medial-lateral talar neck wire also is inserted and fixed to the U-plate. Next, 2 1.8 mm stirrup wires are inserted through the osseous segment just proximal and distal to the CN joint(s). Stirrup wires are bent 90 degrees just outside the skin to extend and attach but are not tensioned to their respective external fixation rings distant from the point of fixation. These stirrup wires capture osseous segments that are far from an external fixation ring, thereby providing accurate and precise CN joint distraction. A full external fixation ring is then mounted to the forefoot with 2 1.8 mm crossing metatarsal wires and the aforementioned distal stirrup wire. Toe(s) pinning often is required whereby the toe(s) wires (1.5 or 1.8 mm) are attached to the forefoot ring. Smooth wires in the foot are preferred in the diabetic neuropathic population. Finally, the 6 TSF struts are placed, and final radiographs are obtained (anteroposterior and lateral views of the foot to include the tibia).

Orthogonal anteroposterior and lateral view fluoroscopic images are obtained of the reference ring; the images provide the mounting parameters that are needed for the computer planning. The choice of which ring (distal or proximal) to use as the reference ring is the surgeon's preference (typically, a distal reference is chosen for foot deformity correction). Superimposition of the reference ring on the final films is critical for accurate postoperative computer deformity planning (http://www.spatialframe.com). It is important to fully understand the TSF planning before attempting this procedure. In synopsis, the surgeon enters the deformity and mounting parameters into an Internet-based software program that produces a daily schedule for the patient to perform adjustments on each of the 6 TSF struts. The rate and duration of the patient's schedule is controlled by the surgeon's data entry. The patient is clinically and radiographically followed in a clinical setting weekly or biweekly.

Fixation construction is creative because of the small pedal anatomy, which renders it difficult to apply external fixation. When applying the forefoot 6 × 6 butt frame, it is important to mount the U-plate on the hindfoot and

the full ring on the forefoot as posterior and anterior as possible, respectively. The greatest distance between the forefoot and hindfoot ring is critical to accommodate the TSF struts. Bone segment fixation is important; otherwise, failure of osteotomy separation or incomplete anatomic reduction occurs. Small wire fixation is preferred in the foot because of the size and consistency of the bones. When treating a patient with CN, building extremely stable constructs is exceptionally important. CN deformity correction with external fixation should include a distal tibial ring with a closed foot ring.

After gradual distraction with the TSF has realigned the anatomy of the foot, the second stage of correction is performed. Gradual distraction for realignment of the dislocated CN joint(s) is obtained in approximately 1 to 2 months. In the second stage, the external fixation device is removed while simultaneously minimally invasive arthrodesis of the affected joints with percutaneous insertion of internal fixation is performed. Before the external fixation device is removed, small transverse incisions (2 to 3 cm in length) overlying the appropriate joint(s) are made to perform cartilage removal and joint(s) preparation for arthrodesis. Minimally invasive arthrodesis is easily preformed because the CN joint(s) are already distracted. Under fluoroscopic guidance, the guidewires for the large-diameter cannulated screws are inserted percutaneously through the plantar skin incision into the metatarsal heads by dorsiflexing the hallux. After the lateral and medial column guidewires are inserted to maintain the corrected foot position, the TSF is removed and the foot is re-prepped in a sterile fashion. Typically, 3 large-diameter cannulated intramedullary metatarsal screws are inserted; medial and lateral column partial threaded screws for compression of the arthrodesis site(s) and one central fully threaded screw for additional stabilization. These intramedullary screws span the entire length of the metatarsals to the calcaneus and talus, provide compression across the minimally invasive arthrodesis site, and stabilize adjacent joints. The intramedullary metatarsal screws cross an unaffected joint, the Lisfranc joint, thereby protecting the Lisfranc joint from experiencing a future CN event. The minimally invasive incisions are then closed, and a well-padded U and L lower extremity splint is applied. Before hospital discharge (length of hospital stay ranges from 1 to 4 days), the patient's operative splint and dressings are removed and a short leg cast is applied. A non–weight-bearing short leg cast is maintained for 2 to 3 months and then gradual progression to weight bearing is achieved. Therefore, the entire treatment is completed in 4 to 5 months with good to excellent success (18). Short-term results are promising considering that neither recurrent ulceration nor deep infections have occurred in previous reports (7). The advantages of this minimally invasive surgical approach to acute CN deformities are preservation of foot length and restoration of the soft tissue and osseous anatomy (Fig. 17.2).

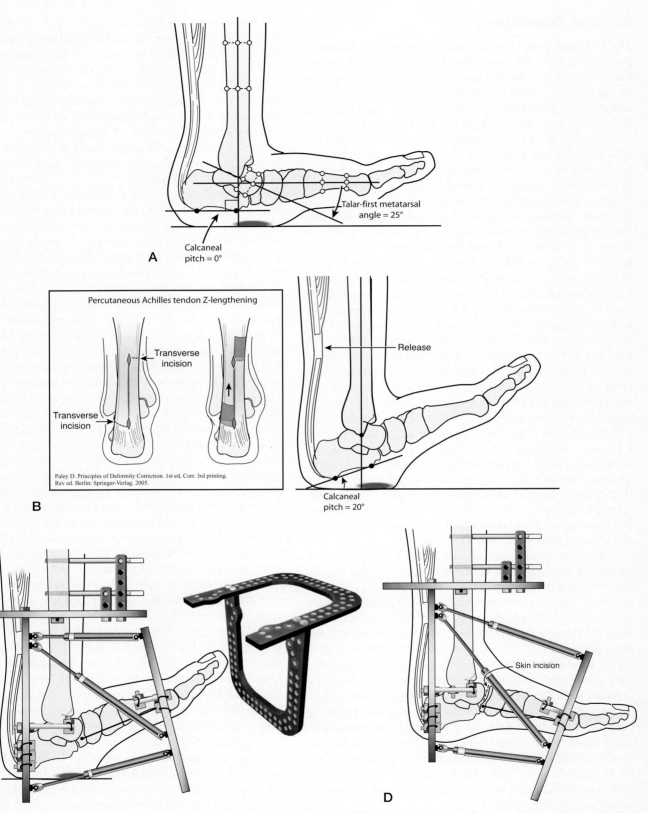

FIGURE 17.2 Schematic illustration of a Charcot neuroarthropathy of the midfoot with equinus deformity (Eichenholtz stage 2 or 3, with ulceration). **A.** Lateral view shows equinus (calcaneal pitch, 0 degree) and rocker bottom deformity (talar-first metatarsal angle, 25 degrees). **B.** Percutaneous Achilles tendon Z-lengthening is performed to acutely correct the equinus deformity. (*Inset* modified with permission from Springer-Verlag [9]) **C.** The hindfoot and ankle are then fixed in the corrected position with the Taylor spatial frame (TSF) (forefoot 6 × 6 butt). Note the initial forefoot position **D.** Gradual distraction (5 to 15 mm) and realignment of the forefoot to the hindfoot are performed with the TSF. Just before the TSF removal, a minimally invasive arthrodesis of the midtarsal joint(s) is performed. *(continued)*

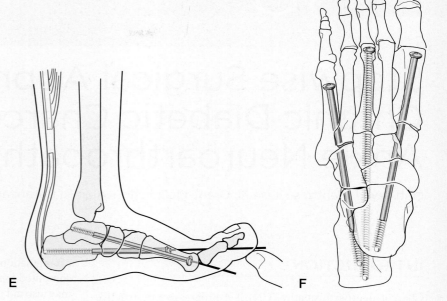

FIGURE 17.2 *(Continued)* **E.** After inserting the percutaneous guidewires for the large-diameter cannulated screws, the TSF is removed. Partially threaded intramedullary metatarsal cannulated screws are inserted beneath the metatarsal heads percutaneously to compress both the medial and lateral columns of the foot. **F.** Anteroposterior view shows a third fully threaded screw inserted to increase midfoot stability. (Illustrations A, C, D, E, and F are used with permission from Sinai Hospital of Baltimore, MD [Rubin Institute for Advanced Orthopedics].)

Conclusion

Identifying the stage and location of the CN foot and/or ankle allows the surgeon to choose the appropriate treatment plan. Many surgical and nonsurgical options exist with the aim of improving the patient's quality of life and preventing amputation. It is critical for the surgeon to choose the best option for the patient from the aforementioned list of treatments.

Acknowledgments

The authors would like to thank Alvien Lee for his excellent photography and Joy Marlowe, MA, for her superb illustrations.

References

1. Brodsky JW, Rouse AM. Exostectomy for symptomatic bony prominences in diabetic Charcot feet. Clin Orthop Relat Res 1993;296:21–26.

2. Catanzariti AR, Mendicino R, Haverstock B. Ostectomy for diabetic neuroarthropathy involving the midfoot. J Foot Ankle Surg 2000;39:291–300.

3. Cooper PS. Application of external fixators for management of Charcot deformities of the foot and ankle. Foot Ankle Clin 2002;7:207–254.

4. Eichenholtz SN. Charcot joints. Springfield, IL: Charles C. Thomas, 1966.

5. Frykberg RG, ed. The high risk foot in diabetes mellitus. New York: Churchill Livingstone, 1991.

6. Jolly GP, Zgonis T, Polyzois V. External fixation in the management of Charcot neuroarthropathy. Clin Podiatr Med Surg 2003;20:741–756.

7. Lamm BM, Paley D. Charcot neuroarthropathy of the foot and ankle. In: Rozbruch RS, Ilizarov S, eds. Limb lengthening and reconstruction surgery. New York: Informa Healthcare, 2006:221–231.

8. McCrory JL, Morag E, Norkitis AJ, et al. Healing of Charcot fractures: skin temperature and radiographic correlates. The Foot 1998;8:158–165.

9. Paley D. Principles of deformity correction. Rev ed. Berlin, Germany: Springer-Verlag, 2005.

10. Petrova NL, Dew TK, Musto RL, et al. Inflammatory and bone turnover markers in a cross-sectional and prospective study of acute Charcot osteoarthropathy. Diabet Med 2015;32:267–273.

11. Petrova NL, Edmonds ME. Acute Charcot neuro-osteoarthropathy. Diabetes Metab Res Rev 2016;32(suppl 1):281–286.

12. Petrova NL, Moniz C, Elias DA, et al. Is there a systemic inflammatory response in the acute Charcot foot? Diabetes Care 2007;30:997–998.

13. Schon LC, Easley ME, Weinfeld SB. Charcot neuroarthropathy of the foot and ankle. Clin Orthop Relat Res 1998;349:116–131.

14. Shibata T, Tada K, Hashizume C. The results of arthrodesis of the ankle for leprotic neuroarthropathy. J Bone Joint Surg Am 1990;72:749–756.

15. Simon SR, Tejwani SG, Wilson DL, et al. Arthrodesis as an early alternative to nonoperative management of Charcot arthropathy of the diabetic foot. J Bone Joint Surg Am 2000;82:939–950.

16. Trepman E, Nihal A, Pinzur MS. Current topics review: Charcot neuroarthropathy of the foot and ankle. Foot Ankle Int 2005;26:46–63.

17. Wang JC, Le AW, Tsukuda RK. A new technique for Charcot's foot reconstruction. J Am Podiatr Med Assoc 2002;92:429–436.

18. Zampa V, Bargellini I, Rizzo L, et al. Role of dynamic MRI in the follow-up of acute Charcot foot in patients with diabetes mellitus. Skeletal Radiol 2011;40:991–999.

CHAPTER 18

Stepwise Surgical Approach to Chronic Diabetic Charcot Foot and Ankle Neuroarthropathy

Matthew J. Hentges • Lisa M. Grant-McDonald • Alan R. Catanzariti

INTRODUCTION

Charcot neuroarthropathy (CN) is a progressive destructive inflammatory process that can affect both the insensate foot and ankle, placing the affected extremity at risk for limb loss. Early diagnosis of the disease process is critical to managing and reducing complications related to deformity and ulceration. Nonoperative management with therapeutic footwear and custom bracing can be successful in greater than 50% of patients (22,30). Nonetheless, ulceration, soft tissue infection, and osteomyelitis are frequent complications associated with CN. These are often the result of aberrant weight bearing forces and altered muscle–tendon balance due to the deformed CN foot or ankle position (17). Early intervention when treating the CN foot and/or ankle deformity often achieves the best results. The goals of surgical intervention for the CN foot and ankle are to restore anatomic alignment, impart stability, preserve osseous anatomy, prevent recurrence of deformity, prevent ulceration/infection (or the recurrence of ulceration/infection), prevent amputation, and allow for the patient to remain ambulatory.

PREOPERATIVE CONSIDERATIONS FOR CHRONIC DIABETIC CHARCOT FOOT AND ANKLE SURGERY

A thorough understanding of the patient's deformity is required prior to operative reconstruction. The physical examination should include non–weight-bearing examination of the foot, ankle, and lower extremity as well as weight bearing examination and observing the patient's gait and stance. Radiographic examination should include foot, ankle, and lower extremity evaluation to assess alignment. Axial imaging for evaluation of the frontal plane alignment of the foot to lower leg is also important (15,16). The radiographic evaluation is essential for determining the apex of the deformity, or center of rotation of angulation (CORA). Additional imaging studies, such as computed tomography or magnetic resonance imaging (MRI), may also aid in preoperative assessment and surgical planning. In the presence of a chronic ulceration or suspected osteomyelitis, obtaining an MRI or bone scan may help identify the extent of bone infection. Additional laboratory studies, such as C-reactive protein or erythrocyte sedimentation rate, may be helpful in diagnosing or identifying osteomyelitis (7).

A comprehensive preoperative medical examination, including cardiac assessment if indicated, is mandatory. Optimization of the patient's nutrition and blood glucose management prior to intervention is important for minimizing postoperative complications (24,26). This should include hemoglobin A_{1c} (HbA_{1c}) and vitamin D evaluation. The incidence of postoperative complications has been shown to increase dramatically with HbA_{1c} levels greater than 8.0% (13,29,32,34,36). Uncontrolled diabetes mellitus and malnutrition are contraindications to surgery. A thorough evaluation of lower extremity arterial disease may identify the need for vascular intervention prior to surgical reconstruction of the foot or ankle. Although noninvasive vascular testing can accurately diagnose macrovascular disease in diabetic patients with CN (37), the presence of microvascular disease is difficult to diagnose and can result in postoperative complications. Vascular consultation should be obtained prior to surgical reconstruction if there is concern regarding healing potential. In the presence of a deep or chronic ulceration, there should be a high index of suspicion for osteomyelitis. A staged surgical approach may be required to ensure a clean surgical environment if internal fixation is to be utilized. Preoperative evaluation by physical therapy may be warranted if there is concern regarding a patient's ability to comply with weight bearing restrictions following surgery. In order to maximize the chances of success in these difficult foot and ankle reconstructions, it is necessary to impart a multidisciplinary team approach.

The decision to undergo major foot and/or ankle reconstruction for limb salvage should be a joint decision made between the patient, family, caregivers, medical, and surgical teams.

A thorough understanding of the patient's family and social circumstances is especially helpful in determining appropriate care. A preoperative discussion regarding goals and expectations should take place with the patient and family. The possibility of limb loss, lifestyle modification, and potential disability should be understood by the patient and family. The family and social environment play a critical role in the success of a patient's limb salvage effort. An ideal candidate has a supportive social network, is committed to the treatment plan, and has a full understanding of goals and expectations.

STEPWISE SURGICAL APPROACH TO CHRONIC DIABETIC CHARCOT FOOT RECONSTRUCTION

The goal of surgical intervention for the chronic diabetic CN foot and ankle is to create a stable and plantigrade foot that can be properly accommodated in therapeutic footwear. This is accomplished through negating the major deforming force on the midfoot (equinus), restoring anatomic alignment of the foot, and imparting stability through extended arthrodesis procedures.

Management of Ankle Equinus

Equinus deformity of the ankle is a major deforming force on the midfoot. It is well known that lengthening of the posterior muscle group greatly reduces plantar pressures of the forefoot and midfoot in the neuropathic patient (1,19). This concept is a fundamental part of the midfoot reconstruction. Posterior muscle group lengthening reduces the deforming force on the midfoot and is an integral part of the reconstruction.

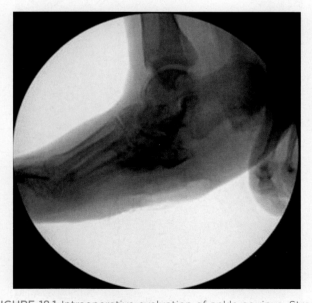

FIGURE 18.1 Intraoperative evaluation of ankle equinus. Stress examination prior to posterior muscle group lengthening can assist the surgeon in the decision of performing a tendo-Achilles lengthening versus gastrosoleal recession.

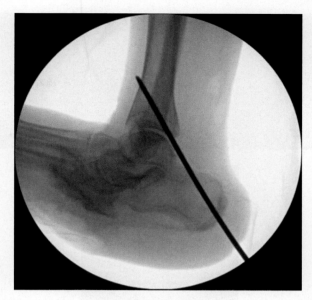

FIGURE 18.2 Correction of ankle equinus with tendo-Achilles lengthening and extra-articular pin ankle stabilization.

The authors' preference is to perform a gastrosoleal recession due to the decreased risk of overlengthening and causing a calcaneus gate. However, there are cases in which tendo-Achilles lengthening is performed. In this case, the authors perform a percutaneous triple hemisection procedure. The decision to proceed with gastrosoleal recession versus tendo-Achilles lengthening is made intraoperatively with the patient under anesthesia. Lengthening can be verified under fluoroscopy comparing prelengthening and postlengthening lateral imaging (Fig. 18.1). The ankle and hindfoot can then be maintained in proper position during and following the midfoot reconstruction by performing temporary extra-articular ankle stabilization (Fig. 18.2). This extra-articular pin can remain in place while the patient is either immobilized in a cast or an external fixation device. The extra-articular pin is removed prior to transitioning the patient to weight bearing to prevent hardware complications or fracture.

Midfoot Deformity Correction with Acute Realignment

The exact location and magnitude of deformity secondary to CN can vary. However, sagittal plane collapse of the midfoot with abduction of the forefoot on the hindfoot is common. A translational deformity, where the forefoot dislocates dorsally on the hindfoot, is frequently observed. It is also important to identify and address the hindfoot deformity. The clinical appearance of hindfoot valgus deformity can be misleading. There are some patients who in fact have hindfoot varus deformity, which is underappreciated and may in fact be detrimental to the stability of the foot if not addressed (Fig. 18.3). Realignment subtalar joint arthrodesis is sometimes necessary to correct for hindfoot deformity or instability.

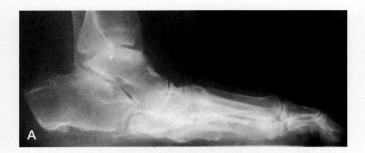

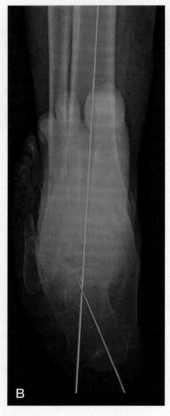

FIGURE 18.3 Charcot neuroarthropathy deformity of the midfoot **(A)** with concomitant hindfoot varus deformity **(B)**.

Acute midfoot deformity correction is performed through a medial or lateral longitudinal incision or combined medial and lateral incisions. Incision placement is dependent on the extent and apex of the deformity. Small incisions with minimal soft tissue stripping are performed to minimize wound healing complications. Periosteal stripping is avoided to preserve vascularity to the osseous segments (33). Smooth wires are inserted as axis guides and later used as osteotomy guides for bone resection (Fig. 18.4). Bone resection is performed perpendicular to the sagittal and transverse plane deformity. Additional translation or rotation of the bony segments is often necessary to obtain full reduction of the deformity. Preparation of unaffected joints proximal and distal to the osteotomy is performed to increase the arthrodesis mass and stability of the construct. This often includes the talonavicular joint and/or the first tarsometatarsal joint, depending on

the apex of the deformity. Bone graft is then utilized to fill any voids within the osteotomy and arthrodesis sites. This is typically a combination of autogenous and allogenic bone as well as osteobiologics. Stem cell preparations and bone morphogenic protein preparations have been used with much success in high-risk patients to enhance arthrodesis (2,8,28,31). Provisional fixation is then delivered in the form of smooth wires or Steinmann pins to hold the reduction of the deformity.

The authors prefer to utilize intramedullary foot fixation (IMFF) or "beaming," for formal fixation and stabilization of the midfoot deformity correction (9,10,12,18). This form of fixation maximizes the strength of the construct and provides a mechanical advantage against ground reactive forces as a load sharing device. IMFF is ideal because it can span beyond the area of diseased bone. Fixation of the medial and lateral columns is typical, with additional fixation of the central column considered if added stability is needed (Fig. 18.5). Special attention is made to reconstruct the Meary's (lateral talo-first metatarsal) angle in both the sagittal and transverse planes. IMFF across the medial column of the foot requires accurate realignment of the deformity in order to ensure proper placement of the fixation. The largest diameter intramedullary (IM) screw possible is utilized to ensure long-term stability, often a 7.0 mm or 8.0 mm screw.

Medial or lateral column plate techniques often require more extensive exposure for placement of the hardware. The robust nature of these plates, even "low-profile" plates, can place increased tension on the soft tissue envelope leading

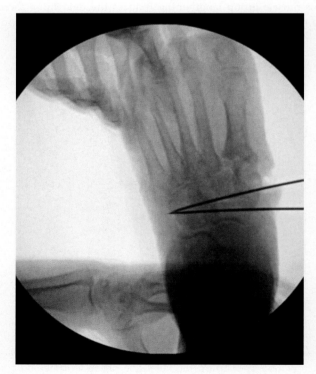

FIGURE 18.4 Placement of smooth wires used as axis/osteotomy guides for acute midfoot osteotomy.

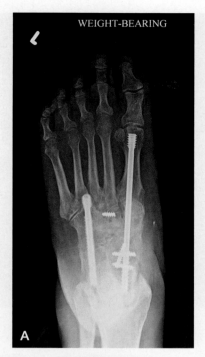

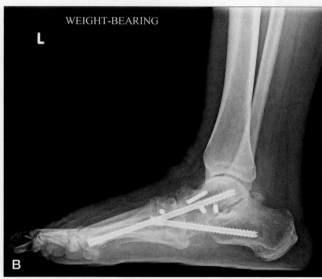

FIGURE 18.5 **A,B.** Use of intramedullary foot fixation (IMFF) for beaming of medial and lateral columns for arthrodesis and stabilization of Charcot neuroarthropathy midfoot deformity correction.

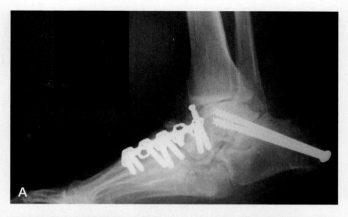

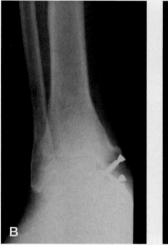

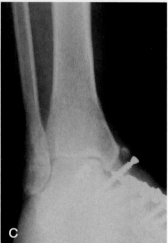

FIGURE 18.6 Failure of medial column plate fixation for Charcot neuroarthropathy midfoot reconstruction shown in foot **(A)** and ankle **(B,C)** radiographic views.

to wound healing complications in this high-risk patient population. Plate fixation is also at risk for failure due to its load-bearing nature and dependency on adequate screw purchase (Fig. 18.6). This form of fixation is not preferred by the authors. However, it should be noted that plate fixation has been used with success in CN (3).

Circular external fixation can be used in combination with IMFF for increased stability. The circular external fixator is used to neutralize weight bearing forces and increase compression across the midfoot osteotomy/arthrodesis (11).

Circular external fixation can also be used in the setting of bone and/or soft tissue infection as the fixation can be placed remotely from the site of infection while maintaining the deformity correction in a single-stage reconstruction (21,23). Two-stage approaches have also been described utilizing circular external fixation in the setting of infection and/or for gradual correction of severe deformity (14,21,23).

STEPWISE SURGICAL APPROACH TO CHRONIC DIABETIC CHARCOT ANKLE RECONSTRUCTION

Patients with chronic diabetic CN of the hindfoot and ankle often present with considerable deformity placing the lower limb at risk for ulceration and amputation (Fig. 18.7). These deformities can be difficult to brace due to the magnitude of deformity and concomitant hindfoot and ankle instability. Primary indications for surgery include a nonreducible deformity with increased plantar pressure and a severe deformity with instability that is not amenable to bracing. Realignment and stabilization through surgical reconstruction is often

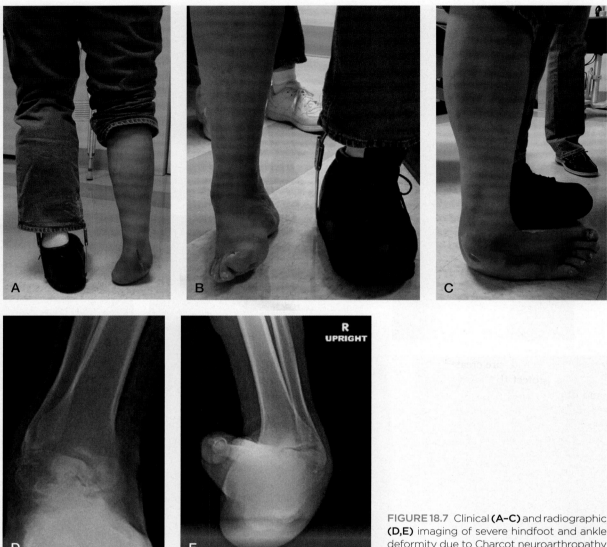

FIGURE 18.7 Clinical **(A–C)** and radiographic **(D,E)** imaging of severe hindfoot and ankle deformity due to Charcot neuroarthropathy and resultant joint instability.

required to create a stable lower extremity, allowing the patient to transfer or remain a short-distance ambulator. A realigned hindfoot and ankle maintained by a stable arthrodesis should be the ultimate goal of surgical reconstruction (5). The authors typically apply internal fixation techniques in most cases of hindfoot and ankle reconstruction. However, in the presence of chronic ulceration, osseous defects, osteomyelitis, or poor bone quality, the authors will utilize circular external fixation.

A thorough understanding of the patient's existing deformity is paramount to surgical planning. Clinical and radiographic evaluation often reveals significant frontal/axial plane deformity of the hindfoot and/or ankle. The authors employ long-leg calcaneal axial and hindfoot alignment radiographs to evaluate the deformity (15,16). These radiographic views demonstrate the relationship of the hindfoot and ankle to the axis of the lower leg, allowing for objective evaluation of angular and translational deformities (Fig. 18.8).

Hindfoot and Ankle Arthrodesis with Intramedullary Nail Fixation

Hindfoot and ankle arthrodesis in the diabetic patient with CN and severe and/or unstable deformity is performed through a lateral transfibular approach (Fig. 18.9). A medial or anteromedial incision can also be made to assist in resection of the medial malleolus or removal of cartilage from the medial gutter if the medial malleolus is to be maintained. A posterior trans-Achilles approach can also be performed if there are concerns regarding soft tissue healing laterally. In cases with lesser amounts of deformity, an anterior approach to the ankle joint can be performed with supplemental lateral sinus tarsi approach to the subtalar joint. The authors typically perform the transfibular approach in these CN cases. However, the incisional approach is dependent on the apex and magnitude of deformity.

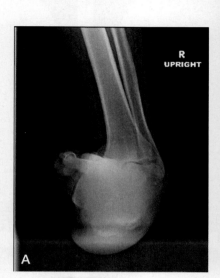
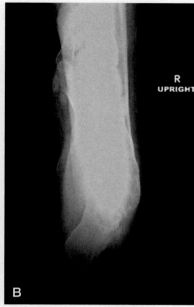

FIGURE 18.8 **A,B.** Hindfoot alignment and long-leg calcaneal axial radiographs used to evaluate frontal (axial) plane hindfoot and ankle deformity.

Full-thickness skin flaps are created, and only deep retraction is utilized to protect the soft tissue. The distal fibula is resected and often utilized for autogenous bone graft and/or placed as an onlay graft. The ankle and subtalar joints are prepared for arthrodesis using a combination of joint curettage and saw resection. In order to anatomically reduce large deformities, wedge resection of the ankle and/or subtalar joints may be required to ensure collinear realignment of the osseous segments. Avascular bone and diseased soft tissue must be thoroughly resected. A healthy cancellous bone substrate should be created to enhance primary union between bone segments. It is also important not to accept residual deformity in order to

maintain limb length. In the authors' experience, shortening is acceptable and well tolerated in the majority of patients when the foot is in a plantigrade and stable position.

Following joint resection and preparation, the osseous segments are realigned. The goal is collinear alignment between the tibia, talus, and calcaneus (Fig. 18.10). This is achieved through medialization of the talus and calcaneus. Correctly positioning the foot under the leg to achieve collinear alignment is the most critical aspect of the procedure. Medialization of the foot may require resection of a portion of the medial malleolus to achieve collinear realignment. Optimal position of the hindfoot is neutral frontal plane rotation,

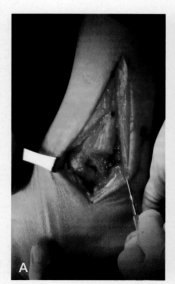
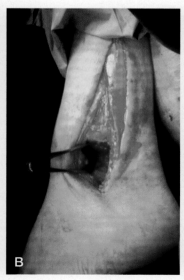
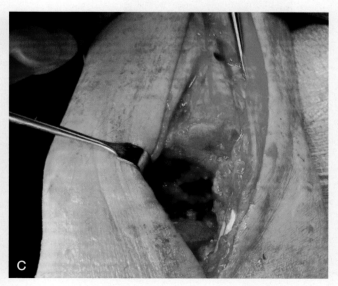

FIGURE 18.9 **A-C.** Lateral transfibular approach for Charcot neuroarthropathy ankle and hindfoot arthrodesis.

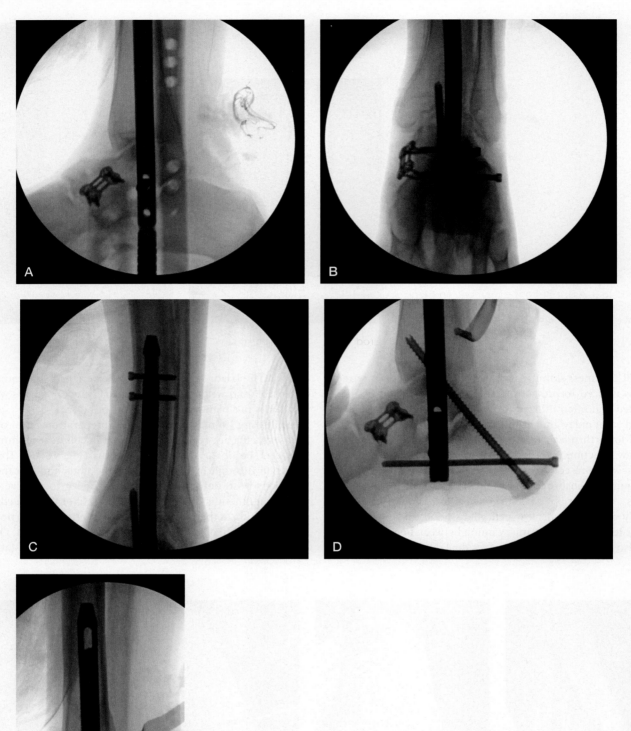

FIGURE 18.10 **A-E.** Collinear alignment of the tibia-talus-calcaneus with tibiota-localcaneal arthrodesis and intramedullary nail fixation.

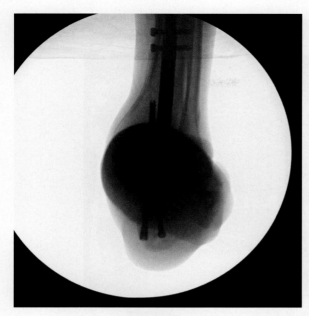

FIGURE 18.11 Utilizing intraoperative axial imaging to verify alignment of the hindfoot during tibiotalocalcaneal arthrodesis.

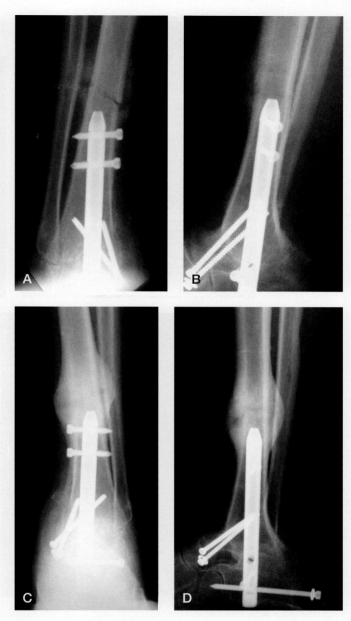

FIGURE 18.12 A,B. Stress fracture of tibia due to placement of intramedullary nail fixation of improper length. **C,D.** Stress fracture healed with extended immobilization and non–weight-bearing.

neutral sagittal plane alignment, and 10 to 15 degrees of external rotation. Provisional fixation is then delivered in the form of Steinmann pins, and position is objectively evaluated with fluoroscopic imaging. Alignment is confirmed with anteroposterior and lateral radiographic views of the ankle and a hindfoot axial view (Fig. 18.11). Failure to properly medialize the foot may result in fracture of the medial calcaneal cortex or damage to the neurovascular structures as well as placement of the IM nail in a valgus angle which may result in a stress riser along the tibial cortex. Improper length of the IM nail may also create increased stress loads on the tibia resulting in a tibial stress fracture (Fig. 18.12).

The IM nail is inserted in standard fashion and to the manufacturer's technique protocol. The exact steps for IM nail delivery is dependent on the type of IM nail that is being used. The insertion site for the IM nail is anterior to the weight bearing surface of the heel and slightly lateral to avoid the neurovascular structures (27). The longest IM nail possible should be utilized to provide additional stability when neuropathy and osteopenia are pronounced. The IM nail must extend beyond the distal isthmus of the tibia. The use of a longer IM nail reduces the risk of stress risers of the tibia, especially in patients with neuropathy or osteopenia. Local autogenous bone graft from the fibula, as well as osteobiologics, is routinely used to augment the arthrodesis sites. In instances where structural bone graft is necessary, the authors will use fresh frozen femoral head allograft. The arthrodesis sites are then compressed and the IM nail is locked. The authors do not routinely use the dynamic hole in the proximal IM nail and prefer a locked construct for added stability. An IM nail serves as a rigid, load-sharing device, which is especially advantageous in CN patients with poor bone quality (4,20,25).

Large-diameter cannulated screws can be used to supplement the IM nail construct to increase stiffness and stability. A static circular external fixator can also be applied to neutralize the hindfoot and ankle arthrodesis. Although there has not been a significant difference in the limb salvage rate when circular external fixation has been added (6), the authors believe it increases stability of the arthrodesis sites. The surgeon must ensure that the circular external fixation spans an appropriate amount of distance above the IM nail so that it does not place increased stress on the tibia and result in a stress riser or tibia fracture (Fig. 18.13).

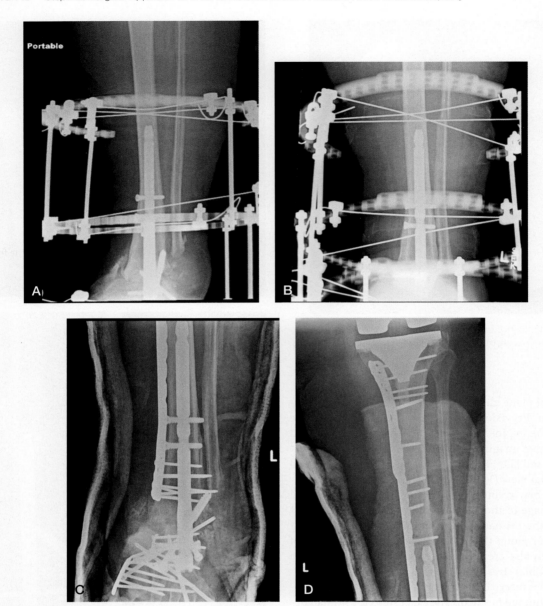

FIGURE 18.13 **A,B.** Placing circular external fixation in close proximity to proximal aspect of intramedullary nail fixation can cause increased stress on the tibia resulting in tibial stress fracture or fracture. **C,D.** Tibia fracture was revised with minimally invasive plate osteosynthesis technique using locking plate fixation.

Conclusion

Ultimately, the decision to proceed with surgical reconstruction of the chronic diabetic CN foot and/or ankle deformity is a combined decision between the surgeon and patient. It is important to ensure that the patient has a supportive social network and that everyone involved fully understands the realistic goals of limb salvage as well as the possible risks and complications that can occur. It is well known that limb loss negatively affects quality of life. However, in some patients, limb loss can improve survival and self-reported quality of life (35). The unique circumstances surrounding each diabetic patient with foot and/or ankle deformity secondary to CN should be taken into account prior to surgical intervention.

References

1. Armstrong DG, Stacpoole-Shea S, Nguyen H, et al. Lengthening of the Achilles tendon in diabetic patients who are at high risk for ulceration of the foot. J Bone Joint Surg Am 1999;81:535–538.

2. Bibbo C, Patel DV, Haskell MD. Recombinant bone morphogenetic protein-2 (rhBMP-2) in high-risk ankle and hindfoot fusions. Foot Ankle Int 2009;30:597–603.

3. Capobianco CM, Stapleton JJ, Zgonis T. The role of an extended medial column arthrodesis for Charcot midfoot neuroarthropathy. Diabetic Foot Ankle 2010;1.

4. Catanzariti AR, Mendicino RW. Intramedullary nail fixation for reconstruction of the hindfoot and ankle in Charcot neuroarthropathy. In: Zgonis T, ed. Surgical reconstruction of the

diabetic foot and ankle. Philadelphia: Lippincott Williams & Wilkins, 2009:241–254.

5. Catanzariti AR, Mendicino RW, Child B. Rearfoot and ankle fusions. In: Frykberg RG, ed. The diabetic Charcot foot: principles and management. Brooklandville, MD: Data Trace, 2010:209–229.

6. DeVries JG, Berlet GC, Hyer CF. A retrospective comparative analysis of Charcot ankle stabilization using an intramedullary rod with or without application of circular external fixator—utilization of the retrograde arthrodesis intramedullary nail database. J Foot Ankle Surg 2012;51:420–425.

7. Fleischer AE, Didyk AA, Woods JB, et al. Combined clinical and laboratory testing improves diagnostic accuracy for osteomyelitis in the diabetic foot. J Foot Ankle Surg 2009;48:39–46.

8. Fourman MS, Borst EW, Bogner E, et al. Recombinant human BMP-2 increases the incidence and rate of healing in complex ankle arthrodesis. Clin Orthop Relat Res 2014;472:732–739.

9. Grant WP, Garcia-Lavin S, Sabo R. Beaming the columns for Charcot diabetic foot reconstruction: a retrospective analysis. J Foot Ankle Surg 2011;50:182–189.

10. Grant WP, Garcia-Lavin SE, Sabo RT, et al. A retrospective analysis of 50 consecutive Charcot diabetic salvage reconstructions. J Foot Ankle Surg 2009;48:30–38.

11. Grant WP, Rubin LG, Pupp GR, et al. Mechanical testing of seven fixation methods for generation of compression across a midtarsal osteotomy: a comparison of internal and external fixation devices. J Foot Ankle Surg 2007;46:325–335.

12. Grant WP, Weinraub GM. Surgical reconstruction and stepwise approach to chronic Charcot neuroarthropathy. In: Zgonis T, ed. Surgical reconstruction of the diabetic foot and ankle. Philadelphia: Lippincott Williams & Wilkins, 2009:230–240.

13. Jupiter DC, Humphers JM, Shibuya N. Trends in postoperative infection rates and their relationship to glycosylated hemoglobin levels in diabetic patients undergoing foot and ankle surgery. J Foot Ankle Surg 2014;53:307–311.

14. Lamm BM, Gottlieb HD, Paley D. A two-stage percutaneous approach to Charcot diabetic foot reconstruction. J Foot Ankle Surg 2010;49:517–522.

15. Lamm BM, Mendicino RW, Catanzariti AR, et al. Static rearfoot alignment: a comparison of clinical and radiographic measures. J Am Podiatr Med Assoc 2005;95:26–33.

16. Lamm BM, Paley D. Deformity correction planning for hindfoot, ankle, and lower limb. Clin Podiatr Med Surg 2004;21:305–326.

17. Lamm BM, Paley D. Reduction of neuropathic foot deformity with gradual external fixation distraction and midfoot fusion. In: Frykberg RG, ed. The diabetic Charcot foot: principles and management. Brooklandville, MD: Data Trace, 2010:195–208.

18. Lamm BM, Siddiqui NA, Nair K, et al. Intramedullary foot fixation for midfoot Charcot neuroarthropathy. J Foot Ankle Surg 2012;51:531–536.

19. Maluf KS, Mueller MJ, Strube MJ, et al. Tendon Achilles lengthening for the treatment of neuropathic ulcers causes a temporary reduction in forefoot pressure associated with changes in plantar flexor power rather than ankle motion during gait. J Biomech 2004;37:897–906.

20. Mendicino RW, Catanzariti AR, Saltrick KR, et al. Tibiotalocalcaneal arthrodesis with retrograde intramedullary nailing. J Foot Ankle Surg 2004;43:82–86.

21. Pinzur MS. Neutral ring fixation for high-risk nonplantigrade Charcot midfoot deformity. Foot Ankle Int 2007;28:961–966.

22. Pinzur M. Surgical versus accommodative treatment for Charcot arthropathy of the midfoot. Foot Ankle Int 2004;25:545–549.

23. Pinzur MS, Gil J, Belmares J. Treatment of osteomyelitis in Charcot foot with single-stage resection of infection, correction of deformity, and maintenance with ring fixation. Foot Ankle Int 2012;33:1069–1074.

24. Pinzur MS, Gurza E, Kristopaitis T, et al. Hospitalist-orthopedic co-management of high-risk patients undergoing lower extremity reconstruction surgery. Orthopedics 2009;32:495.

25. Pinzur MS, Noonan T. Ankle arthrodesis with a retrograde femoral nail for Charcot ankle arthropathy. Foot Ankle Int 2005;26:545–549.

26. Pinzur MS, Sage R, Stuck R, et al. Transcutaneous oxygen as a predictor of wound healing in amputations of the foot and ankle. Foot Ankle 1992;13:271–272.

27. Roukis TS. Determining the insertion site for retrograde intramedullary nail fixation of tibiotalocalcaneal arthrodesis: a radiographic and intraoperative anatomical landmark analysis. J Foot Ankle Surg 2006;45:227–234.

28. Rush SM, Hamilton GA, Ackerson LM. Mesenchymal stem cell allograft in revision foot and ankle surgery: a clinical and radiographic analysis. J Foot Ankle Surg 2009;48:163–169.

29. Sadoskas D, Suder NC, Wukich DK. Perioperative glycemic control and the effect on surgical site infections in diabetic patients undergoing foot and ankle surgery. Foot Ankle Spec 2016;9:24–30.

30. Saltzman CL, Hagy ML, Zimmerman B, et al. How effective is intensive nonoperative initial treatment of patients with diabetes and Charcot arthropathy of the feet? Clin Orthop Relat Res 2005;435:185–190.

31. Schuberth JM, DiDomenico LA, Mendicino RW. The utility and effectiveness of bone morphogenetic protein in foot and ankle surgery. J Foot Ankle Surg 2009;48:309–314.

32. Shibuya N, Humphers JM, Fluhman BL, et al. Factors associated with nonunion, delayed union, and malunion in foot and ankle surgery in diabetic patients. J Foot Ankle Surg 2013;52:207–211.

33. Whiteside LA, Ogata K, Lesker BS, et al. The acute effects of periosteal stripping and medullary reaming on regional bone blood flow. Clin Orthop Relat Res 1978;131:266–272.

34. Wukich DK, Crim BE, Frykberg RG, et al. Neuropathy and poorly controlled diabetes increase the rate of surgical site infection after foot and ankle surgery. J Bone Joint Surg Am 2014;96:832–839.

35. Wukich DK, Pearson KT. Self-reported outcomes of trans-tibial amputations for non-reconstructable Charcot neuroarthropathy in patients with diabetes: a preliminary report. Diabet Med 2013;30:e87–e90.

36. Wukich DK, Raspovic KM, Hobizal KB, et al. Surgical management of Charcot neuroarthropathy of the ankle and hindfoot in patients with diabetes. Diabetes Metab Res Rev 2016;32(suppl 1):292–296.

37. Wukich DK, Raspovic KM, Suder NC. Prevalence of peripheral arterial disease in patients with diabetic Charcot neuroarthropathy. J Foot Ankle Surg 2016;55:727–731.

CHAPTER 19

Stepwise Surgical Approach to Diabetic Charcot Foot and Ankle Neuroarthropathy with Concomitant Osteomyelitis

John J. Stapleton • Thomas Zgonis

INTRODUCTION

Soft tissue and osseous infection is more frequently encountered in the diabetic lower extremity, and once established in patients with Charcot neuroarthropathy (CN) of the foot and ankle, it becomes more difficult to manage. In most cases, the host is compromised with poor metabolic control, vascular insufficiency, and multiple medical comorbidities that further complicate the clinical scenario. The presence of osteomyelitis in the diabetic foot and/or ankle is one of the major clinical pathways that lead into a major lower extremity amputation. For this reason, an experienced specialized medical and surgical team with an interest in the management of diabetes mellitus and diabetic lower extremity reconstruction is essential in order to prevent and minimize the need for amputation. In addition, the role of lower extremity amputation needs to also be understood and recommended in clinical scenarios of lower extremity and/or life-threatening infections with severe peripheral arterial disease, diabetic patients in which a stable metabolic status cannot be re-established, and/or if a dysfunctional and nonambulatory lower extremity is likely the end result.

DIFFERENTIAL DIAGNOSIS

Diagnosis of concomitant osteomyelitis in diabetic patients with CN becomes a great challenge in the presence of acute or chronic open wounds. In most cases, the presence of deep soft tissue and/or osseous infection is obvious and associated with purulent drainage, deep abscess, sinus tracts, exposed bone, elevated inflammatory markers, and/or systemic response. The difficulty arises in diabetic patients with chronic nonhealing open wounds and underlying CN, acute CN with systemic signs of infection, and previously failed CN surgeries with retained hardware. Identifying the presence of concomitant osteomyelitis in

the diabetic patient with CN of the lower extremity is extremely challenging and often diagnosed by surgical bone biopsy and cultures for histopathologic and microbiologic analysis in addition to clinical, laboratory, and medical imaging assessment. Deep intraoperative osseous curettage, soft tissue cultures, and bone biopsies are most representative of the causative bacterial and/or fungal pathogens.

When the diabetic CN of the foot and/or ankle is associated with a chronic ulcer, abscess, osteomyelitis, or failed previous internal fixation, staged surgical reconstruction is planned after the existing wounds and osseous structures are free of infection and ready for the definitive surgical procedure. Surgical resection of osteomyelitis is based on the clinical, laboratory, intraoperative, and medical imaging studies. Oral and parenteral antibiotic coverage is administered based on the infectious disease team assessment and recommendations.

Several medical imaging studies exist and are available for differentiating the diabetic CN from osteomyelitis in the absence of an open wound or previous history of surgical intervention in the lower extremity. Plain radiographs of the foot, ankle, and lower extremity are the first line of treatment and in identifying concomitant osteomyelitis in diabetic patients with CN. Magnetic resonance imaging (MRI) and computed tomography are effective diagnostic tools that can further provide details in bone marrow abnormalities, septic arthritis, and/or associated soft tissue emphysema. MRI alone as a medical imaging study in differentiating osteomyelitis from diabetic CN should be cautiously ordered because it can provide false-positive findings of osteomyelitis in the acute CN stages and in the absence of open wounds. In clinical scenarios where the MRI diagnosis of osteomyelitis is established in a diabetic patient with CN but no clinical, laboratory, or radiographic findings are present and consistent for infection, advanced nuclear medicine imaging may then be considered for further assessment and before any surgical procedures are encountered. Nuclear medicine musculoskeletal radiologists are highly recommended in the clinical scenarios of diabetic CN with concomitant osteomyelitis where surgery may not be required and further determining the presence of osteomyelitis by performing the studies including, but not limited to, technetium-99m methylene diphosphonate bone scan followed by indium-111-labeled leukocyte and technetium-99m sulfur colloid scans. These studies vary in sensitivity and specificity and are dependent on the underlying deformity, infection, lower extremity vascularity, renal function, and patient's multiple medical comorbidities (4).

PREOPERATIVE CONSIDERATIONS

Concomitant osteomyelitis in the diabetic patient with CN of the foot and/or ankle is usually encountered secondary to underlying osseous deformity, soft tissue contracture, ulcer formation, retained hardware, and/or from previous postoperative infections. Ultimate management of osteomyelitis requires surgical resection either by staged reconstructive procedures or through amputation. Osteomyelitis associated with diabetic CN cannot be addressed with antibiotic therapy alone, and failure is commonly encountered if residual bone infection remains. For these reasons, it is essential to adequately surgically resect the infected bone in order to eradicate infection and promote healing. Medical optimization and infectious disease consultation for the management, administration, and duration of oral and/or parenteral antibiotic therapy combined with surgical resection of osteomyelitis is also initiated throughout the patient's treatment.

Diabetic CN forefoot/midfoot deformities with concomitant osteomyelitis are usually managed with midfoot osseous resection(s) followed by staged reconstruction to a shortening and/or global midfoot arthrodesis (Figs. 19.1 to 19.5). In the presence of multiple forefoot locations with osteomyelitis and abscess, a transmetatarsal amputation may be indicated. Similarly, diabetic CN hindfoot/ankle deformities with concomitant osteomyelitis are usually managed with a talectomy and osseous resection(s) of the infected tibia/fibula followed by a staged tibiocalcaneal arthrodesis. In most cases, it is preferred to convert actively infected wounds to clean wounds prior to definitive lower extremity surgery. Antibiotic-impregnated polymethylmethacrylate (PMMA) cemented beads and/or spacers can be utilized during the staged reconstructive procedures (3) and in the presence of large resected osseous and/or soft tissue defects (Figs. 19.6 and 19.7). Circular external fixation can also be utilized as initial temporary spanning device and later modified to achieve compression and osseous stability for the definitive arthrodesis procedure(s).

Single- or multiple-joint salvage arthrodesis is successful when the deformity correction is achieved and the foot and lower extremity are realigned. The foot is required to be aligned to the lower extremity in a plantigrade position, free of soft tissue breakdown, and braceable to allow functional ambulation. Often, a stable pseudoarthrosis as oppose to a successful

osseous union can accomplish the same goals especially in diabetic patients with CN of the midfoot. A pseudoarthrosis of the hindfoot/ankle is usually more difficult to brace and is less predictable in long-term lower extremity salvage as oppose to a successful osseous union. Technical considerations to achieve a successful osseous union require adequate resection of the infected and nonviable bone, meticulous resection of cartilage and osseous fragments, excisional débridement and/or resection to bleeding subchondral bone, bone contouring to achieve maximum surface contact while correcting the underlying deformity, and stable external and/or internal fixation constructs when complete eradication of the infection has been achieved.

The choice of fixation depends on the surrounding soft tissue envelope, bone quality, osseous/soft tissue defect, and infectious process. Circular external fixation typically becomes the most favorable choice when reconstructing diabetic CN foot and/or ankle deformities associated with concomitant wounds and osteomyelitis (2). Although other surgical techniques are advocating the utilization of internal fixation after management of active infection, the authors prefer to avoid internal fixation in diabetic CN patients with osteomyelitis when feasible. However, morbidly obese diabetic patients and/or patients who have failed previous external fixation devices may benefit from internal fixation and/or combined external and internal fixation if no clinical signs of active infection are present.

Soft tissue management must be combined and considered with osseous resection and reconstruction of diabetic CN deformities and osteomyelitis. Understanding the placement of surgical incisions that relieve tension on the wound after bone resection and arthrodesis is paramount to achieving wound closure and a successful outcome. Large CN midfoot wounds with underlying osteomyelitis and deformity can be closed at the time of bone resection and arthrodesis either by primary closure through bone resection and shortening or with local random, muscle, and pedicle flaps. Conversion of preexisting soft tissue defects into triangular- or rhomboid-shaped excisions that are incorporated with the extensile surgical incisions can allow necessary exposure for bone resection, joint preparation, deformity correction, and wound closure. In addition, bone resection can create wound tension on more traditionally placed incisions and must be considered and altered in order to provide tension-free surgical closures.

Finally, primary or delayed below-the-knee amputation is a valid and recommended choice for certain clinical scenarios. The presence of a non-reconstructable lower extremity with an associated severe vascular disease/ischemia, extensive soft tissue and/or osseous compromise, nonambulatory status with multiple uncontrolled medical comorbidities and severe lower extremity and/or life-threatening infection are considered for indications of lower extremity amputation. In addition, some patients may not elect to proceed with multiple invasive surgical procedures and prolonged immobilization and may decide to proceed with a major lower extremity amputation and prosthetic devices as oppose to reconstructive surgery.

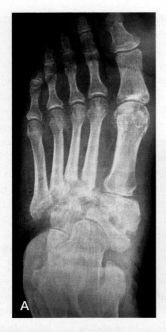

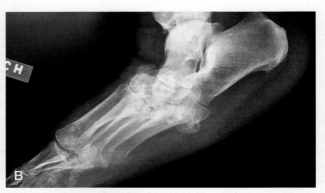

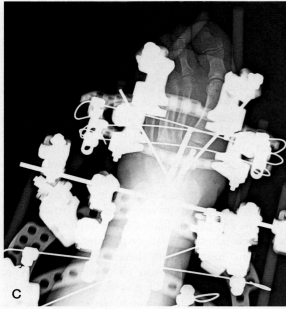

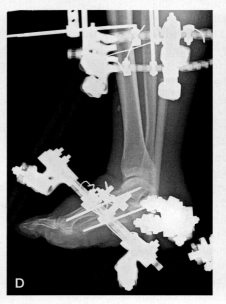

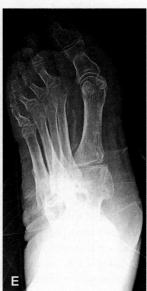

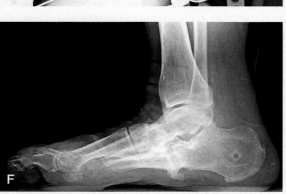

FIGURE 19.1 A,B. Preoperative radiographic views of a left midfoot unstable diabetic Charcot neuroarthropathy with a plantar ulceration, active infection, sepsis, and osteomyelitis. Patient underwent an initial deep incision and drainage procedure and obtaining of intraoperative bone and soft tissue cultures and biopsy followed by an infectious disease team consultation. The patient returned to the operating room 5 days after the first surgery for a wide midfoot resection, deformity correction, and arthrodesis. Delayed primary closure of the plantar wound was performed after shortening of the midfoot. **C,D.** Postoperative radiographic views at 4 weeks reveal osseous stabilization and alignment of the foot to the lower extremity with a circular external fixation device. The circular external fixation device was removed at 16 weeks, and the patient was transitioned to a non–weight-bearing lower extremity cast immobilization for 4 weeks. **E,F.** Final postoperative radiographic views at 1 year follow-up showing successful osseous consolidation and a plantigrade foot without recurrent ulceration or infection.

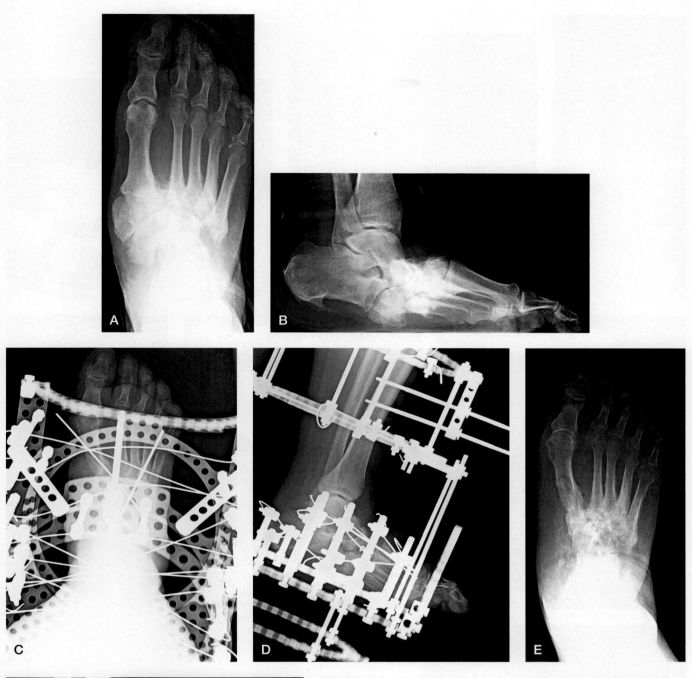

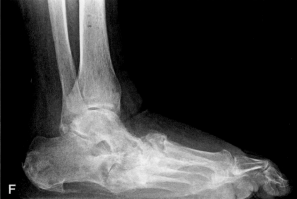

FIGURE 19.2 A,B. Preoperative radiographic views of a right midfoot unstable diabetic Charcot neuroarthropathy with a plantar lateral ulceration, exposed bone, and active deep infection. Patient underwent an initial deep incision and drainage procedure and obtaining of intraoperative bone and soft tissue cultures and biopsy followed by an infectious disease team consultation. The patient returned to the operating room 11 days after the first surgery for a wide midfoot resection, deformity correction, and arthrodesis. Delayed primary closure of the plantar wound was performed after shortening of the midfoot. **C,D.** Postoperative radiographic views at 4 weeks reveal osseous stabilization and alignment of the foot to the lower extremity with a circular external fixation device. The circular external fixation device was removed at 12 weeks, and the patient was transitioned to a non–weight-bearing lower extremity cast immobilization for 6 weeks. **E,F.** Final postoperative radiographic views at 1 year follow-up showing successful osseous consolidation and a plantigrade foot without recurrent ulceration or infection.

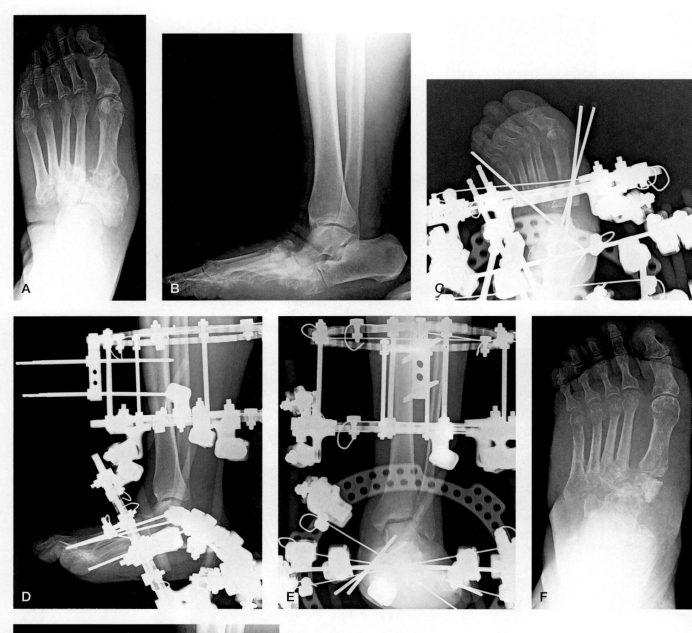

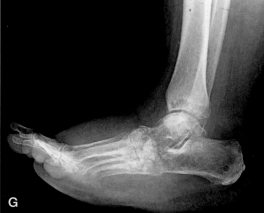

FIGURE 19.3 A,B. Preoperative radiographic views of a left midfoot unstable diabetic Charcot neuroarthropathy with a plantar ulceration and a chronic draining sinus tract infection. **C–E.** Patient underwent reconstruction with a wide midfoot resection, deformity correction, and arthrodesis with the utilization of a circular external fixation device. The circular external fixation device was removed at 13 weeks, and the patient was transitioned to a non–weight-bearing lower extremity cast immobilization for 4 weeks. **F,G.** Final postoperative radiographic views at 1 year follow-up showing a stable midfoot arthrodesis without recurrent ulceration or infection.

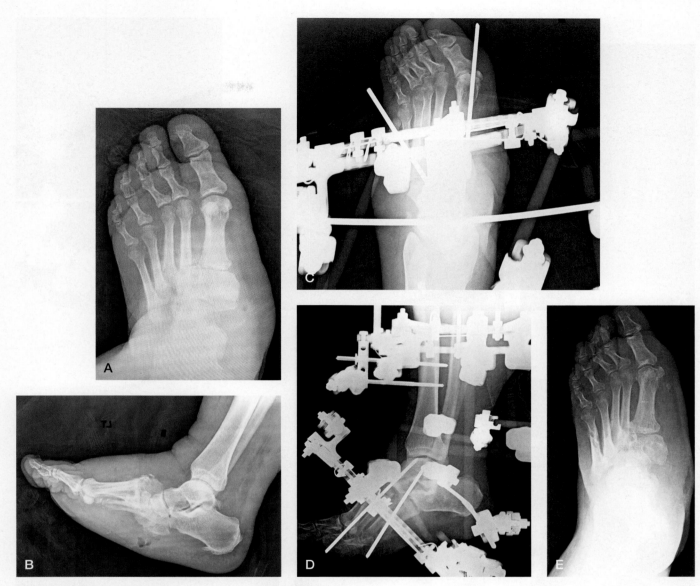

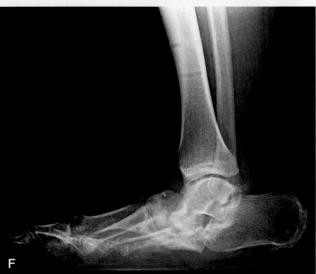

FIGURE 19.4 **A,B.** Preoperative radiographic views of a left midfoot unstable diabetic Charcot neuroarthropathy with a plantar ulceration, active infection, sepsis, necrotizing fasciitis, and osteomyelitis. Patient underwent an initial deep incision and drainage procedure and obtaining of intraoperative bone and soft tissue cultures and biopsy followed by an infectious disease team consultation. The patient returned to the operating room for the staged wide midfoot resection, deformity correction, and arthrodesis. **C,D.** Postoperative radiographic views at 6 weeks reveal osseous stabilization and alignment of the foot to the lower extremity with a circular external fixation device. The circular external fixation device was removed at 14 weeks, and the patient was transitioned to a non–weight-bearing lower extremity cast immobilization for 6 weeks. **E,F.** Final postoperative radiographic views at 15 months follow-up showing successful osseous consolidation and a plantigrade foot.

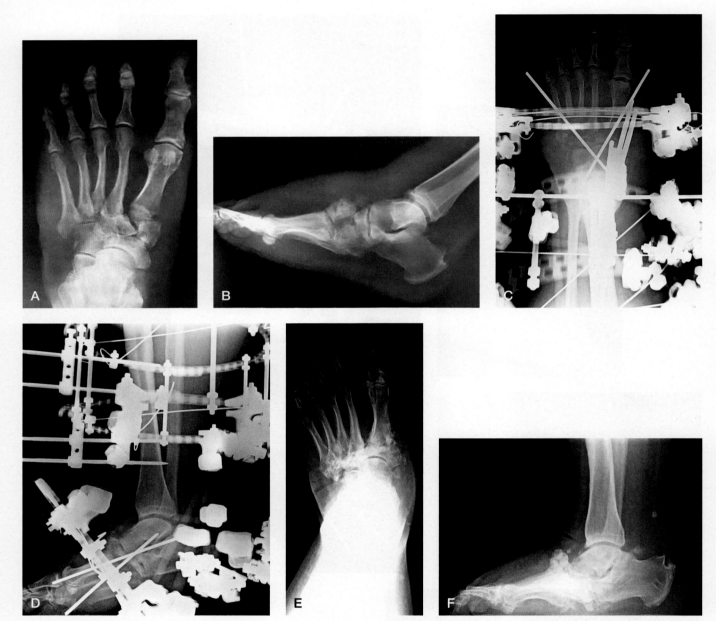

FIGURE 19.5 A,B. Preoperative radiographic views of an acute left midfoot unstable diabetic Charcot neuroarthropathy with a septic joint and osteomyelitis. Patient underwent an initial multiple deep incision and drainage procedure and obtaining of intraoperative bone and soft tissue cultures and biopsy followed by an infectious disease team consultation. The surgical wounds were initially packed with normal saline dressings followed by a lower extremity posterior splint application. Negative pressure wound therapy was then continued with a non–weight-bearing status and until the patient was medically optimized to proceed with the definitive surgical reconstruction. **C,D.** The patient returned to the operating room 14 days after the first surgery for a wide midfoot resection, deformity correction, and arthrodesis with a circular external fixation device. Delayed primary closure of the surgical wounds was performed after shortening of the midfoot. The circular external fixation device was removed at 14 weeks, and the patient was transitioned to a non–weight-bearing lower extremity cast immobilization for 6 weeks. **E,F.** Final postoperative radiographic views at 1 year follow-up showing successful midfoot shortening, osseous consolidation, and a plantigrade foot without recurrent ulceration or infection.

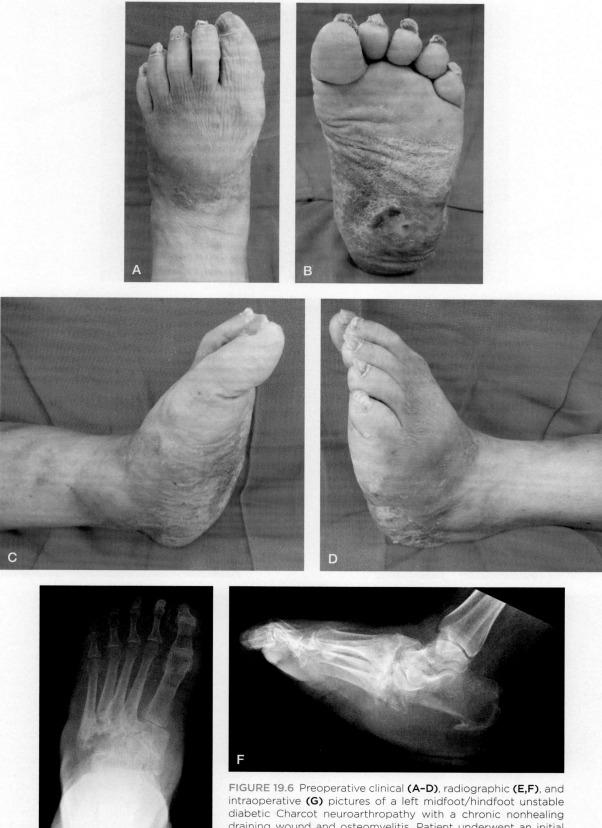

FIGURE 19.6 Preoperative clinical **(A-D)**, radiographic **(E,F)**, and intraoperative **(G)** pictures of a left midfoot/hindfoot unstable diabetic Charcot neuroarthropathy with a chronic nonhealing draining wound and osteomyelitis. Patient underwent an initial deep incision and drainage procedure and obtaining of intraoperative bone and soft tissue cultures and biopsy followed by an infectious disease team consultation. *(continued)*

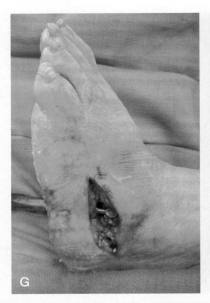
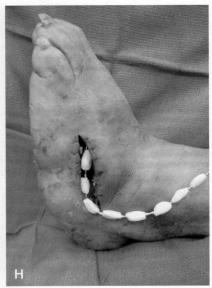
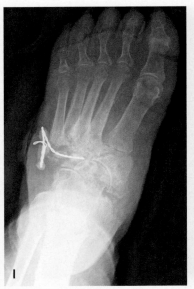
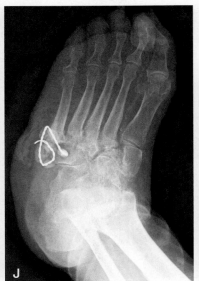
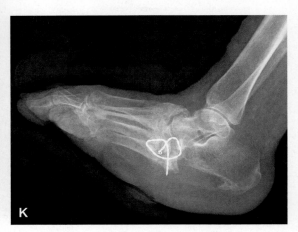
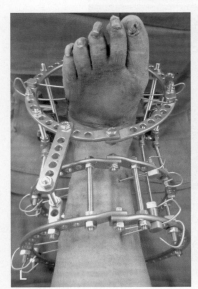
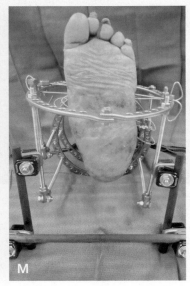

FIGURE 19.6 *(Continued)* The patient returned to the operating room 2 days after the first surgery for a revisional deep excisional débridement to the level of lateral tarsometatarsal joints and insertion of nonbiodegradable antibiotic-impregnated polymethylmethacrylate (PMMA) cemented beads **(H–K)**. At approximately 11 weeks later, the patient returned to the operating room for removal of the retained nonbiodegradable antibiotic-impregnated PMMA cemented beads and further obtaining of intraoperative cultures. The final staged reconstructive procedure was performed at approximately 6 weeks later with a lateral column arthrodesis, allogenic bone grafting, and utilization of a circular external fixation device **(L–R)**. The circular external fixation device was removed at approximately 7.5 weeks, and the patient was transitioned to a non–weight-bearing lower extremity cast immobilization followed by a fracture boot and accommodative devices. *(continued)*

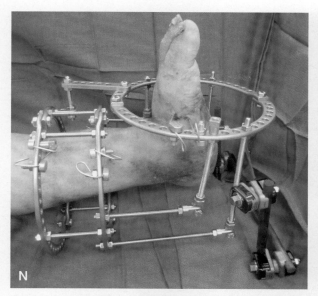

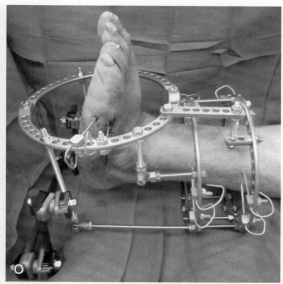

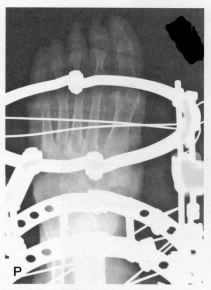

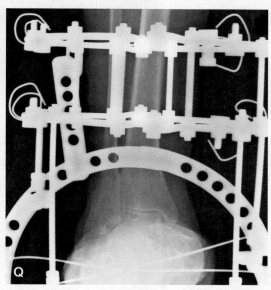

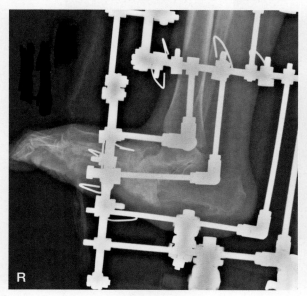

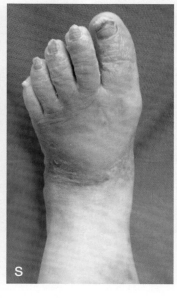

FIGURE 19.6 *(Continued)* Final clinical **(S–V)** and radiographic **(W–Y)** pictures at 9 months follow-up since the first surgery showing osseous consolidation and a plantigrade foot without recurrent ulceration or infection. *(continued)*

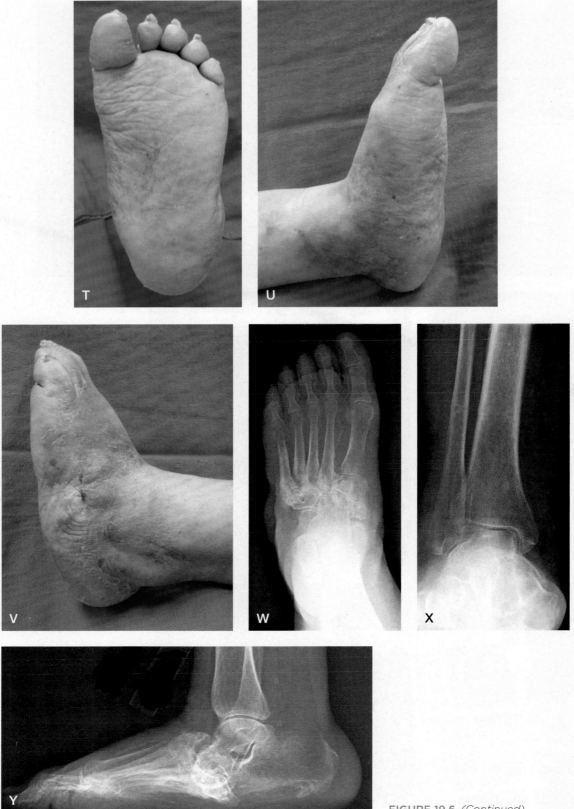

FIGURE 19.6 *(Continued)*

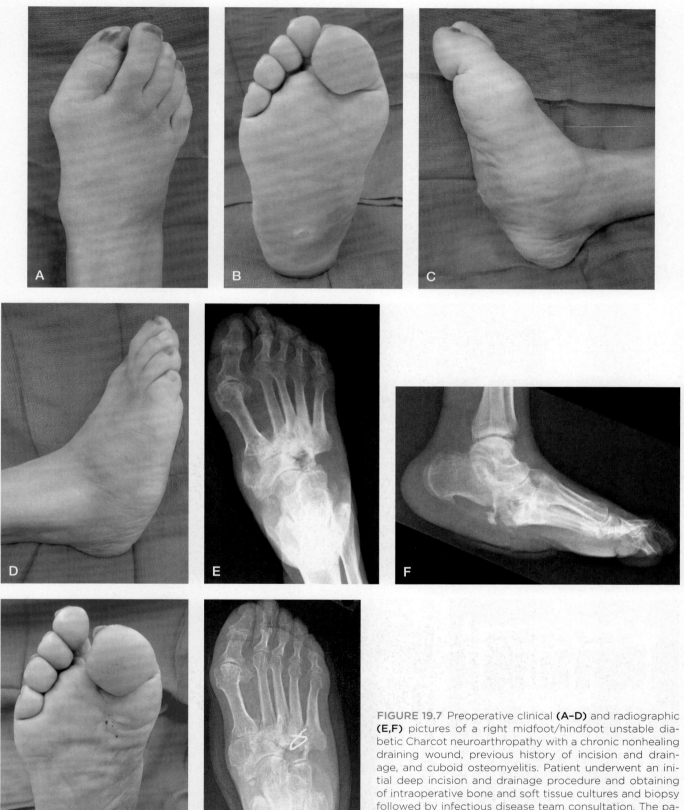

FIGURE 19.7 Preoperative clinical **(A–D)** and radiographic **(E,F)** pictures of a right midfoot/hindfoot unstable diabetic Charcot neuroarthropathy with a chronic nonhealing draining wound, previous history of incision and drainage, and cuboid osteomyelitis. Patient underwent an initial deep incision and drainage procedure and obtaining of intraoperative bone and soft tissue cultures and biopsy followed by infectious disease team consultation. The patient returned to the operating room 2 days after the first surgery for a revisional deep excisional débridement of all nonviable tissues and insertion of nonbiodegradable antibiotic-impregnated polymethylmethacrylate (PMMA) cemented beads **(G,H)**. *(continued)*

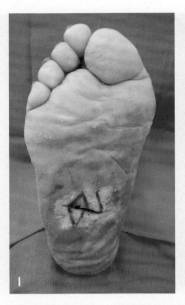
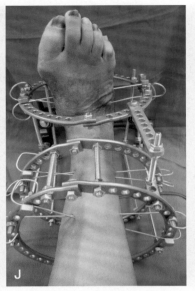
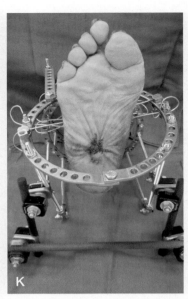

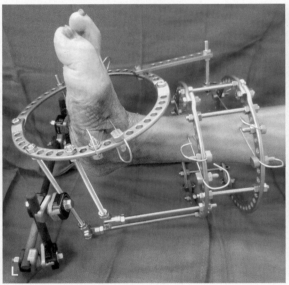
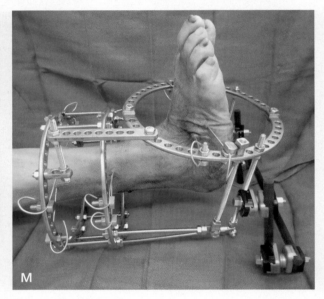

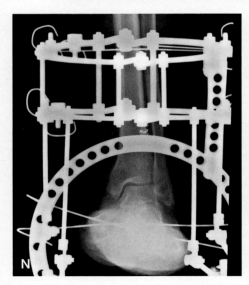
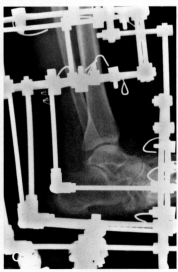

FIGURE 19.7 *(Continued)* At approximately 9.5 weeks later, the patient returned back to the operating room for removal of the retained non-biodegradable antibiotic-impregnated PMMA cemented beads, revisional excisional débridement, lower extremity gastrocnemius recession, local random rhomboid advancement flap closure and circular external fixation for simultaneous surgical off-loading, lower extremity stabilization, and equinus correction **(I–O)**. *(continued)*

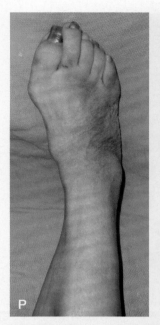
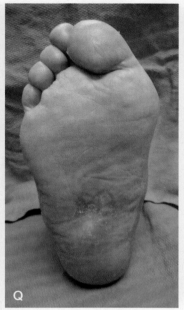
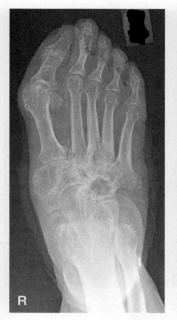
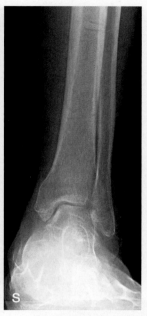

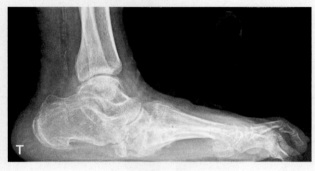

FIGURE 19.7 *(Continued)* The circular external fixation device was removed at approximately 7.5 weeks, and the patient was transitioned to a non–weight-bearing lower extremity cast immobilization followed by a fracture boot and accommodative devices. Final clinical **(P,Q)** and radiographic **(R–T)** pictures at 6.5 months follow-up since the first surgery showing a plantigrade foot without recurrent ulceration or infection.

SURGICAL PRINCIPLES

Excisional débridement of osteomyelitis is paramount to overall successful diabetic lower extremity reconstruction. Ulcers if present should be fully excised to viable skin edges with removal of the hypergranulation, fibrotic, and/or necrotic tissue. In diabetic CN foot and/or ankle deformities, the presence of adventitious bursa is often encountered and needs to be adequately excised. Fibrous joint interposition must also be excisionally débrided and removed from any fragmented and diseased bone.

Surgical techniques for diabetic CN midfoot resections can be performed with large oscillating saws and completed with an osteotome and a mallet as needed. The goal of such a technique is to achieve bleeding from noninfected bone surfaces present at the proximal and distal arthrodesis sites that will allow the deformity to be corrected and wounds to be closed. Often, after wide resection of the tarsal bones, the foot is amenable to be repositioned and stabilized with the utilization of Steinmann pins. Fine adjustments and bone resections can then be performed as needed in order to achieve well-contoured bone surfaces without prominent plantar exostosis. Commonly in the diabetic CN population, the cuboid bone is found to be dislocated in a plantar direction, and release of the plantar tissues or direct approach

through the plantar ulceration will allow for a partial resection or cuboidectomy to be performed (Figs. 19.8 and 19.9). The remaining tarsal bones can also be resected to re-establish equal length to the medial and lateral columns of the foot. Complete resection of the entire midfoot is feasible with shortening of the metatarsals to the talus and calcaneus if required.

Peritalar diabetic CN deformities often present with an unstable deformity about the hindfoot and ankle. The talus bone is often found to be avascular and dislocated with very little soft tissue attachments. A partial or total talectomy can be performed with a direct lateral or medial approach and based on the anatomic position of the hindfoot/ankle (Fig. 19.10). Associated wounds can be excised with a direct approach to the talectomy and closed primarily or by the utilization of negative pressure wound therapy and/or plastic surgery closure techniques. The hindfoot and ankle are destabilized after a talectomy, and considerable amount of dead space is encountered that can be managed with staged bone grafting, arthrodesis, and circular external or internal fixation devices. Staged tibiocalcaneal arthrodesis may also be initially managed with the application of antibiotic-impregnated PMMA cemented beads and/or spacers (Fig. 19.11).

Difficulty usually arises from neglected diabetic CN ankle fractures that present with open wounds and active deep

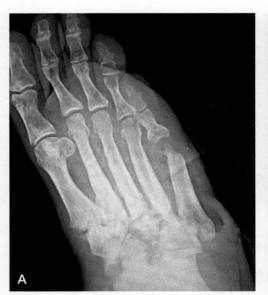

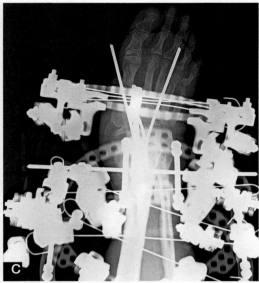

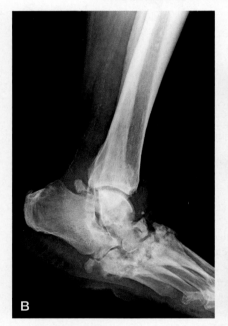

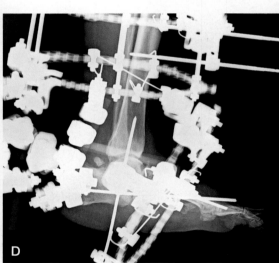

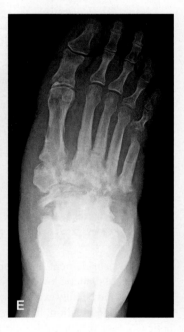

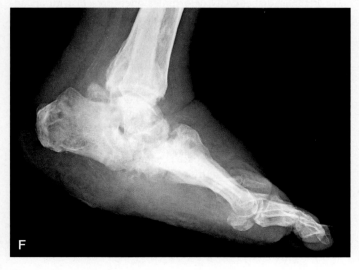

FIGURE 19.8 A,B. Preoperative radiographic views of a right midfoot unstable diabetic Charcot neuroarthropathy with a plantar lateral ulceration, gas gangrene, and osteomyelitis of the midfoot and cuboid bones. Patient underwent an initial deep incision and drainage procedure, cuboidectomy, and obtaining of intraoperative bone and soft tissue cultures and biopsy followed by infectious disease team consultation. **C,D.** The patient returned to the operating room 7 days after the first surgery for a wide midfoot resection, deformity correction, and arthrodesis with a circular external fixation device. The plantar wound was closed by a local random flap after shortening of the midfoot was performed. The circular external fixation device was removed at 12 weeks, and the patient was transitioned to a non–weight-bearing lower extremity cast immobilization for 6 weeks. **E,F.** Final postoperative radiographic views at 8 months follow-up showing osseous consolidation of the midfoot and a plantigrade foot.

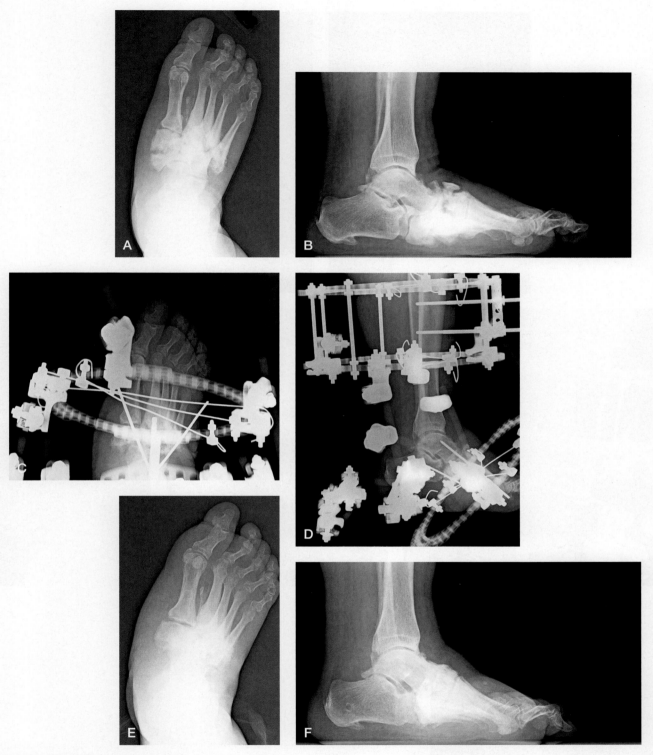

FIGURE 19.9 A,B. Preoperative radiographic views of a right midfoot unstable diabetic Charcot neuroarthropathy with a plantar lateral ulceration and osteomyelitis. Patient underwent an initial deep incision and drainage procedure and obtaining of intraoperative bone and soft tissue cultures and biopsy. **C,D.** The patient returned to the operating room 4 days after the first surgery for a cuboidectomy, osteotomy of the remaining tarsal bones with global midfoot arthrodesis and circular external fixation, and delayed primary closure of the plantar wound. The circular external fixation device was removed at 12 weeks, and the patient was transitioned to a non–weight-bearing lower extremity cast immobilization for 4 weeks. **E,F.** Final postoperative radiographic views at 10 months follow-up showing osseous union and a plantigrade foot.

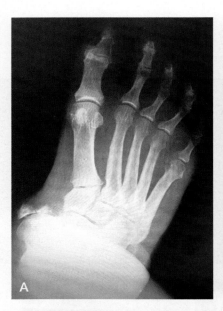
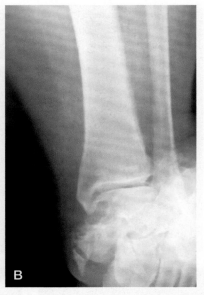
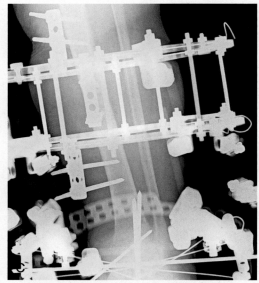
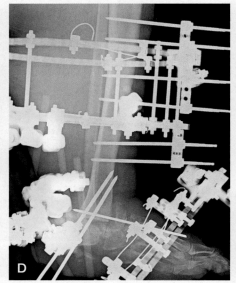
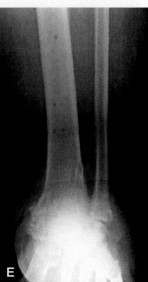
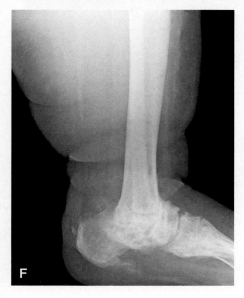

FIGURE 19.10 A,B. Preoperative radiographic views of a right hinfoot/ankle severely unstable diabetic Charcot neuroarthropathy, necrotic/infected wound, and venous stasis dermatitis. **C,D.** Patient underwent a total talectomy with staged tibiocalcaneal arthrodesis and a hybrid external fixation device with the utilization of multiple half pins, transcalcaneal pin fixation, and midfoot circular ring fixation for simultaneous compression, osseous stabilization of the lower extremity, and surgical off-loading. The hybrid external fixation device was removed at 16 weeks, and the patient was transitioned to a non–weight-compressing dressing and lower extremity posterior splint immobilization followed by bracing and custom-made shoes. **E,F.** Final postoperative radiographic views at 14 months follow-up showing a successful tibiocalcaneal arthrodesis.

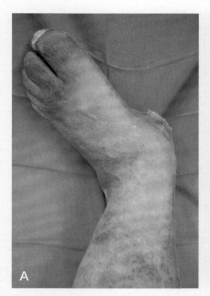

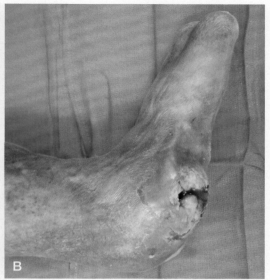

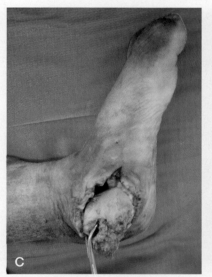

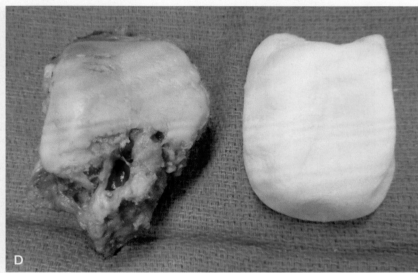

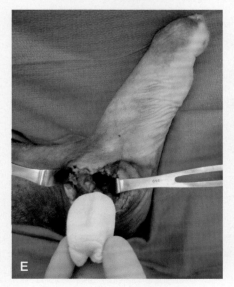

FIGURE 19.11 **A.** Preoperative clinical picture of a left hindfoot/ankle severely unstable diabetic Charcot neuroarthropathy with a chronic nonhealing draining wound and osteomyelitis. Patient underwent an initial deep incision and drainage procedure and obtaining of intraoperative bone and soft tissue cultures and biopsy **(B)** followed by an infectious disease team consultation. The bone cultures were positive for osteomyelitis even though the preoperative medical imaging and intraoperative histopathologic analysis were negative for bone infection. The patient returned to the operating room 4 days after the first surgery for a revisional deep excisional débridement, total talectomy **(C,D)**, and insertion of a nonbiodegradable antibiotic-impregnated polymethylmethacrylate (PMMA) cemented spacer **(D,E)**. Note that the nonbiodegradable antibiotic-impregnated PMMA cemented spacer is similarly contoured to the shape of the resected talus **(D)** before insertion into the large osseous and soft tissue recipient defect **(E)**. *(continued)*

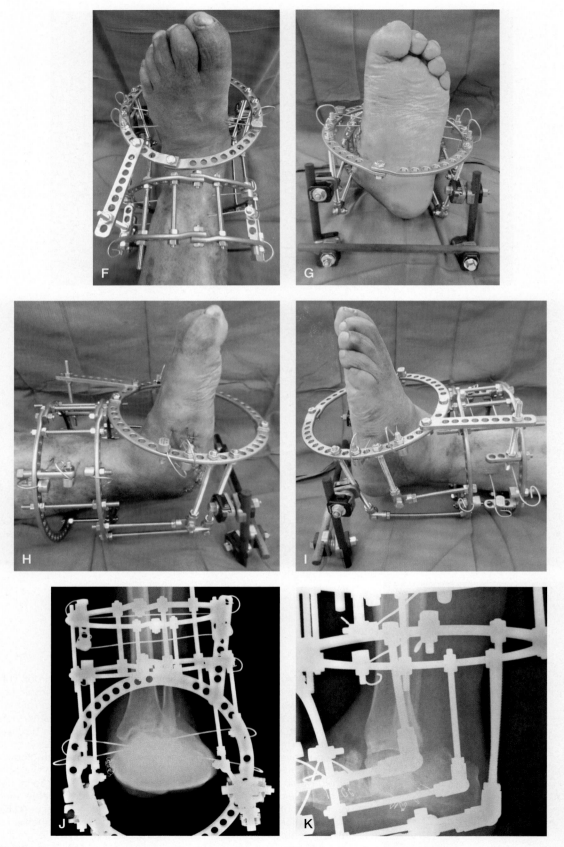

FIGURE 19.11 *(Continued)* A circular external fixation device was utilized for simultaneous osseous and soft tissue stabilization and surgical off-loading **(F–K)**. *(continued)*

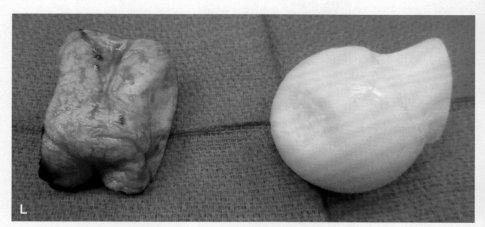

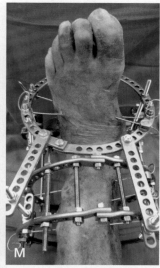

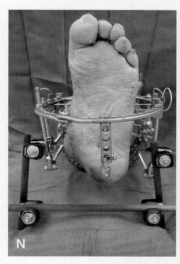

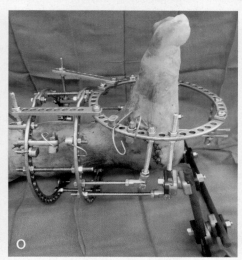

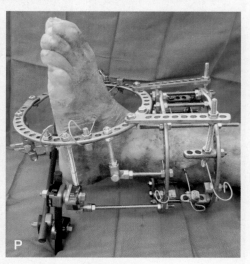

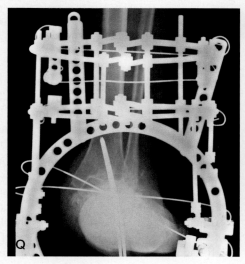

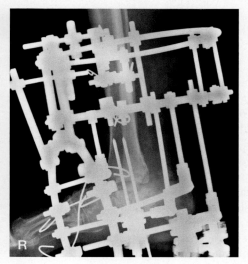

FIGURE 19.11 *(Continued)* At 8 weeks later, the patient returned back to the operating room for removal of the retained non-biodegradable antibiotic-impregnated PMMA cemented spacer and tibiocalcaneal arthrodesis with allogenic bone grafting **(L)** and modification of the preexisting circular external fixation device **(M–R)**. Note the removed nonbiodegradable antibiotic-impregnated PMMA cemented spacer next to the fresh frozen femoral head allograft that is shaped and prepared accordingly for the tibiocalcaneal arthrodesis **(L)**. The circular external fixation device was removed at 9 weeks, and the patient was transitioned to a non–weight-bearing lower extremity cast immobilization followed by a fracture boot and accommodative devices. *(continued)*

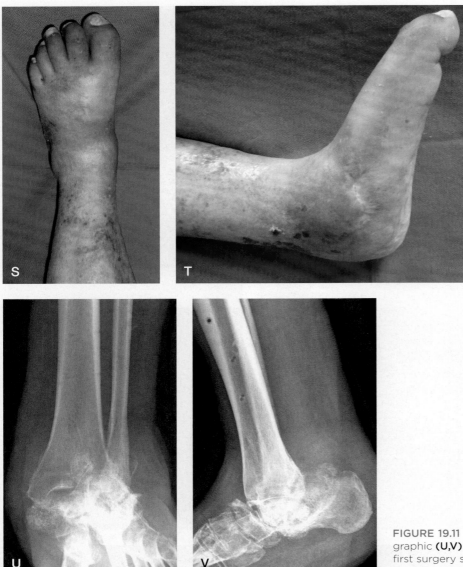

FIGURE 19.11 *(Continued)* Final clinical **(S,T)** and radiographic **(U,V)** pictures at 5.5 months follow-up since the first surgery showing osseous consolidation without recurrent ulceration or infection.

infection. The wounds need to be fully excised in parallel fashion to the joint or area of exposed bone by resecting any associated infected osseous structures. Temporary reduction can be performed with Steinmann pins and/or a spanning external fixation device until the definitive arthrodesis procedure is planned after eradication of the present infection. The reason for this is that associated wounds can be closed in a delayed primary closure fashion after the infected bone is resected and ankle, tibiotalocalcaneal, and/or tibiocalcaneal arthrodesis is performed.

The utilization of smooth and/or threaded Steinmann pins allows for realignment of the foot and lower extremity after adequate bone resection and joint preparation. This is a simple and inexpensive technique that provides temporary osseous stability to facilitate wound closure and external fixation application. Placing Steinmann pins from the posterior inferior aspect of the calcaneus and purchasing the anterior cortex

of the tibia provides increased stability and prevents rotation of a tibiocalcaneal arthrodesis in addition to Steinmann pins placed into the medullary canal of the tibia (Fig. 19.12). Application of Steinmann pins after a wide midfoot resection is typically placed from medial and lateral direction aimed toward the talus and/or anterior process of the calcaneus, respectively.

Wound closure is often performed in delayed primary closure fashion and at the time of definitive bone resection, arthrodesis, and osseous reconstruction. Creating surgical incisions that incorporate preexisting wounds if properly placed can allow for necessary surgical exposures and removal of retained hardware with staged arthrodesis and also permit direct primary closure by reducing wound tension. Reduction of wound tension is paramount to approximate large wounds while preventing postoperative surgical wound dehiscence and infection. Local random muscle and/or pedicle flaps are commonly utilized to address wounds that cannot be closed primarily (1).

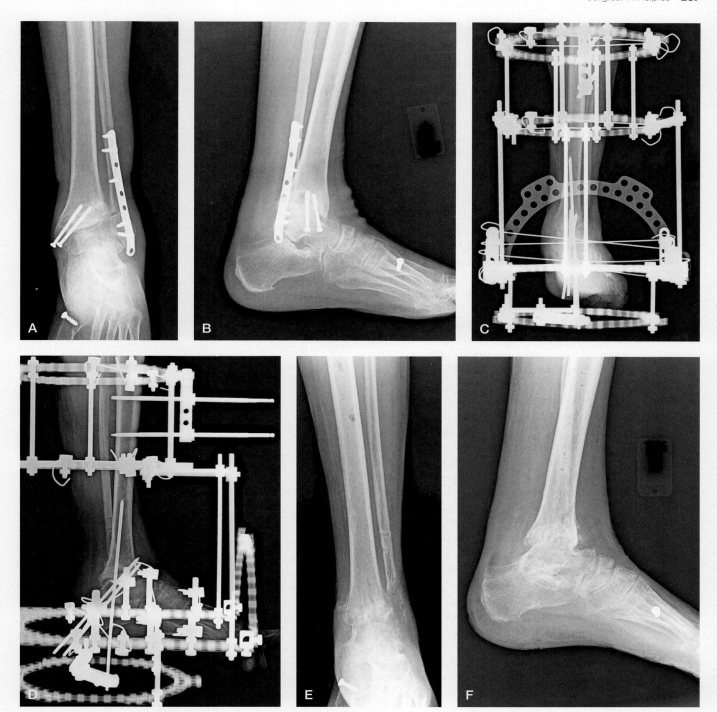

FIGURE 19.12 A,B. Preoperative radiographic views of a right ankle infected nonunion, retained hardware, and unstable diabetic Charcot neuroarthropathy. Patient underwent an initial deep incision and drainage procedure, removal of retained hardware, and obtaining of intraoperative bone and soft tissue cultures and biopsy followed by an infectious disease team consultation. **C,D.** The patient returned to the operating room 7 days after the first surgery for deformity correction and tibiocalcaneal arthrodesis with a circular external fixation device. The circular external fixation device was removed at 16 weeks, and the patient was transitioned to a non–weight-bearing lower extremity cast immobilization for 4 weeks. Patient resumed functional ambulation with a custom-made shoe and bracing at 5 months postoperatively. **E,F.** Final postoperative radiographic views at 6 months follow-up showing successful arthrodesis and lower extremity alignment.

POSTOPERATIVE MANAGEMENT

Postoperative management in this complex diabetic population with CN and concomitant osteomyelitis requires a multidisciplinary team effort. Along with the surgical team, hospitalists, primary care physicians, endocrinologists, nephrologists, vascular surgeons, infectious disease specialists, nutritionists, physical therapists, and social workers are all involved in the postoperative and rehabilitation process of the patient. Close medical observation is paramount because this diabetic population presents with multiple medical comorbidities that require intervention and in order to prevent and minimize any postoperative complications or mortality incidence. Deep vein thrombosis prophylaxis must be coordinated and monitored with other types of anticoagulation that the diabetic patients may be on for cardiac or peripheral arterial disease reasons. The operative lower extremity should be kept elevated and without any weight bearing status at the initial postoperative period. In the presence of a flap closure, its viability and/or further wound management is assessed during the patient's hospitalization by allowing enough space around the circular external fixation device for the wounds to be inspected and/or treated as necessary.

Advancement to the next phase of postoperative care is established once the patient is medically optimized, has stable wound closure without any signs of infection, is able to transfer without any weight bearing status to the operative lower extremity and the antibiotic regimen and dosage has been established by the infectious disease team. Antibiotic therapy and duration is based on clinical, laboratory, medical imaging, and surgical findings. The management of concomitant osteomyelitis in diabetic CN patients if amputation is not performed requires the additional involvement of infectious disease specialists despite the aggressive bone resection and débridement. Residual infection can be detrimental to an arthrodesis site and often result in latent infections and/or infected nonunion that can lead to amputation. For these reasons, prolonged antibiotic therapy is commonly recommended and administered for the management of osteomyelitis in diabetic CN foot and/or ankle deformities.

Before hospital discharge, the patient is assessed for home or extended health care facility placement for rehabilitation and further medical optimization. Postoperative care after hospital discharge typically involves follow-up visits every 2 to 3 weeks until the wounds are healed and are extended longer until osseous union is achieved. After removal of the circular external fixation device, the patient is placed in a non–weight-bearing lower extremity cast until the wound closure has been achieved. Continuous non–weight-bearing status is maintained throughout the postoperative period with frequent lower extremity below-the-knee casting applications and advancement into a fracture boot based on the arthrodesis healing. The patient is then referred to a pedorthotist for proper diabetic shoe fitting, custom inlays, and lower extremity bracing to allow functional ambulation. Diabetic patients with osteomyelitis and CN reconstruction of the foot and/or ankle are followed for a long period of time and are continuously educated on any recurrent clinical and/or medical imaging signs of infection.

Conclusion

As with any surgical treatment algorithm, the surgeon must weigh the benefits and risks when considering reconstruction or amputation in the diabetic CN patient with osteomyelitis. Decision making can be difficult but is ultimately based on the patient's particular condition and associated medical comorbidities, patient, family and surgeon's expectations, and multidisciplinary team efforts. Diabetic lower extremity reconstruction may not be considered if patients are not willing to commit to the prolonged postoperative recovery, when the condition is life threatening, and/or if a functional lower extremity as the end result does not seem feasible.

References

1. Capobianco CM, Zgonis T. Abductor hallucis muscle flap and staged medial column arthrodesis for the chronic ulcerated Charcot foot with concomitant osteomyelitis. Foot Ankle Spec 2010;3:269–273.
2. Dalla Paola L, Brocco E, Ceccacci T, et al. Limb salvage in Charcot foot and ankle osteomyelitis: combined use single stage/double stage of arthrodesis and external fixation. Foot Ankle Int 2009;30:1065–1070.
3. Ramanujam CL, Zgonis T. Antibiotic-loaded cement beads for Charcot ankle osteomyelitis. Foot Ankle Spec 2010;3:274–277.
4. Rodriguez RH, Jeffries LC, Zgonis T. Stepwise approach to foot and ankle osteomyelitis and external fixation. In: Cooper PS, Polyzois VD, Zgonis T, eds. External fixators of the foot and ankle. Philadelphia: Lippincott Williams & Wilkins, 2013;341–359.

CHAPTER 20

Internal, External, and/or Combined Surgical Fixation for the Diabetic Charcot Foot and Ankle Deformity

Patrick R. Burns • Spencer J. Monaco

INTRODUCTION

Surgical interventions and techniques continue to evolve for the treatment of Charcot neuroarthropathy (CN) as the pathology and natural history is better understood. CN is a complicated process of inflammation, fracture, and distortion of anatomy in a medically immunocompromised host. Because of these issues, surgical treatment of CN will test the surgeon's understanding and skill of technique and fixation principles. Comprehensive treatment requires knowledge and experience in many other areas including medicine, biology, physiology, psychology, and biomechanics. Addressing the patient's blood glucose levels, nutrition, vascular status, infection, and social issues is extremely important and should not be neglected. Although these issues are essential to improved outcomes, this chapter focuses on surgical fixation methods.

The basic principles of internal and external fixation need to be well understood when dealing with CN in the active (acute) stage or the inactive (chronic) stage in the presence or absence of ulceration. In each stage, the deformity location is considered because it plays a significant role in the surgical approach. Foot and ankle deformities from CN can be addressed with primary internal fixation, primary external fixation, a combination of both internal fixation and external fixation, or a staged reconstruction approach utilizing internal fixation after the initial treatment with external fixation.

DECISIONS ON CHARCOT NEUROARTHROPATHY TREATMENT (ACTIVE VERSUS INACTIVE)

On initial presentation, there are a few important factors to be distinguished which help decide on treatment and if surgical, which type of fixation. Certain types of fixation may be best utilized in firm circumstances, with the surgeon being able to choose the fixation that may be most advantageous.

One of the first objectives is to divide the CN into either the active or inactive stage (Fig. 20.1). There is a certain controversy among surgeons about timing of surgical intervention. Some believe that the active stage may lead to increased complications, in particular with soft tissue healing and infection. There seems to be no question; in the active phase, there is an increased inflammatory process, leading to amplified edema and irritation of local soft tissue. This clinical case scenario can be one of the reasons that surgery in the active CN may not tolerate large incisions and prominent hardware. However, there is literature to support early intervention in select active CN cases (1,5). For example, significant dislocations are most likely going to be an issue with gross instability and a non-plantigrade foot which becomes challenging to brace. In these clinical case scenarios, it may be more reasonable to intervene early versus waiting for consolidation (Case Study 1). If early surgical intervention is not achieved in the active CN stage, many of these severe dislocations and deformities will have a wound or infection that compounds the existing pathologic entity. Even though without the presence of a wound, it can still be more difficult to surgically correct an inactive consolidated deformity.

In some cases, a concept similar to the evolution of surgical treatment of pilon injuries, a more staged surgical approach may be beneficial (Fig. 20.2). A significant deformity in the active CN stage can be addressed with surgery to achieve better osseous alignment and stabilization until it becomes inactive with the use of external fixation. It can then be converted to more permanent internal fixation construct in the inactive stage (Case Studies 2 and 3). This will allow the soft tissue envelope to improve as well as making the staged procedure much more straightforward as the foot and ankle are held in a more anatomic position. The index operation maintains reduction with the external fixation device and will likely aid in the CN process to become inactive by not allowing for continued fracture, dislocation, and collapse. This also allows the diabetic patient to be medically optimized from a local and systemic standpoint.

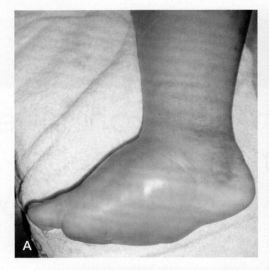

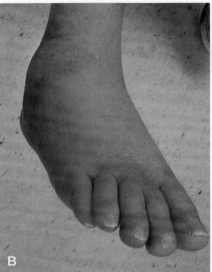

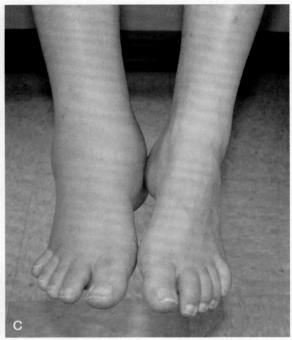

FIGURE 20.1 Clinical examples of active **(A)** and inactive **(B)** Charcot neuroarthropathy (CN) as well as a comparison of both feet of a single patient **(C)**. Note the edema and erythema that accompanies the active CN stage **(A)**.

Charcot Neuroarthropathy with or without Ulceration

A second piece of information on the initial CN presentation is the presence or absence of ulceration. In general, most surgical procedures should be performed in the context of a closed soft tissue envelope. Attempts must be made to heal a wound prior to any surgical intervention. Wounds that are stable and in a location that can be conservatively off-loaded should be the first treatment option when feasible. A wound that can be healed without surgery is the best clinical case scenario (Fig. 20.3). Once the wound is healed, fixation is usually internal or a combination of internal and external fixation with less concern about deep infection as it relates to the wound and fixation. If the wound is unable to be healed without surgical intervention, the surgery itself becomes much more complicated from an infection risk standpoint. These diabetic patients are either in the active stage with a significant deformity and acute wound or inactive stage with a nonhealing chronic wound. Either case

may be complicated by osteomyelitis and will need a staged protocol as mentioned earlier. With the deformity reduced, the external fixator not only allows for decreased tension on the ulceration but also allows access for local wound care and infection management. Osseous stability clearly aids in infection control and soft tissue healing. This surgical protocol is similar to severe traumatic injuries where an external fixation device is utilized for staged treatments stabilizing the soft tissue and osseous structures and thus minimizing continued inflammation from instability. Osseous instability leads to constant movement of the soft tissues which can then lead to delayed wound healing and infection.

Charcot Neuroarthropathy with Ulceration and Osteomyelitis

In the setting of inactive CN with a nonhealing or recurrent wound, the fixation may vary (3). Surgical reconstruction many times is staged with external fixation similar to active

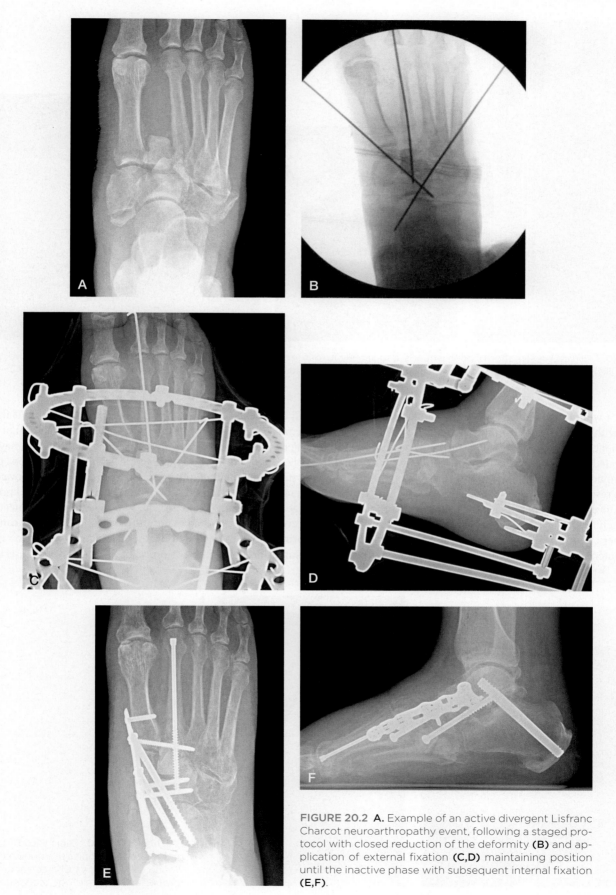

FIGURE 20.2 A. Example of an active divergent Lisfranc Charcot neuroarthropathy event, following a staged protocol with closed reduction of the deformity **(B)** and application of external fixation **(C,D)** maintaining position until the inactive phase with subsequent internal fixation **(E,F)**.

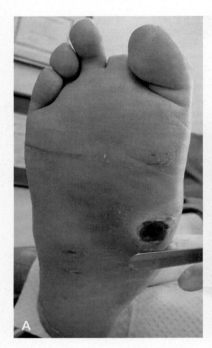
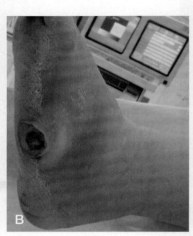
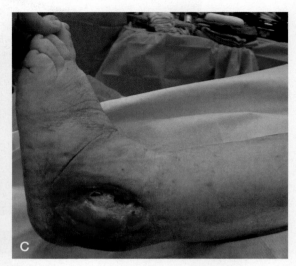

FIGURE 20.3 Clinical presentation of open wounds associated with deformities secondary to Charcot neuroarthropathy. Some wounds are more likely to heal with nonsurgical means **(A)**, whereas others are more likely to be unstable and fail nonsurgical care **(B,C)**.

CN with a wound for similar reasons. This is useful in those patients with longstanding wounds and osteomyelitis. As part of treatment, the bone is débrided and/or removed. While being treated with appropriate antibiotic therapy, an external fixator provides stability and maintains reduction until the infection is resolved (Case Study 4). The external fixation device is then converted to a more permanent internal fixation construct when feasible.

Another option in this particular clinical case scenario is immediate internal fixation. According to the surgeon's preference and experience, the wound and bone may be excised. If there are no clinical signs of infection present after the removal of the potential areas of concern, immediate internal fixation may be utilized (Fig. 20.4). This is also a time where some surgeons perform a combination of internal and external fixation. However, there are a few arguments for combined fixation. One is knowledge of infection. There is a question whether bone infection is ever completely eradicated and pockets of infection can lie dormant only to be stirred by internal fixation. A surgeon may assume that the entire osteomyelitis with the wedge resection

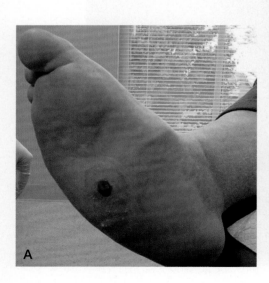
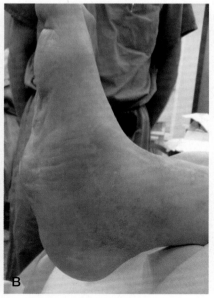

FIGURE 20.4 A–C. Clinical and radiographic case examples of a noninfected wound secondary to Charcot neuroarthropathy of the midfoot. *(continued)*

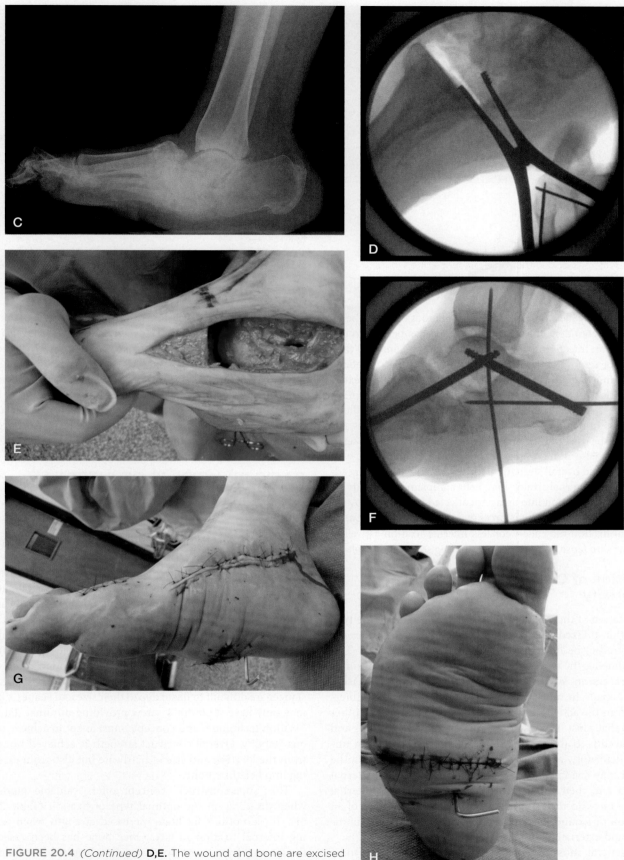

FIGURE 20.4 *(Continued)* **D,E.** The wound and bone are excised during surgery and internal fixation is placed **(F–H)**. *(continued)*

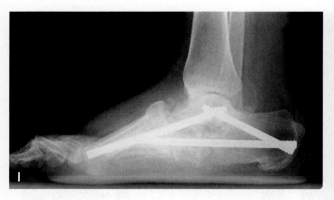

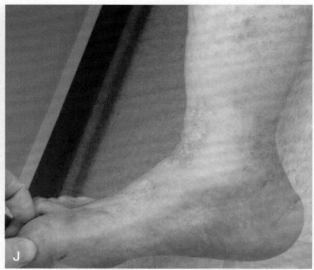

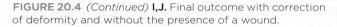

FIGURE 20.4 *(Continued)* **I,J.** Final outcome with correction of deformity and without the presence of a wound.

osteotomy may have been removed, but there is difficulty being completely confident that all infected bone has been resected. If there is an infection that activates after surgery, internal fixation can be removed but the external fixator remains for stability and continued treatment. The combination of internal and external fixation may also be useful in the patient with CN to improve and increase overall stability. These CN deformities are difficult to address in many ways; in the case of fixation principles, the bone may be osteoporotic and space is limited both in the sense of bone but also skin coverage. These factors may interfere with placement and overall strength of local internal fixation. The addition of an external fixator may help complement stability by extending the fixation into areas not affected by the local osteoporosis of CN and distribute forces over a greater anatomic area. External fixation may allow for less internal fixation as well as decrease skin tension from the surrounding soft tissue envelope.

Location of Charcot Neuroarthropathy Deformity

The location of the CN deformity also plays a role in the type of fixation utilized. Some CN foot and ankle deformities are considered to be more unstable than others (Fig. 20.5). This may influence the type of fixation and also the timing of surgical intervention. With a grossly unstable deformity, a decision may be made to move forward with an early surgical intervention in the active stage. Following this decision, the other factors that must be considered are concomitant wounds and osteomyelitis. If there is a wound in the presence of an unstable deformity, a more rapid intervention is required. The patient may need to undergo a staged protocol with external fixation and then converted to a more permanent internal fixation once deemed more appropriate. In the absence of an infection or wound, internal fixation or a combination of internal and external fixation may be all that is required.

In general, most surgeons consider CN of the ankle to be more unstable and therefore more likely to go on to significant

deformity and the development of ulceration earlier than in cases involving the midfoot. However, there are certainly midfoot events that dislocate and cause skin tenting which would fall into the urgent category as well (2). It takes an understanding of the natural history of CN and surgeon experience to assist in the decision making process. The overall goal is to understand the patient with CN that would benefit from surgical intervention and those that would do well with nonsurgical management (Case Studies 5–8).

BASIC PRINCIPLES OF INTERNAL FIXATION FOR CHARCOT NEUROARTHROPATHY

When addressing deformities associated with CN, the type of internal fixation chosen is dictated by the location of the deformity and the local bone anatomy. Internal fixation is much more technically difficult in this condition. Normal anatomy is often distorted from the CN process. Furthermore, local osteoporosis results from the physiology of CN and the fact that many patients have been non–weight-bearing for an extended period of time. Bones may be fragmented or even missing in these deformities, making traditional plates and fixation techniques quite challenging. Many foot bones in the best circumstances are difficult to fixate due to their size and shape. A bone may only have room for 1 screw providing minimal stability. Fixation techniques and concepts must adapt to achieve osseous stability. Overall construct strength is achieved not only from the location and size of hardware but also from extending into healthier bone.

The "superconstruct" concept offers valuable guidance when deciding on the optimal type of fixation (Table 20.1) (4). These notions facilitate increased strength when utilizing internal fixation in CN. Once bone has been resected, the internal fixation employed needs to be placed in the most mechanically advantageous position. For midfoot CN, some

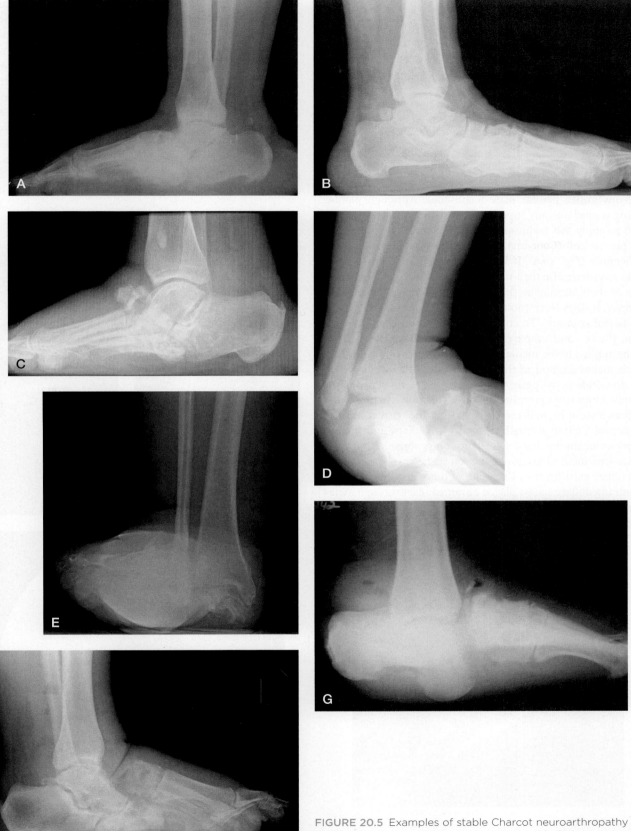

FIGURE 20.5 Examples of stable Charcot neuroarthropathy deformities that may not require surgery **(A–C)** in contrast to more unstable deformities that most likely will require surgical intervention **(D–G)**.

TABLE 20.1
Superconstruct Concept for Charcot Neuroarthropathy Fixation
Resect enough bone to allow reduction of deformity and reduce skin tension
Extend the fixation/arthrodesis beyond the zone of injury
Utilize the strongest fixation devices in the most mechanically sound way permitted by the local skin and soft tissues

surgeons utilize plantar plate techniques. Although plantar plating is mechanically superior for resisting tension, it is difficult to apply this technique in most of the CN deformities. The plantar soft tissue makes placement of plates technically challenging (Fig. 20.6). It is also extremely difficult to place plates anywhere else than the medial column. The medial column of the foot may be the most important area to address; however, it does leave room for improvement for the central and lateral columns. To combat these issues, plates have become thicker and employ locking technology. These plates can be applied to the medial and dorsal surface of the midfoot which makes fixation of these deformities technically easier. The downside is the potential for soft tissue and skin-related complications from prominent internal fixation hardware. The surgeon should be well-versed in finding the correct balance of internal fixation strength from size and shape and the appropriate location to limit soft tissue compromise.

Another method to address the soft tissue envelope concern is to utilize axial fixation. Examples of this category of fixation are intramedullary screws placed intramedullary through metatarsals and midfoot bones or even intramedullary devices of the ankle (Fig. 20.7). This allows a mechanically superior form of fixation, with compression generated directly across the prepared surfaces without the soft tissue impingement associated with more traditional plates and screws. The drawback may be the potential for rotation if axial fixation is the only form employed. To counteract rotational issues, some surgeons employ a technique referred to as "locking the beam." Smaller locking plates or at times just additional screws are added to the construct before or after the intramedullary device. Having fixation in differing planes is biomechanically more complete (Fig. 20.8).

The next concept in internal fixation of gaining mechanical strength with relation to the limitations of bone size, shape, and quality is by extending the fixation past the zone of injury.

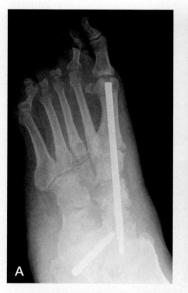
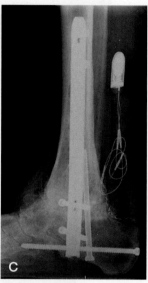
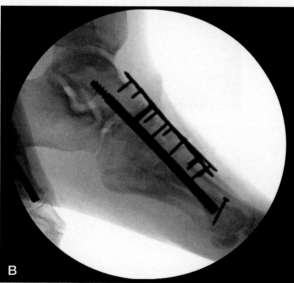

FIGURE 20.6 Example of a plantar plate application along the medial column for reconstruction of Charcot neuroarthropathy. Although plantar plate fixation is more biomechanically advantageous, it can be a difficult form of fixation to employ.

FIGURE 20.7 **A–C.** Different clinical case scenarios of a superconstruct technique of intramedullary fixation which provides axial compression with limited or no compromise to the soft tissue.

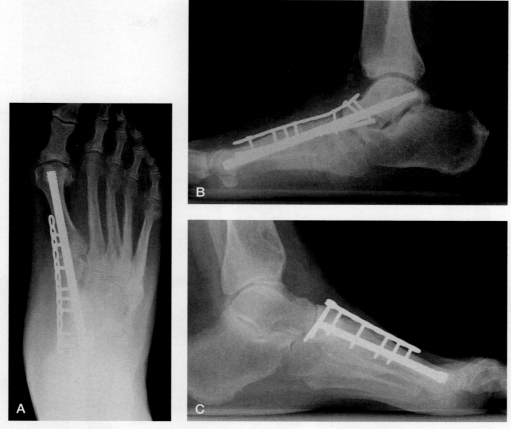

FIGURE 20.8 A–C. Different clinical case scenarios of "locking the beam" concept to add rotational stability to the axial compression generated by the intramedullary fixation.

This seems to be one of the most important concepts when addressing fixation in CN foot and ankle deformities. This concept describes the principle of extending the arthrodesis and fixation for at least 1, if not more, joints distal and proximal to the injured zone. Extending the zone of injury allows for more fixations as well as distributing the stress of the surgical site over a larger anatomic area. This technique may also help limit certain movement or motion from adjacent joints which can be detrimental in this particular population. In lieu of not being able to apply fixation in the best mechanical orientation, extending past the zone of injury is a reasonable method to achieve increased strength. This technique also helps control other local potentially detrimental forces coming from adjacent joints. For certain deformities, it may mean including the ankle joint might be necessary when extending from the zone of injury (Fig. 20.9).

BASIC PRINCIPLES OF EXTERNAL FIXATION FOR CHARCOT NEUROARTHROPATHY

Utilizing circular external fixation is a mandatory skill if treating patients with CN deformities. Many standard principles of external fixation can be applied when managing midfoot, hindfoot, or ankle deformities. However, there are some potential differences concerning weight bearing when compared to a more traditional patient and procedure. The first concept to remember is the difficulty with distal fixation in the foot. The external fixator can be made extremely strong more proximal in the tibia and ankle. In the leg, there is adequate space for fixation with added fixation of drop wires and half-pins to augment the strength. However, in the midfoot and distal part of the foot, there are issues with the amount of space for fixation wires as well as the amount of tension tolerated, making the distal part of the external fixator less robust. Therefore, in patients with surgical correction through the midfoot, one of the limiting factors is the distal fixation. The other consideration concerning with midfoot deformities is the biomechanical forces. In the ankle, it is an axial force that is tolerated well in an external fixator. In the midfoot, it is more of a shear force that can be more difficult to control, especially with a reduced amount of fixation as previously stated. For these reasons, weight bearing with external fixation in midfoot CN may not be tolerated well. This is in contrast to most ankle constructs that do not have the same limitations. The other concern regarding weight bearing in patients with external fixation and CN, is the immunocompromised host itself. It has been shown that although most are minor, complications rates with external fixation in patients with diabetes mellitus and neuropathy are as a whole more frequent.

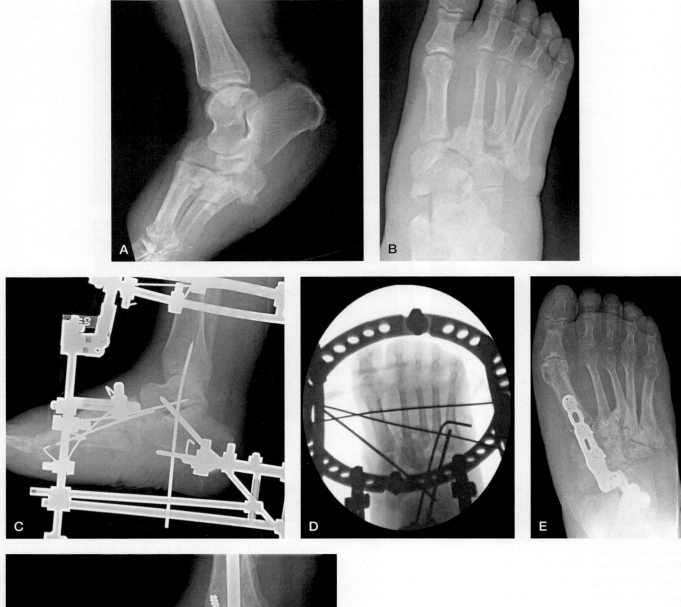

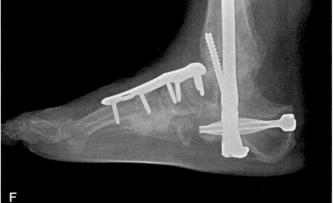

FIGURE 20.9 **A,B.** Clinical case scenario of extending the arthrodesis past the zone of injury. A staged reconstruction of a divergent Lisfranc Charcot neuroarthropathy with associated midfoot and navicular fractures **C,D.** The circular external fixator was used for the initial stage followed by an extended arthrodesis to include the ankle joint in order to gain increased fixation and biomechanical control in the inactive phase **(E,F).**

For many surgeons, there are 2 main constructs of external fixation for CN reconstruction but certainly can depend on the deformity and goal of fixation. Most external fixation in this patient population is utilized for off-loading wounds, infection management, deformity reduction, and maintenance of position. The first and most common form of external fixator is useful for distal tibia, ankle, and subtalar CN. It consists of a tibial "block" of 2 rings and a foot plate (Fig. 20.10). This configuration depending on the deformity may allow the foot to be exposed plantarly or an additional plate to be applied for heel touch weight bearing. There is also the ability to compress axially, if the deformity and treatment plan is such and it can be tolerated. External fixation can be a useful technique in the cases of a septic joint or a patient with osteomyelitis. The external fixator can be continually compressed over the weeks to achieve an arthrodesis which may negate the need for further surgery.

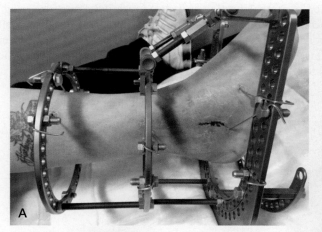
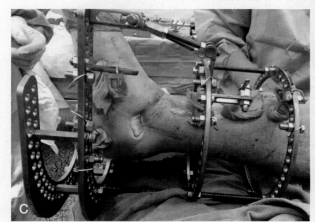
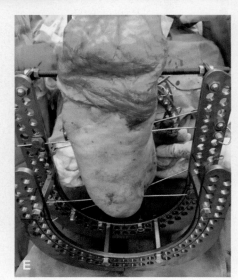
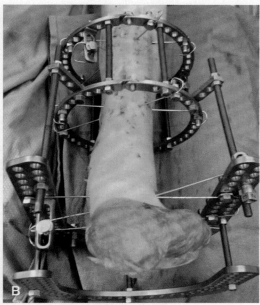
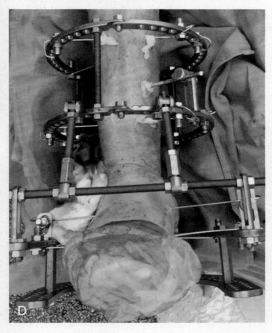

FIGURE 20.10 A–E. Examples of one of the most common circular external fixators used for ankle Charcot neuroarthropathy, showing the tibial "block" of 2 rings, a foot plate, and an additional plantar foot plate protecting the plantar surface of the foot.

The second basic external fixator configuration for CN starts with the same tibial "block," but the foot component is modified (Fig. 20.11). A smaller, half ring replaces the larger foot plate around the heel. Another full ring is then placed around the midfoot and forefoot zone in an axial position. This ring is then connected proximally to the tibial block. The midfoot/forefoot ring allows for increased fixation in the difficult midfoot and forefoot region, increasing strength. It can also be manipulated with respect to the hindfoot and ankle, assisting in reduction. A traditional foot plate in midfoot CN limits the surgeon to the correction performed with joint preparation and osteotomies. There is usually no surgical space to adjust or improve once the foot is connected to the traditional foot plate. The midfoot/forefoot ring construct on the other hand, gives the surgeon the potential to

adjust if desired. This construct also makes the external fixator unique in its design with the patient being unable to bear weight which may be beneficial in this type of reconstruction.

Once the type and configuration of external fixation is decided, proper implementation is essential. Inappropriate assembly or application of the circular external fixator can even damage more an otherwise well-maintained reconstruction. The external fixator in any form must be itself strong enough to withhold any biomechanical forces. Knowing the basic external fixation principles regarding ring size, ring number, amount of connecting elements, and proper placement will improve outcomes. It is also recommended to add more connecting elements, fixation wires, and half-pins to these external fixation constructs as well.

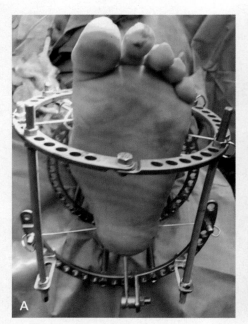
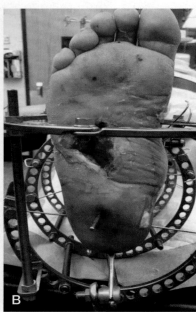
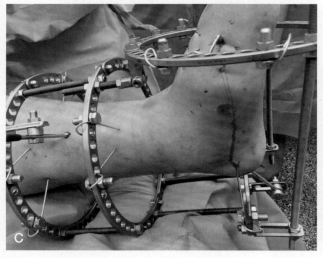
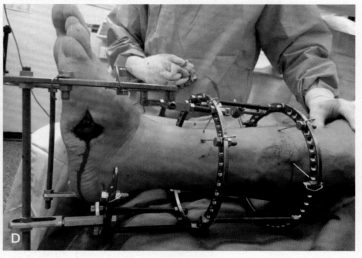

FIGURE 20.11 A–F. Examples of one type of circular external fixator used for midfoot Charcot neuroarthropathy. Note the ring around the foot; to improve fixation and control over the midfoot deformity, allow for better compression and completely off-load the pressure areas. *(continued)*

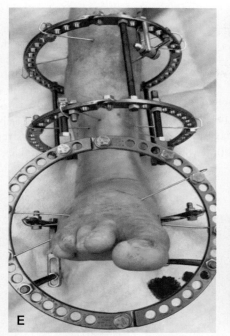
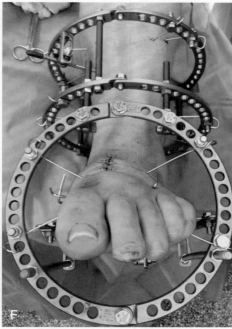

FIGURE 20.11 *(Continued)*

Once the circular external fixator is applied, postoperative care is just as important. Patients must adhere to the surgeon's weight bearing guidelines as well as wire/pin care (Fig. 20.12). It is generally accepted that there will be a wire/pin or 2 during the process that will become locally infected (6). This is dealt with proper local care and, at times, adjustment of the external fixator in the operating room. It is generally accepted that just once or twice a week cleaning with mild soap and water or similar is all that is required. More frequent cleaning and more aggressive agents may actually irritate and cause issues at the wire/pin skin interface. If on the other hand it is multiple pin sites that are becoming irritated or infected, the surgeon needs to concentrate at the stability of the external fixator or the application as the main cause. If the external fixator is not strong enough or if there is too much movement, the skin will be irritated against the wires/pins resulting in infection. Wire/pin tract irritations or infections may also be due to increased heat generated while applying the external fixator or leaving tension on the skin secondary to improper wire/pin placement. All of these factors will lead to irritation and local skin necrosis compromising the wire/pin skin interface.

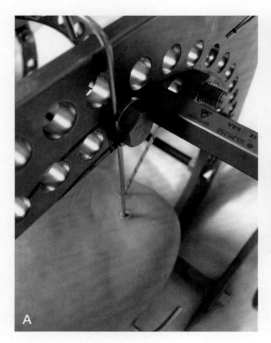
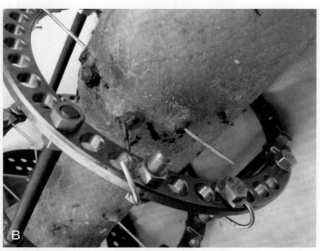

FIGURE 20.12 Clinical case examples of clean **(A)** and irritated/infected **(B)** transosseous wire surgical sites. Proper application of wires/half-pins and aftercare is extremely important in this high-risk diabetic population.

COMBINED INTERNAL AND EXTERNAL FIXATION FOR CHARCOT NEUROARTHROPATHY

In some CN cases, internal fixation itself may not be adequate enough for the surgical correction and anatomic alignment. In addition, there may not be enough bone or the bones may be severely dislocated for adequate internal fixation. In these cases, placing an external fixator in conjunction with the internal fixation may provide additional stability and anatomic correction. It also may be an extension of the internal fixation concept of extending the fixation beyond the zone of injury and immediate surgery. For example, in some CN reconstructions, there can be very little bone left behind after reaming and débridement, so internal fixation may be inadequate for the desired arthrodesis. A surgeon can place limited internal fixation when feasible and also add an external fixator to provide stability and strength by allowing extension of the fixation to the ankle and leg (Fig. 20.13).

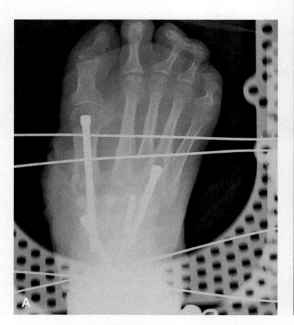
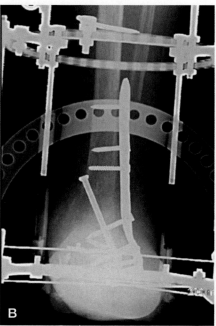
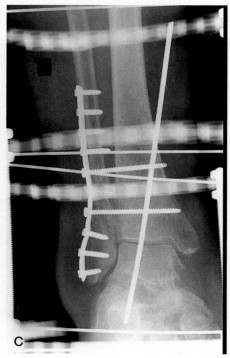

FIGURE 20.13 A–H. Different clinical case examples of combined internal and external fixation for Charcot neuroarthropathy of the foot and ankle. In certain cases, this allows for improved fixation, fixation extended beyond the zone of injury, and essential fixation in this high-risk diabetic population. *(continued)*

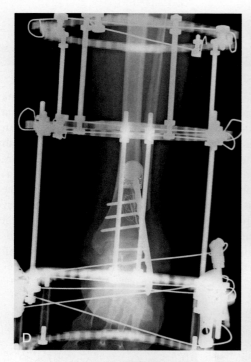
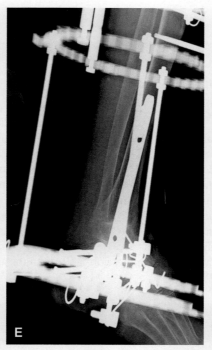
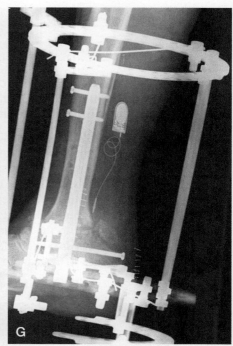
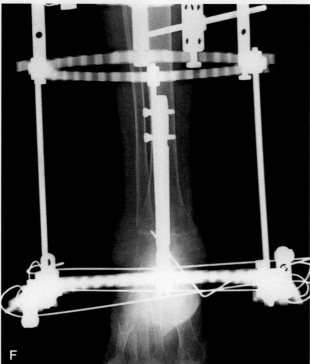
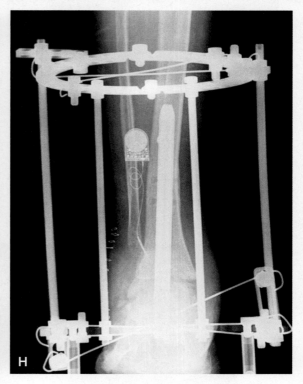

FIGURE 20.13 *(Continued)*

The combination of fixation, in particular for CN reconstruction may allow for adequate control of biomechanical forces and earlier weight bearing, although this has not been shown. However, internal fixation in an axial form, plantar plate, or some of the other methods discussed earlier may help battle the axial forces the external fixator may otherwise not be able to withstand alone. The combined fixation construct may work to permit at least some weight bearing, making the entire process somewhat more tolerable for the patient. Having both internal and external fixation may also be beneficial in CN because if something were to happen to one type of fixation, the other one can still remain.

CLINICAL CASES

Active Charcot Neuroarthropathy of the Midfoot without Ulceration; Surgical Fixation Choice: Internal Fixation

A 36-year-old male with a history of diabetes mellitus, peripheral neuropathy, and a recent injury at work to his left foot was referred to our center with a swollen, red left foot. His injury was 1 week prior, and he was placed into a boot by his work doctor. On physical examination, the patient had peripheral neuropathy, with a swollen, erythematous left foot. The edema and erythema extended to the proximal leg (A). There was no wound, but an obvious midfoot deformity with increased width was evident. He was treated with aggressive compression therapy along with non–weight-bearing consisting of Unna boot and soft cast over the following 2 weeks to reduce edema (B). Plain radiographs revealed a Lisfranc fracture-dislocation with a divergent type injury (C,D). An open reduction with primary arthrodesis was then performed including the entire first and second rays as well as the subtalar joint. Internal fixation was a combination of locking plate and large screws. The arthrodesis was extended beyond the zone of obvious injury to gain access to better bone quality, giving increased fixation strength. The subtalar joint was included to extend past the injury zone to control hindfoot inversion/eversion and to limit stress on the arthrodesis and injury sites (E–G).

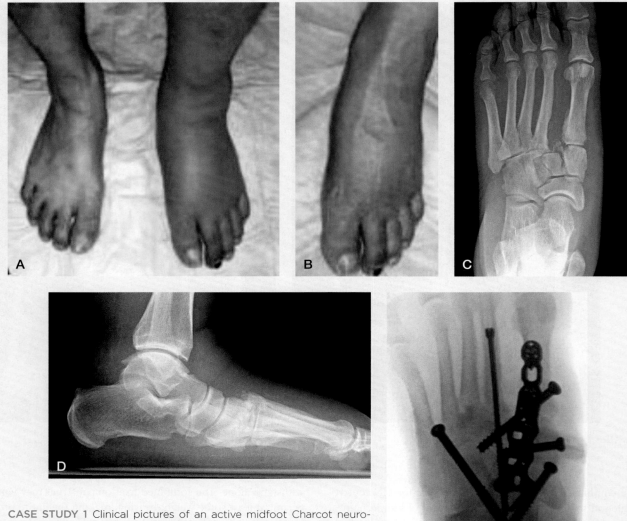

CASE STUDY 1 Clinical pictures of an active midfoot Charcot neuroarthropathy at initial presentation **(A)** and 2 weeks after compression therapy and non–weight-bearing status **(B)**. Preoperative anteroposterior **(C)** and lateral **(D)** radiographic views showing the Lisfranc fracture-dislocation with a divergent type injury. *(continued)*

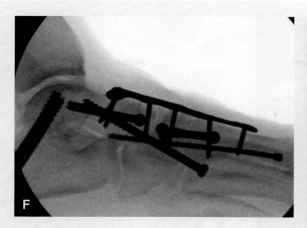

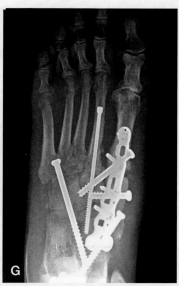

CASE STUDY 1 *(Continued)* Patient underwent an open reduction with primary arthrodesis including the entire first and second rays as well as the subtalar joint extended beyond the zone of injury **(E–G)**.

CASE STUDY 2

Active Charcot Neuroarthropathy of the Midfoot without Ulceration; Surgical Fixation Choice: Staged External to Internal Fixation

A 54-year-old female was referred to our center after 4 weeks of management by another physician. The patient had no specific injury and worked as a nurse. She noticed some swelling and redness on her leg, was treated for cellulitis, and had Doppler studies performed to rule out deep vein thrombosis. Plain radiographs were performed, and she was referred to our center for fracture care. She had a history of longstanding diabetes mellitus and on physical examination had peripheral neuropathy. She had moderate edema and erythema to the left foot and ankle. A preulcerative lesion was present over the medial cuneiform with blanching erythema and obvious gross deformity (A). Plain radiographs revealed a divergent Lisfranc fracture-dislocation with significant shortening and deformity at the medial cuneiform (B,C). In the operating room, the midfoot deformity was reduced with closed techniques and a small incision to aid reduction of the first and second rays. Temporary fixation was applied consisting of Kirschner wires and followed by a circular external fixator (D–F). The circular external fixator provided stability, aiding in reducing the inflammatory process while maintaining reduction. It remained in place for approximately 2 months while the Charcot neuroarthropathy event became more inactive. The injury was then converted to an extended arthrodesis, utilizing locking plates and large screws extending past the zone of injury (G,H).

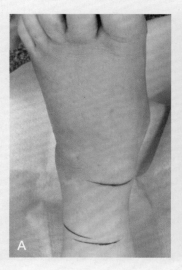

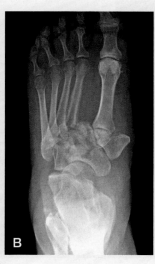

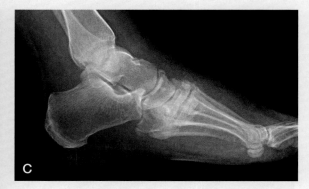

CASE STUDY 2 Clinical **(A)** and radiographic **(B,C)** views of an active midfoot Charcot neuroarthropathy at initial presentation. *(continued)*

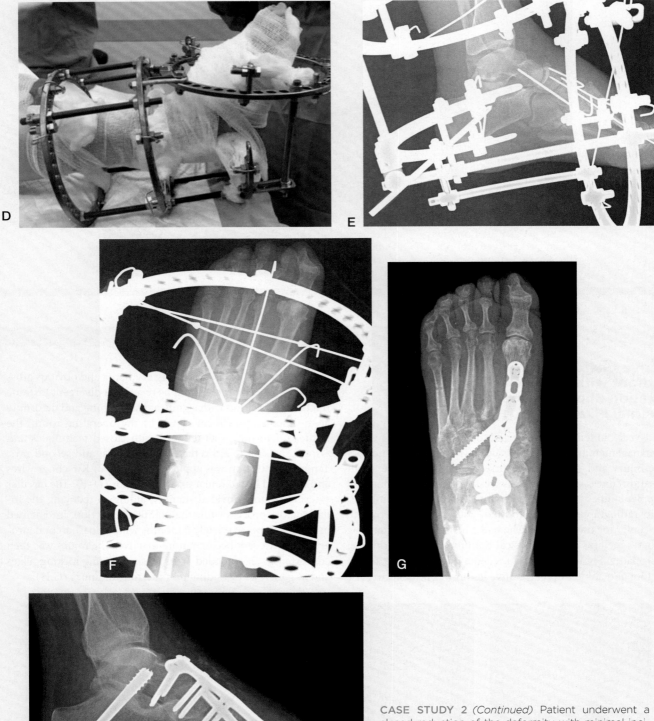

CASE STUDY 2 *(Continued)* Patient underwent a closed reduction of the deformity with minimal incisions, temporary fixation, and application of a circular external fixator **(D–F)**. The circular external fixator remained in place for approximately 2 months, while the Charcot neuroarthropathy event became more inactive. Following the external fixation removal, the initial injury was then converted to an extended arthrodesis, utilizing locking plates and large screws and extending past the zone of injury **(G,H)**.

CASE STUDY 3

Active Charcot Neuroarthropathy of the Ankle without Ulceration; Surgical Fixation Choice: Staged External to Internal Fixation

A 67-year-old male was referred to our center with increasing edema and lower extremity deformity over a period of 2 weeks. The patient had a history of diabetes mellitus with no specific injury. He presented after a recent admission to an outside hospital for this condition, where Doppler studies were performed, and he was started on intravenous antibiotic therapy. Plain radiographs and computed tomography scan were completed. On physical examination, the patient had a severe valgus deformity to the left ankle and foot without any wounds. The deformity was nonreducible and imaging studies demonstrated dislocation of the subtalar joint with local debris

(A–C). Patient was taken urgently to the operation room for closed reduction with a small incision near the sinus tarsi to aid in reduction. The deformity could not be manually reduced and a femoral distractor was needed. A half-pin was inserted in the tibia as well as the calcaneus to help distract and realign the dislocation. These half-pins were then maintained once the femoral distractor was removed and were incorporated into the circular external fixator (D,E). The circular external fixator maintained reduction over the following 2 months, whereas the Charcot neuroarthropathy event became less active. Once the edema and erythema resolved, the external fixation was removed and converted to internal fixation consisting of an intramedullary nail and compression screws (F,G). This method allowed for a rigid intramedullary fixation and extended past the zone of injury to gain increased fixation and stability.

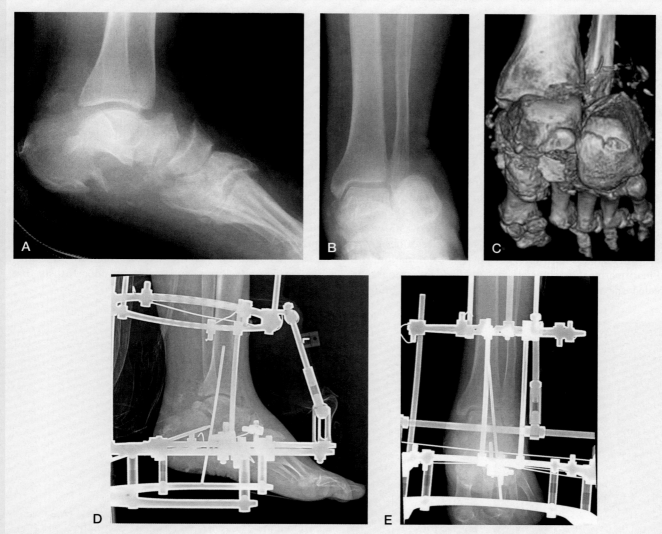

CASE STUDY 3 Radiographic **(A,B)** and medical imaging **(C)** views of an active ankle Charcot neuroarthropathy with fracture-dislocation. Patient underwent a closed reduction of the deformity with minimal incisions, temporary fixation, and application of a circular external fixator **(D,E)**. *(continued)*

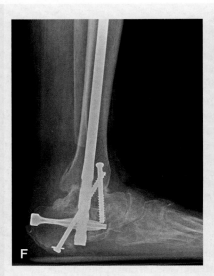

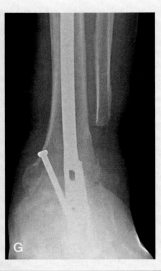

CASE STUDY 3 *(Continued)* Following the external fixation removal, the initial injury was then converted to internal fixation, utilizing a rigid intramedullary fixation and compressions screws being extended past the zone of injury to gain increased fixation and stability **(F,G)**.

CASE STUDY | **4**

Active Charcot Neuroarthropathy of the Ankle with Ulceration and Infection; Surgical Fixation Choice: External Fixation

A 71-year-old female with idiopathic neuropathy and a history of a low-energy pilon fracture was referred to our center with increasing lower extremity deformity and exposed hardware. The patient was initially treated with a spanning external fixator followed by open reduction and internal fixation (ORIF) of the pilon fracture 1 week after the initial surgery. At her clinical visit in our center, she was 3 weeks postoperative with open wounds on both sides of her ankle along with exposed hardware. On physical examination, she had neuropathy and an unstable left ankle. Plain radiographs revealed the recently performed ORIF with new findings of ankle subluxation, destruction, and some fragmentation consistent with active Charcot neuroarthropathy (A,B). Patient was taken urgently to the operating room for surgical débridement and internal fixation hardware removal. Intraoperative cultures were obtained, and a circular external fixator was applied (C–G). Because the talus and tibia were essentially prepared for arthrodesis, the circular external fixator not only could maintain position and aid in inflammation reduction and infection management but also could be utilized to potentially achieve the ankle arthrodesis. Appropriate guided antibiotic therapy and consults were placed. The patient continued with the circular fixator for 3 months, achieving wound closure and stable pseudoarthrosis that could be managed with bracing (H–K).

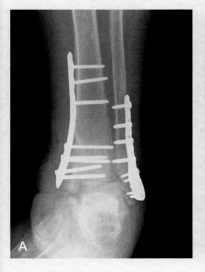

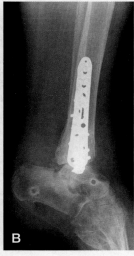

CASE STUDY 4 Preoperative radiographic ankle **(A,B)** views showing findings of ankle subluxation, destruction, and fragmentation consistent with an infected active Charcot neuroarthropathy after a failed open reduction and internal fixation of an ankle fracture. *(continued)*

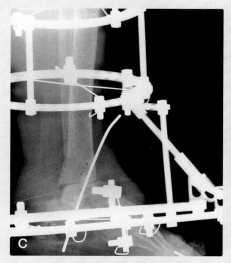

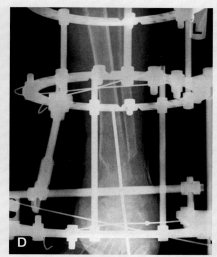

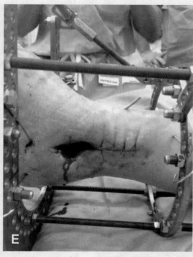

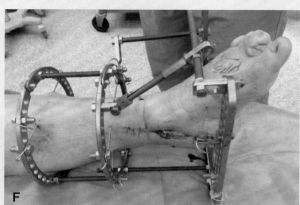

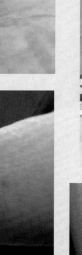

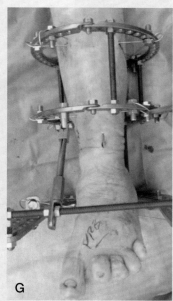

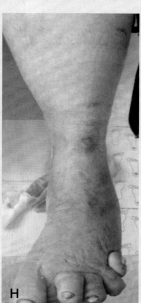

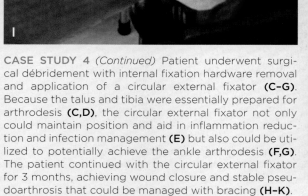

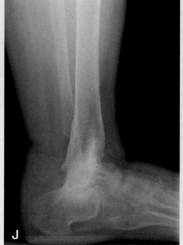

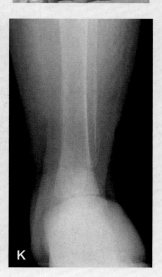

CASE STUDY 4 *(Continued)* Patient underwent surgical débridement with internal fixation hardware removal and application of a circular external fixator **(C–G)**. Because the talus and tibia were essentially prepared for arthrodesis **(C,D)**, the circular external fixator not only could maintain position and aid in inflammation reduction and infection management **(E)** but also could be utilized to potentially achieve the ankle arthrodesis **(F,G)**. The patient continued with the circular external fixator for 3 months, achieving wound closure and stable pseudoarthrosis that could be managed with bracing **(H–K)**.

Inactive Charcot Neuroarthropathy of the Midfoot without Ulceration; Surgical Fixation Choice: Internal Fixation

A 55-year-old female with a history of diabetes mellitus and chronic midfoot Charcot neuroarthropathy deformity was referred to our center after previous attempted conservative treatment options had failed. On physical examination, the patient had peripheral neuropathy with a multiplanar midfoot Charcot neuroarthropathy deformity (A). No open wounds were present at the time of initial presentation. Plain radiographs revealed chronic changes to the Lisfranc joint, forefoot abduction, and sagittal plane deformity (B,C). Laboratory values were within normal levels, and the patient decided to proceed with surgical correction. A single-stage procedure consisting of an extended arthrodesis was performed. A wedge osteotomy was performed from a medial approach, correcting both sagittal and transverse planes (D). Intramedullary fixation was placed which allowed fixation across all joints with direct axial compression. This technique also allowed the fixation to be "hidden," limiting any hardware prominence with the patient's thin soft tissue envelope (E,F). Arthrodesis was extended to the entire first and second rays in order to achieve increased stability and fixation (G).

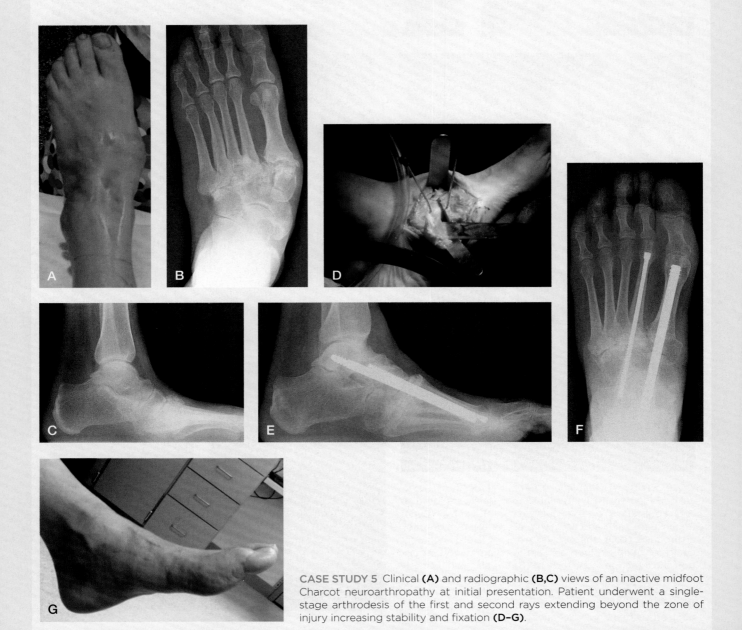

CASE STUDY 5 Clinical **(A)** and radiographic **(B,C)** views of an inactive midfoot Charcot neuroarthropathy at initial presentation. Patient underwent a single-stage arthrodesis of the first and second rays extending beyond the zone of injury increasing stability and fixation **(D–G)**.

Inactive Charcot Neuroarthropathy of the Ankle without Ulceration; Surgical Fixation Choice: Internal Fixation

A 70-year-old female with a history of diabetes mellitus and peripheral neuropathy presented to our center with increasing deformity of her left ankle. She had a reported fracture treated by another physician conservatively for 1 year due to the patient's past medical history. The patient was unable to be braced on her left lower extremity, her deformity was progressing, and a discussion about a below-the-knee amputation was mentioned.

On physical examination, the patient had no open wounds and her lower extremity deformity was nonreducible with loss of height and a varus component (A). Plain radiographs revealed a prior pilon type injury and subsequent deformity secondary to a Charcot neuroarthropathy event (B,C). Decision was made to reduce the deformity with osteotomies of the talus and distal tibia with a femoral head allograft placement to aid in reduction and height loss. Intramedullary fixation with the resected fibula bone was utilized to augment the arthrodesis site as an onlay autograft and "biologic" plate fixation (D–G).

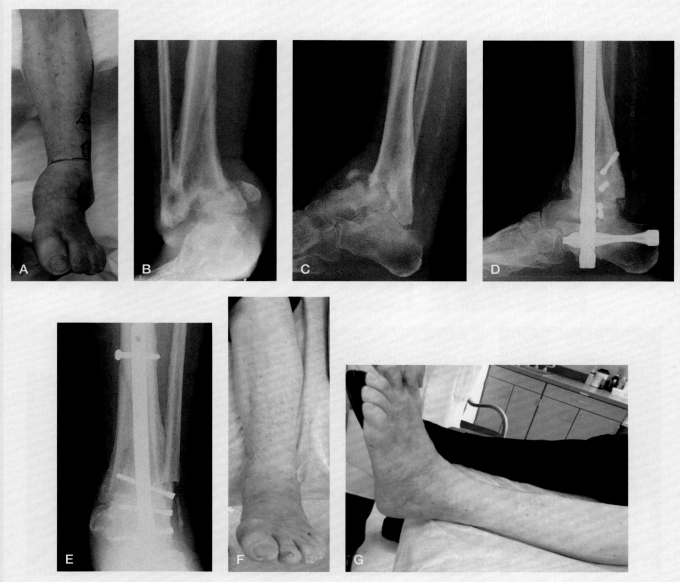

CASE STUDY 6 Clinical **(A)** and radiographic **(B,C)** views of an inactive ankle Charcot neuroarthropathy at initial presentation. Patient underwent a single-stage ankle arthrodesis with a femoral head allograft placement to aid in reduction and height loss. Intramedullary fixation with the resected fibula bone was utilized to augment the arthrodesis site as an onlay autograft and "biologic" plate fixation **(D–G)**.

Inactive Charcot Neuroarthropathy of the Midfoot with Ulceration and Infection; Surgical Fixation Choice: Staged External to Internal Fixation

A 43-year-old male with morbid obesity was referred to our center with a chronic Charcot neuroarthropathy deformity and open wound to the plantar aspect of the right foot. The patient had idiopathic neuropathy and no history of diabetes mellitus. Patient was in a walking boot but with a consistent open wound after attempts at all treatments including skin grafting. He had laboratory and magnetic resonance findings of osteomyelitis as well as findings of an inactive Charcot neuroarthropathy of the midfoot (A). Plain radiographs revealed an inactive Charcot neuroarthropathy of the midfoot with significant equinus (B,C). Patient underwent staged surgical

management with initial wedge resection of the midfoot to remove osteomyelitic bone and reduce the deformity. A circular external fixator was applied to maintain reduction and stability of the lower extremity (D,E). Appropriate consults and guided antibiotic therapy was also initiated. The plantar foot wound healed over the following 5 weeks (F–H). His foot was in a more anatomic position but required permanent fixation (I). Once laboratory values reached to normal levels, the patient's external fixation was removed and converted to a "global" internal fixation arthrodesis with intramedullary nailing, locking plates, and large screws. The internal fixation was carried past the zone of injury and osteotomy to gain improved fixation and control the lower extremity deformity. The ankle arthrodesis would prevent recurrence of the equinus deformity to protect the midfoot (J,K).

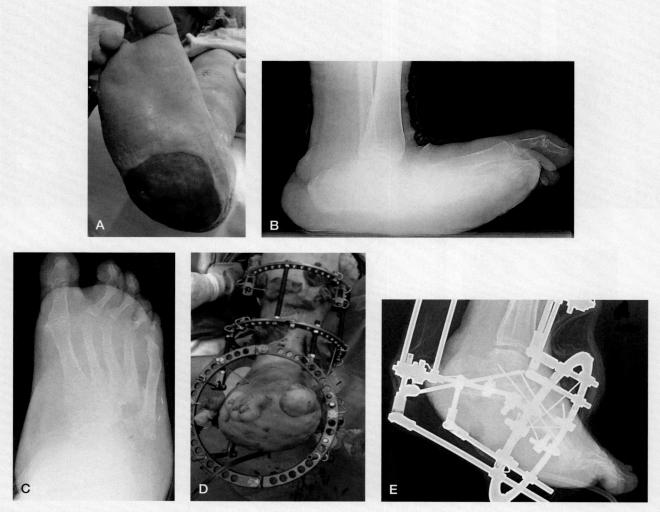

CASE STUDY 7 Preoperative clinical **(A)** and radiographic **(B,C)** views showing an infected inactive midfoot Charcot neuroarthropathy at initial presentation. Patient underwent staged surgical management with initial wedge resection of the midfoot to remove osteomyelitic bone and reduce the deformity. A circular external fixator was applied to maintain reduction and stability of the lower extremity **(D,E)**. *(continued)*

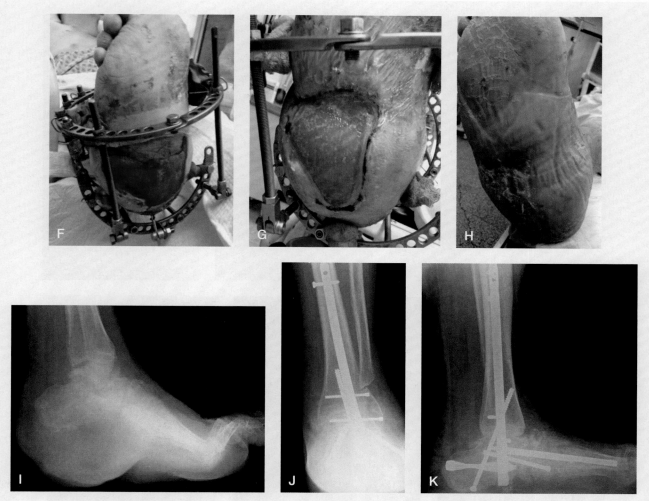

CASE STUDY 7 *(Continued)* The plantar foot wound healed over the following 5 weeks **(F–I)**. Following external fixation removal, a "global" internal fixation arthrodesis with intramedullary nailing and large screws was performed. The internal fixation was carried past the zone of injury and osteotomy to gain improved fixation and control the lower extremity deformity **(J,K)**.

CASE STUDY   8

Inactive Charcot Neuroarthropathy of the Ankle with Ulceration and Infection; Surgical Fixation Choice: Staged External to Internal Fixation

A 63-year-old male presented to our center with an ankle Charcot neuroarthropathy and idiopathic neuropathy. He was being treated conservatively prior to his presentation for an ankle sprain type of injury for over 1 year duration. He subsequently developed a wound over the medial malleolus from attempts at bracing. On physical examination, the patient had an unstable valgus ankle deformity with an open wound probing to bone over the medial malleolus (A,B). The wound had a sinus tract with serous drainage and erythema 1 cm surrounding. Plain radiographs revealed an inactive Charcot neuroarthropathy event

with a severe valgus deformity, destruction of the distal tibia and fibula from abnormal biomechanics and probable osteomyelitis (C,D). The patient underwent staged reconstruction with initial resection of bone and attaining proper alignment. Intraoperative cultures were taken, a cemented antibiotic spacer was placed, and a circular external fixator was applied to maintain reduction and aid in the healing process to limit motion and inflammation (E–G). After appropriate consults, antibiotic therapy, and local wound care, the patient had a closed soft tissue envelope with improved laboratory values and clinical appearance (H). After removal of the circular external fixation, internal fixation consisted of an intramedullary nailing and compression screws with a femoral head allograft to fill the void was utilized to aid in deformity correction and anatomic length (I–L).

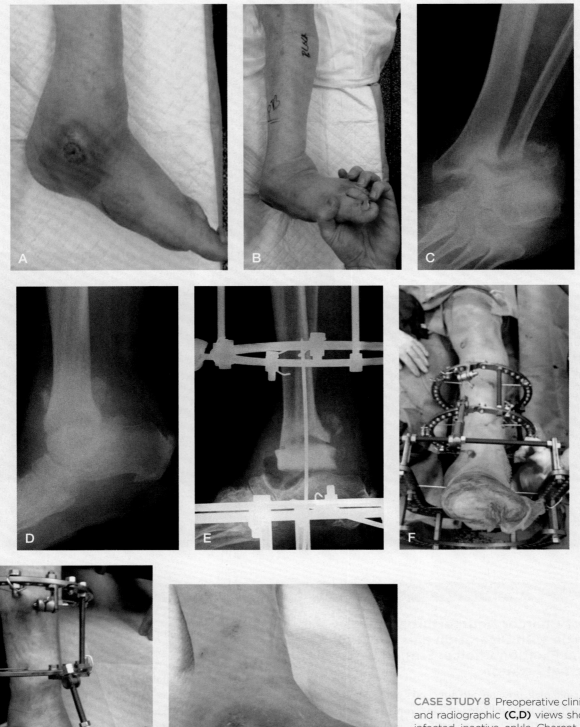

CASE STUDY 8 Preoperative clinical **(A,B)** and radiographic **(C,D)** views showing an infected inactive ankle Charcot neuroarthropathy at initial presentation. Patient underwent staged reconstruction with initial resection of bone and attaining proper alignment. An ankle cemented antibiotic spacer was placed, and a circular external fixator was applied to maintain reduction and aid in the healing process to limit motion and inflammation **(E–G)**. *(continued)*

CASE STUDY 8 *(Continued)* After removal of the circular external fixation, internal fixation consisted of an intramedullary nailing and compression screws with a femoral head allograft to fill the void was utilized to aid in deformity correction and anatomic length **(H–L)**.

Conclusion

This chapter has reviewed and presented clinical case studies in which internal fixation, external fixation, or combined fixation has been used for the surgical correction and anatomic alignment of patients with active and inactive CN foot and ankle deformities. Surgical knowledge and experience in these types of devastating injuries will lead to the patients' overall successful outcome.

References

1. Mittlmeier T, Klaue K, Haar P, et al. Should one consider primary surgical reconstruction in Charcot arthropathy of the feet? Clin Orthop Relat Res 2010;468:1002–1011.

2. Myerson MS, Henderson MR, Saxby T, et al. Management of midfoot diabetic neuroarthropathy. Foot Ankle Int 1994;15:233–241.

3. Pinzur MS, Gil J, Belmares J. Treatment of osteomyelitis in Charcot foot with single-stage resection of infection, correction of deformity, and maintenance with ring fixation. Foot Ankle Int 2012;33:1069–1074.

4. Sammarco VJ. Superconstructs in the treatment of Charcot foot deformity: plantar plating, locked plating, and axial screw fixation. Foot Ankle Clin 2009;14:393–407.

5. Simon SR, Tejwani SG, Wilson DL, et al. Arthrodesis as an early alternative to nonoperative management of Charcot arthropathy of the diabetic foot. J Bone Joint Surg Am 2000;82-A:939–950.

6. Wukich DK, Belczyk RJ, Burns PR, et al. Complications encountered with circular ring fixation in persons with diabetes mellitus. Foot Ankle Int 2008;29:994–1000.

CHAPTER 21

Stepwise Surgical Approach to Diabetic Foot and Ankle Nonunions and Malunions

Jeffrey M. Manway • Patrick R. Burns

INTRODUCTION

Although Charcot neuroarthropathy (CN) remains one of the most challenging problems in foot and ankle surgery, this disease process is often further complicated by delayed union, nonunion, as well as malunion. The causes of nonunion and malunion are often multifactorial, secondary to infection and open wounds, avascular nonunion and peripheral arterial disease, insufficient hardware, patient noncompliance, musculoskeletal imbalance, nutritional compromise, smoking, and altered bone metabolism. Many times, determining the cause of nonunion or malunion may be as challenging as the ultimate treatment. Treatment requires coordination across multiple specialties and frequently staged surgery. This task can be very demanding for the patient as well as the treating physician and surgeon. This chapter reviews the probable etiologic factors for diabetic CN nonunion and malunion as well as the overall management of this very difficult subset of diabetic patients.

INDICATIONS AND CONTRAINDICATIONS

Understanding the appropriate indications for proceeding with surgical correction of CN nonunion and/or malunion cases is paramount to successful management. Similarly, recognizing diabetic patients who are poor candidates for CN reconstruction is imperative.

Indications for surgical reconstruction of the diabetic neuropathic lower extremity have expanded in recent years. Previously, aversion to surgery on the "at-risk" diabetic patients ultimately has led to poor overall outcomes, decreased quality of life, and major amputation. Reconstruction has taken on an expanded role, endeavoring to increase both quality of life and lower extremity preservation. Although surgical indications have not been firmly defined in the literature, relative absolute indications for surgery include unstable or nonbraceable deformity of the CN foot or ankle, impending or nonhealing ulceration of the lower extremity, and pain relief.

Relative contraindications for surgical management are highly debated. These include acute CN, active ulceration, morbid obesity, smoking, and uncontrolled hyperglycemia. These issues are particularly debated among multidisciplinary health care providers. Although historical views suggest that surgery in the setting of acute CN should be avoided, increasing anecdotal and clinical evidence suggest that ultimate diabetic limb salvage may be facilitated by earlier surgical intervention where early fixation may prevent catastrophic collapse and subsequent massive bone loss (21). Similarly, the presence of an open wound has long been viewed as an absolute contraindication for internal fixation; however, literature does exist illustrating the safety of internal fixation in the setting of an ulcer (19). Planned internal fixation in the setting of a clean wound may limit the overall risks of suffering infected hardware, although delayed hardware removal may be necessary in certain clinical scenarios. Surgeons managing nonunion and malunion of the diabetic neuropathic foot must use their best judgment, contemplating the risks of potential complications of preoperative choices versus the risks of short- and long-term complications.

Absolute contraindications for surgical reconstruction of the diabetic foot and ankle include medical comorbidities precluding surgery, nonreconstructible deformity, severe diabetic foot infection, peripheral arterial disease, and a host of other factors. In these clinical presentations, the overall outcomes of each scenario must be particularly assessed. Often, it may be in the patient's best interest to proceed with supportive care or, even in select scenarios, consider major amputation.

INFECTION

Diagnosis of Infection and Suspected Nonunion

Of primary importance in the management of nonunion and malunion of the diabetic neuropathic foot is the diagnosis and treatment of infection. Whether during the primary surgery addressing the CN deformity and ulceration or as a secondary surgery addressing subsequent nonunion and/or malunion, infection may complicate recovery and ultimately lead to failure. The failure of standard laboratory testing to detect infection combined with the compromised immune system of the host significantly complicates the diagnosis and management of infection in the diabetic population (1). Often, diabetic patients will present with a white blood cell count within normal limits, and elevation of inflammatory markers may be nonspecific. The determination of deep infection in the clinical setting of the diabetic neuropathic foot is one of the greatest challenges a foot and ankle specialist can encounter.

Although leukocytosis is the most obvious diagnostic abnormality indicating infection, the use of white blood cell count in diabetic patients is often unreliable. For this reason, the use of acute and chronic inflammatory markers, C-reactive protein, and erythrocyte sedimentation rate have become mainstays in the evaluation for infection. Unfortunately, no universal benchmarks exist for these values to define what may constitute whether infection is present or what depth of infection may exist. Furthermore, use of these inflammatory markers in isolation to diagnose infection is nonspecific. A variety of other factors may influence these values including both acute and chronic inflammatory conditions. Although C-reactive protein levels greater than 3.2 mg/L and erythrocyte sedimentation rates greater than 70 mm/hr are often attributed to deep infection and osteomyelitis, these may be errors in interpretation (8,11). In fact, erythrocyte sedimentation rate is >25 mm/hr in nearly all patients with end-stage renal disease (ESRD) and nephrotic syndrome. Further complicating the diagnosis, about 60% of patients with ESRD will have an erythrocyte sedimentation rate about 60 mm/hr, and 20% of patients with ESRD on hemodialysis will have extreme elevation of erythrocyte sedimentation rate (values >100 mm/hr) (7). It is also unclear the effect of diabetic peripheral neuropathy on these laboratory values; as it clearly affects white cell function, there may be similar effects on other values.

Because laboratory values alone are not 100% sensitive or specific for detection of infection, clinicians must use their clinical judgment in conjunction with laboratory, clinical examination, and medical imaging studies to determine whether infection is present. The ability of medical imaging to aid in the determination of infection in the setting of recent surgery is often limited. Computed tomography (CT), magnetic resonance imaging (MRI), nuclear imaging, and plain radiographs may all have some role; however, each may have their own drawbacks.

CT has become the gold standard for diagnosis of nonunion. However, this study has limited utility in the diagnosis of infection. CT may detect evidence of severe infection such as subcutaneous gas and can also detect cortical disruption that can be seen with osteomyelitis. However, features such as cortical disruption and periosteal reaction may also be seen with recent surgery, history of arthrodesis surgery or fracture, and CN itself. Benefits of CT include its ability to make

adequate observations in the setting of implanted hardware. Although CT artifact is somewhat limiting, both contrast and noncontrast CT may adequately identify fluid collections that may otherwise be obscured by MRI metal artifacts. Nevertheless, in the authors' opinion, CT is best utilized for determining the presence of infected union versus nonunion. Studies of foot and ankle hindfoot arthrodesis suggest that patients may have acceptable functional and subjective outcomes with an arthrodesis mass of 25% to 50% (5,9). Although these numbers cannot be directly applied to fractures, it stands to reason that if more than 50% bridging exists on CT imaging, infected hardware may possibly be removed without necessity of further revision or supplemental fixation.

The role of MRI in the diagnosis of nonunion may be more limited than CT. In the context of CN or neuropathic trauma, MRI is generally utilized to determine the presence of deep infection. Particularly, T1 imaging with marrow fibrosis and replacement is highly specific for osteomyelitis. For this reason, MRI may be of some utility with a staged protocol or in clinical scenarios where external fixation or nonoperative therapies have been previously utilized. MRI in the setting of implanted hardware for the evaluation of nonunion is not recommended by the authors. Rather, this modality is more helpful in an adjunctive capacity. Previous surgery in close relation to the site of interest may elicit false-positive findings for approximately 6 months or more. Although it may detect a nonunion, visualization of bone with MRI is generally not preferred because CT more specifically may quantify percentage of healing. However, MRI may detect other tendon or ligament pathology as well as infection in the absence of other diagnoses.

Nuclear imaging has been shown to have a role in the diagnosis of CN with the addition of a sulfur colloid study. Conversely, this exam has not been traditionally used to evaluate for nonunion given its relative lack of specificity. Although an indium-111–labeled leukocyte nuclear imaging may detect infection, this may have a high false-positive rate and is a relatively poor study regarding its ability to evaluate of nonunion. A frank atrophic nonunion may be detected with a "cold spot" on nuclear imaging; however, this would generally only be evident after an extended period. For this reason, nuclear imaging is not a commonly utilized study for evaluation of nonunion or infection in the setting of CN.

Plain radiographs are of high utility in the evaluation of infection and nonunion as well as deformity. Deep infection may manifest subcutaneous gas or aggressive periosteal bone formation that is far more evident than other methods of imaging. Although hypertrophic nonunion may exhibit localized periosteal reaction, osteomyelitic periosteal reaction tends to be more diffuse and readily evident on plain radiographs. Other indicators of nonunion are also evident on plain radiographs including sclerosis at the fracture or arthrodesis site, periprosthetic loosening (such as "windshield wiper" or "halo effect"), as well as hardware fracture. These may all be signs of aseptic or infectious nonunion.

In addition, conventional plain radiographs have extreme importance because they play a large role in deformity planning.

Plain radiographs are the basis of surgical reconstruction, utilized to reestablish the normal anatomic relationships of bone and joint, as well as relative angles and measurements. Conventional plain radiographs are the beginning of the planning process. They give insight in the revision setting of nonunion and malunion as to the type and level of deformity as well as possible hardware types and location that may be utilized.

Management of Infection

Management of infection in conjunction with nonunion can present a unique challenge. Chronic instability of bone certainly leads to continued inflammation, and at best, this may mimic infection. More likely, the constant inflammation of soft tissue structures in the surrounding area may potentiate, perpetuate, or lead to infection. This process poses a particular challenge for management of osseous healing and maintenance of stability. In trauma patients, it has been shown that in the setting of infection or wounds with exposed hardware, maintenance of hardware may still be possible, with the final goal of late removal and débridement of infected union, or even long-term or lifetime suppression of infection (2). Indeed, the risks of long-term antibiotic management must be carefully weighed against costs of loss of stability or further bone loss. In some cases, chronic infection may be the lesser of the 2 challenges. Although the management of deep infection with 6 weeks of intravenous antibiotics has been the standard of care, there is little evidence basis to support this duration of therapy, whereas there is an increasing trend for longer therapy or suppressive therapy after intravenous antibiotic management has ceased. It is also not clear how the immunocompromised diabetic neuropathic patient fits this standard with antibiotic treatment.

If acute surgical management of nonunion in the setting of infection is deemed necessary, a stepwise staged surgical approach is the most accepted. Generally, the presence of infection is established during the preoperative assessment or intraoperatively by means of pathology and microbiology results. If presence of infection is uncertain, a surgeon may perform an intraoperative frozen section. This has been utilized primarily for the evaluation of deep infection in the setting of total joint replacement surgery (14). Greater than 5 neutrophils per high-powered field has been shown to be equivocal, or possibly suggestive of infection, whereas greater than 10 neutrophils per high-powered field has been shown to be more highly suggestive of infection. This method should be used only as an adjunctive test and should not be relied on solely to determine the presence of infection, especially in the cases of diabetic CN process. If there is doubt as to the presence of infection, staged surgical protocol should be undertaken.

Serial surgical débridement in conjunction with proper antibiotics is the cornerstone of infection management in the setting of nonunion. Relative lower extremity stability in this clinical setting can be achieved through various means while infection is managed and is often imperative for the success of diabetic limb salvage. First and foremost, resection of frankly nonviable tissue including bone must be performed. Preservation of questionable bone should be considered as overabundant resection may limit salvage options. Once resections of nonviable soft tissue and bone have been achieved, stabilization is undertaken. Stabilization should allow access to the soft tissue for frequent evaluation and be planned in such fashion as to not limit ultimate fixation options. Commonly used techniques for stabilization include Kirschner wires, Steinmann pins, antibiotic-impregnated polymethylmethacrylate (PMMA) cemented beads, rods, and spacers as well as external fixators (Fig. 21.1). Often, multiple modalities are incorporated simultaneously and are frequently modified throughout the treatment course because evolution of edema may preclude or facilitate fixation options as time progresses.

Once the soft tissue envelope has been stabilized and the infectious process has been controlled, definitive surgical fixation can be considered. In some instances, adequate arthrodesis or stable pseudoarthrosis has been achieved and patients may proceed with long-term bracing. In the authors' experience, revision to stable internal surgical fixation is required. This may again be supplemented with the use of implanted antibiotic-impregnated PMMA cemented beads, rods, and spacers being followed by staged arthrodesis procedures (Case Studies 1 and 2). The goal as in any diabetic CN surgery is to achieve an infection-free arthrodesis that is well consolidated with a plantigrade foot and minimal bracing. In these difficult nonunion and malunion cases, however, a stable pseudoarthrosis or stable nonunion that has no wound with a braceable and plantigrade foot is an acceptable outcome.

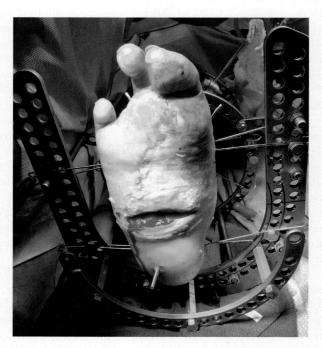

FIGURE 21.1 Surgical management of a diabetic Charcot neuroarthropathy with concomitant plantar foot ulceration undergoing reconstruction and application of a circular external fixation system.

A 43-year-old female was referred to our institution with a history of prior surgical attempt at a Charcot neuroarthropathy midfoot reconstruction. She had wound complications following with progressive radiographic changes and hardware failure. She subsequently had increasing deformity and was failing conservative treatment and bracing. On clinical examination, she had no current open wounds but had increased edema and erythema to the lateral ankle and foot around the previous subtalar joint incision. She had obvious unstable varus deformity of the ankle, and plain radiographs revealed broken hardware, destruction of the talus, and a significant deformity (A,B). Patient wished to proceed with an attempt at lower extremity preservation and had appropriate laboratory work up. The initial surgery consisted of surgical débridement, intraoperative cultures, frozen sections, reduction of the unstable deformity, placement of an antibiotic-impregnated polymethylmethacrylate cemented spacer at the hindfoot/ankle, and circular external fixation to maintain alignment and aid in soft tissue healing (C). She was treated with appropriate intravenous antibiotics coordinated by infectious disease specialists. At 8 weeks postoperatively, the circular external fixator was removed in the clinical setting and a cast applied to allow the pin/wire sites to heal. The patient returned to the operating room for internal fixation with an intramedullary nail device to maintain the anatomic reduction and stability. Intraoperative frozen sections revealed resolution of an acute inflammatory state, new cultures were taken, and intramedullary nailing along with a femoral head allograft was utilized to aid in the management of osseous defect and length (D,E). The patient had an uneventful postoperative course, was non–weight-bearing for 3 months, and finally transitioned into a custom walking boot. She maintained a stable pseudoarthrosis of the lower extremity being free of any recurrent wounds.

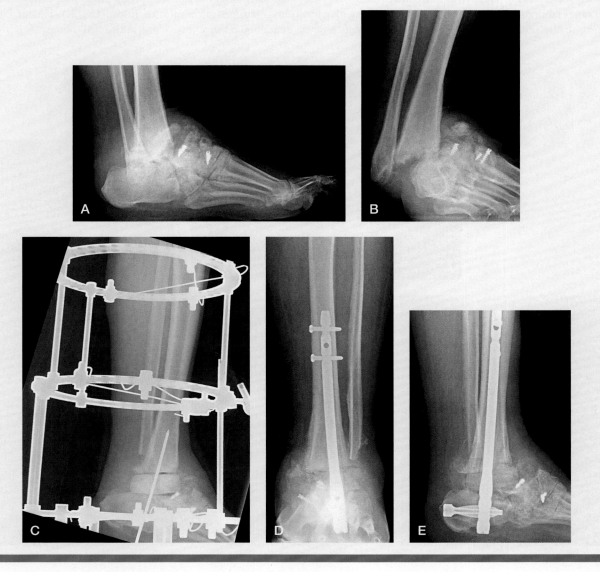

A 72-year-old female presented to the emergency department with a concern of bleeding from her left ankle. She related a twisting injury about 1 week prior and noticed some swelling but was prompted to go to the emergency department upon developing bleeding. She had a medical history of diabetes mellitus treated with insulin, congestive heart failure, history of partial foot amputation, peripheral neuropathy, and chronic renal insufficiency. She was found to have an open trimalleolar fracture of her left ankle (A,B). She was taken emergently to the operating room for surgical débridement and provisional fixation. She underwent repeated irrigation and surgical débridement procedures and provisional immobilization for 1 month with a pin-to-bar external fixation (C). Once bacterial cultures were negative, primary ankle arthrodesis was performed (D–F). Intraoperatively, the medial malleolus was resected and sent for culture. One month postoperatively, bone cultures from the medial malleolus came back positive for yeast infection. The patient was evaluated by infectious disease specialists, and all other laboratory and clinical findings were negative for infection. In the setting of her worsening renal insufficiency,

infectious disease specialists opted to continue without antibiotic therapy. Five months postoperatively, she presented with severe swelling and redness with pain to her left lower extremity and hardware failure. Attempt was made to remove her medial fixation and dynamize her intramedullary nail. Intravenous antibiotic therapy and antifungal therapy were initiated. At this time, the patient had begun hemodialysis as well. Subsequently, complete hardware removal was undertaken, and placement of an intramedullary antibiotic-impregnated polymethylmethacrylate (PMMA) cemented rod was performed after intramedullary reaming and débridement of her tibia and medial ankle site (G). She underwent an additional 3 months of immobilization of her lower extremity with antifungal suppression. All infectious symptoms resolved, and she ultimately had the antibiotic-impregnated PMMA cemented rod removed secondary to persistent plantar irritation. At 18 months after her initial injury (H,I), she was able to ambulate with a plantigrade foot and a double upright ankle foot orthosis without any recurrent ulceration or infection (J,K). Patient had also remained on suppressive oral antifungal therapy.

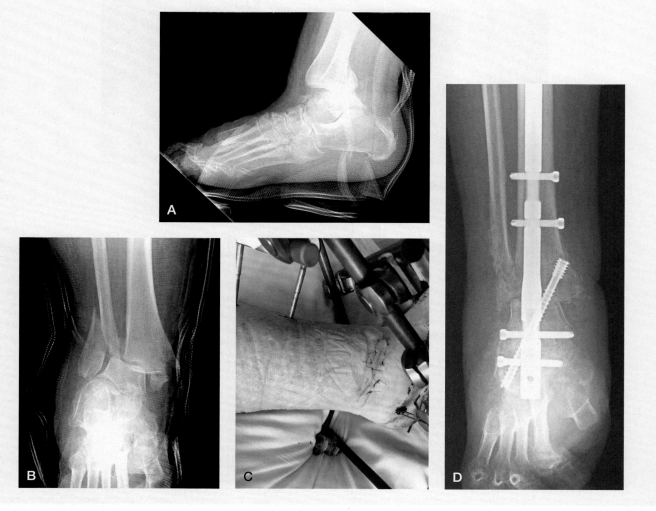

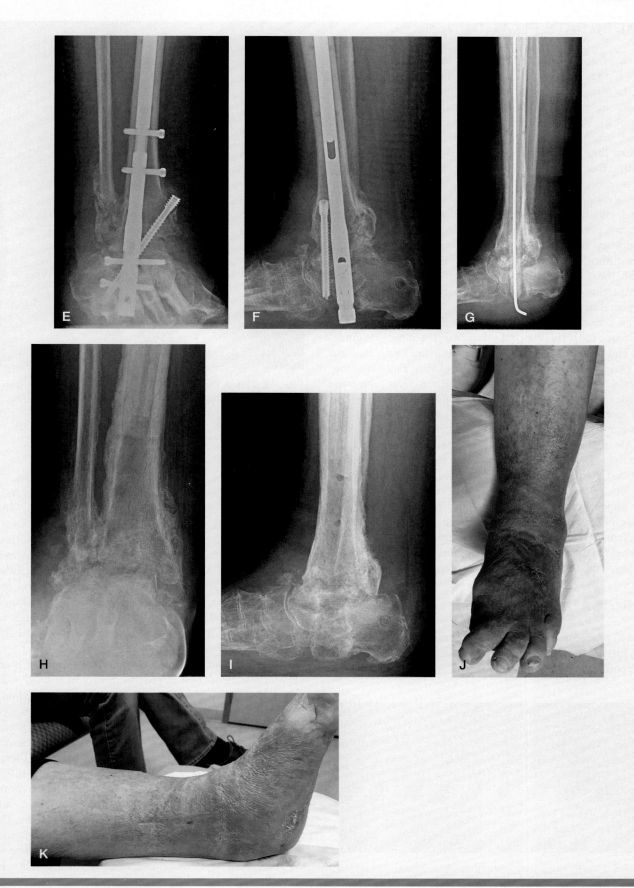

INADEQUATE FIXATION

Although nonunion of the diabetic neuropathic foot and ankle is often complicated by infection, this is not always the rule. In many cases, insufficient fixation in the setting of peripheral neuropathy is often the primary cause of nonunion (Fig. 21.2). This clinical case scenario may be avoidable with proper preoperative planning. Historically, the impetus has been to limit approaches and fixation to the diabetic neuropathic foot for fear of infectious complications or perioperative morbidity/mortality. However, more recent trends have advocated more substantial fixation methods. This has been facilitated by lower profile fixation products, specialty anatomic plating, intramedullary nailing, and locked plating technology. In the setting of acute neuropathic fractures, it is the authors' suggestion that an attempt should be made to double the standard amount of fixation that would otherwise be utilized to repair comparable fractures in patients without peripheral neuropathy (Fig. 21.3).

The concept of "superconstructs" was first presented by Sammarco (20). This concept was developed to provide guidelines and fixation suggestions for the difficulties with anatomy and biology seen in CN patients. To qualify as a superconstruct, fixation should extend beyond the zone of injury and include unaffected bones/joints, allow for reduction of deformity so as not to place undue tension on the skin, utilize the strongest device that soft tissue will tolerate, and utilize devices that are applied in such a way as to maximize their mechanical stability (20). In the setting of acute fractures, for example, extended plating, locked plating, utilization of multiple syndesmotic screws, and plating technique (i.e., antiglide plating) may improve fixation strength. For some cases, primary arthrodesis should be considered to maximize surgical stability. For diabetic CN reconstruction, utilization of plantar plating, external fixation, locked plating, intramedullary fixation, and combined fixation should all be considered (Case Study 3).

SURGICAL PLANNING

Prior to proceeding with the surgical management of diabetic foot and ankle nonunion and malunion, extensive presurgical planning should be undertaken. Careful preoperative

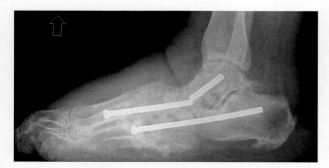

FIGURE 21.2 Example of inadequate and failed fixation for Charcot neuroarthropathy midfoot reconstruction.

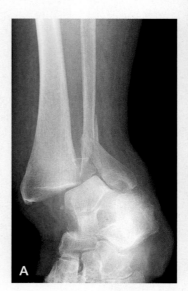
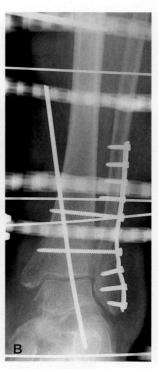

FIGURE 21.3 A,B. Example of increased fixation utilized in a case of a diabetic neuropathic ankle fracture. Note the use of the transarticular hindfoot/ankle Steinmann pin fixation, fibular locking plate, multiple syndesmotic screws, and the circular external fixation system **(B)**.

assessment may help to avoid complications or failures. Comprehensive evaluation may also illuminate risk factors and may ultimately predict failure or prognosis. For diabetic patients who are proceeding with surgery electively (patients without infection), it is important for them to be medically optimized, correcting modifiable risk factors and recognizing nonmodifiable risk factors. Nonmodifiable risk factors may include age, ESRD, peripheral neuropathy, transplant status, and overall patient debilitation. Modifiable risk factors that should be considered include glycemic control, nutritional status, active tobacco use, obesity, cardiovascular status, peripheral arterial disease, or metabolic/endocrine disorders.

In planning for nonunion or malunion surgery, it is generally in the patient's best interest to control modifiable risk factors or eliminate undesirable behavior prior to proceeding with surgery. Probably the most infamous of these factors is tobacco use. Regarding foot and ankle surgery, it has been shown that active tobacco use portends a notably higher complication rate than nonsmoking or previously smoking patients. There is a known increased rate of nonunion or delayed union, infection, and wound healing complications (3,12). Glycemic control is also of interest in surgical planning. A hemoglobin A_{1c} of less than 8% is preferable prior to proceeding with surgery. The effect of glycemic control is multifactorial. In countless studies, proper glycemic control does limit general perioperative surgical risk including cardiogenic morbidity and mortality. However, the pathophysiology of poor glycemic control has yet to

A 58-year-old male with a history of diabetic Charcot neuroarthropathy showed increasing deformity at the midfoot level (A,B) with an associated equinus (C). An attempt was made to address the deformity with multiple joint arthrodesis and internal fixation. There was an uneventful postoperative course, but several months post-surgery, the foot had continued edema and increasing deformity once again. Plain radiographs showed hardware failure, increasing deformity, including increased equinus, and talar declination angle (D,E). Laboratory values were unremarkable, and a decision was made to attempt revision of the Charcot neuroarthropathy nonunion. Intraoperative frozen sections showed no acute inflammation, and subsequent cultures were negative. During surgery, the surgical sites appeared to be evident of a nonunion with no signs of infection. The decision was then made to proceed with an augmented revision arthrodesis. The joints were débrided thoroughly to a healthy bone and extended to include the ankle joint (F,G). Extending the arthrodesis zone would helped control the force from the equinus and allow for increased fixation for an area that was earlier compromised with nonunion and previous fixation. The postoperative course after the revisional surgery was uneventful, and the foot remained in a plantigrade position without any wounds. He ambulated in a diabetic extra depth shoe.

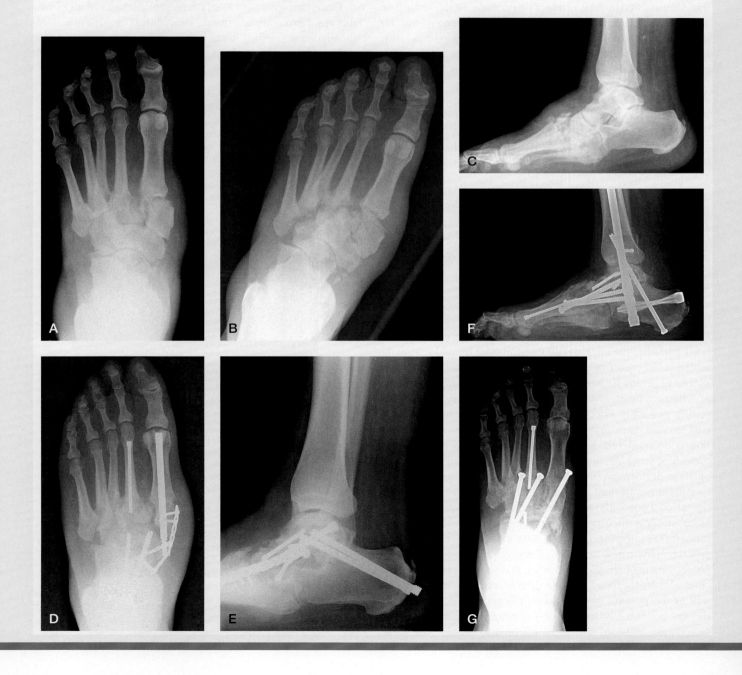

be completely elucidated of whether antihyperglycemic agents themselves, lack of insulin, impaired leukocyte recruitment, or a combination of all factors may play a role in the patient's outcome. In a study by Simpson et al. (22), it was interestingly shown that all antihyperglycemic agents, particularly sulphonyl-ureas, showed anti-osteogenic effects. Conversely, insulin and insulin-like growth factors have been shown to positively affect bone formation in diabetic and nondiabetic modeling (13). In correlation, Myers et al. (16) found that impaired short- and long-term glycemic control (hemoglobin A_{1c} >7%) portended an increased overall complication rate in hindfoot/ankle arthrodesis with both infectious and noninfectious complications.

Finally, of equal importance to the foot and ankle surgeon should be the vascular status of the diabetic patient's lower extremities. Although in the acute setting preemptive vascular intervention may not be prudent or possible, in the setting of a chronic nonunion, it is imperative to have adequate vascular assessment and/or intervention prior to surgery, especially if avascular nonunion is suspected. Appropriate noninvasive arterial studies should include toe pressures and toe-brachial index (TBI) values as an ankle-brachial index may be unreliable in the diabetic population. Although there is no accepted standard established, a TBI >0.7 has generally been found to be conducive with healing. If substantial or suspected impairment exists (i.e., toe pressure <50 mmHg or TBI <0.7), a vascular surgery consultation should be pursued and a diagnostic angiogram should be considered.

BASIC PRINCIPLES OF NONUNION SURGERY

After a thorough preoperative assessment has been completed and the patient has been medically optimized, surgery can proceed. A systematic approach to nonunion should be undertaken with each case to ensure reproducibility of results as well as patient's safety. Preoperative planning is essential. The surgeon should plan for unexpected intraoperative complications and have the appropriate instrumentation and materials available. Revision of nonunions in the diabetic population should generally be performed in a hospital setting regardless of whether inpatient stay is ultimately necessary. A hospital setting generally offers immediate availability of pathology staff and ancillary materials if unsuspected evidence of infection is encountered. Surgery centers may be ill-equipped to provide appropriate materials and seldom have on-site pathologists to perform an immediate Gram stain or frozen section.

Patient positioning and incisional planning are also of particular concern with nonunion cases. If there have been previous surgical incision healing complications, the previous incision(s) or approach should potentially be avoided. However, in many cases, necessity of exposure exceeds the risk of proceeding through these intervals. It is wise to preoperatively counsel patients about possible delayed skin healing events as well as the possible need for use of negative pressure wound therapy or even closure with the assistance of plastic surgery techniques. Incisions should be planned to provide complete

exposure of the surgical site. In general, the previous incision must be opened, and if present, all previous hardware should be removed. As a general rule, these previous incisions must be extended beyond their original course because skin is often far less mobile and accumulation of scar tissue often limits visualization and access to the nonunion site and implanted hardware. It is generally not necessary, in the authors' experience, to bone graft previous hardware sites unless these are felt to be substantial. Often, accessory incisions are then created to facilitate access to the nonunion site and to facilitate new hardware placement. Unfortunately, failed hardware is often encountered. In these clinical scenarios, the surgeon must carefully consider whether the destruction caused by hardware extraction is justified. In the setting of aseptic nonunion, inaccessible failed hardware is often left in place unless it precludes revision fixation.

Once the nonunion site is accessed, excision of all nonviable and fibrous tissues should be undertaken. This is systematically accomplished with the use of osteotomes, curettes, and burrs (Fig. 21.4). It should be noted that despite visible

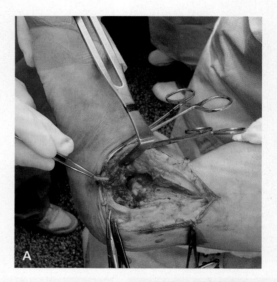

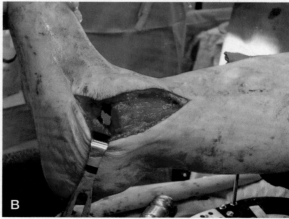

FIGURE 21.4 Example of a combined medial and lateral approach to a revisional Charcot neuroarthropathy nonunion of the hindfoot and ankle **(A)**. Note the healthy bone and soft tissue after proper surgical débridement **(B)**.

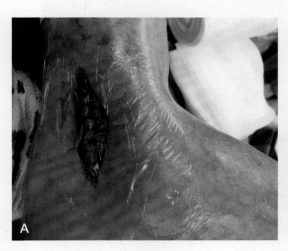 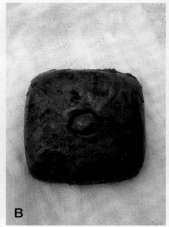 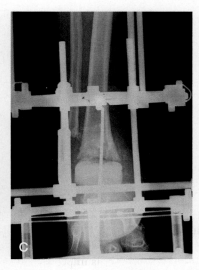

FIGURE 21.5 Examples of different types of antibiotic-impregnated polymethylmethacrylate (PMMA) cemented delivery systems **(A,B)** that can be fabricated to deliver local antibiotics and fill dead space during staged reconstruction in infected Charcot neuroarthropathy cases. Note the antibiotic-impregnated PMMA cemented spacer **(C)** employed during staged reconstruction of an infected Charcot neuroarthropathy ankle malunion surgery.

radiographic nonunion, the nonunion site will often appear quite stable with overlying bone formation on initial surgical inspection. The initial inclination may be to proceed more cautiously with resection; however, once the outermost surface area has been resected, this generally reveals the preoperatively expected nonunion site. The surgeon should not be falsely encouraged by the initial appearance of the nonunion site "at a glance." Once the surgical site is accessed and initial decortication is performed, the site should be mobilized to allow for complete resection of interposed tissue and, if this is a long bone, allow access to the medullary canal. At all times, a high index of suspicion for infection should be maintained. At this point in the procedure, it is often encouraged to send interposed fibrous debris from the nonunion site for immediate frozen section and culture specimens. The use of immediate Gram stain has not been shown to be an adequate intraoperative determinant of deep infection (26). If infection is clinically suspected or frozen section returns an unexpected result, the resection of the interposed nonunion site should be completed with removal of nonviable appearing bone and soft tissue, and the remainder of the procedure may be aborted or alternative fixation elements may need to be selected.

In most cases, infection will generally have been dealt with prior to proceeding with the anticipated definitive surgical revision. However, it is not uncommon to unexpectedly encounter infection in this high-risk diabetic population. Infection may be of low grade or remain latent and suppressed for extended periods of time. Appropriate preplanning should be undertaken to account for this process. In most cases, external fixation devices provide great versatility, and the surgeon should be aware of what products are available at his or her particular facility. For midfoot and hindfoot/ankle procedures, a circular external fixator is generally preferred due to its durability, but pin-to-bar external fixation may be appropriate in certain cir-

cumstances. It is the authors' opinion that the circular external fixator has more versatility and greater stability, allowing it to remain in place longer than pin-to-bar external fixation devices. Whenever possible, intraosseous wire placement for the circular external fixation systems should be avoided in any area where infection is suspected. Once the nonunion site has been prepared and the lower extremity has been stabilized, the surgeon may desire to incorporate an antibiotic-impregnated PMMA cemented spacer. In some instances, use of an antibiotic-impregnated PMMA cemented spacer may function as both temporary fixation and a local antibiotic delivery device (Fig. 21.5). Antibiotic-impregnated PMMA cemented spacers often fulfill multiple roles. They may serve to increase local stability at the nonunion site and have the obvious advantage of eluting antibiotics locally for infection management. Furthermore, use of an induced membrane technique, as described by Masquelet, has been shown to induce secretion of growth factors which may ultimately improve the local environment which has generally matured 4 to 6 weeks after the antibiotic-impregnated PMMA cemented spacer placement (23).

If infection has been excluded or staged surgery has been completed, the definitive surgery can be undertaken. First, the medullary canal must be re-established. This can be accomplished with the use of curettes, burrs, or drilling. If power instrumentation is utilized, attention should be paid to the generation of local heat. Copious use of saline should be employed to prevent burning and necrosis of the operative site. Once the surgical site has been recanalized, healthy bleeding from the intramedullary canal should be noted. At this point, bone graft or bone void filler is generally necessary. In general, a combination of structural and nonstructural bone graft is necessary for maintenance of large voids where small voids may be sufficiently managed with nonstructural bone grafting (Fig. 21.6). Historically, the use of structural

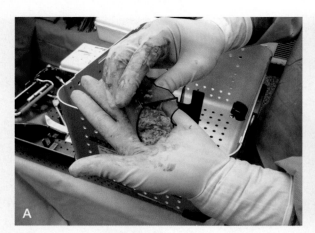 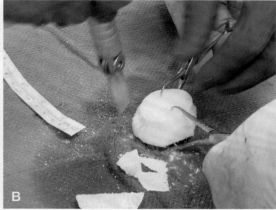

FIGURE 21.6 Types of bone graft that can be utilized during revision of Charcot neuroarthropathy nonunion and malunion surgery. Morselized bone graft **(A)** for small osseous defects and osteogenic properties as well as femoral head allograft **(B)** for structural support are options depending on the surgical procedure(s).

bone autograft has been preferred over allograft; however, in many cases, this may not be feasible. Autogenous iliac crest has been the typical donor bone graft site selected, although this site has well-documented associated complications including chronic pain, infection, and fracture. Conversely, there is increasing evidence that utilization of allograft may yield acceptable arthrodesis rates in the management of foot and ankle nonunions (6,10,15). The authors typically utilize structural femoral head allografts for the management of large osseous defects, whereas autograft cancellous bone from the distal tibia and calcaneus as well as allograft bone chips/putty are utilized to augment large allografts and small osseous defects (Fig. 21.7). Alternatively, a large amount of

cancellous autograft may easily be obtained through reaming of the tibia. This can be accomplished with or without a reamer irrigation aspirator system (Fig. 21.8).

In contrary, although the use of femoral head allografts for hindfoot/ankle arthrodesis and revisions is well documented, it should be noted that there may be a substantially increased risk of complications in patients where this is utilized (25). The authors do not recommend the use of allograft for grafting deficits greater than 2 cm in length. Rather, attempt should be made to truncate the foot or ankle to decrease the bone void as it is the authors' opinion that bone grafts greater than 2 cm are more likely to have significant complications and failure.

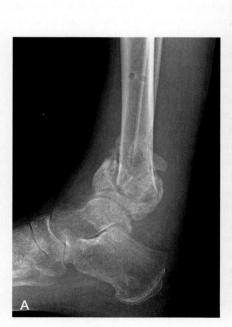 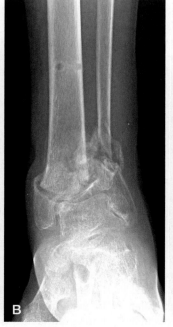 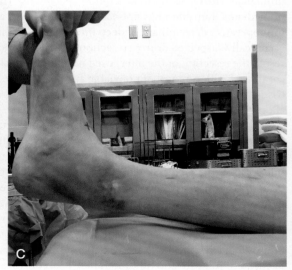

FIGURE 21.7 Surgical management of a neglected and malunited pilon fracture **(A–C)** with intramedullary nail fixation and femoral head allograft **(D,E)**. *(continued)*

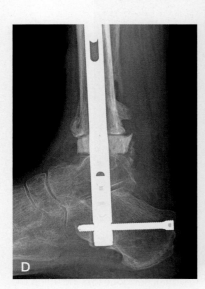
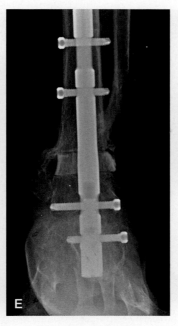
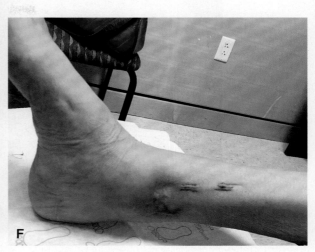

FIGURE 21.7 *(Continued)* **F.** Postoperative clinical outcome after surgical treatment with femoral head allograft.

Once bone grafting is completed, final instrumentation is performed. This can be complicated by necessity for avoiding bone grafts and voids, avoiding fragmented hardware, preventing stress riser formation, and maximizing the arthrodesis surface area. Surgical débridement and bone grafting with replacement of similar or identical hardware is seldom successful and not recommended. Rather, the fixation area should be extended well beyond the previous arthrodesis or fracture site. At the level of the foot and ankle, this often will require incorporating more proximal and distal bones in the fixation construct. This allows for extension to bone of substantially increased quality and support. The inclination is to create a construct that allows for maximum stability, especially in the setting of large structural allografts that will heal slowly through creeping substitution. The surgeon must be creative with fixation choices and must have adequate foresight so that any desired hardware is available at the time of surgery (Fig. 21.9). Locked variable angle plating is of significant utility in this diabetic population.

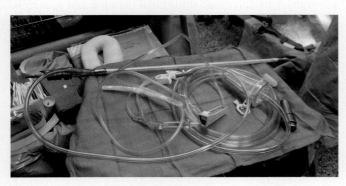

FIGURE 21.8 The reamer irrigation aspirator system may be used to harvest bone graft from long bones.

Carefully understanding the differences between hardware choices is also paramount. Differences such as screw size, core diameter of screws, use of cannulated screws, screw pitch, and plate versatility should all be considered. Because many diabetic neuropathic nonunions result from insufficient stability, construct stiffness is of primary concern. Locked specialty plating now exists for management of CN; however, this hardware fixation seldom fits perfectly as every patient presents with his or her own unique deformity and bone loss. Particularly, the authors have frequently employed hardware designed for the contralateral extremity or alternative bone surfaces to achieve better anatomic fit and increased or improved fixation. These cases will challenge the surgeon's ability to maximize hardware over a small volume of bone in some areas and extend hardware over a large surface area in others. As a general rule, plate and construct length should be at least 3 times the zone of injury when possible, and fixation should extend at least 2 bone diameter lengths beyond previous fixation sites to prevent formation of a stress riser or fracture.

Intramedullary nail fixation of the ankle and subtalar joint has become an increasingly common procedure for management of nonunited diabetic ankle fractures and CN. There is an expanding hardware variety that makes this procedure increasingly attractive surgery for diabetic neuropathic nonunions and/or malunions. Many intramedullary nails now incorporate both internal and external compression devices to assist with the arthrodesis procedures. Furthermore, this ability of the intramedullary nail to extend outside the zone of injury is limited only by the manufacturer's supplied length and the length of the patient's extremity. As the length of the intramedullary nail is increased, the total fixation surface area increases proportionately and thus increasing the overall construct stability. In most cases, use

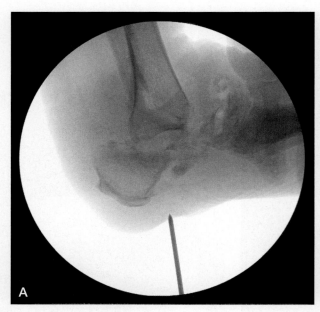
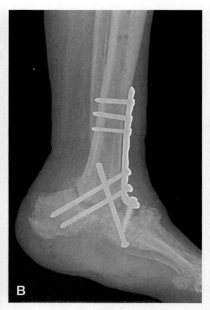

FIGURE 21.9 **A.** Intraoperative image of a Charcot neuroarthropathy of the hindfoot showing the significant bone loss including the anterior calcaneus. One must be familiar with and consider other types of fixation **(B)** in these types of cases where an intramedullary nail device may not be feasible.

of an intramedullary device does not preclude concomitant plating or augmentation; thus, it may be used as an adjunct. Augmentation of the intramedullary nail by means of a "derotational screw" has also been shown to increase construct stiffness and load to failure (18). The authors routinely utilize screw fixation to augment the intramedullary nail fixation (Fig. 21.10). In a comparative cadaveric study, O'Neill et al. (17) concluded that augmented intramedullary nail fixation exhibited similar rigidity. Thus, intramedullary nail fixation

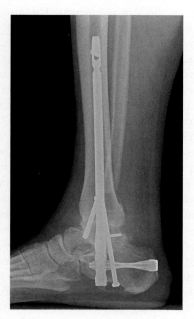

FIGURE 21.10 Example of supplemental screws with an intramedullary nail device to aid in compression and resist rotation.

may be indicated where locked plate fixation is precluded. Similarly, Chodos et al. (4) found in a cadaveric study that intramedullary nail fixation had higher initial stiffness and load to failure than blade plate fixation.

When placing an intramedullary nail in the setting of nonunion or revisional surgery, a few special circumstances should be considered. First, intramedullary nail fixation should be avoided if there is insufficient calcaneal fixation available. This will ultimately result in failure and extrusion of the device inferiorly. Next, optimal intramedullary nail length should be selected based on the zone of injury as well as previous intraosseous fixation points. Often, patients will have a history of previous external fixation. Failure to exceed previous external fixation pin/wire sites by 2 bone diameter lengths may ultimately result in tibia fracture (Fig. 21.11). If this occurs, surgery can be revised with the use of a longer intramedullary nail fixation. If the intramedullary nail device is to be placed in conjunction with a large structural allograft (i.e., femoral head allograft), particular care with initial reaming and sequential reaming should be taken. Overaggressive opening and canal expansion with reamers and drills may result in intraoperative bone graft fracture. Thus, stepwise sequential opening and reaming should be undertaken. Furthermore, in the setting of large allograft, excessive compression across the bone graft and arthrodesis sites is often avoided to limit the risk of bone graft collapse because little literature exists for guidance on this particular topic (Fig. 21.12). Finally, in the setting of previous infection, the surgeon may consider augmentation of the intramedullary nail with antibiotic-impregnated PMMA cemented coating. This can complicate the intramedullary nail placement but can increase overall contact area as well as having the added benefit of short-term elution of antibiotics (24).

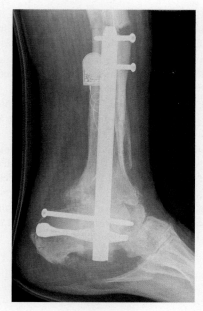

FIGURE 21.11 Example of a broken tibia at the proximal intramedullary nail site. In this clinical case scenario, there had been a previous external fixator pin in the fractured area. For prevention of the occurrence, the intramedullary nail should have been longer, at least 2 diameters proximal to the prior external fixation pin site, to prevent the stress riser and eventual fracture.

Conclusion

Management of nonunion and malunion in the diabetic neuropathic patient will challenge even the most experienced surgeon. Creativity, attention to detail, and patience are all paramount to achieving successful outcomes. The surgeon will require intimate coordination with infectious disease specialists, vascular surgery, endocrinology, and internal medicine services to achieve successful outcomes. Poor bone quality and limited volume often challenges the limits of current orthopedic hardware, and therefore, the surgeon must be well versed in multiple fixation techniques to successfully manage this high-risk diabetic population.

References

1. Armstrong DG, Perales TA, Murff RT, et al. Value of white blood cell count with differential in the acute diabetic foot infection. J Am Podiatr Med Assoc 1996;86:224–227.

2. Berkes M, Obremskey WT, Scannell B, et al. Maintenance of hardware after early postoperative infection following fracture internal fixation. J Bone Joint Surg Am 2010;92:823–828.

3. Bettin CC, Gower K, McCormick K, et al. Cigarette smoking increases complication rate in forefoot surgery. Foot Ankle Int 2015;36:488–493.

4. Chodos MD, Parks BG, Schon LC, et al. Blade plate compared with locking plate for tibiotalocalcaneal arthrodesis: a cadaver study. Foot Ankle Int 2008;29:219–224.

5. Coughlin MJ, Grimes JS, Traughber PD, et al. Comparison of radiographs and CT scans in the prospective evaluation of the fusion of hindfoot arthrodesis. Foot Ankle Int 2006;27:780–787.

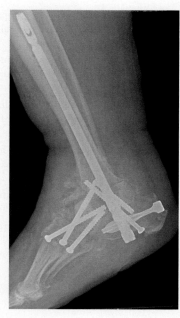

FIGURE 21.12 Example of a broken femoral head allograft due to excessive hardware.

6. Dekker TJ, White P, Adams SB. Efficacy of a cellular bone allograft for foot and ankle arthrodesis and revision nonunion procedures. Foot Ankle Int 2017;38(3):277–282.

7. Fincher RM, Page MI. Clinical significance of extreme elevation of the erythrocyte sedimentation rate. Arch Intern Med 1986;146:1581–1583.

8. Fleischer AE, Didyk AA, Woods JB, et al. Combined clinical and laboratory testing improves diagnostic accuracy for osteomyelitis in the diabetic foot. J Foot Ankle Surg 2009;48:39–46.

9. Glazebrook M, Beasley W, Daniels T, et al. Establishing the relationship between clinical outcome and extent of osseous bridging between computed tomography assessment in isolated hindfoot and ankle fusions. Foot Ankle Int 2013;34:1612–1618.

10. Jones CP, Loveland J, Atkinson BL, et al. Prospective, multicenter evaluation of allogeneic bone matrix containing viable osteogenic cells in foot and/or ankle arthrodesis. Foot Ankle Int 2015;36:1129–1137.

11. Kaleta JL, Fleischli JW, Reilly CH. The diagnosis of osteomyelitis in diabetes using erythrocyte sedimentation rate: a pilot study. J Am Podiatr Med Assoc 2001;91:445–450.

12. Krause F, Younger AS, Baumhauer JF, et al. Clinical outcomes of nonunions of hindfoot and ankle fusions. J Bone Joint Surg Am 2016;98:2006–2016.

13. Malekzadeh B, Tengvall P, Öhrnell L-O, et al. Effects of locally administered insulin on bone formation in non-diabetic rats. J Biomed Mater Res A 2013;101:132–137.

14. Mirra JM, Marder RA, Amstutz HC. The pathology of failed total joint arthroplasty. Clin Orthop Relat Res 1982;170:175–183.

15. Monaco SJ, Brandao RA, Manway JM, et al. Subtalar distraction arthrodesis with fresh frozen femoral neck allograft: a retrospective case series. Foot Ankle Spec 2016;9:423–428.

16. Myers TG, Lowery NJ, Frykberg RG, et al. Ankle and hindfoot fusions: comparison of outcomes in patients with and without diabetes. Foot Ankle Int 2012;33:20–28.

17. O'Neill PJ, Logel KJ, Parks BG, et al. Rigidity comparison of locking plate and intramedullary fixation for tibiotalocalcaneal arthrodesis. Foot Ankle Int 2008;29:581–586.

18. O'Neill PJ, Parks BG, Walsh R, et al. Biomechanical analysis of screw-augmented intramedullary fixation for tibiotalocalcaneal arthrodesis. Foot Ankle Int 2007;28:804–809.

19. Papa J, Myerson M, Girard P. Salvage, with arthrodesis, in intractable diabetic neuropathic arthropathy of the foot and ankle. J Bone Joint Surg Am 1993;75:1056–1066.

20. Sammarco VJ. Superconstructs in the treatment of Charcot foot deformity: plantar plating, locked plating, and axial screw fixation. Foot Ankle Clin 2009;14:393–407.

21. Simon SR, Tejwani SG, Wilson DL, et al. Arthrodesis as an early alternative to nonoperative management of Charcot arthropathy of the diabetic foot. J Bone Joint Surg Am 2000;82:939–950.

22. Simpson C, Jayaramaraju D, Agraharam D, et al. The effects of diabetes medications on post-operative long bone fracture healing. Eur J Orthop Surg Traumatol 2015;25:1239–1243.

23. Wang X, Wei F, Luo F, et al. Induction of granulation tissue for the secretion of growth factors and the promotion of bone defect repair. J Orthop Surg Res 2015;10:147.

24. Woods JB, Lowery NJ, Burns PR. Permanent antibiotic impregnated intramedullary nail in diabetic limb salvage: a case report and literature review. Diabet Foot Ankle 2012;3.

25. Wukich DK, Mallory BR, Suder NC, et al. Tibiotalocalcaneal arthrodesis using retrograde intramedullary nail fixation: comparison of patients with and without diabetes mellitus. J Foot Ankle Surg 2015;54:876–882.

26. Zywiel MG, Stroh DA, Johnson AJ, et al. Gram stains have limited application in the diagnosis of infected total knee arthroplasty. Int J Infect Dis 2011;15:e702–e705.

CHAPTER 22

Autogenous Bone Grafting and Osteobiologics for the Diabetic Lower Extremity

John Joseph Anderson • Devin Bland

INTRODUCTION

During the last decade, bone grafting products, applications, and techniques have become available at a torrid pace. A myriad of bone graft products are now available including growth factors and stem cells with different bone harvesting and processing techniques. Bone grafting is a valuable tool that will aid in obtaining positive results in the complex diabetic lower extremity reconstruction. This chapter reviews in detail both clinical and surgical applications of bone grafting concepts and osteobiologics in the diabetic population.

AUTOGENOUS BONE GRAFTS

Autogenous bone graft (autograft) is harvested from the same person and has been considered by many authors as the gold standard for bone grafting and bony union results. Autogenous bone grafts lack the immunologic reactions that may be encountered with allogenic (same species, allograft) or xenogenic (another species, xenograft) bone grafts while providing great donor site availability and ideal cellular characteristics to enhance bone healing. However, some technical challenges in harvesting autogenous bone grafts may include the limiting amounts available at the donor site as well as the morbidity of the autogenous bone graft sites including, but not limited to, pain, edema, bleeding, fracture, and infection.

Continuous advancements in stem cell research, osteobiologics, and orthobiologics mimic the autogenous bone graft characteristics and will continue to challenge the standards in bone grafting (3–7,9,16,18,24–26,32,34,38,44,61,105). Orthobiologically enhanced allogenic bone materials have allowed many of the same benefits as that of autogenous bone grafts. A combination of autogenous and allogenic bone grafts retains some of the ideal characteristics of bone grafting and allows the smallest amounts harvested for the autogenous bone grafting (Fig. 22.1).

Iliac Crest Bone Graft Harvest

Iliac crest autogenous bone grafting has been well described in the literature for its applications in reconstructive and traumatic lower extremity injuries. The harvested bone graft is obtained with a lateral incision directly over the anterior superior iliac spine (ASIS) in a tricortical fashion and provides great living cell characteristics for bone healing in reconstructive surgery of the lower extremity. Upon harvesting, care should be taken to avoid the lateral femoral cutaneous nerve (1,10,18,37). These bone grafts are well incorporated in the recipient defect sites and can be contoured based on the application needs (24,32,44,105).

Most patients have minimal donor site tenderness past the usual postoperative course, and this concurs with multiple studies (1,10,18,37,71,87,90,105). However, some of the most common complications of the harvested iliac crest autogenous bone graft donor site include bleeding, fracture, infection, neuritis, and invasion into surrounding soft tissue and osseous structures, such as the abdomen and hip joint (Fig. 22.2).

If a greater amount of autogenous bone graft is needed, it can be harvested from the posterior superior iliac spine (PSIS). This approach can be quite challenging by increasing the operative time and repositioning the patient for the definitive reconstructive surgery. Special attention is given to preventing damage of the cluneal and superior gluteal nerves during the dissection technique (1,10,18). Unless a great amount of autogenous bone graft is needed, the proximal and distal tibia can serve as excellent donor sites for most of the foot, ankle, and lower extremity reconstructions.

Proximal Tibia Bone Graft Harvest

The proximal tibia autogenous bone graft is harvested from the anteromedial tibial face where minimal neurovascular structures are encountered (15,34,48,87,102). This is an excellent site for autogenous bone graft harvesting because the donor site is readily available and easy to access in limited

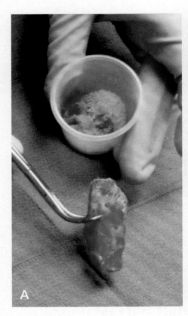
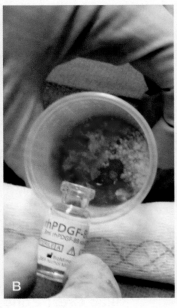
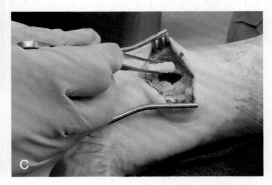

FIGURE 22.1 **A.** Intraoperative picture of a recombinant human platelet-derived growth factor-BB (rhPDGF-BB) mixed with β-tricalcium phosphate (β-TCP) matrix (Augment Bone Graft, Wright Medical Group, Memphis, TN) and a harvested autogenous distal fibula shaped as fibular strut for an onlay bone graft application. **B.** Intraoperative picture of a recombinant human platelet-derived growth factor-BB (rhPDGF-BB) mixed with β-TCP matrix (Augment Bone Graft, Wright Medical Group, Memphis, TN), tibia autogenous bone graft, and demineralized bone matrix (DBM) putty. **C.** Intraoperative picture of a distal tibia autogenous bone graft donor site filled a DBM sponge.

surgical time. Usually, 5 to 25 cm² of excellent cancellous bone graft can be harvested from this region, whereas in older patients or in patients with decreased bone mineral density, the amount of bone graft harvest may be limited to less than 10 to 15 cc. The harvested proximal tibia bone graft is used to nearly any nonstructural weight bearing region as with any other cancellous type of bone grafting.

Some of the most common limitations and complications of harvesting a proximal tibia bone graft include pain at the donor site, fracture into the knee joint, and infection (41,42,48,105). Other complications include hematoma when

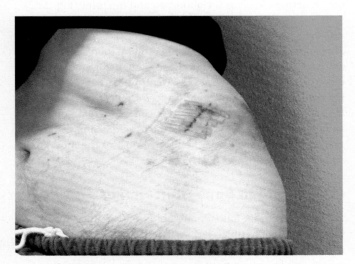

FIGURE 22.2 Postoperative picture of an iliac crest autogenous bone graft donor site.

the resected tibia cortical cap is not replaced and wound dehiscence when the bone void fillers such as calcium sulfate or calcium phosphate have leaked into the surrounding soft tissues at the donor site. Another limitation of harvesting the proximal tibia bone graft is a lack of true tricortical graft strut and its availability in this region. Special attention is given when the harvesting of the proximal tibia bone graft is performed at the same time a lower extremity external fixation device is applied because a stress riser in the tibia can lead into a potential fracture. Bone void filler to the donor site of the proximal tibia is used when the harvested bone grafts are greater than 5 cm² (Figs. 22.3 and 22.4).

Most common applications for the harvested proximal tibia autogenous bone graft include complex pilon and/or ankle fractures, ankle arthrodesis, distal lower extremity malunions and nonunions, and especially midfoot or hindfoot/ankle reconstructions in patients with diabetes mellitus and peripheral neuropathy. In theory, harvesting autogenous bone graft from the proximal tibia is distant to the reconstructive procedures of the foot and ankle and is more likely to heal the harvest site in the diabetic population with already impaired distal wound and osseous healing potential (Figs. 22.5 and 22.6).

Distal Tibia Bone Graft Harvest

The distal tibia autogenous bone graft is harvested from the anteromedial tibial face proximal to the ankle joint taking care to avoid any neurovascular structures encountered. The distal tibia is an excellent source of harvesting cancellous bone (15,20,77,78,83), and the resected tibia cortical cap may also be applied to the recipient site in various midfoot/

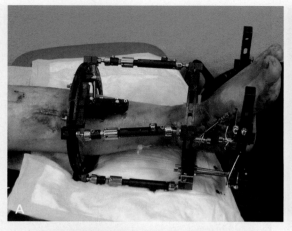
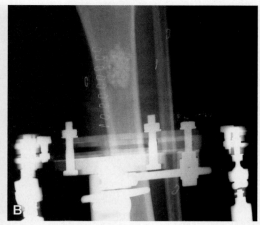
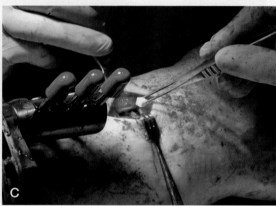

FIGURE 22.3 **A.** Postoperative picture showing the proximal tibia bone graft harvesting site superior to the circular external fixator. **B.** Postoperative anteroposterior leg radiograph showing the proximal tibia donor site filled with calcium phosphate and allogenic bone void filler. **C.** Intraoperative picture of a proximal tibia harvest site filled with allogenic bone chips.

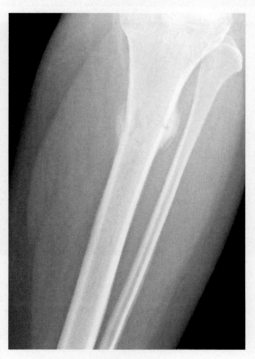

FIGURE 22.4 Postoperative anteroposterior leg radiograph showing a fracture created due to stress riser in the proximal tibia as a result from a non-drilled donor site.

hindfoot arthrodesis procedures if structural support is needed (Fig. 22.7). Its size is also ideal for repair to metatarsal malunions and/or nonunions in which the nonunited metatarsal portion is resected and the distal tibia cortical cap along with the harvested cancellous underlying bone can be inserted directly in the recipient osseous defect area and overlaid with fixation. Harvesting the distal tibia autogenous bone graft is a reliable procedure with minimal operative time and complications.

Some of the most common limitations in harvesting the distal tibia autogenous bone graft include its proximity to the ankle joint if an ankle arthrodesis or other distal tibia or fibula type of surgery is to be performed. Other reported limitations and complications are availability of bone, which is typically limited between 10 and 20 cc of cancellous bone grafting, fracture, entrance into the ankle joint, neurovascular injury, pain, neuritis, and saphenous nerve entrapment (77,78,83,105) (Fig. 22.8).

The donor site is usually filled with either calcium phosphate or a mixed calcium ceramic and allogenic bone void filler to provide an osteoconductive bridge allowing regrowth and filling in the tibia medullary canal. Allogenic bone grafts are preferable for bone void filling at the donor site because they provide immediate support with less time to incorporate. The resected distal tibia cortical cap should also be replaced over the harvest site, unless it is being used in the reconstructive procedures.

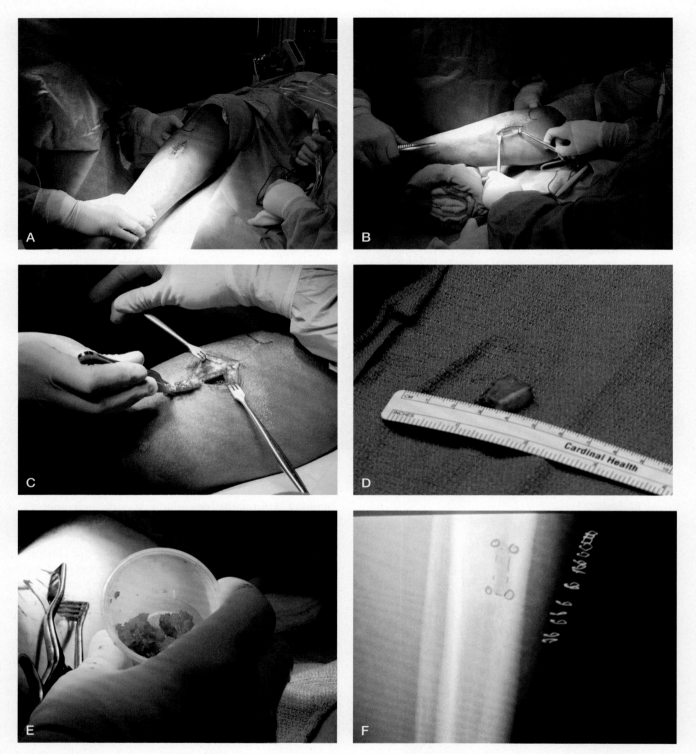

FIGURE 22.5 A. Example of a proximal tibia autogenous bone graft harvest. An incision about 5 cm in length is made over the antero-medial tibial face at approximately 2 to 3 cm below the tibial tubercle. **B.** Sharp periosteal dissection is made, and care is taken to avoid any anomalous neurovascular structures. A small drill is then used to provide unicortical stress relief to the 4 corners of the entrance site into the tibia. Next, a small saw is used to connect the premade drill holes. Care is taken not to burn the bone with the saw, and an osteotome may then be used to finish the cuts once started. **C,D.** The resected tibia cortical cap is lifted, which is saved for replacement later or for use in the reconstructive procedure if needed. **E.** A round Bruns bone curette is used to harvest the cancellous bone graft proximally toward the knee. The desired amount of bone graft is harvested. **F.** The surgical wound at the donor site is irrigated, and the donor site bone void may be filled with allogenic bone chips, calcium phosphate, or a mixture of bone void fillers. The resected tibia cortical cap is then replaced at the donor site. Care is taken to avoid any bone void filler or allogenic bone grafts from leaking into the surrounding soft tissues at the donor site. Meticulous periosteal flap closure is made, followed by irrigation and layered closure.

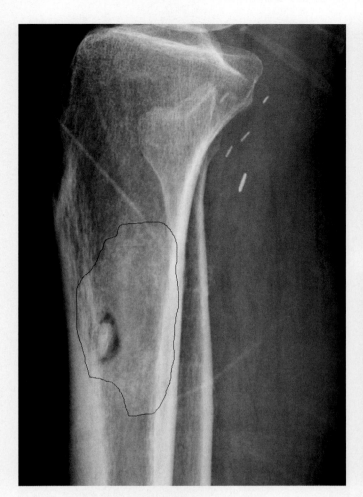

FIGURE 22.6 Postoperative lateral leg radiograph showing a proximal tibia autogenous bone graft harvest in a diamond-shaped cortical window which is superior to the rectangular-shaped window as shown in Figure 22.5F, allowing for better access with a curette into the proximal and distal tibia medullary canal.

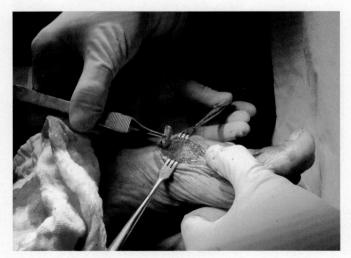

FIGURE 22.7 Intraoperative picture showing the application of a harvested distal tibia autogenous corticocancellous bone graft at the first metatarsocuneiform joint arthrodesis site.

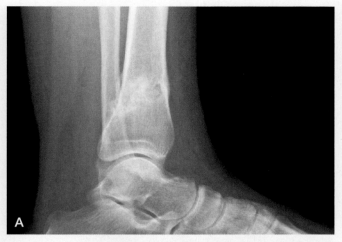

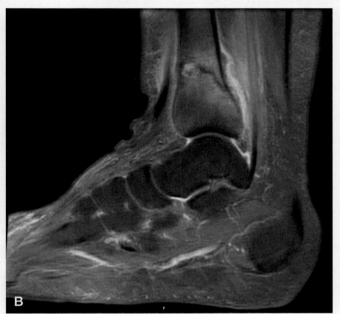

FIGURE 22.8 **A.** Postoperative lateral ankle radiograph showing a fracture at the distal tibia autogenous bone graft harvest site. **B.** Magnetic resonance imaging showing a stress fracture through the distal tibia autogenous bone graft harvest site.

Oversewing the periosteal flap is necessary as well in order to prevent the bone void filler from leaking into the surrounding soft tissues at the harvest site (Figs. 22.9 and 22.10).

Fibula Bone Graft Harvest

The fibula autogenous bone graft provides an excellent source for harvesting especially when a vascularized bone graft is needed. In these cases, the central third of the fibula is harvested with significant reported morbidity at the donor site (8,11,41,105). This autogenous bone graft is harvested when a cortical strut is needed for the reconstructive procedure, but it has limitations in the length and the total amount of harvested bone. It is generally accepted that the distal third of the fibula should be allowed to remain for adequate stability

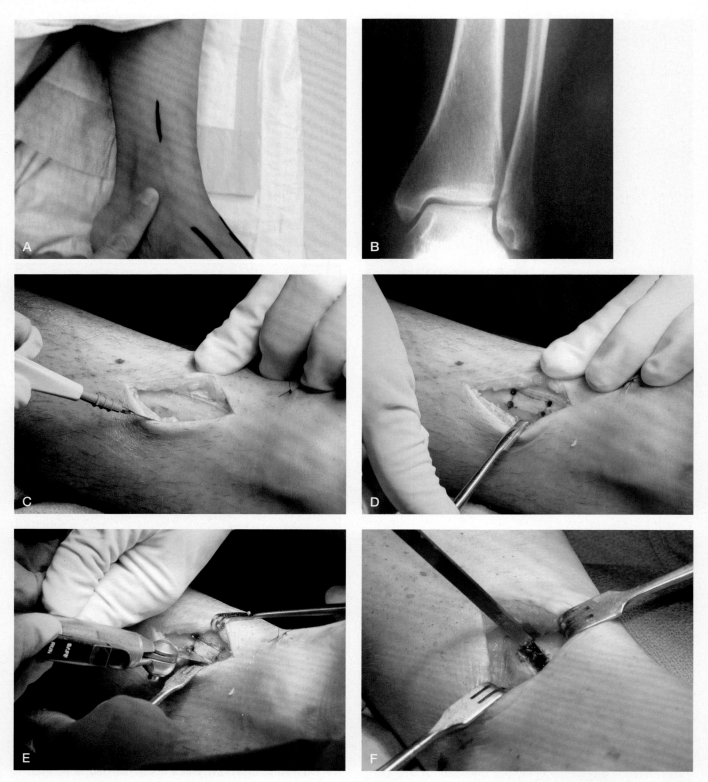

FIGURE 22.9 **A,B.** Example of a distal tibia autogenous bone graft harvest. A 3 to 5 cm incision in length is made over the antero-medial tibial face at approximately 4 to 6 cm above the medial malleolus and parallel to the central line of the tibial shaft. **C.** Sharp periosteal dissection is made, and care is taken to avoid the most common neurovascular structures encountered, being the saphe-nous nerve and vein. **D.** If the saphenous vein or branches are cut, they may be ligated as necessary. Close proximity to the ankle joint may be confirmed via an intraoperative C-arm fluoroscopy, but this may not be necessary. A small drill is then used to provide unicortical stress relief to the 4 corners of the entrance site into the distal tibia. **E.** Next, a small saw is used to connect the premade drill holes. **F.** Care is taken not to burn the bone with the saw, and an osteotome may then be used to finish the cuts once started. *(continued)*

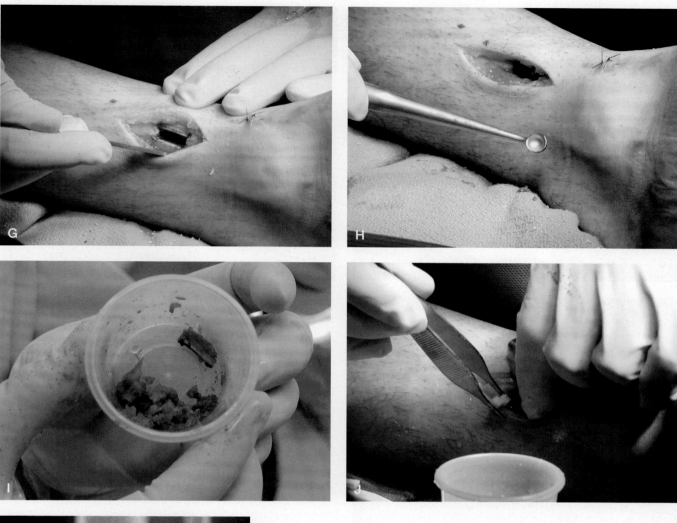

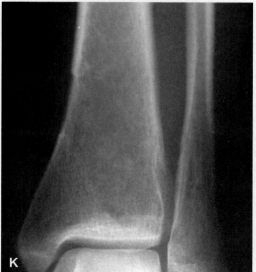

FIGURE 22.9 *(Continued)* **G.** The resected distal tibia cortical cap is lifted, which is saved for replacement later or for use in the reconstructive procedure if needed. **H.** A round Bruns bone curette is used to harvest the cancellous bone graft distally toward the ankle. **I.** The desired amount of bone graft is harvested. Care is taken in bone with decreased bone mineral density not to enter into the ankle joint. **J.** The surgical wound at the donor site is irrigated, and the donor site void may be filled with allogenic bone chips, calcium phosphate, or a mixture of bone void fillers. **K.** The resected distal tibia cortical cap is then replaced at the donor site or used in the reconstructive procedure. Care is taken to avoid any bone void filler or allogenic bone grafts from leaking into the surrounding soft tissues at the donor site. Meticulous periosteal flap closure is made, followed by irrigation and layered closure.

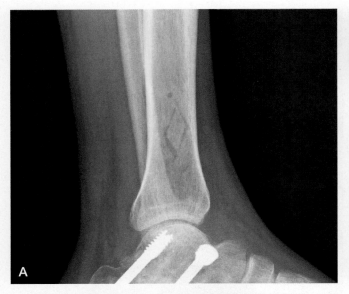

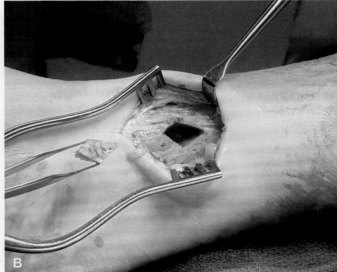

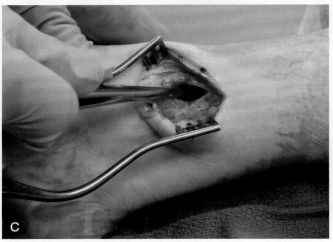

FIGURE 22.10 **A.** Postoperative lateral leg radiograph showing a distal tibia autogenous bone graft harvest in a diamond-shaped cortical window. **B.** Intraoperative picture showing the removal of the distal tibia cortical cap from a diamond-shaped cortical window. **C.** Intraoperative picture showing a greater access into the medullary canal of the distal tibia through a diamond shaped cortical window.

to the ankle joint, but this concept may be altered in cases of ankle or pantalar arthrodesis procedures.

The distal third of the fibula is an excellent source to be used either as a ground corticocancellous bone graft or a partial fibula onlay strut graft. The amount of bone that can be harvested usually depends on the quality of the central medullary canal of the fibula and whether the fibula has been operated on previously (as is the case in many ankle fractures). The distal fibula is resected and can be used as an onlay strut graft, transecting it in half and shortening it, in ankle/pantalar arthrodesis procedures. The partial fibula onlay strut graft is fixated proximally or distally with the remaining portions of the bone graft ground up within the prepared joint(s) to help compensate for the shortening that occurs with multiple-joint arthrodeses (Fig. 22.11). The distal fibula may also be used as an in situ bone graft when performing a synostosis of the tibia to the fibula in tibia–fibula malunions as well as in syndesmotic arthrodesis procedures in cases of nonunion, malunion, and syndesmotic instability (Figs. 22.12 and 22.13).

Fibula autogenous bone grafts are usually limited because the quality of the graft is often poor. In many cases when resecting the fibula as either a vascularized strut graft or onlay strut graft, the central medullary canal is very poor in cancellous stock, and the major portion of the bone itself is cortical. High donor-site morbidity in this region has been reported, and care must be taken to avoid injury to the peroneal tendons, sural nerve, bleeding, and/or fracture at the harvest site. Lastly, in some clinical scenarios, sparing the fibula during an ankle arthrodesis may be feasible and therefore minimizing any complications associated with the fibula bone graft harvesting (Fig. 22.14).

Calcaneus Bone Graft Harvest

The calcaneus autogenous bone graft provides an excellent source of harvesting cancellous bone. The donor site of the calcaneus can provide 5 cc or less of cancellous bone but has at times taken up to 25 cc of bone harvesting. The harvested

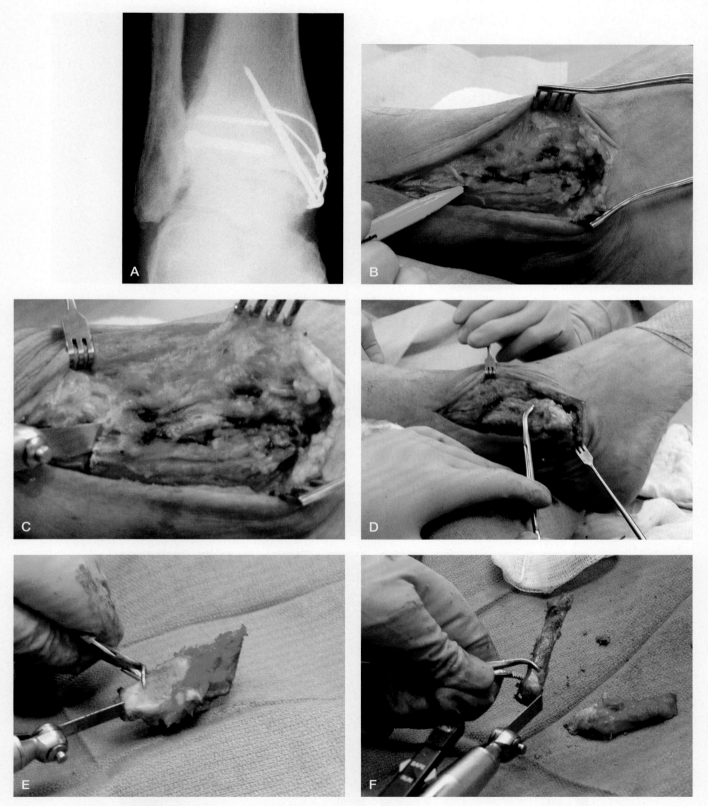

FIGURE 22.11 A,B. Example of a fibula autogenous bone graft harvest. A 5 to 10 cm incision in length is made over the lateral aspect of the distal fibula. **B.** Sharp periosteal dissection is made, and care is taken to avoid the sural nerve posteriorly and the more medial branches of the peroneal nerve above the ankle. The peroneal tendons are identified and retracted posteriorly. **C.** The distal fibula is resected with power saw instrumentation and is then removed **(D)** distally. **E.** Any fibrotic tissue and distal ligament attachments are removed from the harvested fibula bone graft which is then held firmly with a bone forceps **(F)** and transected in the middle. *(continued)*

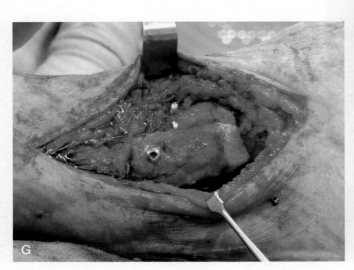
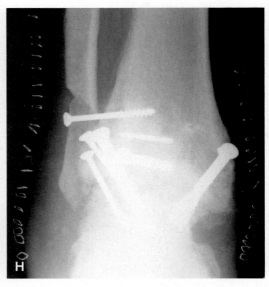

FIGURE 22.11 *(Continued)* **G,H.** The remaining portions are shaped to fit the application as an onlay strut graft at the arthrodesis site. Use of the split fibula autogenous bone graft can be used as an onlay strut graft, or viable bone graft portions may be morselized and applied in the arthrodesis site.

calcaneus autogenous bone graft seems to always be of fair quality, even in the poorest bone stock. The harvest sites in this region have minimal morbidity, and the incisional tenderness tends to be no more than the surrounding surgical sites (15,16,18,34,48,105).

The main calcaneal harvest sites have been described as the medial instep of the calcaneus and more often the lateral wall of the calcaneus. Incisional entrapment of the medial calcaneal nerve and above the sural nerve regions has been described with the above calcaneal harvest sites (16,18,34,48). Some of the most common limitations and complications

in harvesting a calcaneus autogenous bone graft especially in the diabetic population is that the amount of blood flow in the distal extremities can potentially interfere with the surgical wound healing. In addition, harvesting bone graft through the calcaneus can impair surgical correction, such as in simultaneous hindfoot arthrodesis, unless used in the midfoot and/or forefoot surgical sites. In contrary, the calcaneus may be an excellent source of cancellous bone harvesting if a calcaneal osteotomy and midfoot or forefoot arthrodesis is performed in the same patient where some of the harvested bone graft from the calcaneal osteotomy site

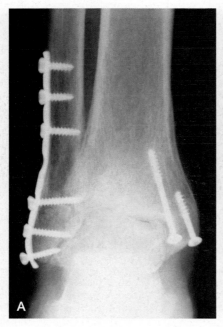
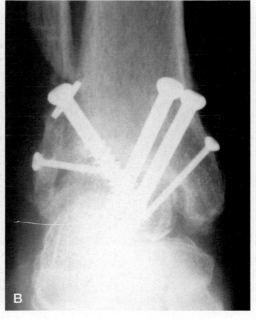

FIGURE 22.12 **A.** Preoperative anteroposterior ankle radiograph of an ankle fracture with retained hardware and ankle posttraumatic arthritis. **B.** Postoperative anteroposterior ankle radiograph showing the ankle arthrodesis with a partial fibula onlay strut graft.

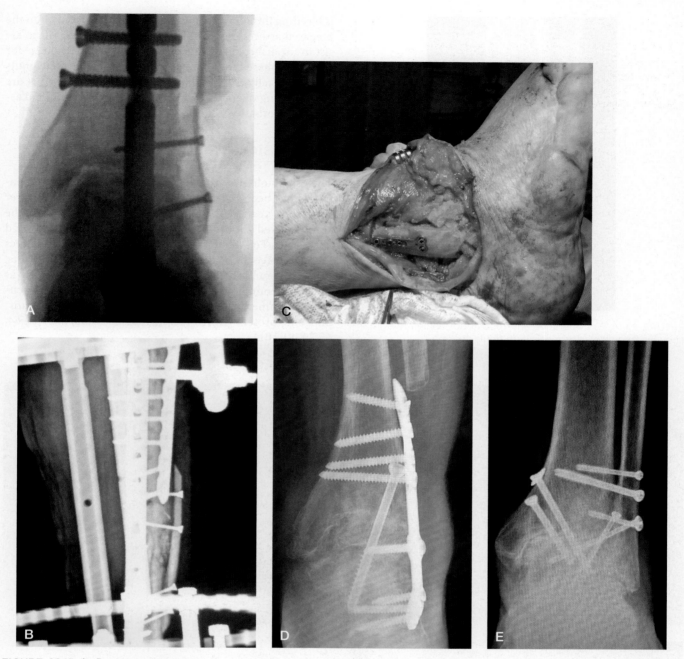

FIGURE 22.13 A. Postoperative anteroposterior ankle radiograph showing a tibiotalocalcaneal arthrodesis with an autogenous fibula onlay strut graft and intramedullary nailing. **B.** Postoperative lateral leg radiograph showing the application of an allogenic fibula onlay strut graft in comminuted fracture. **C.** Intraoperative picture showing an autogenous fibula onlay strut graft fixated in the ankle arthrodesis site. **D.** Postoperative anteroposterior ankle radiograph showing a tibiotalocalcaneal arthrodesis with the distal fibula autogenous bone graft harvest morselized and applied into the tibiotalocalcaneal arthrodesis site. **E.** Postoperative anteroposterior ankle radiograph showing an ankle and tibia–fibula syndesmosis arthrodesis with the fibula being used as in situ bone graft and after the medial aspect of the fibula was prepared for the arthrodesis.

can be utilized in the distal foot arthrodesis sites (Figs. 22.15 and 22.16).

Alternative Autogenous Bone Graft Sites

Some of the most common alternative autogenous bone graft sites may include the phalangeal heads from toe joint arthroplasties, the medial eminence after a hallux

abducto valgus correction, and portions of the navicular after a resection of an accessory or hypertrophic navicular tuberosity (Fig. 22.17). In addition, hypertrophic bone formation following a Charcot neuroarthropathy foot and/or ankle reconstruction can be harvested and prepared for the arthrodesis site(s). However, this type of bone quality is usually marginal, with a significant amount of soft periosteal and mixed fibrous tissue. If the harvested bone is viable and

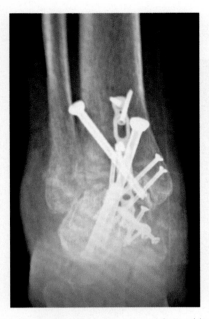

FIGURE 22.14 Postoperative anteroposterior ankle radiograph showing an ankle arthrodesis with fibula sparing.

is bleeding intraoperatively, it could be used directly into the prepared arthrodesis site(s) or as an onlay bone graft to assist in the arthrodesis procedure(s). The main advantage for the use of these types of alternative autogenous bone grafts is that typically they are harvested from local sites that are already being operated on or close by and have minimal associated morbidity.

OSTEOBIOLOGICS

The osteobiologics group of graft or graft type implant materials has been redefined, reinvented, and reapplied over the last 30 years. For this reason, bone grafting cannot be simply talked about in terms of autografts, allografts, and xenografts. For the purpose of this chapter, osteobiologics includes osteoconductive materials such as bone allografts, calcium ceramics, hydroxyapatite (HA), and collagen as well as osteoinductive materials such as platelet gel concentrates, demineralized bone matrix (DBM), and bone morphogenic protein (BMP) (2,19,21–23,28,29,33,47,57,62,64, 65,79–81,101).

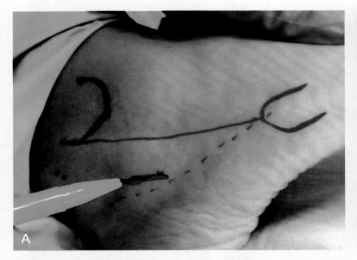

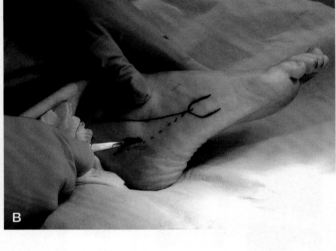

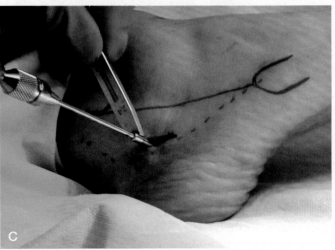

FIGURE 22.15 A. Example of a calcaneus autogenous bone graft harvest (lateral side). The distal tip of the lateral malleolus and the base of the fifth metatarsal are marked and the course of the peroneal tendons is visualized. **B.** A skin incision is made 2 to 3 cm inferior and parallel to the peroneal tendons on the lateral calcaneal wall making sure to avoid the lateral dorsal cutaneous/sural nerve. A hemostat is used to spread the soft tissues bluntly to the level of the calcaneal periosteum which is then incised. **C.** A small drill is used to make a unicortical entrance on the lateral side of the calcaneal wall. *(continued)*

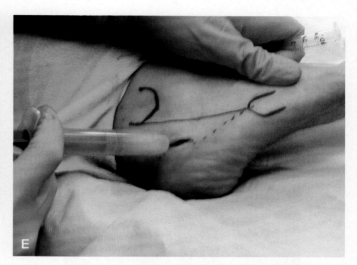

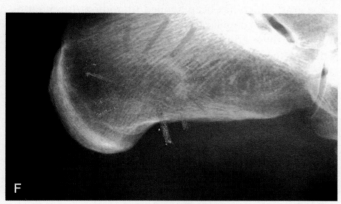

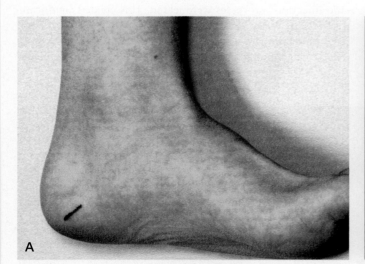

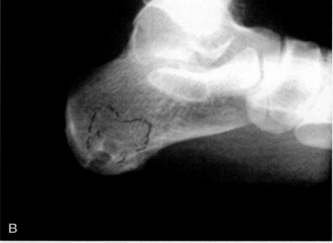

FIGURE 22.15 *(Continued)* **D.** A round Bruns bone curette is used to harvest the desired calcaneal cancellous bone graft. Care is taken not to enter the subtalar joint or opposite side of the calcaneal wall. **E.** Bone void filler such as allograft bone chips or calcium ceramics may be used at the harvest site. The periosteum is then closed followed by skin closure. Care is taken to avoid entrapment of the lateral dorsal cutaneous/sural nerve. **F.** Postoperative lateral foot radiograph showing the calcaneal lateral wall and harvested calcaneus autogenous bone graft site.

FIGURE 22.16 A. Example of a calcaneus autogenous bone graft harvest (medial side). A posterior medial instep incision is made. Care is taken to avoid the medial neurovascular bundle and specifically the medial calcaneal nerve. This medial approach is useful if less bone is needed via a small 1 to 2 cm incision. No bone void filler is usually needed for the calcaneal-harvested site, and skin closure is only performed. **B.** Postoperative lateral foot radiograph showing the calcaneal wall and harvested medial calcaneus autogenous bone graft site.

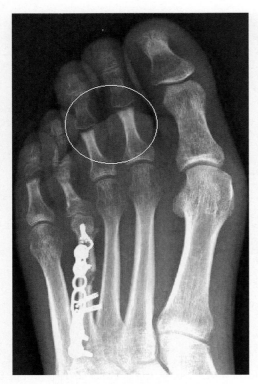

FIGURE 22.17 Postoperative anteroposterior foot radiograph showing the second and third toe proximal interphalangeal arthroplasties being used as harvested autogenous bone graft sites for surgical repair of a short fourth metatarsal.

Osteoconductive Agents and Materials

Allogenic bone grafts are excellent bone graft substitutes for most applications in foot and ankle reconstructive surgery. Many times, unless they are coupled with a significant amount of osteoinductive products or combined with autogenous bone graft, their usefulness for diabetic reconstructive surgery can be limited. Because of the variable processing with allogenic bone grafts, they also carry some additional risk of immunologic reactions. The most common methods for processing allogenic bone grafts are freeze-drying, liquid nitrogen freezing, and demineralization. The closest type of bone graft to one's own bone is through the fresh frozen technique; however, these also have the most associated immunologic reactions. The main advantage to fresh frozen bone grafts is their retention of some osteogenic potential and properties (8,34,44,56,71).

For most diabetic foot and ankle reconstructive surgeries, the additional threat posed by fresh frozen bone grafts by an immune reaction, when other viable and predictable bone graft options are available, has limited the use of this particular type of bone grafting. These allogenic bone grafts have mostly consisted of fresh frozen iliac crest tricortical bone graft which has been applied to midfoot/hindfoot osteotomies and some large resected osteomyelitic defects. In addition, these bone grafts can be particularly useful when other methods of bone graft harvesting are either unavailable or have failed. Most facilities will have a freezer and cold storage available for these types of allogenic bone grafts (Fig. 22.18).

Freeze-dried Allografts

Freeze-dried allografts, excluding DBM, do not contain the same osteogenic potential as the autogenous bone grafts. These types of bone products are excellent for autograft bone extenders and can be combined with other osteoinductive agents. The main fear through mid-1980s through the 1990s was the transmission of disease through a same-species donor. Human immunodeficiency virus, hepatitis C, other prions, and infectious processes were feared. This created significant restrictions in the acceptance of donors and also standardized guidelines for tissue banks. However, this process has effectively eliminated fear for most surgeons and patients.

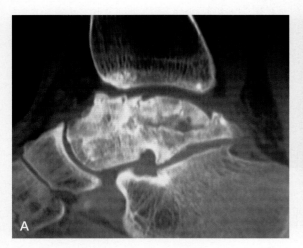
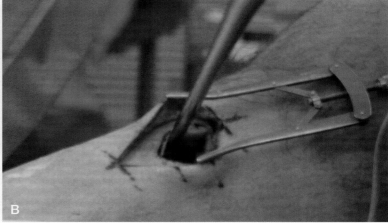

FIGURE 22.18 **A.** Preoperative computed tomography showing fracture of the talus with associated collapse. **B.** A proximal tibia autogenous bone graft was harvested to be combined with the allogenic talar bone graft. *(continued)*

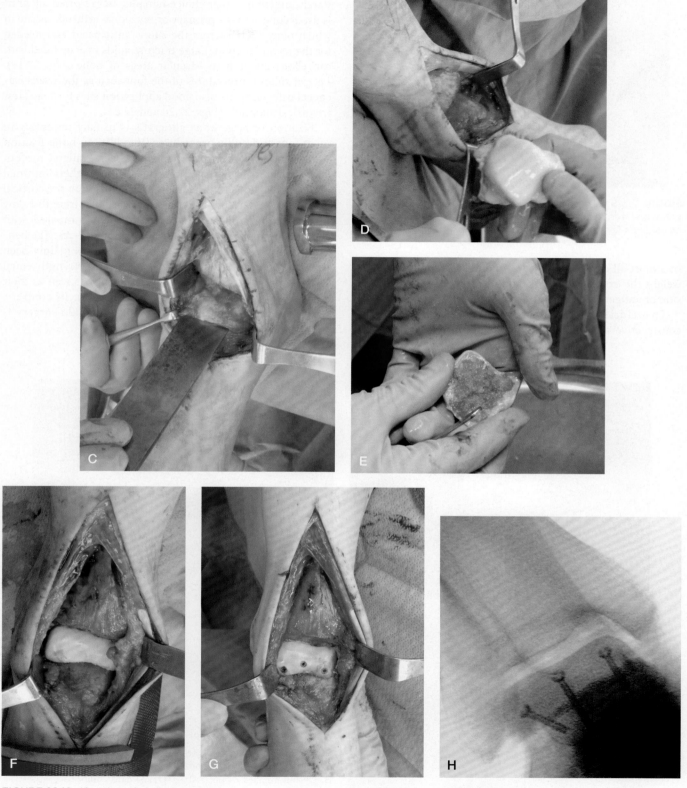

FIGURE 22.18 *(Continued)* **C.** Exostectomy and excisional débridement of the nonviable superior aspect of the talus was performed. **D.** Measuring the fresh donor talus before application into the ankle joint. **E.** Harvested proximal tibia autogenous bone graft application on the underside of the prepped donor talus. **F.** Insertion and fixation of the allogenic bone graft with internal fixation **(G)** at the ankle joint. **H.** Postoperative anteroposterior ankle radiograph showing the application of allogenic bone graft.

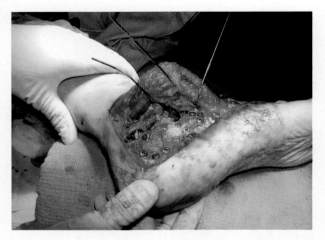

FIGURE 22.19 Intraoperative picture of a calcaneal fracture repair with internal fixation and application of allograft cancellous bone chips for the calcaneal fracture void.

In almost all cases, the benefit of bone graft application outweighs the extremely low likelihood of any disease transmission or antigenic reaction (19,34,44,56,71,93).

Freeze-dried allografts have mainly been used during reconstructive surgery for large bone voids. In large resolved osteomyelitic voids or nonunions, freeze-dried allograft in combination with DBM gel or autograft is sometimes used. Rarely, unless no other choice remains, freeze-dried allograft is used alone across a primary or revisional arthrodesis site in which bony union across the site is anticipated and needed for the reconstruction. Large fracture voids may be filled with cancellous allograft in vascular areas of bone (Fig. 22.19). Lateral column procedures of the foot such as the Evans calcaneal osteotomy are also good application sites for iliac crest tricortical allografts (Figs. 22.20 and 22.21).

Fixation of large bone allografts is usually necessary in most foot and ankle procedures. In addition, bone fixation devices made from cortical bone have been available for foot and ankle reconstructive procedures due to their minimal antigenicity. However, the main limitations with the cortical bone fixation devices have been their variable strengths, slow incorporation, and lack of strength when compared with standard rigid internal or external fixation devices. The benefit of these cortical bone fixation devices has mainly been the lack of need for removal, density, and strength equal to the bone that they are being placed into as well as their general availability (19,28,46,71,81,91,93,102). In contrary, their use in the field of diabetic foot and ankle surgery is very limited.

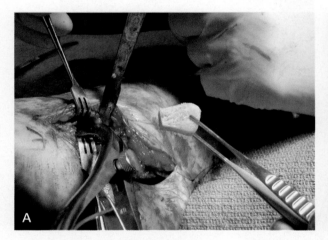

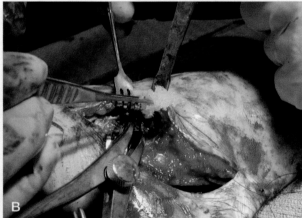

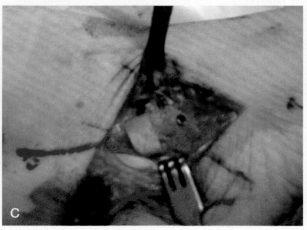

FIGURE 22.20 **A.** Intraoperative picture showing an iliac crest tricortical allograft for an Evans calcaneal osteotomy. **B.** Demineralized bone matrix (DBM) putty allograft was also applied around the iliac crest tricortical allograft and within the calcaneal osteotomy site. **C.** Internal fixation was utilized at the surgical site with the iliac crest tricortical allograft and DBM putty.

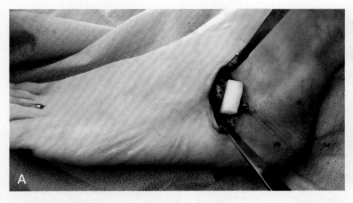
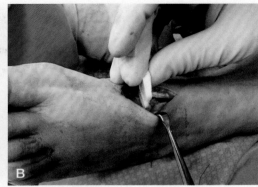
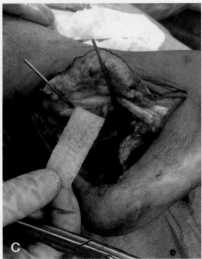
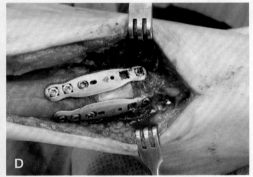

FIGURE 22.21 Examples of freeze-dried allografts in reconstructive foot surgery. **A.** Evans calcaneal osteotomy procedure carried out with the use of a tricortical wedge allograft placement. **B.** Cotton medial cuneiform osteotomy procedure carried out with the use of an allograft. **C.** Allograft usage for severe subtalar joint depression after a calcaneal fracture. **D.** First metatarsocuneiform joint arthrodesis carried out with the use of a tricortical allograft.

Hydroxyapatite Xenografts

HA grafts are considered xenografts because they are composed of the *Goniopora* coral species. These grafts are purely osteoconductive bridges that may be used to fill minimally load-bearing or protected voids in bone. HA come in a 200- and 500-μg pore size. This approximately mimics cortical and cancellous bone, respectively (Pro Osteon 200R and 500R, Interpore Cross Int., Irvine, CA). The structure of HA makes it excellent for large bone voids and cysts, and its use may be widened when mixed with a DBM autograft or osteoinductive agent.

HA is useful as a building block or structure to add to, in large voids after pilon fractures, severe calcaneal void fractures, and after resecting large tibia defects (Fig. 22.22). It is also beneficial for filling the bone void at the majority of autograft harvest sites. At most sites, the application of HA must be rigidly protected by both surrounding bone and fixation. The slow osteoclastic breakdown of HA prevents any significant usefulness at arthrodesis sites (22,23,30,34,49,52,68,85,89,104).

Biocompatible Porous Metals

Biocompatible porous metals are used as an interface between implants or as an isolated implant themselves, where the metal structure mimics cancellous bone with the desired outcome for partial or complete bony ingrowth. On the undersurface of a tibial or talar tray of a total ankle joint replacement or on some stems of first metatarsal joint implants, it is desirable to have a partial ingrowth of the implant to hold the joint replacement in optimal position. In other areas, such as an Evans- or Cotton-type porous metal wedge, it may be desirable to have the porous metal completely incorporate with the surrounding bone. In addition, there have also been wedge plates and other arthrodesis devices that utilize some of this same technology (12,45,51,63,66,94,99).

Calcium Phosphate Ceramics

Calcium phosphates have been used in their various forms in filling large bony voids and autogenous bone graft donor sites. The main drawback of calcium phosphate, as with other ceramics, is that they are clearly osteoconductive. They are also useful in filling tumor voids when mixed with allografts (Fig. 22.23). Another potential drawback with calcium phosphate is that when it does get into the surrounding soft tissues, it can create a soft tissue sterile abscess that can develop into a surgical wound dehiscence. There have also been studies in which calcium phosphate mixtures have been useful in calcaneal fracture repairs, allowing early weight bearing and

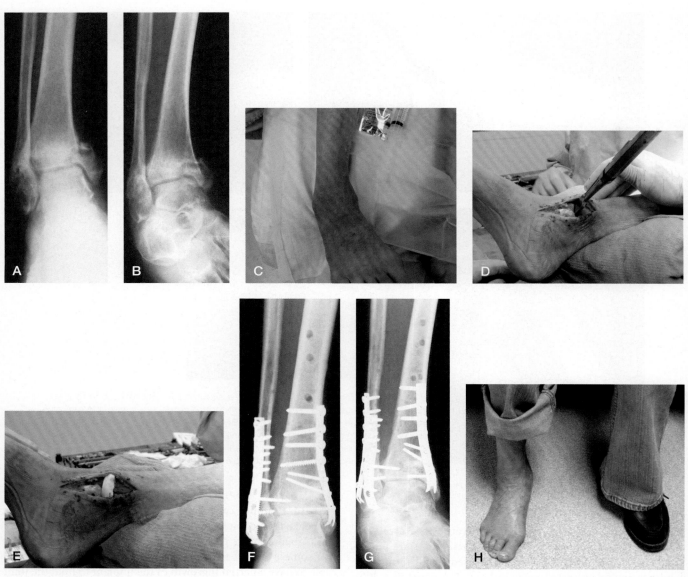

FIGURE 22.22 **A.** Preoperative anteroposterior, medial oblique **(B)** radiographic, and clinical **(C)** views of a diabetic neuropathic distal tibia malunion with varus deformity. **D,E.** Intraoperative distal tibia osteotomy and deformity correction followed by the application of a hydroxyapatite bone graft wedge mixed with allograft bone cancellous chips and demineralized bone matrix paste. **F.** Postoperative anteroposterior, medial oblique **(G)** radiographic, and clinical **(H)** views after the lower extremity deformity correction.

mobilization (92). However, most of the calcium ceramics are used for filling large bony voids (22,30,31,39,53,54,58,62,65,67, 70,73,81,83,86,103,104).

Calcium Sulfate Ceramics

Calcium sulfates are usually in the form of pellets and have been useful in filling large bone voids, defects, and donor sites in the proximal tibia, distal tibia, and pelvis. These, like calcium phosphates, can leak into the surrounding soft tissues and have a spontaneous sterile abscess within the site itself. Calcium ceramics are usually avoided at any arthrodesis sites or any other sites where cyclical loading and bone repair would be expected to occur to any reasonable extent beyond the conductive bridge they provide (28,43,57,58,65,75,81,101).

Antibiotic-impregnated calcium phosphate or sulfate products are usually utilized for large osseous and/or soft tissue defects with underlying osteomyelitis. These mixtures have been applied to large defects after resection of osteomyelitis but not for bridging or spanning the bone to facilitate bone healing. These bone healing properties are usually indicated for autogenous or another bone allograft mixture in combination with other bone growth factors or BMP (Fig. 22.24).

Collagen Materials

Collagen has been combined with multiple other materials to help create a better bone graft supplement. Collagen is an excellent carrier of other materials, including calcium phosphate

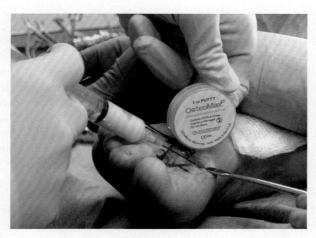

FIGURE 22.23 Intraoperative picture of a mixed calcium ceramic paste and allograft injected into the first metatarsal tumor void.

and calcium sulfate, but its use seems more applicable to irregular defects because it may be shaped, cut, and packed into a variety of clinical applications, especially when combined with an osteoinductive material (28,29,62,65,76,81,102). The main applications in reconstructive surgery have been as bone graft extenders, filling bone voids and non–weight-bearing structural defects of the tibia and calcaneus. They have been used for supplementary overlay grafts in addition to autogenous bone grafts, but they are still combined with DBM or other osteoinductive materials.

Osteoinductive Agents and Materials

There are a variety of osteoinductive agents that are used in reconstructive surgery including, but not limited to, DBM, platelet gel concentrates, BMP, mesenchymal stem cells (MSCs), and human amniotic allografts. Over the last 2 decades, research and technology have allowed an expansion in the number of materials available for surgical use (9,14,17,27,28,33,35,36,47,79,80,82,96–98,101).

Demineralized Bone Matrix

DBM has been used for many years since residual properties of BMPs were originally discovered. DBM is a mixture of cortical and cancellous bone organic material, and because different techniques and processing of DBM are available, it is likely and significant that many products contain variable amounts of different types of BMP. The benefit and ideal properties of various BMPs described are not fully known or realized; however, it is generally accepted that almost all BMPs create a rich environment for osteoinduction, which is beneficial for bone healing (17,65,72,88,102).

In addition to BMP, other growth factors continue to be isolated, and many of these have been shown to be beneficial in bone healing. These include insulin-like growth factor, osteocalcin, osteonectin, and transforming growth factor beta. Most of the carriers with DBM are a glycerol-type gel similar to some of the delivery systems with calcium pellet products. Most of the DBM products vary only in the concentration of protein gels or BMPs (17,33,55,72,88,105).

DBM is very useful across arthrodesis and nonunion sites as well as in Charcot neuroarthropathy reconstruction. DBM has been manufactured in gel, paste, and putty bases and is applied as a primary bone graft or more commonly in combination with allograft bone (Fig. 22.25). DBM is readily available and may be combined with calcium ceramics and other materials to provide osteoinductive capabilities. One of the main disadvantages is their lack of structural integrity, but it can be combined with a structural autograft or allograft.

Platelet Gel Concentrate

Platelet-derived growth factor (PDGF), vasculoendothelial growth factor, insulin-like growth factor, epithelial growth factor, and transforming growth factor have been found to be beneficial in bone, soft tissue, and wound healing. Each of these agents has the variable ability to progress the process of bone, soft tissue, and wound healing in various ways, including stimulation of osteoprogenitor cells and reviving the normal wound healing process (35,36,47,69,74,80,84).

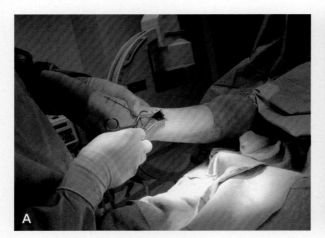
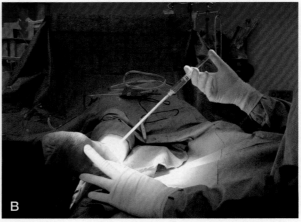

FIGURE 22.24 **A.** Intraoperative picture of a distal tibia autogenous bone graft harvest site filled with calcium sulfate **(B)** at the donor site.

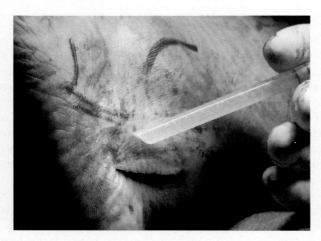

FIGURE 22.25 Intraoperative picture of a medial displacement calcaneal osteotomy in a patient with diabetes mellitus and osteopenic bone filled with demineralized bone matrix.

There have been various platelet aggregates and gel concentrate systems. The main difference in most of these systems is the amount of blood drawn from the patient and the variable amount of yield of platelet growth materials. The platelets become 2 main materials as they are separated: platelet-rich plasma (PRP) and platelet-poor plasma (PPP). The PRP is typically mixed with a thrombin-like material and used with an additional grafting agent or directly on the wound bed, whereas the PPP that contains fibrinogen and other clotting materials has been found to be beneficial in reconstructive surgery and especially when a residual Charcot neuroarthropathy defect or wound remains. PPP is applied directly to the surgical wound area either prior to closure or by applying it to the region after surgical débridement if there is an ulcerative site that is going to granulate by secondary intention. The use of PRP and PPP is becoming more widespread as the benefits of adding them to an osteoconductive bridge, material, or as an adjunct to autogenous or allograft bone materials are seen (35,47,69,80,84).

Bone Morphogenic Protein

BMP serves as the osteoinductive portion of DBM. In tandem with a bone scaffold, BMPs are powerful inducers of new bone formation. They stimulate osteoblast to form and create new bone across arthrodesis and fracture sites (17,33,55,60,79,82,95–98,101). The most commonly used BMPs today are the recombinant human BMP-2 (rhBMP-2) (Infuse, Medtronic Sofamor Danek, Memphis, TN) and BMP-7 (osteogenic protein 1; OP-1) (Stryker Biotech, Hopkinton, MA).

Mesenchymal Stem Cells

MSCs have recently seen a widespread application in bone grafting. MSCs are attached to an allograft scaffold, usually in the form of cancellous bone. MSCs contain separated precursor cells from an adult bone marrow which convert into osteoblasts, osteocytes, and hematopoietic stem cells. New bone is formed directly and indirectly. Osteogenesis occurs through osteoid and matrix production by the osteoblasts and osteocytes. Osteoinduction occurs by signaling host cells to produce more bone and causing further expression of BMPs (9,14,21,27,35,47,76).

MSCs are commercially manufactured and available for use by several industries with main drawbacks of cost and that they must be thawed for a half hour from its storage temperature of −80°C before their use (3,5,13,40,100). MSCs may be mixed with other bone graft products to extend their osteogenesis properties. This is also an excellent product for extending any harvested autograft and has been especially useful in large deformity corrections and Charcot neuroarthropathy reconstruction (3,5) (Figs. 22.26 and 22.27).

Amniotic Tissue Grafts or Human Amniotic Allografts

By definition, these tissues fall into the category of allografts. They come in various forms from freeze-dried sheets, cryopreserved, reconstitutional, and even freshly preserved formulations. The main differences in the tissues are (a) the amount or

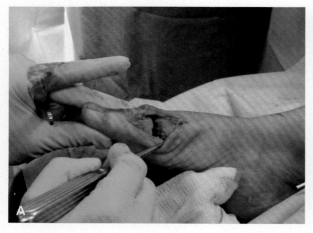
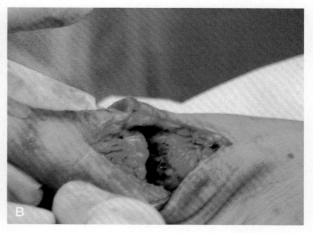

FIGURE 22.26 **A.** Intraoperative picture of a nonunion at the first metatarsophalangeal joint in a patient with diabetes mellitus and peripheral neuropathy. **B.** *(continued)*

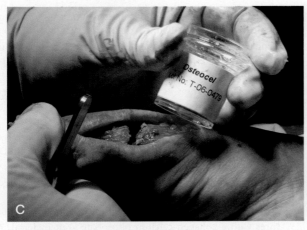

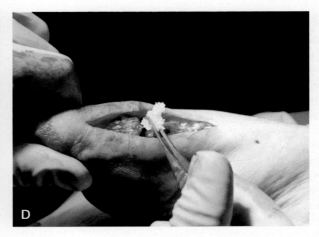

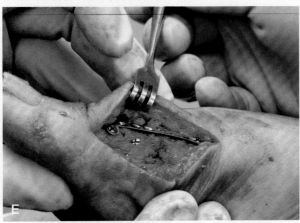

FIGURE 22.26 *(Continued)* Short first metatarsal with void at the prepared arthrodesis site after nonunion resection. **C.** Mesenchymal stem cells (MSCs) at the arthrodesis site to fill the bone void. **D.** MSCs packed into the first metatarsophalangeal joint arthrodesis site. **E.** Rigid internal fixation with incorporated MSCs bone graft.

percentage of amnion and chorion contained, (b) the preparation process including washing and incubation periods, (c) the amount of beneficial characteristics contained in each brand and preparation type, and (d) the differences in form and the manufacturing processes. Evidence of nerve, cartilage, and bone regeneration has been shown in a multitude of these preparations. Wounds, tissue sleeves, open fracture sites, complex arthrodesis sites, exposed bone and tissue, and tendon repairs are plausible areas that have found extensive use in reconstructive surgery. It is both the inherent properties of human amniotic allografts and the secondary effects of the biologic factors that make human amniotic allografts useful in so many applications (4,6,7,50,59).

Conclusion

Understanding the variety of bone grafting and osteobiologics options is an essential component of diabetic lower extremity surgery. Appropriate internal, external, or a combination of both fixation methods may be necessary to the overall success rate of bone grafting with or without osteobiologics. The surgeon and patient need to be aware of all the risks and benefits of these major reconstructive procedures and have an astute knowledge of the bone and wound healing process in the presence of diabetes mellitus, peripheral neuropathy, and associated medical comorbidities.

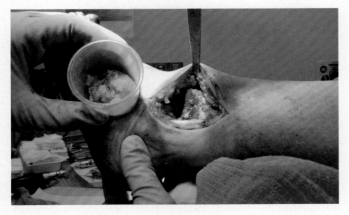

FIGURE 22.27 Mixed mesenchymal stem cells, demineralized bone matrix paste, and allograft bone chips for an ankle arthrodesis in a patient with diabetes mellitus and peripheral neuropathy.

Acknowledgment

Special thanks are given to Zflan Swayzee for all of her hard work with this chapter.

References

1. Ahlmann E, Patzakis M, Roidis N, et al. Comparison of anterior and posterior iliac crest bone grafts in terms of harvest-site morbidity and functional outcomes. J Bone Joint Surg Am 2002;84:716–720.

2. Albee FH. Fundamentals in bone transplantation: experiences in three thousand bone graft operations. JAMA 1923;81:1429–1432.

3. Anderson JJ, Boone JJ, Hansen M, et al. Ankle arthrodesis fusion rates for mesenchymal stem cell bone allograft versus proximal tibia autograft. J Foot Ankle Surg 2014;53:683–686.

4. Anderson JJ, Gough AF, Hansen MH, et al. Initial experience with tricortical iliac crest bone graft and human amniotic allograft in Evans calcaneal osteotomy. Stem Cell Discov 2015;5:11–17.

5. Anderson JJ, Jeppesen NS, Hansen M, et al. First metatarsophalangeal joint arthrodesis: comparison of mesenchymal stem cell allograft versus autogenous bone graft fusion rates. Surg Sci 2013;4:263–267.

6. Anderson JJ, Swayzee Z. The use of human amniotic allograft on osteochondritis dissecans of the talar dome: a comparison with and without allografts in arthroscopically treated ankles. Surg Sci 2015;6:412–417.

7. Anderson JJ, Swayzee Z, Hansen MH. Human amniotic allograft in use on talar dome lesions: a prospective report of 37 patients. Stem Cell Discov 2014;4:55–60.

8. Anthony JP, Rawnsley JD, Benhaim P, et al. Donor leg morbidity and function after fibula free flap mandible reconstruction. Plast Reconstr Surg 1995;96:146–152.

9. Arinzeh TL. Mesenchymal stem cells for bone repair: preclinical studies and potential orthopedic applications. Foot Ankle Clin 2005;10:651–665.

10. Arrington ED, Smith WJ, Chambers HG, et al. Complications of iliac crest bone graft harvesting. Clin Orthop Relat Res 1996;329:300–309.

11. Babovic S, Johnson CH, Finical SJ. Free fibula donor-site morbidity: the Mayo experience with 100 consecutive harvests. J Reconstr Microsurg 2000;16:107–110.

12. Bansiddhi A, Sargeant TD, Stupp SI, et al. Porous NiTi for bone implants: a review. Acta Biomater 2008;4:773–782.

13. Bianco P, Cao X, Frenette PS, et al. The meaning, the sense and the significance: translating the science of mesenchymal stem cells into medicine. Nat Med 2013;19:35–42.

14. Bidula J, Boehm C, Powell K, et al. Osteogenic progenitors in bone marrow aspirates from smokers and nonsmokers. Clin Orthop Rel Res 2006;442:252–259.

15. Blitch EL IV, Pachuda NM, Karlock LG, et al. Bone grafts. In: Banks AS, Downey MS, Martin DE, et al., eds. McGlamry's comprehensive textbook of foot and ankle surgery. 3rd ed. Philadelphia: Lippincott Williams & Wilkins, 2001:1465–1486.

16. Blitch EL, Ricotta PJ. Introduction to bone grafting. J Foot Ankle Surg 1996;35:458–462.

17. Blum B, Moseley J, Miller L, et al. Measurement of bone morphogenetic proteins and other growth factors in demineralized bone matrix. Orthopedics 2004;27(1 suppl):161–165.

18. Boone DW. Complications of iliac crest graft and bone grafting alternatives in foot and ankle surgery. Foot Ankle Clin 2003;8:1–14.

19. Boyce T, Edwards J, Scarborough N. Allograft bone. The influence of processing on safety and performance. Orthop Clin North Am 1999;30:571–581.

20. Brown CH. A technique for distal tibial bone graft for arthrodesis of the foot and ankle. Foot Ankle Int 2000;21:780–781.

21. Bruder SP, Fink DJ, Caplan AI. Mesenchymal stem cells in bone development, bone repair, and skeletal regeneration therapy. J Cell Biochem 1994;56:238–294.

22. Bucholz RW, Carlton A, Holmes RE. Hydroxyapatite and tricalcium phosphate bone graft substitutes. Orthop Clin North Am 1987;18:323–334.

23. Bucholz RW, Carlton A, Holmes RE. Interporous hydroxyapatite as a bone graft substitute in tibial plateau fractures. Clin Orthop Relat Res 1989;240:53–62.

24. Campbell M, Seligson D. The history of bone grafting. Tech Orthop 1992;7:1–6.

25. Chapman MW, Bucholz R, Cornell C. Treatment of acute fractures with a collagen-calcium phosphate graft material. A randomized clinical trial. J Bone Joint Surg Am 1997;79:495–502.

26. Chase SW, Herndon CH. The fate of autogenous and homogenous bone grafts. J Bone Joint Surg Am 1995;37-A:809–841.

27. Chong AK, Ang AD, Goh JC, et al. Bone marrow-derived mesenchymal stem cells influence early tendon-healing in a rabbit Achilles tendon model. J Bone Joint Surg Am 2007;89:74–81.

28. Cornell CN. Osteoconductive materials and their role as substitutes for autogenous bone grafts. Orthop Clin North Am 1999;30:591–598.

29. Cornell CN, Lane JM, Chapman M, et al. Multicenter trial of Collagraft as bone graft substitute. J Orthop Trauma 1991;5:1–8.

30. Cüneyt Tas A, Korkusuz F, Timuçin M, et al. An investigation of the chemical synthesis and high-temperature sintering behavior of calcium hydroxyapatite (HA) and tricalcium phosphate (TCP) bioceramics. J Mater Sci Mater Med 1997;8:91–96.

31. Daculsi G. Biphasic calcium phosphate concept applied to artificial bone, implant coating and injectable bone substitute. Biomaterials 1998;19:1473–1478.

32. de Boer HH. The history of bone grafts. Clin Orthop Relat Res 1988;226:292–298.

33. Derner R, Anderson AC. The bone morphogenic protein. Clin Podiatr Med Surg 2005;22:607–618.

34. Donley BG, Richardson EG. Bone grafting in foot surgery. Foot Ankle Int 1996;17:242.

35. Einhorn TA. The cell and molecular biology of fracture healing. Clin Orthop Relat Res 1998;(355 suppl):S7–S21.

36. Einhorn TA, Lee CA. Bone regeneration: new findings and potential clinical applications. J Am Acad Orthop Surg 2001;9:157–165.

37. Fernyhough JC, Schimandle JJ, Weigel MC, et al. Chronic donor site pain complicating bone graft harvesting from the posterior iliac crest for spinal fusion. Spine 1992;17:1474–1480.

38. Fleming JE Jr, Cornell CN, Muschler GF. Bone cells and matrices in orthopedic tissue engineering. Orthop Clin North Am 2000;31:357–374.

39. Frayssinet P, Gineste L, Conte P, et al. Short-term implantation effects of a DCPD-based calcium phosphate cement. Biomaterials 1998;19:971–977.

40. Frenette PS, Pinho S, Lucas D, et al. Mesenchymal stem cell: keystone of the hematopoietic stem cell niche and a stepping-stone for regenerative medicine. Annu Rev Immunol 2013;31:285–316.

41. Friedlaender GE. Bone grafts. The basic science rationale for clinical applications. J Bone Joint Surg Am 1987;69:786–790.

42. Geideman W, Early JS, Brodsky J. Clinical results of harvesting autogenous cancellous graft from the ipsilateral proximal tibia for use in foot and ankle surgery. Foot Ankle Int 2004;25:451–455.

43. Gitelis S, Piasecki P, Turner T, et al. Use of a calcium sulfate-based bone graft substitute for benign bone lesions. Orthopedics 2001;24:162–166.

44. Goldberg VM, Stevenson S. Natural history of autografts and allografts. Clin Orthop Relat Res 1987;225:7–16.

45. Habibovic P, de Groot K. Osteoinductive biomaterials—properties and relevance in bone repair. J Tissue Eng Regen Med 2007;1:25–32.

46. Hamer AJ, Strachan JR, Black MM, et al. Biomechanical properties of cortical allograft bone using a new method of bone strength measurement. A comparison of fresh, fresh-frozen and irradiated bone. J Bone Joint Surg Br 1996;78:363–368.

47. Hernigou PH, Mathieu G, Poignard A, et al. Percutaneous autologous bone-marrow grafting for nonunions. Surgical technique. J Bone Joint Surg Am 2006;88(suppl 1):322–327.

48. Hofbauer MH, Delmonte RJ, Scripps ML. Autogenous bone grafting. J Foot Ankle Surg 1996;35:386–390.

49. Holmes R, Mooney V, Bucholz R, et al. A coralline hydroxyapatite bone graft substitute. Preliminary report. Clin Orthop Relat Res 1984;188:252–262.

50. Ilic D, Vicovac L, Nikolic M, et al. Human amniotic membrane grafts in therapy of chronic non-healing wounds. Br Med Bull 2016;117:59–67.

51. Imwinkelried T. Mechanical properties of open-pore titanium foam. J Biomed Mater Res A 2007;81:964–970.

52. Irwin RB, Bernhard M, Biddinger A. Coralline hydroxyapatite as bone substitute in orthopedic oncology. Am J Orthop (Belle Mead NJ) 2001;30:544–550.

53. Jansen J, Ooms E, Verdonschot N, et al. Injectable calcium phosphate cement for bone repair and implant fixation. Orthop Clin North Am 2005;36:89–95.

54. Jarcho M. Calcium phosphate ceramics as hard tissue prosthetics. Clin Orthop Relat Res 1981;157:259–278.

55. Joyce ME, Jingushi S, Bolander ME. Transforming growth factor-beta in the regulation of fracture repair. Orthop Clin North Am 1990;21:199–209.

56. Kagan RJ. Standards for tissue banking. McLean, VA: American Association of Tissue Banks, 1998.

57. Kelly C, Wilkins R, Gitelis S, et al. The use of a surgical grade calcium sulfate as bone graft substitute: results of a multicenter trial. Clin Orthop Relat Res 2001;382:42–50.

58. Khan SN, Tomin E, Lane JM. Clinical applications of bone graft substitutes. Orthop Clin North Am 2000;31:389–398.

59. Kim J, Jeong SY, Ju YM, et al. In vitro osteogenic differentiation of human amniotic fluid-derived stem cells on a poly (lactide-co-glycolide) (PLGA)-bladder submucosa matrix (BSM) composite scaffold for bone tissue engineering. Biomed Mater 2013;8:014107.

60. Kloen P, Doty SB, Gordon E, et al. Expression and activation of the BMP-signaling components in human fracture nonunions. J Bone Joint Surg Am 2002;84-A:1909–1918.

61. Kübler A, Neugebauer J, Oh JH, et al. Growth and proliferation of human osteoblasts on different gone graft substitutes: an in vitro study. Implant Dent 2004;131:171–179.

62. Lane JM, Bostrom MP. Bone grafting and new composite biosynthetic graft materials. Instr Course Lect 1998;47:525–534.

63. Levine B. A new era in porous metals: applications in orthopaedics. Adv Eng Mat 2008;10:788–792.

64. Levine BR, Fabi DW. Porous metals in orthopedic applications—a review. Materwiss Werksttech 2010;41:1001–1010.

65. Lewandrowski KU, Gresser JD, Wise DL, et al. Bioresorbable bone graft substitutes of different osteoconductivities: a histologic evaluation of osteointegration of poly(propylene glycol-co-fumaric acid)-based cement implants in rats. Biomaterials 2000;21:757–764.

66. Li JP, Habibovic P, van den Doel M, et al. Bone ingrowth in porous titanium implants produced by 3D fiber deposition. Biomaterials 2007;28:2810–2820.

67. Lobenhoffer P, Gerich T, Witte F, et al. Use of an injectable calcium phosphate bone cement in the treatment of tibial plateau fractures: a prospective study of twenty-six cases with twenty-month mean follow-up. J Orthop Trauma 2002;16:143–149.

68. Martin RB, Chapman MW, Sharkey NA, et al. Bone ingrowth and mechanical properties of coralline hydroxyapatite 1 yr after implantation. Biomaterials 1993;14:341–348.

69. Marx RE, Carlson ER, Eichstaedt RM, et al. Platelet-rich plasma: growth factor enhancement for bone grafts. Oral Surg Oral Med Oral Pathol Oral Radiol Endod 1998;85:638–646.

70. Matsushita N, Terai H, Okada T, et al. A new bone-inducing biodegradable porous beta-tricalcium phosphate. J Biomed Mater Res A 2004;70:450–458.

71. McGarvey WC, Braly WG. Bone graft in hindfoot arthrodesis: allograft vs autograft. Orthopedics 1996;19:389–394.

72. Michelson JD, Curl LA. Use of demineralized bone matrix in hindfoot arthrodesis. Clin Orthop Relat Res 1996;325:203–208.

73. Moore DC, Chapman MW, Manske D. The evaluation of a biphasic calcium phosphate ceramic for use in grafting long bone diaphyseal defects. J Orthop Res 1987;5:356–365.

74. Nash TJ, Howlett CR, Martin C, et al. Effect of platelet-derived growth factor on tibial osteotomies in rabbits. Bone 1994;15:203–208.

75. Nelson CL, McLaren SG, Skinner RA, et al. The treatment of experimental osteomyelitis by surgical débridement and the implantation of calcium sulfate tobramycin pellets. J Orthop Res 2002;20:643–647.

76. Niemeyer P, Krause U, Fellenberg J, et al. Evaluation of mineralized collagen and alpha-tricalcium phosphate as scaffolds for tissue engineering of bone using human mesenchymal stem cells. Cells Tissues Organs 2004;177:68–78.

77. O'Malley DF Jr, Conti SF. Results of distal tibial bone grafting in hindfoot arthrodeses. Foot Ankle Int 1996;17:374–377.

78. Raikin SM, Brislin K. Local bone graft harvested from the distal tibia or calcaneus for surgery of the foot and ankle. Foot Ankle Int 2005;26:449–453.

79. Reddi AH. Bone morphogenetic proteins: from basic science to clinical applications. J Bone Joint Surg Am 2001;83-A(suppl 1 pt 1):1–6.

80. Roukis TS, Zgonis T, Tiernan B. Autologous platelet-rich plasma for wound and osseous healing: a review of the literature and commercially available products. Adv Ther 2006;23:218–237.

81. Rush SM. Bone graft substitutes: osteobiologics. Clin Podiatr Med Surg 2005;22:619–630.

82. Ryaby JT, Fitzsimmons RJ, Khin NA, et al. The role of insulin-like growth factor II in magnetic field regulation of bone formation. Bioelectrochem Bioenerg 1994;35:87–91.

83. Saltrick KR, Caron M, Grossman J. Utilization of autogenous corticocancellous bone graft from the distal tibia for reconstructive surgery of the foot and ankle. J Foot Ankle Surg 1996;35:406–412.

84. Sammarco VJ, Chang L. Modern issues in bone graft substitutes and advances in bone tissue technology. Foot Ankle Clin 2002;7:19–41.

85. Sartoris DJ, Holmes RE, Resnick D. Coralline hydroxyapatite bone graft substitutes: radiographic evaluation. J Foot Surg 1992;31:301–313.

86. Schildhauer TA, Bauer TW, Josten C, et al. Open reduction and augmentation of internal fixation with an injectable skeletal cement for the treatment of complex calcaneal fractures. J Orthop Trauma 2000;14:309–317.

87. Schulhofer SD, Oloff LM. Iliac crest donor site morbidity in foot and ankle surgery. J Foot Ankle Surg 1997;36:155–158.

88. Schwartz Z, Mellonig JT, Carnes DL Jr, et al. Ability of commercial demineralized freeze-dried bone allograft to induce new bone formation. J Periodontol 1996;67:918–926.

89. Shimazaki K, Mooney V. Comparative study of porous hydroxyapatite and tricalcium phosphate as bone substitute. J Orthop Res 1985;3:301–310.

90. Silber JS, Anderson DG, Daffner SD, et al. Donor site morbidity after anterior iliac crest bone harvest for single-level anterior cervical discectomy and fusion. Spine (Phila Pa 1976) 2003;28:134–139.

91. Simonian PT, Conrad EU, Chapman JR, et al. Effect of sterilization and storage treatments on screw pullout strength in human allograft bone. Clin Orthop Relat Res 1994;302:290–296.

92. Thordarson DB, Hedman TP, Yetkinler DN, et al. Superior compressive strength of a calcaneal fracture construct augmented with remodelable cancellous bone cement. J Bone Joint Surg Am 1999;81:239–246.

93. Tomford WW. Transmission of disease through transplantation of musculoskeletal allografts. J Bone Joint Surg Am 1995; 77:1742–1754.

94. Tucker DJ. Lateral column lengthening in adult flatfoot surgery using a titanium metal foam wedge implant. Tech Foot Ankle Surg 2010;9:205–210.

95. Urist MR. Bone: formation by autoinduction. Science 1965; 150:893–899.

96. Urist MR, Dowell TA, Hay PH, et al. Inductive substrates for bone formation. Clin Orthop Relat Res 1968;59:59–96.

97. Urist MR, McLean FC. Osteogenetic potency and new-bone formation by induction in transplants to the anterior chamber of the eye. J Bone Joint Surg Am 1952;34-A:443–467.

98. Urist MR, Silverman BF, Büring K, et al. The bone induction principle. Clin Orthop Relat Res 1967;53:243–283.

99. Wazen RM, Lefebvre LP, Baril E, et al. Initial evaluation of bone ingrowth into a novel porous titanium coating. J Biomed Mater Res B Appl Biomater 2010;94:64–71.

100. Wei CC, Lin AB, Hung SC. Mesenchymal stem cells in regenerative medicine for musculoskeletal diseases: bench, bedside, and industry. Cell Transplant 2014;23:505–512.

101. Weinraub GM. Orthobiologics: a survey of materials and techniques. Clin Podiatr Med Surg 2005;22:509–519.

102. Wright Medical Group. Augment bone graft: technology overview. Memphis, TN: Wright Medical Group, 2016.

103. Xu HH, Takagi S, Quinn JB, et al. Fast-setting calcium phosphate scaffolds with tailored MacroPore formation rates for bone regeneration. J Biomed Mater Res A 2004;68:725–734.

104. Yamada S, Heymann D, Bouler JM, et al. Osteoclastic resorption of calcium phosphate ceramics with different hydroxyapatite/beta-tricalcium phosphate ratios. Biomaterials 1997;18: 1037–1041.

105. Younger EM, Chapman MW. Morbidity at bone graft donor sites. J Orthop Trauma 1989;3:192–195.

Recommended Reading

Danziger MB, Abdo RV, Decker JE. Distal tibia bone graft for arthrodesis of the foot and ankle. Foot Ankle Int 1995;16:187–190.

Huse RO, Quinten Ruhe P, Wolke JG, et al. The use of porous calcium phosphate scaffolds with transforming growth factor beta 1 as an onlay bone graft substitute. Clin Oral Implants Res 2004;15: 741–749.

Moroni A, Aspenberg P, Toksvig-Larsen S, et al. Enhanced fixation with hydroxyapatite coated pins. Clin Orthop Relat Res 1998;346:171–177.

Scranton PE Jr. Results of arthrodesis of the tarsus: talocalcaneal, midtarsal, and subtalar joints. Foot Ankle 1991;12:156–164.

Shors EC. Coralline bone graft substitutes. Orthop Clin North Am 1999;30:599–613.

CHAPTER 23

Revisional Diabetic Foot and Ankle Surgery

John J. Stapleton • Thomas Zgonis

INTRODUCTION

Revisional surgery for the diabetic foot and ankle entails complications from previous surgical procedures including, but not limited to, traumatic, elective, and reconstructive surgery. Most common diabetic complications leading to revisional surgery include deep soft tissue and osseous infections, hardware failure, malunions, nonunions, avascular necrosis, surgical wound dehiscence, and/or surgically induced Charcot neuroarthropathy of the foot and ankle. The use of circular external fixation becomes ideal when managing revisional diabetic foot and ankle surgeries because external fixation can provide simultaneous stabilization and compression of any prepared joint(s) for arthrodesis and surgically off-load the lower extremity when needed.

PREOPERATIVE CONSIDERATIONS

The timing of revisional surgery is dependent on the clinical scenario severity and medical optimization of the diabetic patient. Staged reconstruction may often be necessary in the presence of exposed internal fixation hardware, open nonhealing wounds, and history of osteomyelitis. Intraoperative soft tissue and/or bone cultures and biopsies are required in the presence of an infection along with an appropriate infectious disease consultation for the use of long-term intravenous and/or oral antibiotic therapy.

A thorough clinical, laboratory, and medical imaging evaluation is paramount to determine the etiologic factors that might have led to the failure of the original diabetic foot and/or ankle surgery. In the presence of clinical and systemic signs of deep infection following diabetic fracture care with internal fixation, it is imperative that both surgical and medical management of the patient's comorbidities entails a comprehensive and expedited plan on evidence-based recommendations. Preoperative consultations with medicine, cardiology, nephrology, and infectious disease may be necessary and based on the patient's medical history and clinical evaluation.

Medical optimization of the diabetic patient is required because these patients present with multiple medical comorbidities and are usually undergoing numerous surgical procedures. Laboratory testings that consist of a complete blood count (CBC) with differential, erythrocyte sedimentation rate (ESR), C-reactive protein (CRP), and coagulation studies as well as an electrocardiogram and a chest radiograph are obtained. The presence of a normal CBC with differential but abnormal and elevated inflammatory markers (ESR and CRP) is a quite common finding in the immunocompromised diabetic population. Hemoglobin A_{1c} levels are also important in determining whether the diabetic patient's blood glucose numbers are well-controlled or will require aggressive medical therapy adjustments. In the presence of an obvious deep infection, inflammatory markers are still obtained to help guide antibiotic treatment and determine the effectiveness of infection management. This process is imperative because numerous staged surgical procedures may often need to be performed in order to achieve osseous union and wound healing.

Adequate vascularity to the lower extremity must also be well-established because diabetic patients are susceptible to peripheral arterial disease that could lead to lower extremity amputation. Initial noninvasive arterial studies can be followed by a vascular surgery consultation for further vascular imaging studies and/or intervention when necessary.

The treatment of deep infections with retained hardware becomes a surgical challenge especially when osseous stability is still required, and osseous union is not present. In certain cases, removal of all infected hardware is not always feasible, and surgical débridement along with hardware exchange or limited fixation and chronic antibiotic therapy may be required. In cases where persistent signs of deep infection are present, the internal fixation hardware will typically need to be removed and osseous stabilization may be performed with external fixation.

After the initial surgical débridement and removal of the infected internal fixation hardware, the patient returns to the operating room for further surgical débridement, probable insertion of antibiotic-impregnated polymethylmethacrylate

(PMMA) cement blocks or beads based on the initial intra-operative cultures and probable temporary external fixation for stabilization, spanning, or surgical off-loading if necessary. Most commonly mixed antibiotic-impregnated PMMA cement blocks or beads include gentamicin or tobramycin with the addition of vancomycin when needed (2,3).

Delivery of local antibiotic therapy in the form of antibiotic-impregnated PMMA cement is shaped into beads or spacers and is an excellent way of achieving increased local concentrations of antibiotics to the surgical site. These materials are implanted by placing the antibiotic beads on a nonabsorbable suture or cerclage wire for easier removal and then packed within the osseous or soft tissue defects as required. Often, nonabsorbable antibiotic-impregnated PMMA beads or spacers are exchanged when repeat serial surgical débridements are required and definitely removed once osseous stabilization and bone grafting can be performed. Unlike PMMA beads or spacers that are not absorbable, calcium sulfate mixed antibiotics are metabolized by the body but provide less stability over a larger osseous and soft tissue defect. These revisional staged surgical treatments are combined with systemically administered antibiotic therapy for approximately 6 to 8 weeks and until the final reconstructive procedures are planned for definitive treatment.

Thorough preoperative planning is crucial in regard to surgical incision placement, hardware removal of retained plates, screws, pins, and/or intramedullary nails, soft tissue coverage, and off-loading of the lower extremity. The utilization of circular external fixation can be extremely helpful in addressing any distal tibia and ankle infected nonunions. External fixation is indicated in the stabilization of unstable fractures and/or deformities and the relief of any strain on the soft tissue for subsequent closure. The utilization of circular external fixation may be advantageous in any stage of the previous failed surgery and help in staged arthrodesis procedures if joint salvage is not feasible.

In many cases, infected nonunions can present with a significant bone loss due to avascular necrosis and concomitant osteomyelitis. Bone grafting or bone transport procedures may also be necessary to address the bone loss and/or limb length discrepancy in any malunion or nonunion clinical scenario if indicated. This chapter discusses in detail some of the most common complications encountered in failed surgeries of the diabetic foot and ankle with a rational approach to functional limb salvage. Complex clinical scenarios in the traumatic, elective, and Charcot neuroarthropathy diabetic patients are presented in detail, whereas a stepwise surgical approach is provided for the revisional and reconstructive procedures.

REVISION OF DIABETIC ANKLE FRACTURES

Failed fixation in the management of diabetic ankle fractures can be quite challenging for the treating surgeon. Revisional surgery for diabetic ankle fractures can be considered in certain clinical scenarios where the ankle joint presents with minimal or no evidence of posttraumatic arthritis, is without the presence of associated Charcot neuroarthropathy and when the underlying osseous and soft tissue structures maintain great viability for the revisional ankle fracture reduction (Fig. 23.1). On the other hand, if the patient is not amenable to revisional fracture reduction of the ankle with or without osteotomy and/or bone grafting, then consideration for an ankle, tibiotalocalcaneal, or tibiocalcaneal arthrodesis either for the posttraumatic ankle arthritis or as a salvage procedure is highly considered in this complex diabetic population.

When contemplating revisional surgery for the failed diabetic ankle fracture, certain questions will need to be addressed in the preoperative planning stage. Some of those questions

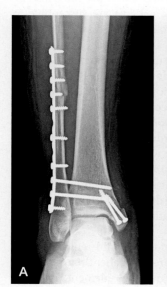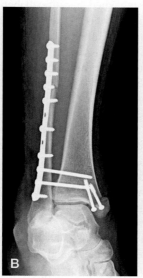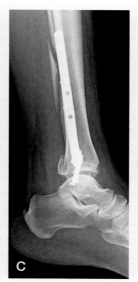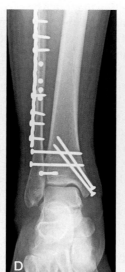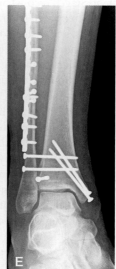

FIGURE 23.1 Preoperative anteroposterior **(A)**, medial oblique **(B)**, and lateral **(C)** radiographic views showing a malreduced ankle fracture 4 weeks from the original surgery on a well-controlled diabetic patient. *(continued)*

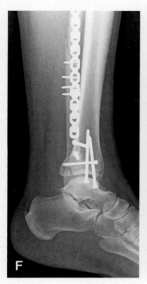
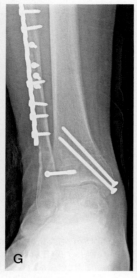
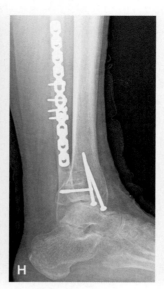

FIGURE 23.1 *(Continued)* Postoperative anteroposterior **(D)**, medial oblique **(E)**, and lateral **(F)** radiographic views at 2 weeks after the revisional ankle fracture reduction and removal of preexisting hardware. Syndesmotic screws were removed at 6 months after the revisional surgery. Final postoperative anteroposterior **(G)** and lateral **(H)** radiographs at 12 months showing satisfactory reduction and osseous union.

may include if the original fracture was malreduced and unstable, if the surgical exposure was sufficient for reduction, if the biologic activity for fracture healing was compromised, if an underlying infection was present, or if there were any signs of noncompliance with treatment. If the original ankle fracture was not properly reduced, the surgeon needs to determine if the fracture can be revisionally reduced and fixated or if an osteotomy must be considered to achieve the desired anatomic reduction.

Revisional surgical incision placements should be generous and located in anatomic sites where it allows necessary exposure to remove preexisting hardware, create full-thickness flaps for mobilization of osseous segments while minimizing soft tissue handling, and facilitate revisional fixation. In many cases, distractors are utilized to mobilize osseous segments and to ensure the ankle mortise is reduced. The utilization of autogenous bone grafting is often required as bone

loss is commonly encountered in the revisional surgery and in order to enhance the osseous biologic activity at the original fracture site.

Nonunion sites are often associated with significant fibrous interposition and scar tissue that will need to be resected along with the avascular bone at the surgical site. Subchondral drilling to ensure viable bleeding bone and to enhance vascular ingrowth is essential to optimize the healing potential at the fracture site. Although allogenic bone grafting and substitutes are promoted for their lack of donor site complications, autogenous bone grafting can provide the required biologic activities for osseous healing and incorporation in the complex diabetic population. Common local donor sites of autogenous bone grafting of the lower extremity include the calcaneus, fibula, distal tibia, and proximal tibia (Figs. 23.2 and 23.3).

Fixation considered for revisional diabetic foot and ankle surgeries must be planned in advance in order to allow

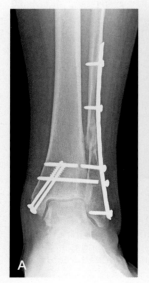
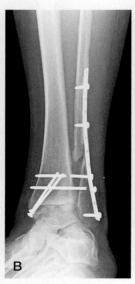
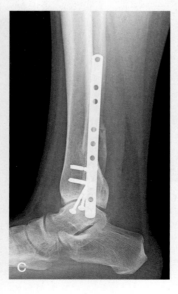

FIGURE 23.2 Preoperative anteroposterior **(A)**, medial oblique **(B)**, and lateral **(C)** radiographic views showing a symptomatic aseptic fibula nonunion 9 months from the original surgery in a well-controlled diabetic patient without peripheral neuropathy. Revisional surgery consisted of preexisting hardware removal by creating a cortical bone window at the medial aspect of the distal tibia to assist in the removal of broken hardware and harvesting of an autogenous bone graft from the tibia metaphysis to augment the fibula nonunion site. The fibula nonunion was revised and new fixation was performed. *(continued)*

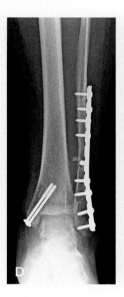 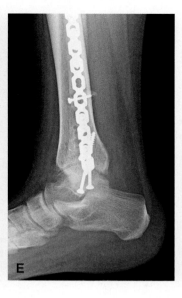

FIGURE 23.2 *(Continued)* Final postoperative antero-posterior **(D)** and lateral **(E)** radiographs at 6 months showing successful fracture healing.

necessary osseous stabilization and healing potential. At times, external fixation may be required especially in cases compromised with infection and those that necessitate additional osseous stability. The decision of whether a revisional diabetic ankle fracture reduction is feasible or whether conversion to diabetic limb salvage ankle arthrodesis is warranted is usually multifactorial and patient-dependent (Fig. 23.4). The presence of Charcot neuroarthropathy after a failed open reduction and internal fixation of a diabetic ankle fracture should

be a contraindication for revisional fracture reduction, and revisional surgery should be focused on salvage arthrodesis or overall improvement in lower extremity alignment that will allow for functional ambulation.

The available bone stock is extremely compromised in diabetic patients with Charcot neuroarthropathy fractures-dislocations, and revisional fracture reduction is not feasible. The presence of avascular bone needs to be surgically removed, and at times, this can be challenging to manage when

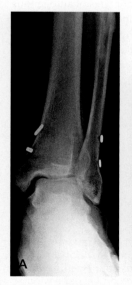 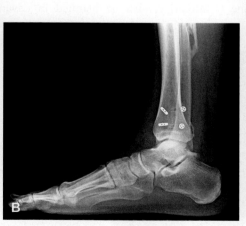 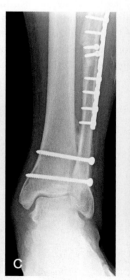 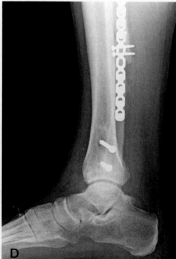

FIGURE 23.3 Preoperative anteroposterior **(A)** and lateral **(B)** radiographic views showing a syndesmotic malreduction with tight-rope fixation in a well-controlled diabetic patient without peripheral neuropathy 6 months from the original surgery. Revisional surgery consisted of tightrope fixation removal, isolated distal syndesmotic arthrodesis augmented with autogenous bone graft harvested from the distal tibia metaphysis, fixation of the malreduced fibula shaft fracture after the rotation, and alignment of the length of the fibula. Final postoperative anteroposterior **(C)** and lateral **(D)** radiographic views at 6 months showing anatomic reduction of the ankle mortise, arthrodesis of the distal tibia–fibula syndesmosis, and osseous healing of the fibula shaft fracture with alignment.

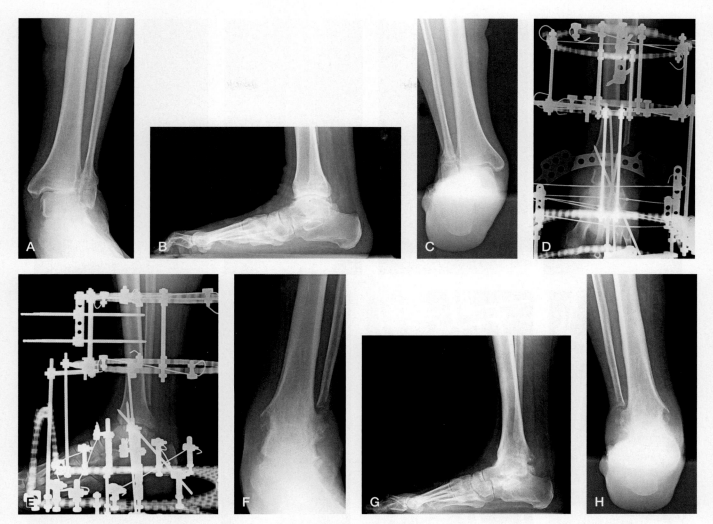

FIGURE 23.4 Preoperative anteroposterior **(A)**, lateral **(B)**, and calcaneal axial **(C)** radiographic views showing a fibula nonunion with a hindfoot/ankle valgus deformity and posttraumatic ankle arthritis. The patient had a history of diabetic peripheral neuropathy and previous open reduction and internal fixation of a lateral malleolus fracture that was complicated with wound dehiscence and deep infection. Early hardware removal was performed at 3 weeks after the original surgery. The patient underwent a tibiotalocalcaneal arthrodesis with the application of a multiplane circular external fixation device **(D,E)**. Final postoperative anteroposterior **(F)**, lateral **(G)**, and calcaneal axial **(H)** radiographic views at 12 months showing successful lower extremity deformity correction and tibiotalocalcaneal arthrodesis.

large osseous segments are excised. If concomitant infection is present after surgical débridement of any nonviable soft tissue and osseous structures, then placement of antibiotic-impregnated PMMA cement blocks or beads along with osseous stabilization is performed and planned for staged bone grafting (Fig. 23.5). In cases involving the hindfoot/ankle, staged bone grafting and/or arthrodesis in the resected osteomyelitic areas might be necessary.

The integrity of the surrounding soft tissues, surgical scars, sinus tracts, and/or nonhealing surgical incisions requires revisional surgical excision and débridement to healthy margins. Deep intraoperative soft tissue and/or bone cultures and bone biopsies when necessary are obtained for guidance of antibiotic therapy. Large soft tissue defects that remain after wide surgical wound margin excisions can be closed with staged revisional procedures by utilizing local random, muscle, pedicle,

perforator, or free tissue transfer flaps. In addition, the use of negative pressure wound therapy and split-thickness skin grafting might also be necessary for soft tissue coverage of previously infected hardware removal and surgical wound dehiscence.

Achieving a successful ankle arthrodesis may be straightforward in a well-controlled diabetic patient with posttraumatic ankle arthritis after fixation of a diabetic ankle fracture. However, the difficulty arises in diabetic patients with dense peripheral neuropathy and/or peripheral arterial disease who have broken hardware, severe deformity, malunions, Charcot neuroarthropathy, bone loss, history or presence of active infection, and poor soft tissue envelope (Fig. 23.6). In these cases, the surgeon needs to be meticulous in placing surgical incisions that are extensile and provide an easy access for hardware removal, joint resection or preparation, and

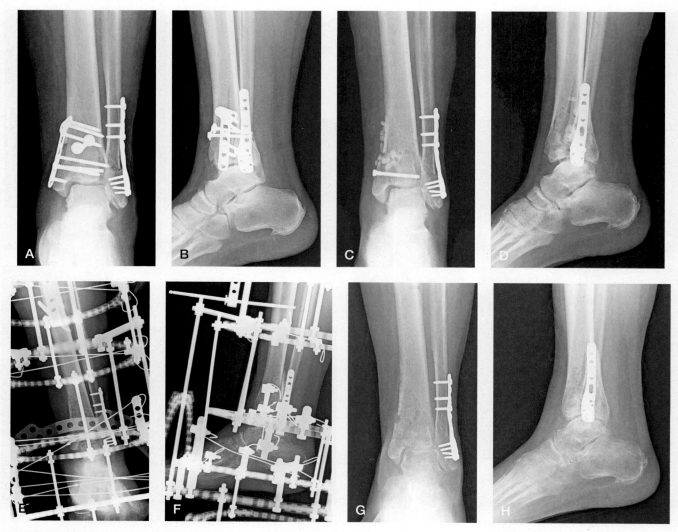

FIGURE 23.5 Preoperative anteroposterior **(A)** and lateral **(B)** radiographic views showing an open reduction and internal fixation of a tibia plafond fracture 16 weeks after the original surgery. Patient presented with a draining abscess and was admitted to the hospital for removal of the hardware medially and surgical débridement but allowing one screw for stabilization of the distal intra-articular fracture with application of antibiotic-impregnated polymethylmethacrylate (PMMA) cemented beads (tobramycin with vancomycin addition) positioned in place with a nonabsorbable suture **(C,D)**. Approximately 6 weeks after the aforementioned surgery, the patient returned to the operating room for removal of the nonabsorbable antibiotic-impregnated PMMA cemented beads along with the retained internal screw medially. An autogenous bone graft was harvested from the proximal tibia metaphysis, and a multiplane circular external fixation device with tensioned olive wires was utilized for osseous stabilization **(E,F)**. The circular external fixation device was removed at approximately 4 months. Final postoperative anteroposterior **(G)** and lateral **(H)** radiographic views at approximately 6 months showing the osseous union without clinical signs of infection.

realignment while minimizing skin tension. The removal of preexisting hardware can be challenging when dealing with broken internal fixation. Preoperative planning and available equipment to extract necessary hardware is required. At times, bone windows or appropriately sized trephines need to be utilized for direct access to remove retained broken hardware that interfere with the revisional surgery. The surgeon should also avoid from removing deeply embedded hardware that do not interfere with the revisional surgical procedures.

Internal fixation constructs such as locking or blade plates and intramedullary nails are commonly utilized for an ankle, tibiotalocalcaneal, or tibiocalcaneal arthrodesis in order to achieve long-term osseous stability and when the infection has been eradicated (4). External fixation constructs are advantageous because they are utilized when concern for infection still remains in the presence of poor bone stock and in order to achieve necessary osseous stabilization for correction of severe deformities. The goal of the aforementioned clinical scenarios is to achieve a diabetic lower extremity that is well

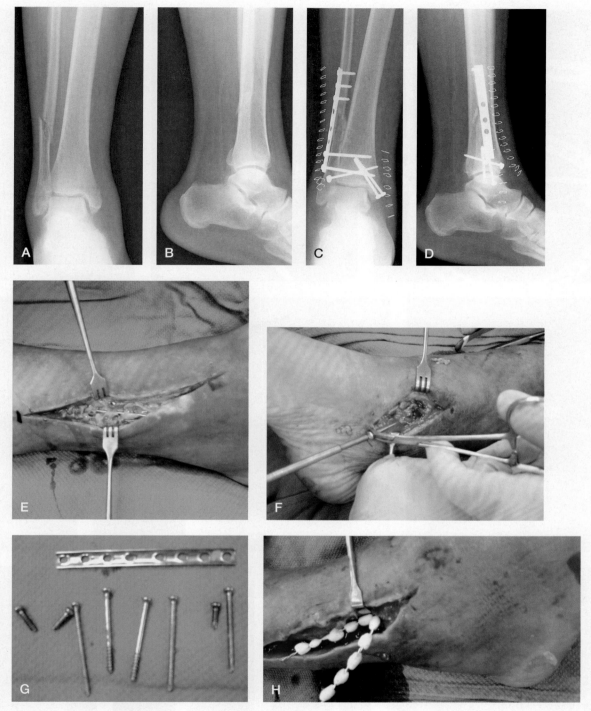

FIGURE 23.6 Preoperative anteroposterior **(A)** and lateral **(B)** radiographic views of diabetic patient with peripheral neuropathy who underwent an open reduction and internal fixation of an ankle fracture with syndesmosis repair **(C,D)**. Patient was referred 8 days after the original surgery for purulence and drainage from the medial and lateral ankle surgical incisions. Patient was admitted to the hospital and brought to the operating room for hardware removal and intraoperative bone biopsy along with bone and soft tissue cultures **(E–G)**. No tourniquet was utilized during the hardware removal, and minimal bleeding was noted intraoperatively. A vascular surgery consultation was initiated and followed by a lower extremity angioplasty procedure. The bone cultures were positive for ankle osteomyelitis, and the patient was then brought back to the operating room for insertion of antibiotic-impregnated polymethylmethacrylate (PMMA) cemented beads and application of a circular external fixation for stabilization and surgical off-loading **(H–M)**. *(continued)*

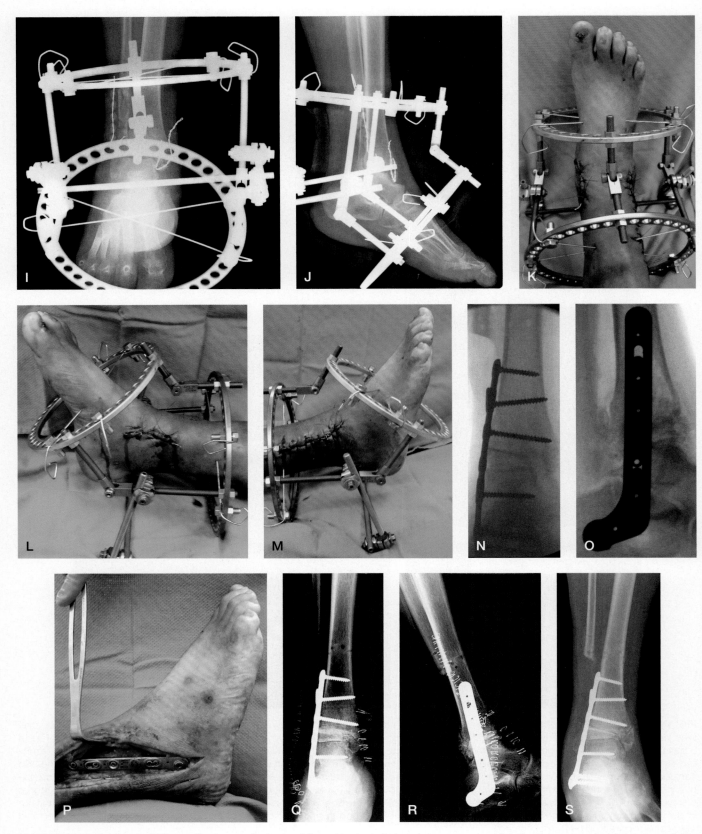

FIGURE 23.6 *(Continued)* The patient was discharged from the hospital on intravenous antibiotic therapy and strict non–weight-bearing status. After 7 weeks, the patient was brought back to the operating room for removal of the antibiotic-impregnated PMMA cemented beads and circular external fixator. Intraoperative bone cultures were negative for osteomyelitis, and the patient underwent a tibiotalocalcaneal arthrodesis with a locking plate fixation due to the patient's osteopenia and morbid obesity **(N–P)**. Postoperative anteroposterior and lateral radiographic views at 5 weeks **(Q,R)** and 12 weeks **(S,T)**. *(continued)*

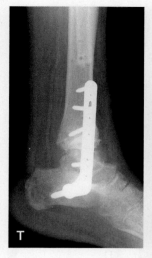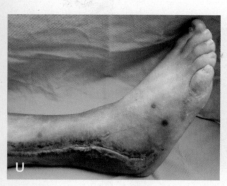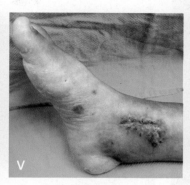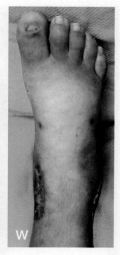

FIGURE 23.6 *(Continued)* Final clinical presentation at 12 weeks postoperatively **(U–W)**.

aligned and stable and allow for functional ambulation without soft tissue compromise or infection. For these reasons, the role of major lower extremity amputation may also be considered instead of extensive diabetic limb salvage surgery with prolonged postoperative recovery periods in certain clinical scenarios.

REVISION OF FAILED DIABETIC FOOT AND ANKLE ARTHRODESIS

Residual deformities, malunions, and nonunions of the diabetic foot and ankle after primary arthrodesis can lead to significant disability, pain, ulceration, infection, and/or amputation. Revisional arthrodesis procedures must be combined with correction of the residual deformity to realign the weight bearing forces of the foot to the leg (Figs. 23.7 and 23.8). The soft tissue envelope has to be evaluated for previous incisions, sinus tracts, pressure callosities, and/or ulcerations. When feasible, it is preferable to incorporate the fully excised ulceration with the planned surgical incision in order to create full-thickness local flaps for closure without tension. In addition, the degree of surgical correction can increase skin tension, and therefore, osseous resection needs to be considered in conjunction with planned incisions in order to minimize skin tension while facilitating wound closure.

In the presence of a diabetic foot or ankle malunion, the correctional osteotomy can be planned through the apex of deformity (Figs. 23.9 and 23.10). However, in diabetic patients who present with a nonunion, the planned osteotomies need to allow sufficient joint resection to achieve osseous union in addition to deformity correction. Often, deformity correction after previous failed arthrodesis in the diabetic population is treated with shortening osteotomies as opposed to large structural bone grafts. The utilization of viable resected bone can be morselized and used to fill any osseous defects to promote osseous healing at the

arthrodesis site. This technique is common with resection of the distal fibula and/or medial malleolus when a revisional ankle, tibiotalocalcaneal, or tibiocalcaneal arthrodesis is performed.

Creating maximum bone apposition after revisional joint resection and/or correctional osteotomy across a malunion and/or nonunion site is paramount for successful arthrodesis. For this reason, it is important for the surgeon to be meticulous with the osteotomy placement and shape of the bone that needs to be resected. Time should be spent ensuring that the planned osteotomy will close with maximum bone apposition. Small ridges of bone or altered bony shapes that prevent bone on bone apposition should be avoided when feasible. Residual bone defects can be managed with autogenous bone graft that is harvested during the revisional surgery or allogenic bone graft if necessary.

Alignment of the foot, ankle, and lower extremity is dependent on the final position after bone resection and prior to stabilization with internal, external, or combined fixation. For this reason, subtle adjustments to the deformity correction and/or fixation constructs should be made intraoperatively if needed. The utilization of intraoperative C-arm fluoroscopy in conjunction with temporary joint stabilization by using Steinmann pin fixation allows the surgeon to achieve deformity correction prior to definitive fixation.

Fixation constructs for revisional diabetic foot and ankle arthrodesis need to provide compression and osseous stability at the arthrodesis site(s). When dealing with revisional hindfoot/ankle arthrodesis, constructs that are most stable include intramedullary nails, locking or blade plates, and/or multiplane circular external fixation. The advantages to multiplane circular external fixation constructs are numerous including the ability to provide additional compression throughout the postoperative period if required. Multiplane circular external fixators are useful when dealing with infected nonunions, poor soft tissue envelope, poor bone

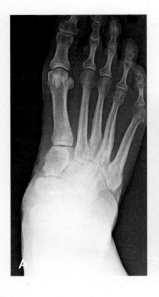

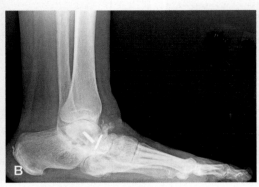

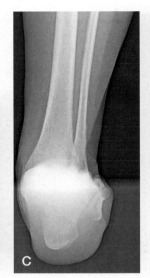

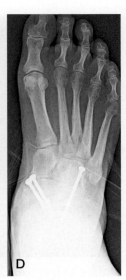

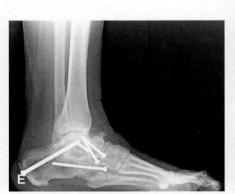

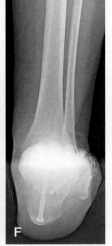

FIGURE 23.7 Preoperative anteroposterior **(A)**, lateral **(B)**, and calcaneal axial **(C)** radiographic views showing a talonavicular nonunion in a well-controlled diabetic patient after 2 previous failed surgical attempts with broken hardware and acquired pes planovalgus deformity. Revisional surgery consisted of gastrocnemius recession and conversion to a triple arthrodesis to promote osseous healing by increasing stability at the nonunion site and for deformity correction. Autogenous bone graft was obtained from the proximal tibia and utilized at the nonunion site. Final postoperative anteroposterior **(D)**, lateral **(E)**, and calcaneal axial **(F)** radiographic views at 12 months showing successful arthrodesis and alignment.

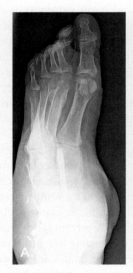

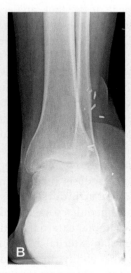

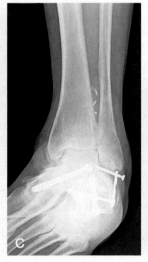

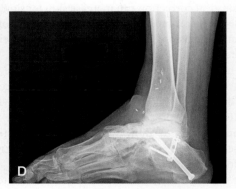

FIGURE 23.8 Preoperative foot **(A)**, ankle **(B)** anteroposterior, medial oblique **(C)**, lateral **(D)**, and calcaneal axial **(E)** radiographic views showing a malunion of a previous triple arthrodesis in a diabetic patient with previous history of high-energy trauma. *(continued)*

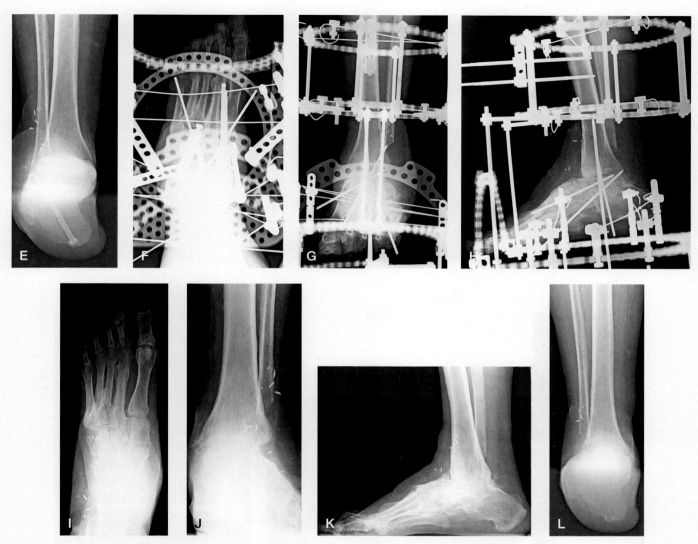

FIGURE 23.8 *(Continued)* Patient had a free flap to the lateral hindfoot/ankle, and intermittent skin breakdown was evident from the varus deformity and malunion. The patient underwent hardware removal and a triplane midfoot osteotomy combined with an ankle arthrodesis and circular external fixation in order to reestablish the alignment of the foot to the leg **(F–H)**. The circular external fixation device was removed at 16 weeks. Final postoperative foot **(I)** and ankle **(J)** anteroposterior, lateral **(K)**, and calcaneal axial **(L)** radiographic views at 12 months showing successful arthrodesis and deformity correction.

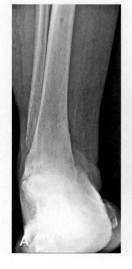
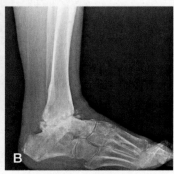

FIGURE 23.9 Preoperative anteroposterior **(A)** and lateral **(B)** radiographic views showing a hindfoot/ankle varus malunion in a diabetic patient with peripheral neuropathy. *(continued)*

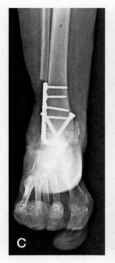
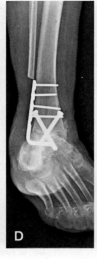
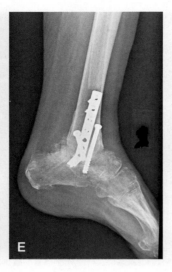

FIGURE 23.9 *(Continued)* The patient had a reported history of a subtalar joint arthrodesis with removal of hardware and subsequent attempted ankle arthrodesis with a unilateral external fixator that resulted in hind-foot/ankle varus malunion. Patient underwent a revisional ankle arthrodesis with a lateral wedge correctional osteotomy at the arthrodesis site and stabilization with a blade plate and internal fixation. Final postoperative anteroposterior **(C)**, medial oblique **(D)**, and lateral **(E)** radiographic views at 6 months showing osseous union and deformity correction.

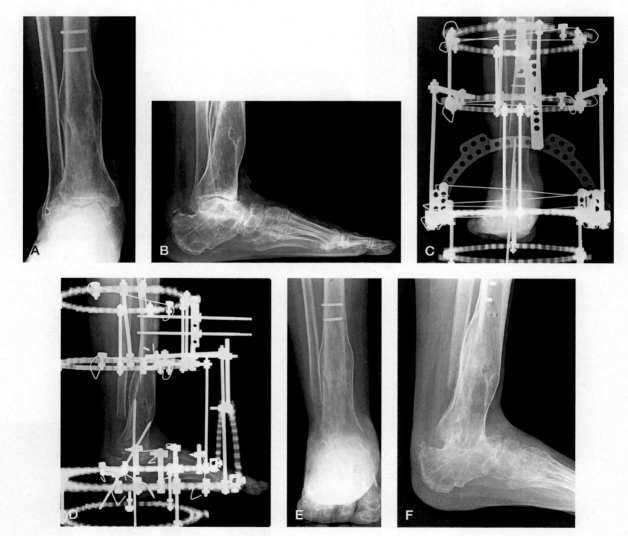

FIGURE 23.10 Preoperative anteroposterior **(A)** and lateral **(B)** radiographic views showing previous multiple surgeries and subtalar joint arthrodesis with avascular necrosis of the talus with history of infections and poor soft tissue envelope. Patient underwent an ankle arthrodesis with circular external fixation **(C,D)**. Final postoperative anteroposterior **(E)** and lateral **(F)** radiographic views at 6 months showing successful alignment and osseous healing.

stock, and instability of the lower extremity (Figs. 23.11 and 23.12).

Revisional arthrodesis procedures often require extensive immobilization periods, and this is especially evident and followed in diabetic patients with peripheral neuropathy. The immobilization period is at times doubled in the diabetic neuropathic population with an end-organ disease to ensure successful arthrodesis and prevent lower extremity amputation.

REVISION OF FAILED CHARCOT NEUROARTHROPATHY RECONSTRUCTION

Attempts at revisional surgical reconstruction of the diabetic Charcot neuroarthropathy foot and/or ankle can range from simple exostectomy procedures to revisional arthrodesis and/or soft tissue coverage of recurrent ulcerations. Open wounds with or without osteomyelitis from heterotopic bone

formation or from stable arthrodesis deformities may be surgically managed with staged soft tissue coverage such as local random, muscle, pedicle, perforator flaps, and osseous reconstruction. Staged surgical procedures with delayed primary closure or soft tissue reconstruction may be performed once the surgical wound is free of infection and the patient is on appropriate antibiotics based on intraoperative cultures, sensitivities, and/or bone biopsies. Circular external fixation devices can then be used as a definitive treatment for revisional arthrodesis and also be modified to surgically off-load the lower extremity to promote simultaneous osseous and wound healing.

Failed internal fixation with nonunion and/or osteomyelitis in the diabetic Charcot neuroarthropathy patient can be quite challenging because multiple surgeries may be required including extensive surgical débridements, removal of hardware, probable insertion of antibiotic-impregnated PMMA cement blocks or beads, and revisional staged deformity correction with arthrodesis (Figs. 23.13 and 23.14). Failed surgery at the Charcot neuroarthropathy midfoot level is usually surgically

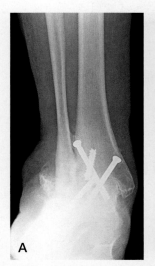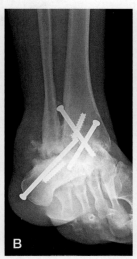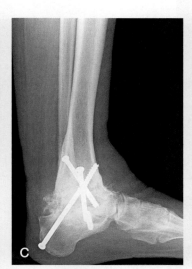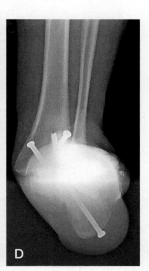
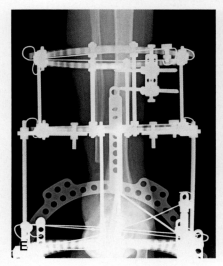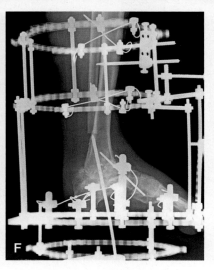

FIGURE 23.11 Preoperative anteroposterior **(A)**, medial oblique **(B)**, lateral **(C)**, and calcaneal axial **(D)** radiographic views showing an infected nonunion at an attempted tibiotalocalcaneal arthrodesis with retained hardware in a diabetic patient with peripheral neuropathy. Patient underwent a staged reconstruction with initial hardware removal, surgical débridement, and intraoperative cultures. After 1 week, the patient returned to the operative room for a revisional tibiotalocalcaneal arthrodesis, delayed primary closure of wounds, and application of a circular external fixation device **(E,F)**. *(continued)*

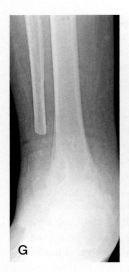
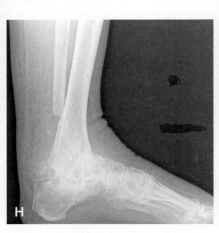
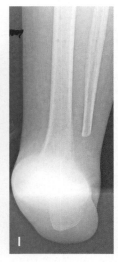

FIGURE 23.11 *(Continued)* Intravenous antibiotic therapy was also initiated by the infectious disease team for 6 weeks based on positive intraoperative cultures. The circular external fixation device was removed at 14 weeks. Final postoperative anteroposterior **(G)**, lateral **(H)**, and calcaneal axial **(I)** radiographic views at 18 months showing successful osseous union and deformity correction.

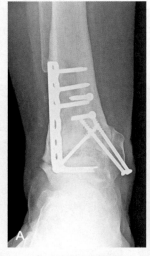
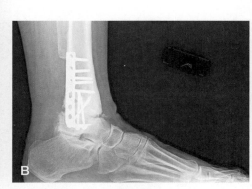
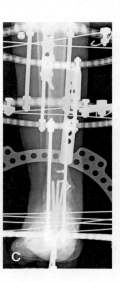
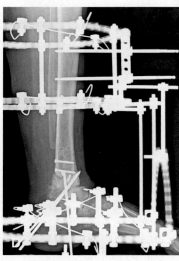
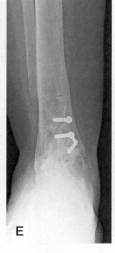
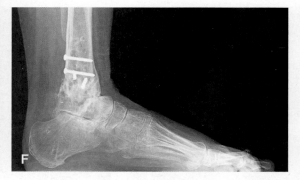

FIGURE 23.12 Preoperative anteroposterior **(A)** and lateral **(B)** radiographic views showing a chronically infected ankle nonunion with blade plate fixation 12 months after the original surgery in a diabetic patient with a smoking history. Patient underwent hardware removal and a revisional ankle arthrodesis with the application of a circular external fixation device and autogenous bone grafting harvested from the proximal tibia **(C,D)**. Intravenous antibiotic therapy was continued for 6 weeks based on positive intraoperative cultures. The circular external fixation device was removed at 16 weeks. Final postoperative anteroposterior **(E)** and lateral **(F)** radiographic views at 18 months showing successful osseous union and alignment.

managed with wide osseous resection and shortening of the midfoot. At times, complete resection of the tarsal bones and removal of all nonviable bone and soft tissues may be required in order to eradicate the infection and achieve the necessary wound closure. Shortening of the midfoot can be stabilized with a multiplane circular external fixation device and bone grafting when necessary. Reapplication of internal fixation is often not sufficient to achieve compression after wide bone resection and should be avoided in infectious cases. Often, patients will develop a stable pseudoarthrosis or osseous union with the foot in a plantigrade position and free of ulceration and infection. The diabetic patient with peripheral neuropathy and a shortened foot after revisional surgery at the midfoot

level can easily be accommodated with custom made shoe gear as long as the foot is in a plantigrade position without osseous prominences and ulcerations.

In contrary, when failed surgery of the Charcot neuroarthropathy hindfoot/ankle deformity is encountered, the treating surgeon needs to determine if sufficient bone is present to allow for diabetic salvage procedures or if the patient may benefit from a lower extremity amputation. If significant bone loss from the calcaneus is present, then lower extremity amputation may be considered as a treatment option. Failed fixation, deformity, and infection can be resolved with staged surgical removal of infected hardware, surgical débridement, applications of antibiotic-

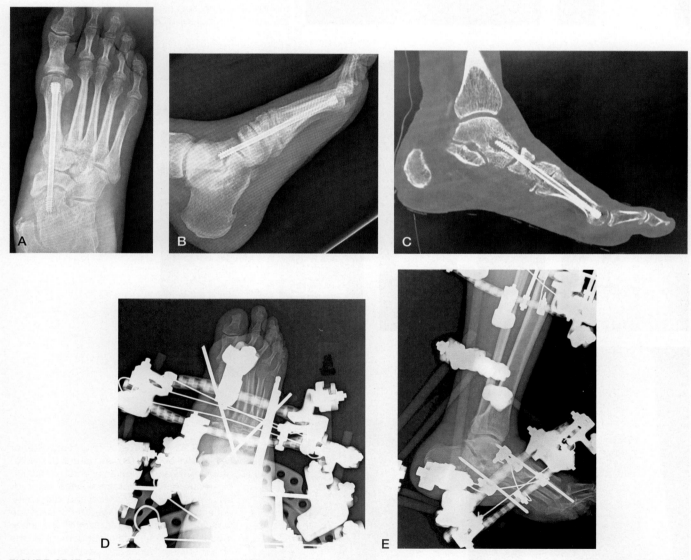

FIGURE 23.13 Preoperative anteroposterior **(A)** radiographic and lateral **(B)** radiographic and computed tomography **(C)** views showing an infected nonunion of an attempted medial column arthrodesis with deep infection, drainage, and nonhealing plantar medial ulceration. After medical optimization, a staged reconstruction with initial hardware removal, surgical débridement, and intraoperative cultures was performed. After 1 week, the patient returned to the operative room for a revisional medial column arthrodesis, local flap closure, and application of a circular external fixation device **(D,E)**. *(continued)*

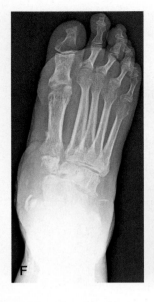

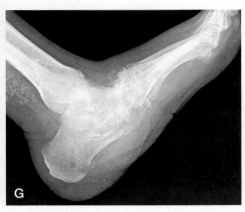

FIGURE 23.13 *(Continued)* Intravenous antibiotic therapy was also initiated by the infectious disease team for 6 weeks based on positive intraoperative cultures. The circular external fixation device was removed at 14 weeks. Final postoperative antero-posterior **(F)** and lateral **(G)** radiographic views at 14 months showing successful osseous healing without recurrent infection or ulceration.

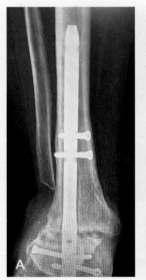

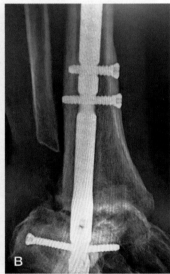

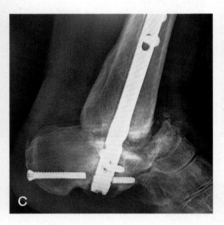

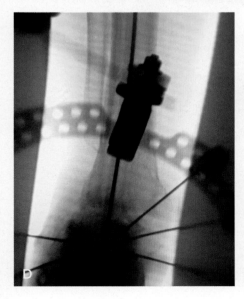

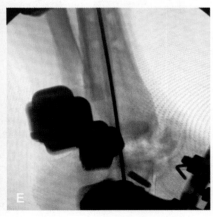

FIGURE 23.14 Preoperative anteroposterior **(A)**, medial oblique **(B)**, and lateral **(C)** radiographic views showing an infected nonunion of an attempted tibiotalocalcaneal arthrodesis with broken hardware and deformity. Patient underwent a staged reconstruction with initial hardware removal of the intramedullary nail, surgical débridement of the tibia medullary canal, and intraoperative cultures. Temporary osseous stabilization was performed with an antibiotic-impregnated polymethylmethacrylate (PMMA) cemented intramedullary nail and circular external fixation **(D,E)**. *(continued)*

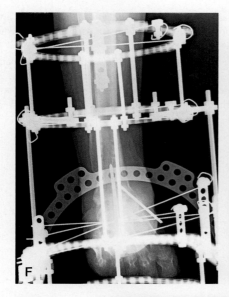
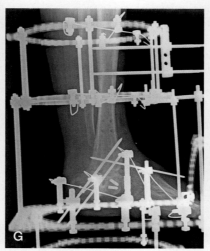
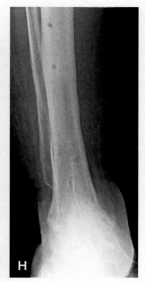
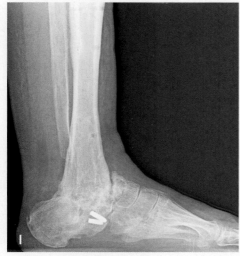

FIGURE 23.14 *(Continued)* Intravenous antibiotic therapy was continued for 6 weeks, at which time the staged revisional arthrodesis was performed with removal of the retained antibiotic-impregnated PMMA cemented intramedullary nail, autogenous bone grafting, and modification of the circular external fixation device **(F,G)**. The circular external fixation device was removed at 16 weeks. Final postoperative anteroposterior **(H)** and lateral **(I)** radiographic views at 12 months showing successful tibiocalcaneal arthrodesis.

impregnated PMMA cement blocks or intramedullary nails and staged revisional joint resection, realignment, and arthrodesis. Failed Charcot neuroarthropathy hindfoot/ankle deformities may benefit from a talectomy and tibiocalcaneal arthrodesis. Wide resection of the distal tibia to enhance the surface area of viable bone and create a docking site for the prepared calcaneus is often required to achieve a successful tibiocalcaneal arthrodesis. Significant revisional Charcot neuroarthropathy hindfoot/ankle deformities can be corrected with this surgical approach while also allowing soft tissue defects to be closed primarily when feasible. Tibiocalcaneal arthrodesis can be stabilized with intramedullary nails and blade plates if the infection has been eradicated. However, multiplane circular external fixation provides excellent osseous stability in the presence of a poor soft tissue envelope, allows for additional compression if desired, and can be utilized when a simultaneous infectious process is being managed (1).

Conclusion

Revisional surgery for diabetic foot and ankle complications with or without concomitant osteomyelitis can present with great challenges. Delayed arthrodesis is highly recommended in patients with failed diabetic ankle fracture repairs and Charcot neuroarthropathy, whereas revisional diabetic ankle fracture repair may be considered in well-controlled diabetic patients without peripheral neuropathy or posttraumatic ankle arthritis. In addition, the utilization of a multiplane circular external fixation device is advantageous in diabetic patients with a poor soft tissue envelope, have an ongoing infectious process, or when managing large bone voids after a midfoot shortening osteotomy or talectomy. Finally, staging revisional procedures such as delayed wound closure techniques and arthrodesis are preferred in the diabetic population with an active soft tissue infection or osteomyelitis.

References

1. Ramanujam CL, Zgonis T. An overview of internal and external fixation methods for the diabetic Charcot foot and ankle. Clin Podiatr Med Surg 2017;34:25–31.

2. Ramanujam CL, Zgonis T. Antibiotic-loaded cement beads for Charcot ankle osteomyelitis. Foot Ankle Spec 2010;3:274–277.

3. Ramanujam CL, Zgonis T. Salvage of Charcot foot neuropathy superimposed with osteomyelitis: a case report. J Wound Care 2010;19:485–487.

4. Zgonis T, Stapleton JJ, Polyzois VD, et al. Revisional and reconstructive surgery for the diabetic foot and ankle. In: Zgonis T, ed. Surgical reconstruction of the diabetic foot and ankle. Philadelphia: Lippincott Williams & Wilkins, 2009:315–343.

CHAPTER 24

Diabetic Neuropathic Midfoot/Hindfoot Fractures and Dislocations

John J. Stapleton • Thomas Zgonis

INTRODUCTION

Midfoot and hindfoot fractures and/or dislocations in the diabetic patient pose a great challenge to the treating physician and surgeon. A broad spectrum of injuries with fractures and/or dislocations can occur, and a well-coordinated treatment plan is necessary to optimize the patient's outcome while minimizing any inherent complications in the diabetic population. The presence of dense peripheral neuropathy and type of injury can further complicate the clinical case scenario of operative management. A differentiation between an initial traumatic injury in a diabetic patient with dense peripheral neuropathy and an acute episode of a diabetic Charcot neuroarthropathy (CN) fracture and/or dislocation needs to be determined because the operative management may significantly differ in the time and type of fixation as well as postoperative treatment.

The role of traditional osteosynthesis in an acute midfoot and hindfoot trauma exists among diabetic patients with or without peripheral neuropathy and cannot be overlooked. The well-controlled diabetic patient without evidence of an end-organ disease (coronary arterial disease, peripheral arterial disease, renal disease) with midfoot and/or hindfoot trauma is usually treated with traditional operative fracture management. In contrary, midfoot and/or hindfoot trauma in the diabetic patient with multiple medical comorbidities and peripheral neuropathy is usually managed operatively with primary joint arthrodesis procedures.

The timing of primary joint arthrodesis is often diverse for a diabetic patient with peripheral neuropathy that has sustained an acute traumatic midfoot/hindfoot fracture and/or dislocation versus a diabetic patient who has developed a CN midfoot/hindfoot fracture and/or dislocation. In the former group, the primary joint arthrodesis is often performed acutely, whereas in the latter group, primary arthrodesis may be performed if conservative treatment options cannot provide a stable and plantigrade foot that allows ambulation without soft tissue compromise.

PREOPERATIVE CONSIDERATIONS

Physical Examination and Imaging

Initial management of the diabetic patient who presents with an acute injury to the midfoot/hindfoot is a combination of a thorough history and physical examination; laboratory; radiographic foot, calcaneal axial, ankle, and lower extremity views; and further medical imaging when necessary. Special emphasis is given to any associated lower extremity or body injuries, history of open wounds, medical comorbidities, ambulatory status, type of anesthesia to be utilized during surgery, and medical optimization if feasible prior to surgical intervention.

Equal attention is specified to the soft tissue envelope and presence of pedal pulses when managing the diabetic midfoot/hindfoot trauma. Acute fractures and/or dislocations of the midfoot/hindfoot may require immediate reduction in order to prevent further injury to the soft tissue envelope and/or neurovascular structures. Midfoot/hindfoot fractures and/or dislocations that result in deformity, compartment syndrome, and skin tension require urgent operative intervention to prevent tissue necrosis and/or probable lower extremity amputation. Closed reduction and percutaneous pinning or spanning external fixation with staged reconstruction can be performed in circumstances in which the soft tissue envelope may not be suitable for an acute open surgical approach.

The lack of pedal pulses is concerning in the diabetic patient who presents with an acute midfoot/hindfoot trauma. Vascular surgery consultation can be initiated when the fracture patterns may allow for delayed surgical intervention. However, high-energy fractures with dislocations may not be amenable to an initial vascular intervention prior to surgical reduction. In these circumstances, the diabetic fractures and/or dislocations may need to be addressed in an expedited manner in order to provide the best chance of lower extremity preservation. Vascular surgery consultation can then be initiated to determine if intervention is required or feasible. In the presence of severe peripheral arterial disease or acute arterial injury in a diabetic patient with significant midfoot and/or hindfoot trauma, an acute or delayed amputation may be required.

Mechanism of Injury

Understanding the initial mechanism of injury is decisive in the management of midfoot/hindfoot trauma in the diabetic patient with or without peripheral neuropathy. Thorough clinical, radiographic, and/or medical imaging of the traumatic injuries can further assist the surgeon to determine if the trauma sustained is related to diabetic CN or follows an expected fracture pattern process. For example, if a diabetic patient with peripheral neuropathy presents with a very low-energy injury but radiographic findings reveal a fracture pattern that is usually sustained with a high-energy injury, this clinical scenario may represent the development of an acute CN process and not the direct result of an acute trauma. In addition, the existence of peripheral neuropathy can be identified when a diabetic patient sustains a high-energy injury with associated fractures and/or dislocations and presents with very little pain.

Evaluating the fracture pattern is critical in order to determine the best surgical approach. Midfoot and hindfoot trauma often requires computed tomography (CT) scans to adequately evaluate the fracture pattern and guide the surgical approach. Detail to surgical incision placement in order to allow necessary fracture and/or joint exposure is paramount in order to achieve fracture reduction and/or joint preparation if a primary arthrodesis is considered.

Operative Fixation Options

Attempt at traditional osteosynthesis for an acute CN of the midfoot/hindfoot after an initial mechanism of injury will likely result in failed reduction, probable broken hardware, malunion, nonunion, and progressive deformity as the CN process continues. For these reasons, an acute CN fracture and/or dislocation may require a delayed arthrodesis in order to obtain joint realignment and deformity correction. The arthrodesis procedure(s) if required are often performed once the CN acute phase has progressed to a coalescent and/or remodeling phase. This is represented by diminished edema, erythema, and normalization of skin temperature to the affected foot. The role of primary arthrodesis is also commonly utilized for pure midfoot/hindfoot dislocations in diabetic patients with dense peripheral neuropathy. In addition, primary arthrodesis has also been utilized in highly comminuted midfoot and/or hindfoot fractures-dislocations where joint reconstruction is not feasible.

In contrary, traditional osteosynthesis techniques for common midfoot/hindfoot fractures and/or dislocations are still utilized in diabetic patients without dense peripheral neuropathy and no evidence of diabetic end-organ disease. Combined internal and external fixation methods might also offer the surgeon an alternate surgical option in the incidence of an acute midfoot/hindfoot traumatic injury in the diabetic patient without peripheral neuropathy.

DIABETIC MIDFOOT FRACTURES AND DISLOCATIONS

Surgical Incisional Approaches

Midfoot trauma involving the tarsometatarsal and associated tarsal joints can be approached through medial, plantar medial, dorsal medial, central, and dorsal lateral incisions. The skin bridge (distance between surgical incisions) should be kept as wide as possible. In addition, extensile incisions when feasible are usually preferred compared to smaller incisions when internal fixation is utilized in order to allow necessary surgical exposure. Frequently, medial column bridge plating is required for high-energy trauma of the midfoot which is best approached with a curvilinear medial incision. Extensile curvilinear incisions if appropriately placed allow excellent exposure of the medial column and facilitate tension-free wound closure over the internal plate fixation if utilized. This surgical approach allows exposure of the entire medial column of the midfoot for reduction, fixation, and/or arthrodesis. Incisions over the dorsum of the foot, when necessary, require careful mobilization of the extensor tendons and muscle along with the neurovascular bundle. Several advantages to a dorsal midfoot incision include reduction of the central tarsometatarsal joint(s), associated tarsal joints, and select navicular fractures and/or dislocations. Dorsal lateral incisions allow internal fixation placement in the lateral column of the tarsometatarsal joint(s) and/or associated comminuted cuboid fractures.

Surgical Techniques

The first step for an acute primary arthrodesis of the tarsometatarsal joint(s) and/or extended medial column arthrodesis begins with appropriate joint(s) preparation and adequate cartilage resection. Maintaining the anatomic shape of the joints in the acute traumatic setting after cartilage resection is usually performed with sharp chisels, osteotomes, and curettes as opposed to joint(s) resection with a sagittal saw. Once the joints are prepared and ready for the arthrodesis procedures, reduction is performed by stabilization and temporary fixation of the tarsometatarsal and tarsal bones with Steinmann pins. Once the tarsal bones are reduced, reduction of the tarsometatarsal joints can then be performed. Reduction and deformity correction is performed from medial to lateral and temporarily stabilized with large point reduction clamps and Steinmann pins. Exchange of the Steinmann pins for interfragmentary screws can be performed when necessary. Additional bridge plating once compression of the joints has been achieved can be applied for further stability (Fig. 24.1). The lateral column of the foot is usually stabilized with large Steinmann pin fixation and/or arthrodesis in very severe cases if necessary (Fig. 24.2).

On the contrary, delayed primary arthrodesis of the midfoot is usually reserved for the reduction and realignment

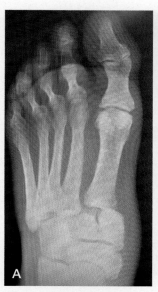
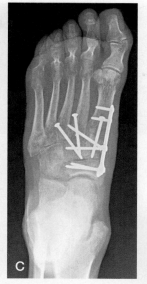
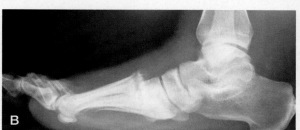
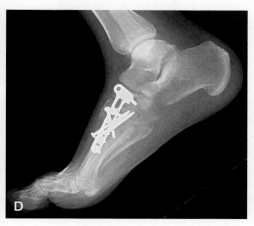

FIGURE 24.1 Preoperative anteroposterior **(A)** and lateral **(B)** left foot radiographic views of a diabetic patient with peripheral neuropathy showing an acute tarsometatarsal fracture and dislocation 5 days after the initial injury. Patient underwent a primary acute midfoot arthrodesis with an open reduction and internal fixation and simultaneous bridge plating stabilization at the medial column of the foot. Postoperative anteroposterior **(C)** and lateral **(D)** left foot radiographic views showing anatomic reduction and primary arthrodesis of the midfoot with bridge plating stabilization of the medial column at 6 months follow-up.

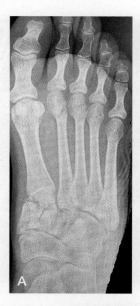
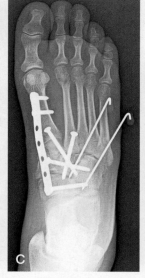
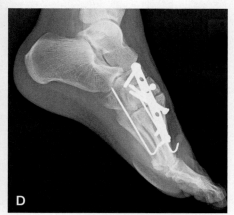
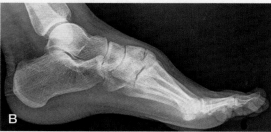

FIGURE 24.2 Preoperative anteroposterior **(A)** and lateral **(B)** right foot radiographic views of a diabetic patient, demonstrating a complex midfoot fracture-dislocation after sustaining a crush injury. Patient underwent a primary acute midfoot arthrodesis with an open reduction and internal fixation and simultaneous bridge plating stabilization at the medial column of the foot. The lateral column of the foot was stabilized with large Steinmann pin fixation **(C,D)**. *(continued)*

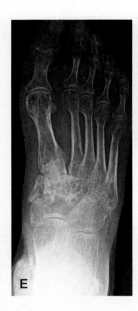

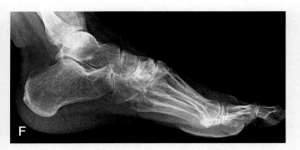

FIGURE 24.2 *(Continued)* Symptomatic retained hardware was removed at 12 months postoperatively. Final postoperative anteroposterior **(E)** and lateral **(F)** right foot radiographic views showing anatomic reduction and osseous consolidation at 14 months follow-up.

of CN fractures and/or dislocations. Joint preparation for this type of surgical reconstruction is usually consisted of bone wedge resection with a sagittal saw because deformity is commonly encountered and the anatomic osseous alignment is altered. The use of circular external fixation for the management of CN midfoot fractures and/or dislocations is usually preferred. In this clinical case scenario, after the joints are resected and properly aligned, they are stabilized with large Steinmann pins and filled with allogenic or autogenous bone grafting when necessary. The surgical incisions are then closed. Stability and compression of the joints are performed through percutaneous placement of smooth wires and/or half-pins and circular external fixation (Fig. 24.3).

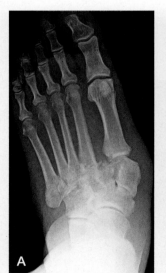

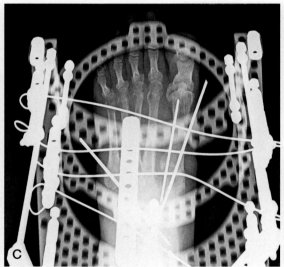

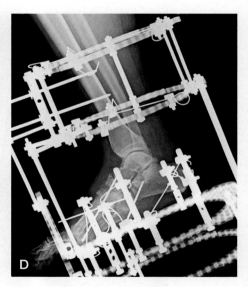

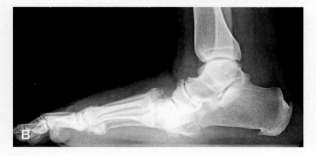

FIGURE 24.3 Preoperative anteroposterior **(A)** and lateral **(B)** left foot radiographic views of a diabetic patient with Charcot neuroarthropathy at the tarsometatarsal joints. Postoperative anteroposterior **(C)** and lateral **(D)** left foot and ankle radiographic views showing the utilization of circular external fixation to achieve deformity correction and arthrodesis of the tarsometatarsal fracture and dislocation. *(continued)*

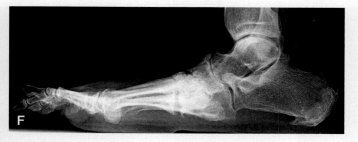

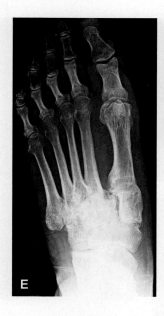

FIGURE 24.3 *(Continued)* Final postoperative anteroposterior **(E)** and lateral **(F)** left foot radiographic views showing the arthrodesis and deformity correction to achieve a stable plantigrade foot at 12 months follow-up.

Additional surgical procedures might be necessary in the acute or delayed type of midfoot arthrodesis procedures when the hindfoot and/or ankle are usually involved in the CN or acute trauma setting. For example, the delayed primary medial column arthrodesis for CN deformity may also be accompanied by a simultaneous lateral column, subtalar, ankle, or tibiotalocalcaneal arthrodesis and/or stabilization when the deformity involves the proximal joints as well. On the other hand, primary subtalar joint arthrodesis may also be necessary to be performed simultaneously in the acute midfoot trauma setting if a severely comminuted calcaneal fracture is also present at the initial time of injury.

DIABETIC HINDFOOT FRACTURES AND DISLOCATIONS

Surgical Incisional Approaches

Surgical incisional approaches for a navicular fracture with or without talonavicular dislocation is best managed by an anteromedial, anterolateral, or medial approach when necessary. In the acute setting of a displaced navicular fracture, open reduction and internal fixation with or without external fixation as an adjunct for stabilizing the medial column might be necessary at the time of injury (Fig. 24.4). Conversely, in the diabetic patient with peripheral neuropathy, comminuted navicular fractures may be delayed for primary arthrodesis of the talonavicular or talonaviculocuneiform joints.

Surgical incisional approaches for talar neck fractures are best managed with medial and lateral incisions to achieve fracture reduction. Often, medial talar comminution is encountered, and confirmation of reduction is achieved through further visualization of the lateral fracture fragments to avoid varus malunion of the talus. Talar body fractures are often approached through a combination of anterior and/or posterior medial and/or lateral approaches (Fig. 24.5). Although rare, a

medial malleolar osteotomy may be required to achieve fracture reduction of talar body fractures. Surgical approaches must be planned by the pattern of the involved fractures represented on CT scans.

Reduction and fixation of diabetic calcaneal fractures are either addressed through a closed reduction with percutaneous pinning (Fig. 24.6), a limited open approach with internal and/or external fixation, or an extensile lateral approach (Fig. 24.7) (4). In the diabetic population, the surgical approach is dependent on the presence and severity of medical comorbidities, vascular compromise, and ambulatory status as well as the type and severity of fracture pattern. Certain fracture patterns are not always amenable to closed reduction with pinning and/or limited open approach with internal fixation. Comminuted and displaced calcaneal fractures often require an extensile lateral approach to achieve anatomic reduction.

At times, a diabetic patient with multiple comorbidities may not be amenable to adequate fracture reduction because the risk of nonhealing wounds, deep infection, and lower extremity amputation are considered to be likely. In these circumstances, the surgeon may consider closed reduction and percutaneous pinning to improve the overall alignment of the calcaneus and/or consider reduction with an external fixator and ligamentotaxis. Often, anatomic reduction is not achieved with these methods, but improvement can be made in the alignment and height of the calcaneus as the fracture heals.

Primary subtalar joint arthrodesis is considered for comminuted intra-articular calcaneal fractures in diabetic patients with peripheral neuropathy (Fig. 24.8) (1,2). Delayed subtalar joint arthrodesis is usually performed for management of painful posttraumatic arthritis, deformity secondary to CN, and salvage of a nonunion and/or malunion of a calcaneal fracture. In the acute traumatic event, primary subtalar joint arthrodesis is typically performed through an extensile

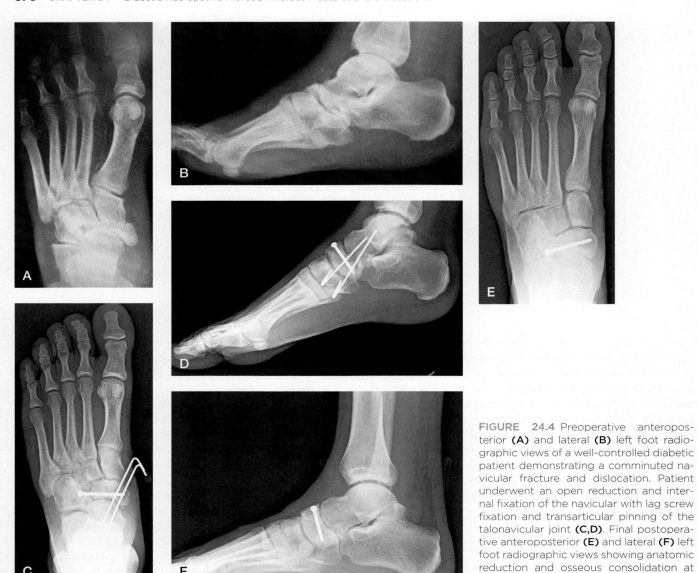

FIGURE 24.4 Preoperative anteroposterior (A) and lateral (B) left foot radiographic views of a well-controlled diabetic patient demonstrating a comminuted navicular fracture and dislocation. Patient underwent an open reduction and internal fixation of the navicular with lag screw fixation and transarticular pinning of the talonavicular joint (C,D). Final postoperative anteroposterior (E) and lateral (F) left foot radiographic views showing anatomic reduction and osseous consolidation at 6 months follow-up.

FIGURE 24.5 Preoperative anteroposterior (A) and lateral (B) right ankle radiographic views demonstrating a comminuted talar body/neck fracture and dislocation with skin tension and potential vascular compromise. *(continued)*

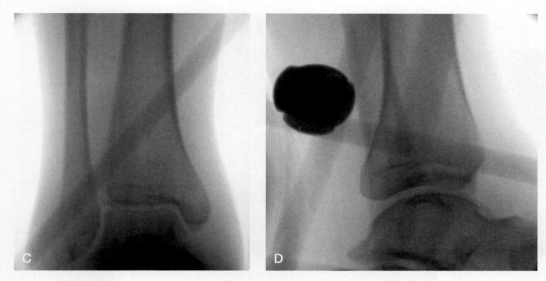

FIGURE 24.5 *(Continued)* Immediate postoperative anteroposterior **(C)** and lateral **(D)** right ankle radiographic views showing reduction through ligamentotaxis and application of a spanning external fixator.

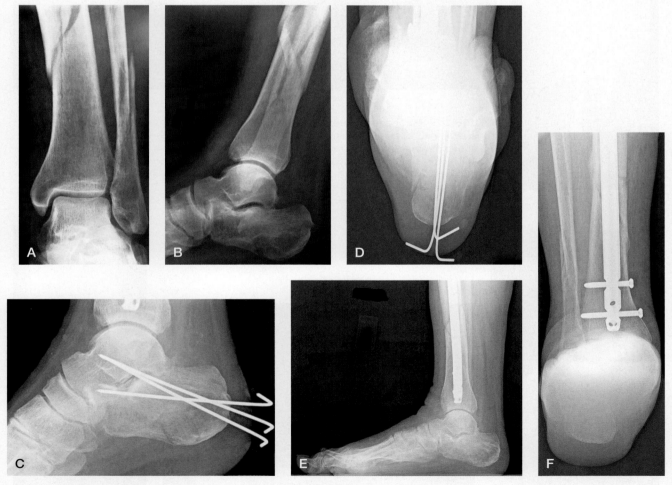

FIGURE 24.6 Preoperative anteroposterior **(A)** and lateral **(B)** left leg radiographic views of a diabetic patient with peripheral neuropathy showing a tongue-type intra-articular joint depressed calcaneal fracture and ipsilateral tibia shaft fracture. Patient underwent a closed reduction and transarticular subtalar joint pinning 3 days after the intramedullary nailing of the tibia shaft fracture was performed by the orthopedic team **(C,D)**. Postoperative lateral **(E)** and calcaneal axial **(F)** left leg radiographic views showing anatomic reduction and osseous consolidation at 4 months follow-up.

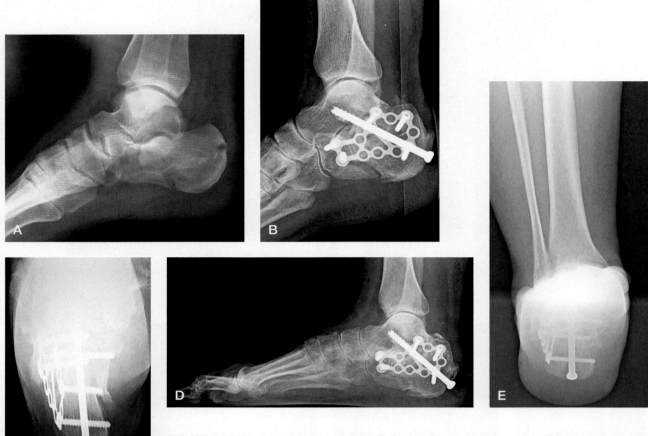

FIGURE 24.7 Preoperative lateral **(A)** left foot radiographic view of a diabetic patient with peripheral neuropathy showing an acute comminuted intra-articular calcaneal fracture. Patient underwent an open reduction and internal fixation of the calcaneus with primary subtalar joint arthrodesis **(B,C)**. One month follow-up **(B,C)** and final postoperative lateral **(D)** and calcaneal axial **(E)** left foot radiographic views showing anatomic reduction and osseous consolidation at 6 months follow-up.

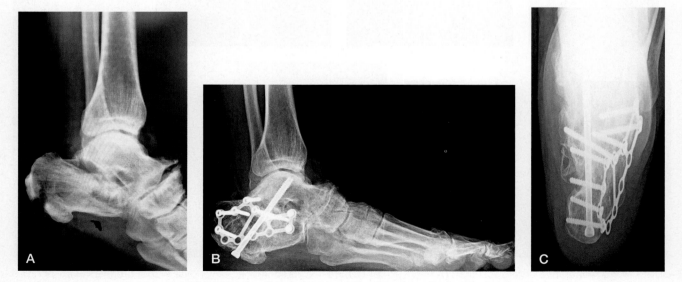

FIGURE 24.8 Preoperative lateral **(A)** right foot radiographic view of a diabetic patient with peripheral neuropathy showing a comminuted intra-articular joint depressed calcaneal fracture with remote history of trauma and hindfoot arthritis. Postoperative lateral **(B)** and calcaneal axial **(C)** right foot radiographic views showing anatomic reduction and osseous consolidation of an open reduction and internal fixation of the calcaneus with primary subtalar joint arthrodesis at 6 months follow-up.

lateral approach. However, delayed subtalar joint arthrodesis in the diabetic patient with peripheral neuropathy is usually performed through either a sinus tarsi incision or a vertical incision posterior to the peroneal tendons. The vertical incision is utilized to manage malunited joint depressed calcaneal fractures that require a large bone block distraction arthrodesis of the subtalar joint. The vertical incision in these cases allows exposure to excise a prominent lateral wall of the calcaneus, realign the posterior tuberosity of the calcaneus, distract the subtalar joint, and address any peroneal tendon pathology while minimizing skin tension on wound closure (Fig. 24.9).

Surgical Techniques

Alternative treatment options other than the extensile lateral approach may be considered for select calcaneal fracture patterns in the diabetic population. Closed reduction and percutaneous pinning of calcaneal fractures are best utilized for tongue-type fracture patterns. Percutaneous pinning is advantageous for comminuted and displaced open calcaneal fractures. Often, a transverse medial open wound is encountered with open calcaneal fractures as a result of displacement across the primary calcaneal fracture line. The open wound should be surgically débrided and reduction can be achieved through the open traumatic wound by transarticular pinning across the subtalar joint (Fig. 24.10). This surgical technique

negates the need for further incisions and hardware placement while providing osseous stability to promote fracture healing. The utilization of a Schanz pin inserted into the calcaneal tuberosity can further assist in fracture reduction.

Minimal surgical incisions can be utilized to assist in fracture reduction and placement of limited internal fixation. A sinus tarsi incision or an incision placed between the interval of the peroneal brevis and longus can be utilized to assist in reduction of the subtalar joint depression and calcaneal lateral wall. The utilization of external fixation for calcaneal fracture reduction can be combined with a limited surgical incision as opposed to transarticular percutaneous pinning.

CIRCULAR EXTERNAL FIXATION FOR DIABETIC MIDFOOT AND/OR HINDFOOT TRAUMA

External fixation is utilized for management of diabetic midfoot and/or hindfoot trauma when additional osseous stability and soft tissue protection are required. Various clinical case scenarios benefit from the utilization of external fixation for management of diabetic midfoot and/or hindfoot trauma. External fixation can range from temporary spanning external fixators that are applied until definitive fracture reduction is performed to circular external fixators that are utilized to achieve definitive fracture reduction, surgical off-loading of

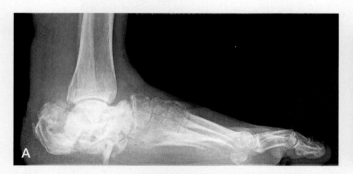
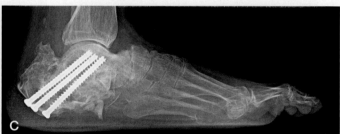
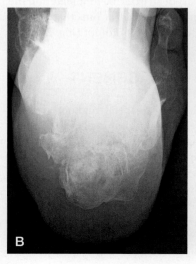
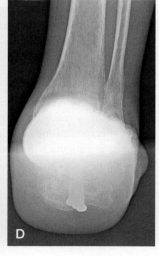

FIGURE 24.9 Preoperative lateral (A) and calcaneal axial (B) right foot radiographic views of a diabetic patient with peripheral neuropathy showing a calcaneal fracture nonunion with significant joint depression and deformity 6 months after a traumatic fall with a contralateral calcaneal, pelvic, and spinal fractures. Patient underwent a delayed subtalar joint distraction bone block arthrodesis that was performed through a vertical incision posterior to the peroneal tendons. Final postoperative lateral (C) and calcaneal axial (D) right foot radiographic views showing near-anatomic reduction and osseous consolidation at 12 months follow-up.

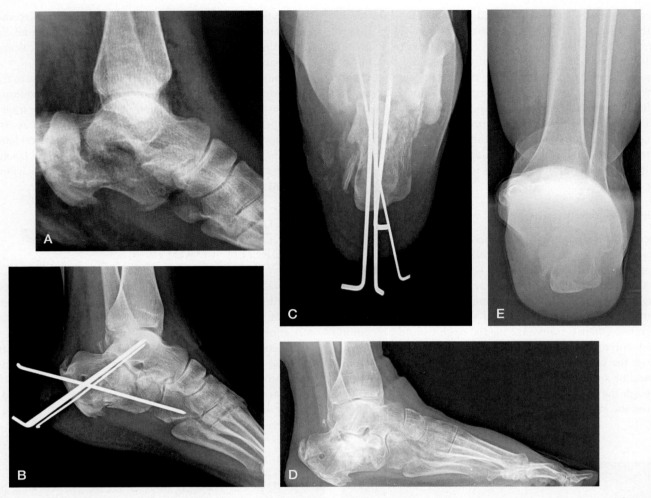

FIGURE 24.10 Preoperative lateral **(A)** right foot radiographic view of a diabetic patient showing an open calcaneal fracture. Patient underwent an open reduction and percutaneous transarticular subtalar and calcaneocuboid joint pinning that was performed through the open fracture wound **(B,C)**. Final postoperative lateral **(D)** and calcaneal axial **(E)** right foot radiographic views showing anatomic reduction and posttraumatic arthritis of the subtalar joint at 9 months follow-up.

soft tissue flaps, deformity correction, and/or primary arthrodesis (Fig. 24.11). External fixation may also be combined with internal fixation when necessary in order to provide additional osseous stability or to protect the traumatic soft tissue envelope.

Stabilization of CN fractures and/or dislocations of the midfoot and/or hindfoot are not usually achieved with simple spanning external fixators. CN fractures and/or dislocations typically require either multiplane circular external fixators or hybrid fixators to achieve stabilization for extended periods of time. Spanning external fixators for temporary fracture reduction may be applied for approximately 1 to 4 weeks until definite surgical treatment, whereas circular external fixators utilized for CN midfoot and/or hindfoot fractures and/or dislocations are applied for approximately 3 to 4 months postoperatively. These types of circular external fixators consist of a tibial "block" (2 circular rings) attached to a transcalcaneal pin and/or forefoot pin(s)/ring that stabilizes the midfoot by

placing multiple smooth wires and/or pins for stability (3). Alternative constructs consist of an external foot plate and the utilization of multiple smooth wires and/or pins that are tensioned to stabilize the midfoot and/or hindfoot (Fig. 24.12).

POSTOPERATIVE MANAGEMENT

Postoperative management of the diabetic midfoot/hindfoot trauma may require a longer period of immobilization, antibiotic therapy, and/or anticoagulation treatment when necessary. Diabetic patients with peripheral neuropathy, peripheral arterial disease, or the presence of CN may require prolonged time to heal compared to a well-controlled diabetic patient without evidence of an end-organ disease. Antibiotic therapy before and after the surgical reconstruction is dependent on the initial type and severity of injury, hardware application, associated medical comorbidities, and/or vascular status. Anticoagulation treatment

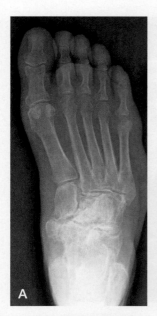
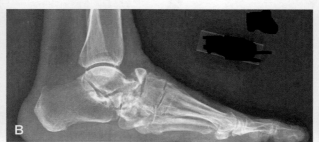
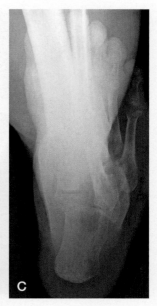
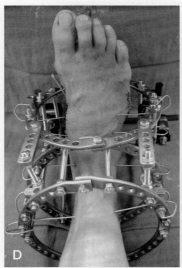
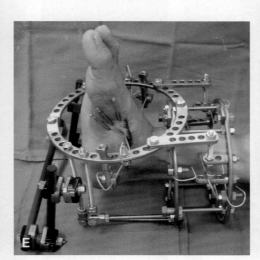
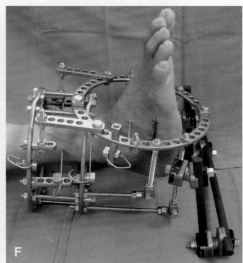
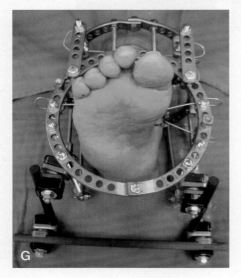

FIGURE 24.11 Preoperative anteroposterior **(A)**, lateral **(B)**, and calcaneal axial **(C)** right foot radiographic views of a diabetic patient with peripheral neuropathy showing an initial navicular fracture and dislocation with subsequent Charcot neuroarthropathy. Patient underwent a partial naviculectomy with medial column arthrodesis **(D–G)**, fifth metatarsal and bursa resection, gastrocnemius recession, and circular external fixation for compression and stability of the lower extremity **(H–J)**. *(continued)*

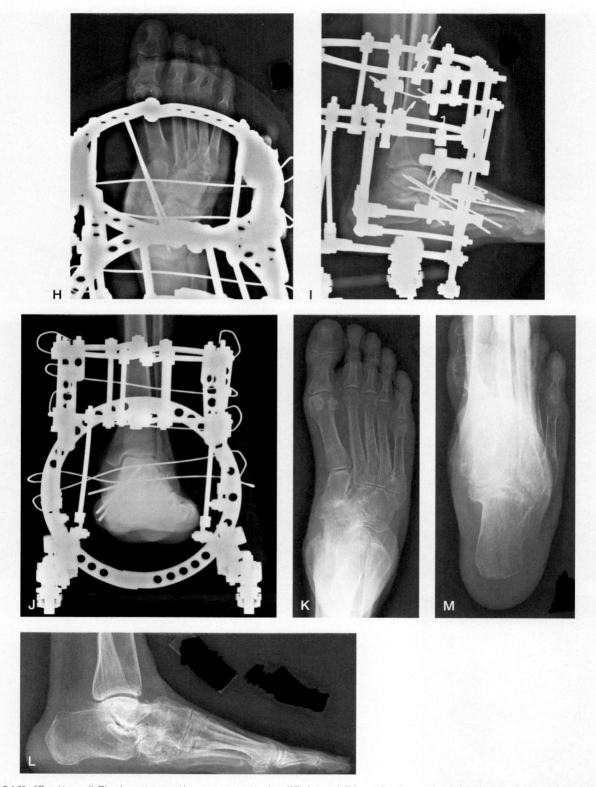

FIGURE 24.11 *(Continued)* Final postoperative anteroposterior **(K)**, lateral **(L)**, and calcaneal axial **(M)** right foot radiographic views showing the arthrodesis and deformity correction to achieve a stable plantigrade foot at approximately 34 months follow-up.

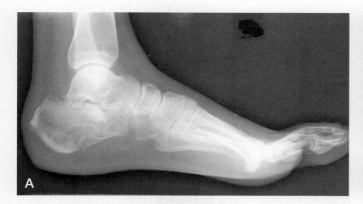
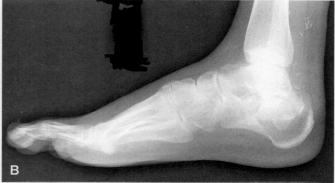
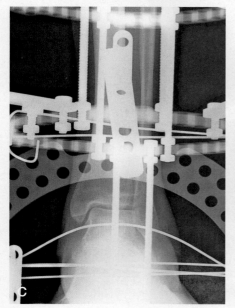
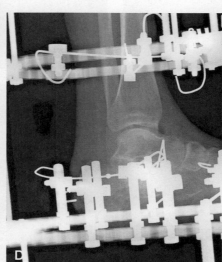
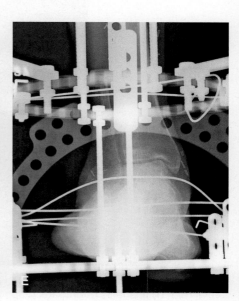
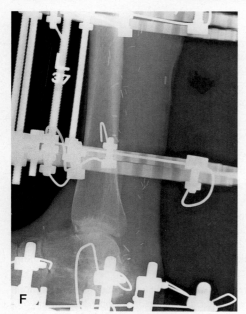

FIGURE 24.12 Preoperative lateral right **(A)** and left **(B)** foot radiographic views of a patient with type 1 diabetes mellitus who presented with multiple injuries and comminuted intra-articular calcaneal fractures. Patient underwent a simultaneous right **(C,D)** and left **(E,F)** calcaneal fracture repair with primary subtalar joint arthrodesis and circular external fixation to both lower extremities. *(continued)*

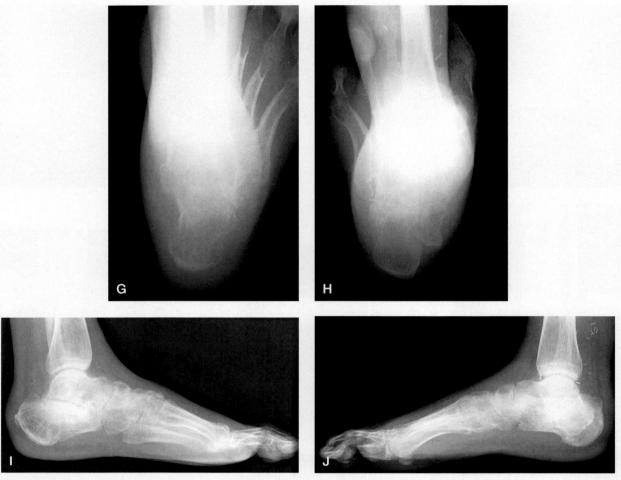

FIGURE 24.12 *(Continued)* Postoperative calcaneal axial right **(G)** and left **(H)** foot radiographic views at 3 months follow-up and lateral right **(I)** and left **(J)** foot radiographic views at approximately 5 months follow-up.

is also dependent on the type and severity of injury, past medical and surgical history, prolonged immobilization, vascular status, and smoking history.

Diabetic patients with peripheral neuropathy may also require physical therapy and rehabilitation in order to maintain a non–weight-bearing status safely or for safety evaluations once a patient begins early transfers or weight bearing. In the presence of peripheral neuropathy, diabetic patients may not be able to sensate or self-protect a traumatic event that can lead to postoperative nonunion, broken hardware, deformity, and/or a CN process. For these reasons, a detailed postoperative course with rehabilitation is necessary in order to minimize any complications.

Conclusion

Identifying traumatic from neuropathic fractures and/or dislocations when dealing with midfoot/hindfoot trauma in the diabetic population is crucial for the patient's overall successful outcome. Many surgical options exist in the management of neuropathic and/or CN fractures and/or dislocations as compared to

routine trauma management in the well-controlled diabetic patient. Understanding this difference is critical in order to choose the best treatment option for the diabetic patient with or without multiple medical comorbidities.

References

1. Facaros Z, Ramanujam CL, Zgonis T. Primary subtalar joint arthrodesis with internal and external fixation for the repair of a diabetic comminuted calcaneal fracture. Clin Podiatr Med Surg 2011;28:203–209.

2. Marin LE, DiDomenico LA, Mandracchia VJ, et al. Diabetic neuropathic forefoot, midfoot, and hindfoot osseous trauma and dislocations. In: Zgonis T, ed. Surgical reconstruction of the diabetic foot and ankle. Philadelphia: Lippincott Williams & Wilkins, 2009:344–356.

3. Stapleton JJ, Polyzois VD, Zgonis T. Stepwise approach to midfoot/hindfoot trauma and external fixation. In: Cooper PS, Polyzois VD, Zgonis T, eds. External fixators of the foot and ankle. Philadelphia: Lippincott Williams & Wilkins, 2013:162–186.

4. Stapleton JJ, Zgonis T. Surgical treatment of intra-articular calcaneal fractures. Clin Podiatr Med Surg 2014;31:539–546.

CHAPTER 25

Diabetic Neuropathic Ankle/Pilon Fractures and Dislocations

John J. Stapleton • Thomas Zgonis

INTRODUCTION

Diabetic ankle and distal tibia (pilon) fractures and/or dislocations can present with various pathologies and associated medical comorbidities. The presence of diabetic peripheral neuropathy, peripheral arterial disease, high-energy trauma, open injuries, and evidence of poorly controlled diabetes mellitus can further complicate the patient's treatment plan.

A well-controlled diabetic patient with an ankle or pilon fracture and without any evidence of an end-stage organ disease such as coronary arterial disease, peripheral arterial disease, and renal disease is typically managed with a traditional open reduction and internal fixation (ORIF) surgical approach because the incidence of postoperative complications may be similar to nondiabetic patients (Fig. 25.1).

On the contrary, poorly controlled diabetic patients with a history of elevated hemoglobin A_{1c} (HbA_{1c}) levels; multiple uncontrolled medical comorbidities including, but not limited to, coronary arterial disease, renal disease, diabetic neuropathy, obesity, smoking, and peripheral arterial disease; and history of previous ulcerations and/or amputations are challenging to treat when an ankle/pilon fracture is encountered. The initial clinical presentation with an acute ankle and/or pilon fracture in this type of diabetic population may require a different surgical approach and protocol in order to minimize any potential surgical complications. In many cases, diabetic patients with peripheral neuropathy can start with an acute ankle fracture that can rapidly progress to Charcot neuroarthropathy (CN) subluxation and gross deformity. Accurate diagnosis, medical optimization, and early treatment are crucial for the patient's successful outcome.

Clinical correlation of higher surgical complication rates in diabetic patients with ankle fractures has been well reported in the literature. In 2015, Cavo et al. (3) in a large study from a nationwide inpatient sample concluded that diabetes mellitus and obesity had higher health care costs and utilization compared to nonobese or nondiabetic patients. In another study by Basques et al. (2) of patients with an ankle fracture treated with an ORIF identified by the American College of Surgeons National Surgical Quality Improvement Program

concluded that insulin-dependent diabetes mellitus patients had an increase rate of surgical complications and hospital readmission determined by the American Society of Anesthesiologists classification ≥ 3. Liu et al. (9) have also retrospectively reviewed 21 diabetic patients and the effects of HbA_{1c} on ankle ORIF procedures and concluded that HbA_{1c} levels $\geq 6.5\%$ were statistically associated with poor radiologic outcomes. Wukich et al. (13) reported on the increased surgical complication rates in patients with complicated versus uncomplicated diabetes mellitus. In this study, the authors have found higher incidence of nonunion, malunion, and CN as well as subsequent revision surgery in the population with complicated diabetes mellitus (13).

Furthermore, a large survey by Rosenbaum et al. (10) on the management of ankle fractures in the diabetic population by the American Orthopaedic Foot and Ankle Society membership concluded that the use of syndesmotic screws in displaced fractures and prolonged non–weight-bearing was advocated by most of the respondents in contrast to casting and non–weight-bearing for the non-displaced ankle fractures. Case reports of combined circular external fixation with pro-syndesmotic screws (5) and arthroscopic reduction with fibula nailing (12) for the high-risk diabetic patient have also been reported in the literature.

Conversely, very limited literature is found on the surgical complication rates in diabetic patients with pilon fractures. Kline et al. (7) in a retrospective review of operative pilon fractures in diabetic and nondiabetic patients concluded that higher rate of surgical complications such as infection, delayed union, and nonunion was encountered in the diabetic population, whereas the surgical wound dehiscence rate was the same in both groups (7). In a case report by Koutsostathis et al. (8), a combination of circular external fixation and Papineau technique was utilized for the treatment of septic distal tibia pseudoarthrosis in a diabetic patient.

The goal of surgical management of acute traumatic diabetic ankle or pilon fractures is to achieve anatomic or near-anatomic fracture reduction and osseous union while minimizing any inherent surgical complications encountered in this population. In the presence of CN secondarily to ankle or pilon fracture

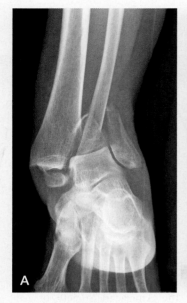
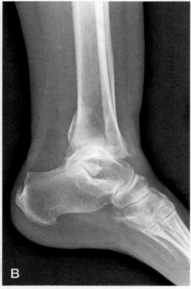
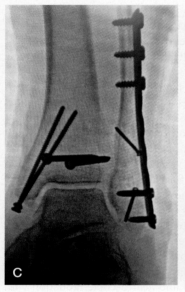
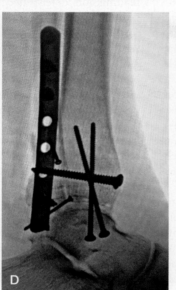
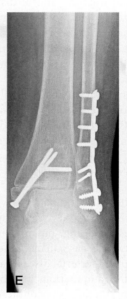
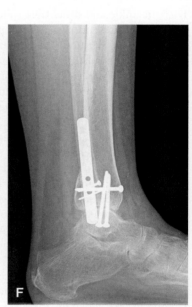

FIGURE 25.1 Preoperative anteroposterior **(A)** and lateral **(B)** right ankle radiographic views of a well-controlled diabetic patient without peripheral neuropathy who sustained a trimalleolar ankle fracture-dislocation. Immediate **(C,D)** and final postoperative anteroposterior **(E)** and lateral **(F)** radiographic views showing osseous union and anatomic alignment at 6 months follow-up.

and/or dislocation, successful outcomes are usually achieved by performing an ankle, tibiocalcaneal, or tibiotalocalcaneal arthrodesis for lower extremity preservation and functional ambulation (Fig. 25.2). The use of isolated osteosynthesis in a diabetic ankle/pilon fracture that have led to CN may not be practical and able to withstand the biomechanical manifestations and inherent instability encountered with the diabetic CN patient.

PREOPERATIVE CONSIDERATIONS

Physical Examination and Imaging

Initial management of the diabetic patient who presents with an acute injury to the ankle and/or pilon begins with a complete history and physical examination as well as determining the type and severity of the fracture-dislocation. Equal attention

is emphasized for the management of any associated body or lower extremity injuries and patient's medical comorbidities. Appropriate lower extremity radiographs, medical imaging, laboratory testing, and medical optimization are paramount in the diabetic patient who will undergo surgical repair of the ankle/pilon fracture.

In the presence of an open ankle/pilon fracture, a temporarily spanning external fixator may be utilized initially until definitive treatment with an ORIF and/or external fixation is feasible. Acute high-energy ankle/pilon fractures may require immediate reduction in order to prevent further injury to the soft tissue envelope and/or neurovascular structures. Associated compartment syndrome and skin tension require urgent operative intervention to prevent soft tissue necrosis and/or probable lower extremity amputation. In the presence of diminished lower extremity pulses, noninvasive arterial studies and/or vascular surgery consultation may be

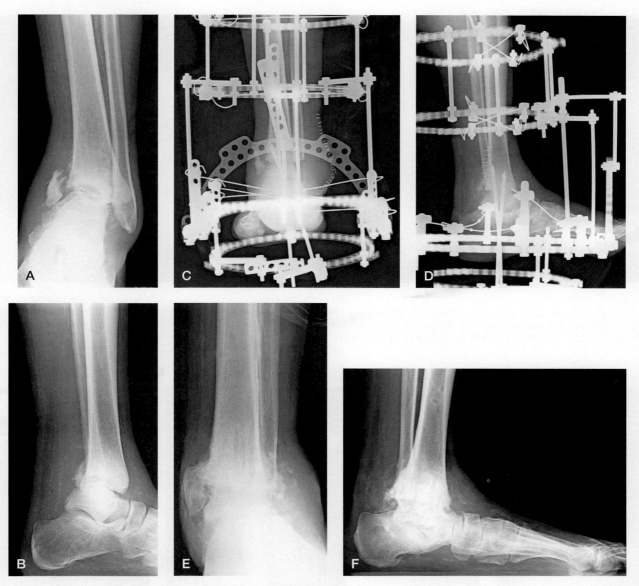

FIGURE 25.2 Preoperative anteroposterior **(A)** and lateral **(B)** right ankle radiographic views of a poorly controlled diabetic patient with multiple medical comorbidities who sustained a distal tibia pilon fracture and Charcot neuroarthropathy. Patient underwent a primary tibiotalocalcaneal arthrodesis with a multiplane circular external fixation device **(C,D)**. Final postoperative anteroposterior **(E)** and lateral **(F)** lower extremity radiographic views showing osseous union and anatomic alignment at 12 months follow-up.

necessary before the definitive reconstruction. External fixation may be initially utilized for the fracture reduction and allow healing of the soft tissue compromise when indicated.

Mechanism of Injury and Treatment Planning

Traumatic dislocations of the ankle joint need to be reduced and immobilized in an expedited manner in order to prevent soft tissue necrosis and minimize the development of fracture blisters. Well-padded lower extremity dressings and splints should be initially applied to stabilize the fracture as well as the closed reduction procedure. The timing of surgery is then dependent based on the overall medical condition of the diabetic patient, fracture pattern and severity as well as

viability of the surrounding soft tissue envelope on initial presentation.

Low-energy rotational ankle/pilon fractures and/or dislocations are usually surgically addressed once the diabetic patient is medically optimized for the operating room without significant delay unless extensive edema and/or fracture blisters are present (Fig. 25.3). Diabetic ankle/pilon fractures that are presenting with skin tension and probable compromise to the neurovascular structures due to persistent joint subluxation/instability after closed reduction are necessary to be addressed in an expedited manner. High-energy pilon fractures usually present with soft tissue complications and initial fracture stabilization is typically fixated with a spanning external fixator until definitive fracture reduction and stabilization can be planned and performed (Figs. 25.4 and 25.5).

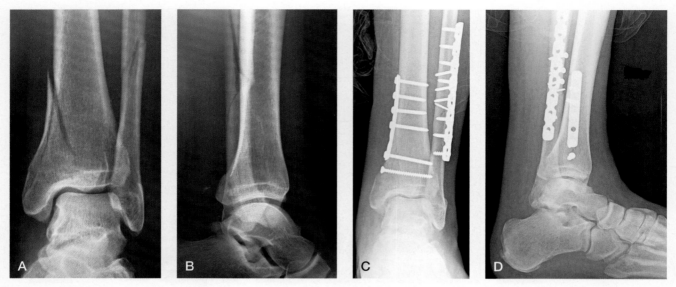

FIGURE 25.3 Preoperative anteroposterior **(A)** and lateral **(B)** right ankle radiographic views of a well-controlled diabetic patient who sustained a low-energy rotational distal tibia and fibula pilon fracture. Final postoperative anteroposterior **(C)** and lateral **(D)** lower extremity radiographic views at 4 months follow-up showing osseous union and anatomic reduction of the tibia and fibula that were fixated in a single stage 2 days after the initial injury.

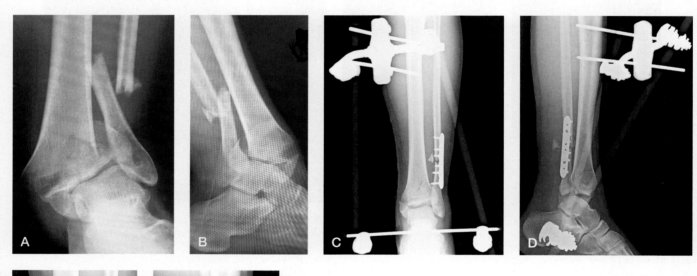

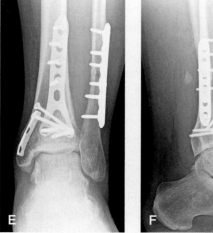

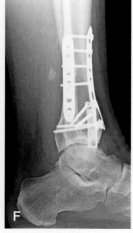

FIGURE 25.4 Preoperative anteroposterior **(A)** and lateral **(B)** right ankle radiographic views of a poorly controlled diabetic patient who sustained a severely displaced distal tibia and fibula pilon fracture with a valgus deformity. Patient underwent an initial open reduction and internal fixation (ORIF) of the fibula and closed reduction and stabilization of the tibia pilon fracture with a spanning external fixation device **(C,D)**. Final postoperative anteroposterior **(E)** and lateral **(F)** lower extremity radiographic views showing osseous union, anatomic alignment, and posttraumatic arthritis of the ankle at 9 months follow-up. Definitive ORIF of the tibia and removal of the spanning external fixator was performed at 14 days after the initial surgery.

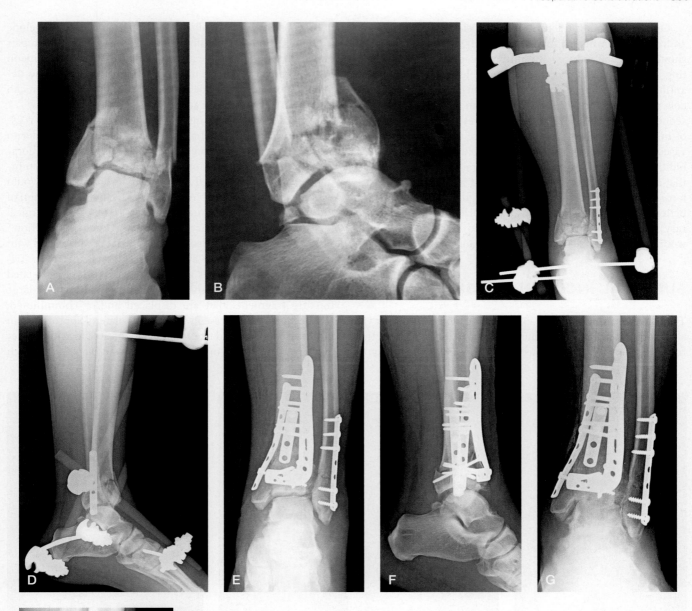

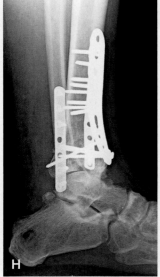

FIGURE 25.5 Preoperative anteroposterior **(A)** and lateral **(B)** right ankle radiographic views of a well-controlled diabetic patient without peripheral neuropathy who sustained a tibia and fibula pilon fracture-dislocation with comminution of the ankle articular surface and varus deformity. Patient underwent an initial open reduction and internal fixation (ORIF) of the fibula and closed reduction and stabilization of the tibia pilon fracture with a spanning external fixation device **(C,D)**. Postoperative anteroposterior **(E)** and lateral **(F)** lower extremity radiographic views showing removal of the spanning external fixator and definitive ORIF of the distal tibia at approximately 10 days after the initial surgical procedure. Final postoperative anteroposterior **(G)** and lateral **(H)** lower extremity radiographic views showing osseous union, near-anatomic reduction, and posttraumatic arthritis of the ankle at 9 months follow-up.

Open ankle/pilon fractures and/or dislocations need to be addressed in an urgent manner. Open fractures of the ankle should be closed reduced and immobilized in the clinical setting and/or operating room when feasible, while intravenous antibiotics start immediately and based on open fracture protocols. Adequate surgical débridement, fixation options, and subsequent wound closure are dependent on the severity and type of initial surgery, soft tissue compromise and contamination, vascular supply, and patient's management of medical comorbidities (Fig. 25.6). Conversely, open fractures with wounds that are heavily contaminated or present with significant skin tension and wounds associated with high-energy trauma are better treated with a staged surgical débridement and temporary spanning external fixation followed by delayed surgical wound closure and definitive fracture reduction (Fig. 25.7).

SURGICAL INCISION CONSIDERATIONS

The compromised soft tissue envelope must be assessed for viability and planned surgical incision approaches to address the fracture pattern are determined based on the severity and type of osseous and associated soft injury. The soft tissue envelope is often one of the most limiting factors to the surgical repair of complex diabetic ankle and/or pilon fractures. The surgeon needs to be aware of the underlying fracture pattern and deforming forces that, if not addressed in a timely manner, can lead to further soft tissue compromise and skin necrosis.

Surgical incision planning cannot be overlooked and is essential to ensure a direct approach when feasible in order to achieve fracture reduction while minimizing soft tissue complications. Surgical incision planning begins with determining if there is a preexisted soft tissue compromise that would preclude further surgical incisions. Next, careful evaluation of the fracture pattern is crucial in order to determine surgical incisions that are necessary to achieve the fracture reduction.

Routine closed bimalleolar ankle fractures are treated with traditional direct lateral and medial surgical incisions. Trimalleolar ankle fractures and in particular those associated with complex posterior malleolar fracture that involves large fracture fragments that are displaced and/or comminuted, may need to be addressed with a posterolateral approach if an indirect reduction and fixation may not be able to achieve adequate fracture reduction (Fig. 25.8). A posterolateral approach

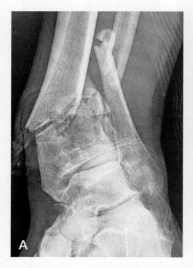
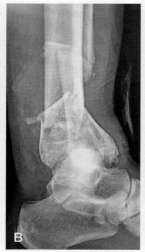
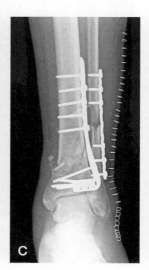
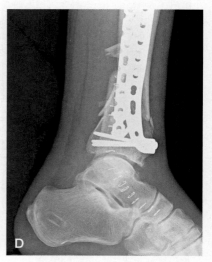
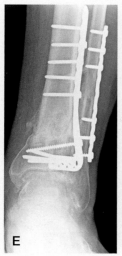
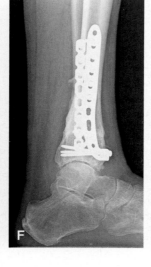

FIGURE 25.6 Preoperative anteroposterior **(A)** and lateral **(B)** right ankle radiographic views of a diabetic patient with peripheral neuropathy who sustained a significant comminution of the tibia metaphysis with a valgus deformity and an approximately 2 cm open clean medial wound that was previously surgically débrided. Immediate postoperative anteroposterior **(C)** and lateral **(D)** lower extremity radiographic views demonstrate definitive fixation of the tibia and fibula through an extensile lateral approach. Final postoperative anteroposterior **(E)** and lateral **(F)** lower extremity radiographic views showing osseous union, anatomic reduction, and posttraumatic arthritis of the ankle at 12 months follow-up.

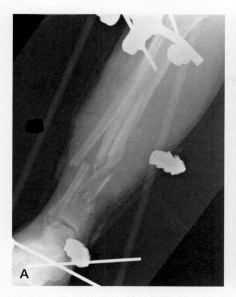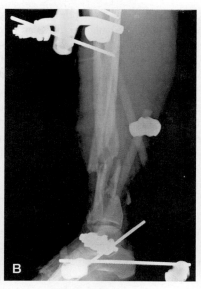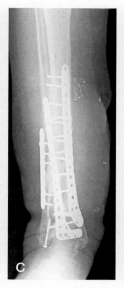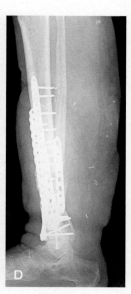

FIGURE 25.7 Preoperative anteroposterior **(A)** and lateral **(B)** left lower extremity radiographic views of a diabetic patient who sustained a high-energy open and comminuted distal tibia and fibula pilon fracture that was initially stabilized with a spanning external fixator with simultaneous surgical débridement and application of a negative pressure wound therapy. Final postoperative anteroposterior **(C)** and lateral **(D)** lower extremity radiographic views showing osseous union and near-anatomic reduction of the ankle at 14 months follow-up. Soft tissue coverage of the lower extremity consisted of a free latissimus dorsi flap and split-thickness skin graft performed by the plastic surgery team.

may allow fixation of both the posterior malleolus and fibular shaft or lateral malleolus fracture. Pilon fractures can be addressed with various surgical incisions that are usually based on the fracture pattern, compromised soft tissue envelope, and the severity of deforming fracture force.

One of the most common surgical incisions for the pilon fracture and/or dislocation is the anteromedial approach. This technique allows for excellent visualization of the anterior and medial aspects of the distal tibia and is extended medially along the course of the tibialis anterior tendon. The surgical incision can also be acutely curved toward the medial malleolus which will allow improved exposure of the lateral portion of the distal tibia articular surface. Full-thickness flap elevation of the anterior compartment allows for lateral plating if required (11). A surgical incision directly over the tibia crest or medial face of the distal tibia will not allow for full-thickness flap elevation

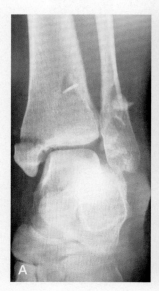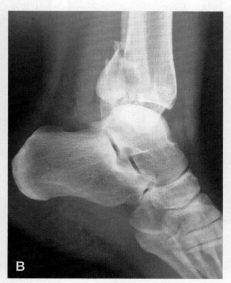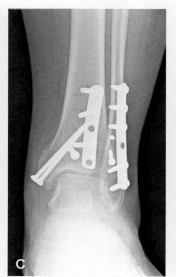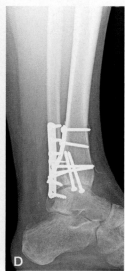

FIGURE 25.8 Preoperative anteroposterior **(A)** and lateral **(B)** right ankle radiographic views of a diabetic patient who sustained a trimalleolar ankle fracture with a significantly comminuted and displaced posterior malleolus fracture **(B)**. Final postoperative anteroposterior **(C)** and lateral **(D)** lower extremity radiographic views showing osseous union and anatomic alignment at 6 months follow-up. Fixation of the fibula and posterior malleolus was performed through a posterolateral approach **(D)**.

and surgical exposure is minimized. In addition, surgical closure over a medially based plate with minimal surgical exposure can lead to surgical wound dehiscence, infection, exposed hardware, need for flap coverage, and probable lower extremity amputation.

Other relatively common surgical incisions for the pilon fracture and/or dislocation include the anterolateral and direct lateral approaches. The anterolateral approach is performed laterally to the ankle joint and for addressing any ankle valgus angulation. In addition, this incision can also be utilized for addressing fracture fragments of the lateral and centrally impacted tibia plafond and/or for indirect reduction of displaced posterolateral fragments. Surgical exposure is usually limited, and if longer anterolateral plates are required, they may need to be tunneled directly along the lateral aspect of the tibia with the most proximal screws being inserted percutaneously. These lateral surgical incisions should be avoided to address any varus angulation of the lower extremity and impaction of the medial tibial plafond (11).

Posteromedial and posterolateral surgical incision approaches can be utilized for complex posterior tibial plafond fracture fragments that would be difficult to reduce indirectly through the aforementioned surgical approaches. A posterolateral approach can be utilized to address distal tibia metaphyseal–diaphyseal nonunions with posterolateral bone grafting and/or additional posterolateral plating (Fig. 25.9). This incision may also be extended proximally with the posterior deep compartment and neurovascular bundle being raised off the posterior tibia to allow posterior plating of the tibia. This technique may be utilized to address distal tibia nonunions that have a poor soft tissue envelope from previous wound complications. Concomitant fibula fractures can be addressed through this surgical approach as well. The posteromedial approach, although not frequently used, can be utilized to address complex posteromedial tibial plafond fractures but with certain limitations due to lack of exposure of the anterior aspect of the tibial plafond.

In the diabetic patient, ankle/pilon fractures and dislocations may present with an underlying untreated peripheral arterial disease that can further compromise the wound healing. Vascular assessment and consultation may be necessary before the surgical reconstruction if it is feasible based on the severity and type of initial injury. However, certain fracture patterns and/or dislocations are not amenable to vascular intervention prior to surgery and vascular surgery consultation can be initiated immediately during the postoperative course. In certain cases, limited surgical incision approaches with circular external fixation in the presence of severe peripheral arterial disease (4) or delayed osseous reconstruction that may require an ankle arthrodesis as opposed to traditional osteosynthesis in order to achieve lower extremity preservation might be necessary (1).

In diabetic patients with multiple medical comorbidities and poorly controlled diabetes mellitus, nonambulatory status, severe peripheral arterial disease without revascularization options, and gross fracture, dislocation, and deformity, lower extremity amputation may also provide the patient with another alternative treatment option. Through the input of a well-established multidisciplinary health care team with great knowledge in the medical and surgical management of the diabetic patient, surgical outcomes can be successful while minimizing inherent complications encountered in this population.

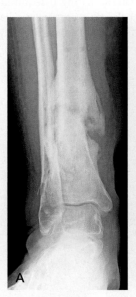 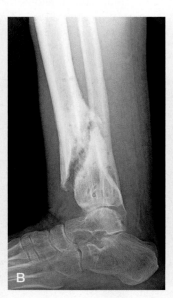 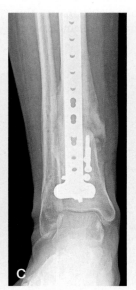 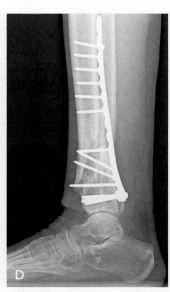

FIGURE 25.9 Preoperative anteroposterior **(A)** and lateral **(B)** left lower extremity radiographic views of a diabetic patient who sustained a distal tibia fracture and osseous nonunion after a tibia open reduction and internal fixation. Patient's internal fixation hardware was removed and the patient received a total of 6 weeks parenteral antibiotics. Patient presented with a compromised soft tissue envelope over the anterior and medial aspect of the tibia. Patient underwent a revisional reconstructive surgery consisted of a posterolateral approach, autogenous bone grafting, and posterior plating of the tibia. Final postoperative anteroposterior **(C)** and lateral **(D)** lower extremity radiographic views showing osseous union and near-anatomic alignment at 6 months follow-up after the revisional surgery.

OPERATIVE FIXATION CONSIDERATIONS

Careful evaluation of lower extremity and foot radiographs as well as computed tomography imaging of the distal tibia and fibula fractures are the basis of ultimate fracture reduction. Given the importance of appropriate surgical incision placement for select fracture patterns, surgeons need to be aware of avoiding unnecessary surgical incisions that can compromise the overall patient's outcome. In many cases, a staged reduction with the application of a spanning external fixator without performing an initial ORIF of the fibula is indicated. The application of a simple spanning external fixator can achieve initial fracture stabilization and allow for better utilization and evaluation of the ankle joint with computed tomography while protecting the soft tissue envelope.

Common bimalleolar and/or trimalleolar ankle fractures in a diabetic patient with multiple medical comorbidities might require alternate surgical methods to avoid surgical complications. Such surgical variations include, but are not limited to, enhanced fixation, pro-syndesmotic screws, transarticular Steinmann pins, and/or additional external fixation. These types of surgical techniques are primarily based on surgical experience dealing with the complicated diabetic population because specific evidence-based protocols do not currently exist. For example, pro-syndesmotic screws may be utilized even if a syndesmotic injury is questionable in the presence of deltoid ligament injury, potential for valgus collapse of the ankle, osteopenia, diabetic peripheral neuropathy, and presence of multiple medical comorbidities. The placement of adjunctive transarticular smooth Steinmann pins and/or circular external fixation is often utilized in the presence of internally fixated ankle fractures that still display significant instability. These techniques are common in diabetic patients with peripheral neuropathy and multiple uncontrolled medical comorbidities where the dislocated ankle/pilon fracture has still a significant capsule and ligament insufficiency even after the ORIF. In contrary, these techniques may not need to be utilized in a well-controlled diabetic patient without any other medical conditions.

Distal pilon fractures in the diabetic neuropathic patient with multiple medical comorbidities and end-stage organ disease present with numerous challenges to avoid devastating surgical complications and lower extremity amputation. These injuries are difficult to manage, and, in the presence of diabetic peripheral neuropathy, the surgical complications are clearly higher despite the minimal scientific evidence among patients with diabetic pilon fractures (7). The literature focuses primarily on diabetic patients with common ankle fractures, and this information is extrapolated to assume that the surgical complication rates are higher in the complex diabetic patient population with pilon fractures.

At times, significantly comminuted pilon fractures that are not amenable to reconstruction are encountered in the diabetic population. In those cases, a primary ankle arthrodesis is considered for lower extremity preservation (Fig. 25.10). Depending on the fracture pattern and severity, achieving a successful ankle arthrodesis is a challenge in these clinical scenarios. Autogenous and/or allogenic bone grafting may also be required. Multiplane circular external fixators, blade plates, and/or intramedullary nailing can be utilized for osseous stabilization and union. Mangled lower extremities with significant soft tissue and osseous defects may be managed with combined internal and external fixation to allow osseous stabilization and surgical off-loading of the soft tissue while avoiding potential complications from frequent casting/splint changes that would otherwise be required (Fig. 25.11).

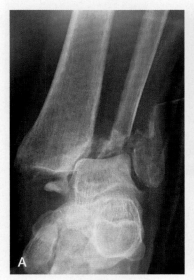 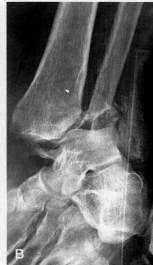 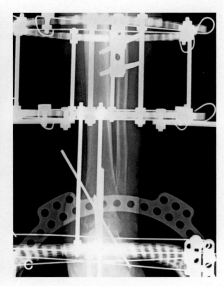

FIGURE 25.10 Preoperative anteroposterior **(A)** and lateral **(B)** right ankle radiographic views of a diabetic patient with peripheral neuropathy who sustained an ankle fracture and dislocation with clinical and systemic signs of infection at initial presentation. Postoperative anteroposterior **(C)** and lateral **(D)** right lower extremity radiographic views showing a primary ankle arthrodesis after surgical débridement and negative pressure wound therapy at 6 weeks follow-up. *(continued)*

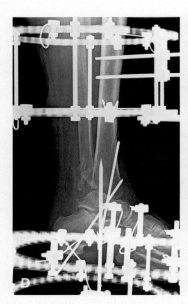
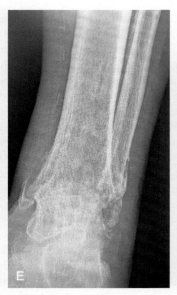
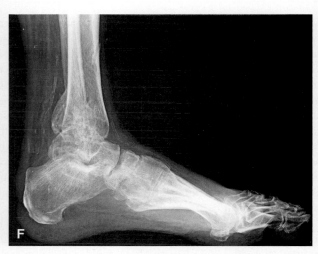

FIGURE 25.10 *(Continued)* Soft tissue coverage of the lower extremity wound was performed by a split-thickness skin graft at 3 months postoperatively. The circular external fixation device was removed at 4 months postoperatively, and the patient remained in a non–weight-bearing status for an additional 1 month. Functional ambulation with a custom-made shoe and a double upright brace initiated at 6 months postoperatively. Final postoperative anteroposterior **(E)** and lateral **(F)** radiographic views showing osseous union and anatomic alignment at 12 months follow-up.

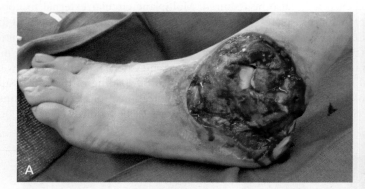

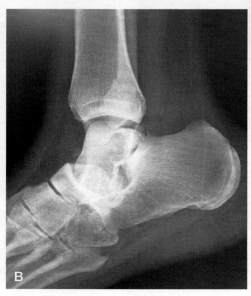

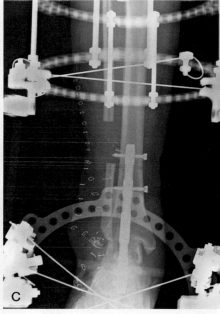

FIGURE 25.11 Preoperative clinical **(A)** and lateral **(B)** left ankle radiographic view of a diabetic patient who sustained an open total talar extrusion with reimplantation upon initial presentation. Patient underwent surgical débridement and staged primary tibiotalocalcaneal arthrodesis with an intramedullary nail **(C)** and anterolateral thigh free tissue transfer 5 days after the initial surgical débridement **(D)**. *(continued)*

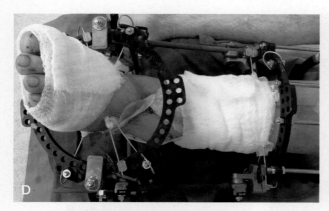

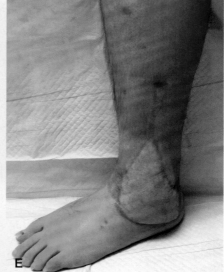

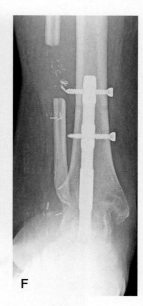

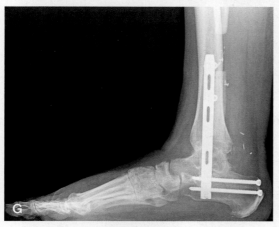

FIGURE 25.11 *(Continued)* A circular external fixation device was utilized for additional osseous stability and for surgical off-loading of the free flap **(C,D)**. Final clinical **(E)** and postoperative anteroposterior **(F)** and lateral **(G)** radiographic views showing osseous union and anatomic alignment at 6 months follow-up.

COMPLICATIONS AND POSTOPERATIVE MANAGEMENT

Surgical wound complications can lead to deep infection with potential lower extremity amputation. The incidence of surgical wound complications and infections may be lessened by expediting the surgical repair for low-energy rotational ankle fractures while delaying definitive surgery for approximately 5 to 14 days for high-energy distal tibia pilon fractures until the edema subsides. The utilization of a spanning external fixator allows temporary osseous stability and healing of the compromised soft tissue envelope. The planning of surgical incisions and approach are paramount to minimize skin tension while achieving fracture reduction.

In the diabetic patient with peripheral neuropathy and multiple medical comorbidities, surgical wound infections may require immediate surgical débridement, laboratory analysis, intraoperative bone, soft tissue cultures, and histopathology testing in order to identify causative pathogens and guide appropriate antibiotics. Infectious disease consultation is highly considered in the diabetic population with severe injuries and infections to the lower extremity. Clinical and/or systemic signs of deep infection often require hardware removal or exchange, antibiotic-impregnated cement spacers and/or beads, delayed osseous, and soft tissue

reconstruction (Fig. 25.12). Large soft tissue defects with exposed hardware and bone often require free tissue transfer for lower extremity preservation.

One of the most common surgical complications for the management of severe trauma in the diabetic lower extremity is the incidence of nonunion. If osseous healing is delayed, close observation until 6 to 9 months postoperatively is required. Nonunion may need to be addressed if the diabetic lower extremity is unstable, and significant hardware failure is evident prior to 6 months. Diabetic fractures that do not demonstrate osseous union at approximately 6 months postoperatively often require revisional surgery to repair the symptomatic nonunion (Figs. 25.13 and 25.14). Asymptomatic and stable nonunion that can be accommodated in a lower extremity brace and orthosis may be suitable for the diabetic neuropathic patient with poorly controlled diabetes mellitus and multiple medical comorbidities.

Late complications such as limited ankle joint range of motion and posttraumatic arthritis correlate with the severity of the initial injury and accuracy of fracture reduction. Loss of motion can be minimized by early range-of-motion exercises after stable fixation has been achieved. However, in the diabetic neuropathic patient, early range of motion is typically avoided while the lower extremity is protected and immobilized for longer time (6).

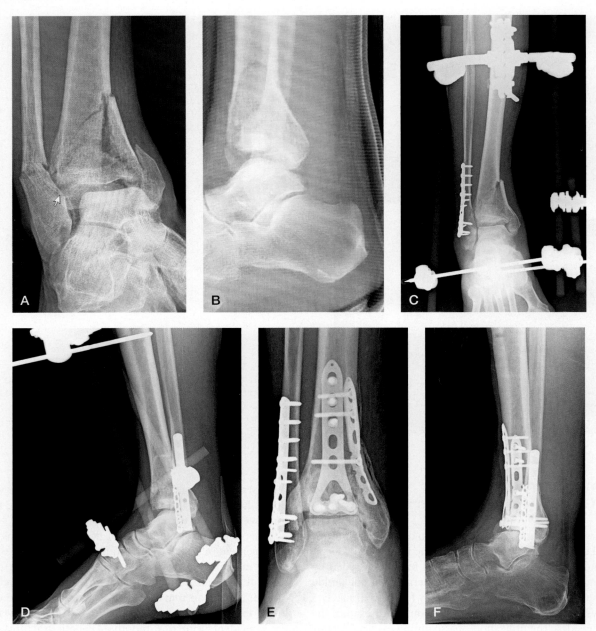

FIGURE 25.12 Preoperative anteroposterior **(A)** and lateral **(B)** left ankle radiographic views of a poorly controlled diabetic patient with multiple comorbidities who sustained a comminuted distal tibia and fibula pilon fracture with ankle varus deformity **(A)**. Patient underwent an initial open reduction and internal fixation (ORIF) of the fibula and closed reduction and stabilization of the tibia pilon fracture with a spanning external fixation device **(C,D)**. Definitive ORIF of the tibia and removal of the spanning external fixator was performed at 14 days after the initial surgery. Following the definitive surgery, the patient sustained a surgical wound dehiscence and postoperative infection that was evident at 12 days after the final procedure. Patient required further surgical débridement with intraoperative cultures for guidance of oral and/or intravenous antibiotic therapy. Repeat surgical débridement and closure of the surgical wound was performed with the application of an incisional negative pressure wound therapy 3 days following the initial surgical débridement. The patient received 6 weeks of culture-specific parenteral antibiotics. Wound healing was evident 3 weeks after the second surgical débridement with no signs of recurrent infection at 16 months postoperatively. Final postoperative anteroposterior **(E)** and lateral **(F)** lower extremity radiographic views showing osseous union, near-anatomic reduction, and posttraumatic arthritis of the ankle at 16 months follow-up.

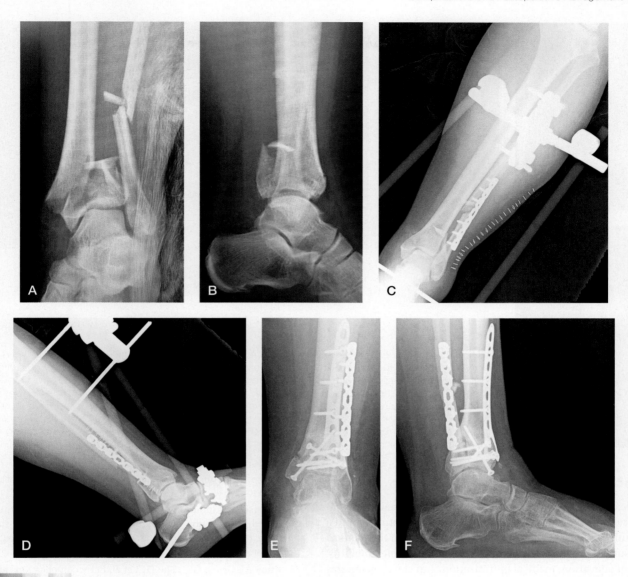

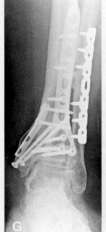
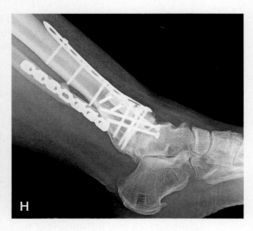

FIGURE 25.13 Preoperative anteroposterior **(A)** and lateral **(B)** right ankle radiographic views of a well-controlled diabetic patient who sustained a severely displaced distal tibia and fibula pilon fracture. Early postoperative anteroposterior **(C)** and lateral **(D)** right lower extremity radiographic views showing the open reduction and internal fixation (ORIF) of the fibula and closed reduction and stabilization of the tibia pilon fracture with a spanning external fixation device. Postoperative anteroposterior **(E)** and lateral **(F)** right lower extremity radiographic views demonstrate an osseous nonunion at the medial malleolus at approximately 6 months after definitive ORIF of the tibia and removal of the spanning external fixator. Patient underwent a revisional reconstructive surgery that consisted of autogenous bone grafting and plating of the medial malleolar fracture fragment. Final postoperative anteroposterior **(G)** and lateral **(H)** lower extremity radiographic views showing osseous union and anatomic reduction at 4 months follow-up after the revisional surgery.

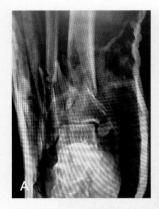
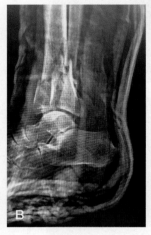
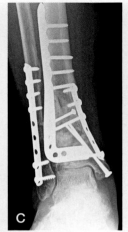
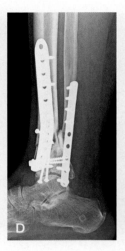
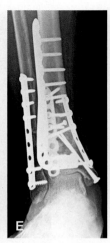
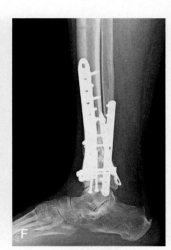

FIGURE 25.14 Preoperative anteroposterior **(A)** and lateral **(B)** left ankle radiographic views of a poorly controlled diabetic patient with peripheral neuropathy who sustained a severely comminuted distal tibia and fibula pilon fracture. Postoperative anteroposterior **(C)** and lateral **(D)** lower extremity radiographic views showing osseous nonunion of the tibia metaphysis at 9 months after definitive fixation of the tibia and fibula. Patient underwent a revisional reconstructive surgery that consisted of a posterolateral approach, autogenous bone grafting, and posterior plating of the distal tibia. Final postoperative anteroposterior **(E)** and lateral **(F)** lower extremity radiographic views showing osseous union and anatomic reduction at 6 months follow-up after the revisional surgery.

Conclusion

Surgical management of diabetic ankle/pilon fractures and dislocations require accurate diagnosis, early treatment, and a multidisciplinary health care team that focuses on the medical and surgical management of patients with diabetes mellitus. Patient education, medical optimization, and close postoperative visits may decrease the overall surgical complication rates in this diabetic population.

References

1. Ayoub MA. Ankle fractures in diabetic neuropathic arthropathy: can tibiotalar arthrodesis salvage the limb? J Bone Joint Surg Br 2008;90:906–914.
2. Basques BA, Miller CP, Golinvaux NS, et al. Morbidity and readmission after open reduction and internal fixation of ankle fractures are associated with preoperative patient characteristics. Clin Orthop Relat Res 2015;473:1133–1139.
3. Cavo MJ, Fox JP, Markert R, et al. Association between diabetes, obesity, and short-term outcomes among patients surgically treated for ankle fracture. J Bone Joint Surg Am 2015;97:987–994.
4. DiDomenico LA, Brown D, Zgonis T. The use of Ilizarov technique as a definitive percutaneous reduction for ankle fractures in patients who have diabetes mellitus and peripheral vascular disease. Clin Podiatr Med Surg 2009;26:141–148.
5. Facaros Z, Ramanujam CL, Stapleton JJ. Combined circular external fixation and open reduction internal fixation with pro-syndesmotic screws for repair of a diabetic ankle fracture. Diabet Foot Ankle 2010;1.
6. Folestad A, Ålund M, Asteberg S, et al. Offloading treatment is linked to activation of proinflammatory cytokines and start of bone repair and remodeling in Charcot arthropathy patients. J Foot Ankle Res 2015;8:72.
7. Kline AJ, Gruen GS, Pape HC, et al. Early complications following the operative treatment of pilon fractures with and without diabetes. Foot Ankle Int 2009;30:1042–1047.
8. Koutsostathis SD, Lepetsos P, Polyzois VD, et al. Combined use of Ilizarov external fixation and Papineau technique for septic pseudoarthrosis of the distal tibia in a patient with diabetes mellitus. Diabet Foot Ankle 2014;5.
9. Liu J, Ludwig T, Ebraheim NA. Effect of the blood HbA1c level on surgical treatment outcomes of diabetics with ankle fractures. Orthop Surg 2013;5:203–208.
10. Rosenbaum AJ, Dellenbaugh SG, Dipreta JA, et al. The management of ankle fractures in diabetics: results of a survey of the American Orthopaedic Foot and Ankle Society membership. Foot Ankle Spec 2013;6:201–205.
11. Stapleton JJ, Zgonis T. Surgical treatment of tibial plafond fractures. Clin Podiatr Med Surg 2014;31:547–564.
12. Thevendran G, Younger A. Arthroscopic reduction and fibula nailing in high-risk diabetic ankle fractures: case reviews and technical tip. Foot Ankle Spec 2012;5:124–127.
13. Wukich DK, Joseph A, Ryan M, et al. Outcomes of ankle fractures in patients with uncomplicated versus complicated diabetes. Foot Ankle Int 2011;32:120–130.

CHAPTER 26

Surgical Management of Postoperative Diabetic Foot and Ankle Complex Wounds

Crystal L. Ramanujam • Thomas Zgonis

INTRODUCTION

As the diabetic population increases worldwide, the amount of diabetic foot and ankle surgeries is also expected to rise. Several studies have shown an increased risk of complications after either elective or nonelective surgeries in diabetic versus nondiabetic patients. From major to minor complications involving wound and/or bone healing, postoperative morbidity in diabetic foot and ankle surgery may impact outcomes significantly, leading to increased lengths of hospital stay, hospital readmissions, revisional surgeries, amputations, and increased mortality rates. Surgeons should approach any diabetic foot and ankle surgery with careful thought to possible postoperative complications, providing patients with reasonable expectations for outcomes and the potential need for further surgery.

This chapter focuses on the surgical management of the most commonly encountered postoperative diabetic foot and ankle complications with emphasis on complex wounds.

LITERATURE REVIEW AND CLINICAL OUTCOMES

Existing studies clearly support the incidence of an increased risk of postoperative complications in diabetic versus nondiabetic patients; however, an in-depth look at the types of complications that occur with particular diabetic foot and ankle surgeries may provide insight on how to better address them.

Elective Foot and Ankle Surgery

Several references cite higher rates of complications in elective foot and ankle surgery compared to many other elective orthopedic procedures (1,17,50,54). Table 26.1 provides a summary of selected studies that include pertinent information on postoperative complications related to diabetes mellitus for elective foot or ankle surgery. Infection represents the most common type of complication for elective foot or ankle

surgery. Surgical site infections (SSIs) are generally divided into mild or severe infections, with the latter requiring hospitalization and/or surgical intervention. A prospective study by Wukich et al. (55) of 2,060 patients who underwent elective foot and/or ankle surgery demonstrated that complicated diabetes mellitus, presence of peripheral neuropathy, and poor long-term glycemic management increased the risk of SSIs. However, this study did not provide information regarding specific types of elective foot or ankle surgery performed. A retrospective study by Domek et al. (21) including 21,854 diabetic patients who underwent elective foot or ankle surgery revealed an overall 3.2% complication rate in which 42.3% were SSIs including both superficial and deep infections. This study mentioned only a few types of elective foot or ankle procedures that were performed including hammertoe correction, bunionectomy, sesamoidectomy, and flatfoot reconstruction, with the authors pointing out that those procedures of lower frequency had greater complication rates (21).

First metatarsophalangeal joint arthrodesis outcomes have been extensively studied in nondiabetic patients, demonstrating a wide range of postoperative complications ranging from wound and bone healing problems to amputation. With the aim of comparing outcomes of diabetic patients with existing outcomes available for nondiabetic patients, Anderson et al. (2) performed a retrospective study on 76 diabetic patients who underwent first metatarsophalangeal joint arthrodesis. They found 5.3% with wound dehiscence and 3.2% with mild SSIs which required only oral antibiotics and local wound care for resolution; additionally, their study had no cases of postoperative osteomyelitis. Nonunion and malunion occurred in 19.7% of their population, with the majority of these diabetic patients having concomitant peripheral neuropathy; only 2 of these subjects required surgical revision.

Surgical management of ankle arthritis in the form of ankle arthrodesis and total ankle arthroplasty has identified diabetic patients at increased risk of postoperative complications. Raikin et al. (42) found a higher risk of minor wound complications in diabetic patients who underwent total ankle

TABLE 26.1	Selected Studies for Complications in Patients with Diabetes Mellitus and Elective Foot and Ankle Surgery	
Authors	**Surgical Procedure(s)**	**Postoperative Complications Related to Diabetes Mellitus**
Anderson et al. (2)	First metatarsophalangeal joint arthrodesis	Superficial infection Wound dehiscence Malposition Malunion Nonunion Hardware failure
Choi et al. (11)	Total ankle replacement	Delayed wound healing Infection requiring débridement Early-onset osteolysis Implant failure
Schipper et al. (47)	Ankle arthrodesis Total ankle arthroplasty	Infection requiring irrigation and débridement Increased length of hospital stay Nonhome discharge
Myers et al. (37)	Hindfoot and/or ankle arthrodesis	Superficial infection Deep infection Delayed union Nonunion Infected nonunion
Mendicino et al. (35)	Tibiotalocalcaneal arthrodesis with intramedullary nail	Wound dehiscence Chronic drainage Ulceration Osteomyelitis Acute Charcot neuroarthropathy Nonunion Hardware failure Wound necrosis
Zarutsky et al. (57)	Ankle arthrodesis with external fixation	Nonunion Below-knee amputation Osteomyelitis and/or deep space infection Malunion
Chahal et al. (9)	Subtalar joint arthrodesis	Malunion Chronic pain

arthroplasty; however, all of the diabetic patients had well-controlled diabetes mellitus and no peripheral neuropathy. Similarly, Choi et al. (11) revealed uncontrolled diabetic patients who underwent total ankle arthroplasty had a higher rate of delayed wound healing as well as early-onset osteolysis and subsequently higher rate of failure compared to nondiabetic patients. Schipper et al. (47) analyzed both ankle arthrodesis (12,122 patients) and total ankle arthroplasty (2,973 patients) outcomes demonstrating overall higher complication rates for both procedures in patients with diabetes mellitus and further showing increased lengths of hospital stay. In the ankle arthrodesis group, diabetes mellitus was also independently associated with increased risk of operative irrigation and débridement.

Arthrodesis can also be utilized in the surgical management of clinical entities in addition to primary osteoarthritis, including, but not limited to, rheumatoid arthritis, gouty arthritis, deformity correction, Charcot neuroarthropathy,

neuromuscular disease, and posttraumatic conditions. A study by Mendicino et al. (35) which compared the outcomes of tibiotalocalcaneal arthrodesis with a retrograde locked intramedullary nail in diabetic patients versus nondiabetic patients also found higher rates of major and minor complications in their diabetic group. Similarly, a retrospective comparative study by Myers et al. (37) including 74 diabetic patients who had underwent hindfoot or ankle arthrodesis found significantly higher rates of both infectious and noninfectious complications in the diabetic group when compared to the matched nondiabetic group. Likewise, Zarutsky et al. (57) found higher rates of major complication in diabetic patients treated with external fixation; however, it should be noted that the indications for these surgeries varied widely. Chahal et al. (9) retrospectively reviewed 88 patients who underwent subtalar joint arthrodesis for primary or secondary osteoarthritis, revealing the poorest outcomes in diabetic patients with the most common complication being malunion.

Although there is limited information focusing on postoperative complications for tendon surgery in diabetic patients, most of the existing literature generally indicates increased risk of tendon rupture and wound healing complications in the diabetic population (3). This presumption has been based on animal studies which have shown that tendon damage and subsequent healing problems are linked to the production of excessive advanced glycation end products leading to collagen changes within diabetic tendons (12,23,36). However, a recent study by Rensing et al. (45) on 1,626 patients who had undergone primary repair of Achilles tendon ruptures, of which 4.9% of the patients had diabetes mellitus, showed an overall 1.7% local complication rate, none of which were related directly to the presence of diabetes mellitus.

Partial Foot Amputations

A variety of partial foot amputations have been described to treat diabetic foot ulcerations, soft tissue infection, osteomyelitis, and/or gangrene. The most common postoperative complications for these procedures include, but are not limited to, wound dehiscence, soft tissue infection, necrosis, osteomyelitis, reulceration, proximal amputation, and hospital readmission (Fig. 26.1). The majority of information on outcomes in diabetic patients has come from studies on transmetatarsal amputation (TMA) (Fig. 26.2). Pollard et al. (41) found no statistically significant difference in healing rates for TMA in diabetic patients versus nondiabetic patients, whereas a study by Younger et al. (56) on 68 diabetic patients who underwent TMA demonstrated blood glucose control as measured by glycosylated hemoglobin (HbA$_{1c}$) was the most important factor predicting success, specifically showing higher HbA$_{1c}$ level in patients with failed TMA subsequently requiring transtibial amputation. In a study by Beaulieu et al. (6) of 717 patients who underwent minor foot amputations, chronic renal insufficiency, and peripheral arterial disease were associated with hospital readmission for 100 patients; furthermore, proximal amputation including below-knee, through-knee, and above-knee occurred in 64 of those readmitted. Regarding primary toe amputations in 92 hospitalized diabetic patients with forefoot sepsis, Nehler et al. (38) found high rates of complications including nonhealing, persistent infection, revisional surgeries, and hospital readmission. A recent systematic review and meta-analysis by Thorud et al. (52) showing high complication rates, particularly reoperation and reamputation rates after TMA, emphasized that the decision between TMA and other minor foot amputations such as toe or partial ray (toe and metatarsal) amputations should be highly patient-specific.

Foot and Ankle Trauma

It is well-established in the literature that diabetic patients undergoing surgical intervention for treatment of foot and/or ankle fractures are at higher risk for postoperative complications. The most data in support of this has resulted from studies on the operative management of ankle fractures in

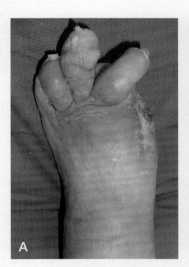
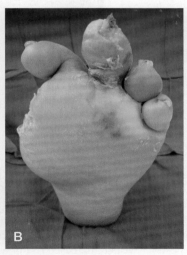
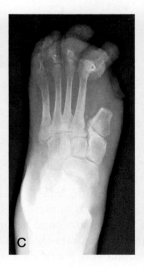
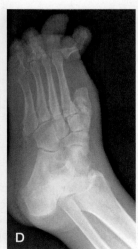
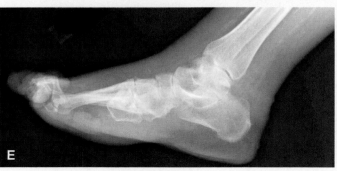

FIGURE 26.1 Preoperative clinical **(A,B)** and radiographic **(C–E)** views showing a previously healed left foot partial first ray (hallux and first metatarsal) amputation with a severe diabetic infection, osteomyelitis of the third toe, and subluxation of multiple toes. *(continued)*

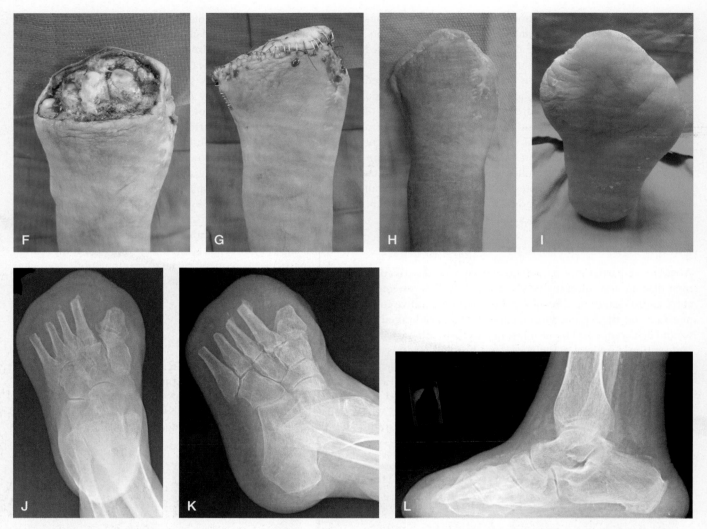

FIGURE 26.1 *(Continued)* Patient underwent an initial open amputation of second, third, fourth, and fifth toes at the metatarsopha-langeal joint articulations with excisional débridement of all nonviable tissues **(F)** being followed by a revisional modified transmeta-tarsal amputation and closure 2 days after the initial surgery **(G)**. Final postoperative clinical **(H,I)** and radiographic **(J–L)** outcomes at approximately 7 months follow-up.

diabetic patients, ranging from small case series to larger retrospective comparative studies (7,13,15,26,28,31,34,51,53). Collectively, postoperative complications in these studies included, but were not limited to, delayed wound healing, infection, delayed union, nonunion, hardware failure, Charcot neuroarthropathy, amputation, and need for revision surgery. More recently, a study by Basques et al. (4) using a registry of 4,412 patients found that insulin-dependent diabetes mellitus was associated with an increased rate of adverse events after ankle fracture open reduction and internal fixation (ORIF) including wound complications, infection, and hospital readmission. Using a large database of over 6,000 patients who underwent ORIF for ankle fractures, Dodd et al. (20) demonstrated that bimalleolar ankle fractures were about 5 times more likely to develop any complication; furthermore, their study found that diabetes mellitus was a predictive factor for postoperative complications.

Similar findings have been reported for calcaneal fractures in diabetic patients. Most reports indicate operative fixation of calcaneal fractures in this population suffer from soft tissue rather than osseous complications. A study by Folk et al. (27) of 179 patients who underwent ORIF of calcaneal fractures revealed increased risk of wound complications in those patients with diabetes mellitus; additionally, smoking history and open fractures cumulatively increased risk of wound dehiscence and infection. Ding et al. (18) also found that diabetes mellitus, Sanders type classification of the fracture, and smoking were the strongest risk factors for postoperative wound complications in a study of 479 patients treated via ORIF using the extensile lateral approach with plate fixation. Recently, a systematic review and meta-analysis of pertinent studies by Zhang et al. (58) identified diabetes mellitus and fracture severity as significant risk factors for postoperative wound complications, whereas smoking made no significant difference.

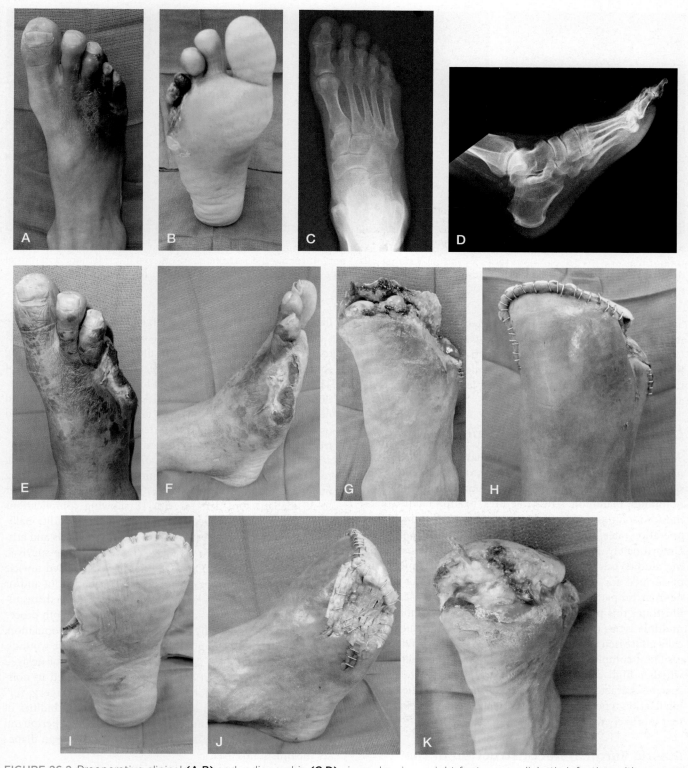

FIGURE 26.2 Preoperative clinical **(A,B)** and radiographic **(C,D)** views showing a right foot severe diabetic infection with gangrenous changes of the fourth and fifth toes as well as soft tissue emphysema at the fifth metatarsophalangeal joint. Patient underwent an initial open partial fourth and fifth ray (toe and metatarsal) amputation with excisional débridement of all nonviable tissues being followed by a selective catheterization of the peroneal artery and anterior tibial artery, percutaneous atherectomy and angioplasty of the posterior tibial artery, and angioplasty of the medial plantar artery approximately 7 weeks after the initial surgery. The patient was followed closely in an outpatient and wound care specialty clinics for local wound care dressings. At approximately 5½ months since the initial foot surgery **(E,F)**, the patient underwent an open modified transmetatarsal amputation (TMA) **(G)** followed by a revisional TMA and application of a dermoconductive acellular dermal replacement **(H–J)** 2 days after the open modified TMA. Five weeks later, the patient developed a severe wound dehiscence **(K)** and returned to the operating room for further excisional débridement, revisional TMA, and application of negative pressure wound therapy **(L,M)**. *(continued)*

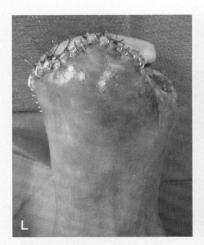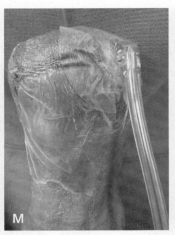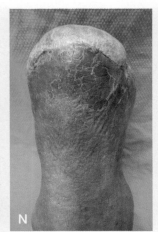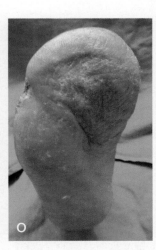

FIGURE 26.2 *(Continued)* Ten weeks later, the patient underwent a revisional percutaneous angioplasty of the posterior tibial, anterior tibial, and medial plantar arteries by vascular surgery. The patient required an additional excisional débridement and partial resection of the first metatarsal stump at approximately 5 weeks after the revisional vascular procedure. **N,O.** Final clinical outcomes at 13 months follow-up after the initial foot surgery.

Similar findings have been extrapolated to other traumatic injuries than the foot and ankle. For example, Basques et al. (5) studied outcomes of 519 patients who underwent ORIF of tibial plateau fractures and found that the presence of diabetes mellitus was associated with extended length of hospital stay and hospital readmission.

Charcot Foot and Ankle Neuroarthropathy

Several postoperative complications have been documented in the treatment of Charcot neuroarthropathy including, but not limited to, delayed wound and/or bone healing, infection, nonunion, malunion, stress fractures, fixation failure, metal-induced soft tissue irritation, pin/wire tract infection, high reoperation rates, and amputation (14,16,24,25,29,39,40,44,49). Unfortunately, it is difficult to analyze and compare existing studies due to the large variety of surgical procedures performed for different clinical manifestations of Charcot neuroarthropathy of the diabetic foot and ankle. Table 26.2 illustrates this point with a sample of studies demonstrating multiple types of diabetic Charcot neuroarthropathy surgically addressed with several different kind of procedures and resultant complications. Although it is yet to be determined whether high complication rates are attributed to patient-specific characteristics or selected surgical techniques including fixation types, most of the evidence available demonstrate that it is likely multifactorial.

Plastic Surgical Reconstruction of the Foot and Ankle

Reconstruction utilizing plastic surgical techniques has become a viable option for complex diabetic foot and ankle wounds that are not amenable to traditional wound closure. Many of these procedures have noted postoperative complications in diabetic patients including, but not limited to, hematoma, seroma, delayed wound healing, infection, and flap necrosis. Yet due to lack of larger cohort and comparative studies, the degree to which diabetes mellitus contributes to such complications is largely unknown. In a study using square random fasciocutaneous plantar flaps for treatment of 21 patients with diabetic plantar foot ulcerations, complications included transfer ulceration, delayed wound healing, and need for revision surgery (8). Sato and Ichioka (46) performed ostectomy and medial plantar artery flap reconstruction for treatment of diabetic Charcot neuroarthropathy foot ulceration in 4 patients, with complication in 1 patient involving recurrent ulceration and concomitant infection requiring major amputation. Lee et al. (33) utilized free flap transfer in 33 diabetic foot defects, with 18 showing complications including partial flap necrosis and flap failure; additionally, these authors found elevated serum creatinine levels and atherosclerotic calcifications as risk factors for free flap survival. Ducic and Attinger (22) analyzed the use of pedicled muscle flaps versus free flaps in 38 patients with diabetic foot and/or ankle defects, noting delayed healing time and need for additional débridements as complications; however, both procedures were found equally effective in their study population. For split-thickness skin grafting of foot and/or ankle wounds, Ramanujam et al. (43) demonstrated higher risk of delayed healing and infection in diabetic patients compared to nondiabetic patients, therefore requiring revisional surgery; furthermore, this higher risk was attributed to comorbidities of diabetes mellitus including cardiovascular disease, peripheral neuropathy, retinopathy, and nephropathy rather than diabetes mellitus status itself.

PREOPERATIVE CONSIDERATIONS

Preoperative medical optimization in patients undergoing surgical management of diabetic foot and ankle complications is critical for successful outcomes. Thorough preoperative medical history with review of all prior surgical

TABLE 26.2	Selected Studies for Complications in Operative Treatment of Diabetic Charcot Foot and Ankle Neuroarthropathy		
Author(s)	Pathology Addressed	Surgical Procedure(s)	Postoperative Complications
Eschler et al. (24)	Unstable Charcot neuroarthropathy deformity midfoot and/or hindfoot, ulceration, osteomyelitis	Débridement, corrective osteotomy, and arthrodesis using internal fixation, autologous bone graft, equinus correction	Wound infection Reulceration Osteomyelitis Hardware breakage Hardware loosening Nonunion Amputation (below-knee, Chopart, toe)
Siebachmeyer et al. (49)	Unstable Charcot neuroarthropathy deformity of hindfoot and/or ankle, ulceration	All with intramedullary hindfoot fusion nail, some with midfoot fusion bolt, equinus correction, autologous and/or allogenic bone graft	Ulceration Nonunion Hardware loosening Amputation (below-knee, Chopart)
Grant et al. (29)	Unstable Charcot neuroarthropathy deformity of midfoot, hindfoot, and/or ankle	Internal (intramedullary screws) and circular external fixation, some bone graft, some implantable bone stimulation, equinus correction	Pin tract infection Wound dehiscence Osteomyelitis Nonunion Hardware failure Amputation (below-knee)
Dalla Paola et al. (16)	Unstable Charcot neuroarthropathy deformity of ankle with osteomyelitis, ulceration	Débridement, talectomy, antibiotic-impregnated cement beads, external fixation, internal fixation, bone graft	Delayed wound healing Amputation (below-knee) Revision surgery
Pinzur (39)	Unstable Charcot neuroarthropathy deformity of midfoot, some osteomyelitis and ulceration	Débridement, circular external fixation	Reulceration Amputation (below-knee) Stress fractures Revision surgery

procedures performed at the affected site with standard laboratory workup should be undertaken. Diabetic patients with renal insufficiency, cardiovascular disease, and history of organ transplant have all shown to have increased risk for surgical complications (10,59). Furthermore, the following preoperative laboratory values have been associated with higher risk of complications and therefore should be addressed if possible: elevated HbA$_{1c}$ showing poor long-term glycemic control, low hemoglobin/hematocrit representing anemia, and decreased albumin indicating poor nutritional status (19,21,45,48). Diagnostic imaging pertinent to the affected lower extremity of complication should be reviewed carefully for preoperative plans to address any soft tissue and/or osseous pathology. If deficiencies in vascular status are clinically suspected, noninvasive arterial studies to the lower extremities with subsequent vascular surgery consultation for further imaging and/or surgical intervention as indicated should be undertaken (30,32). If the foot and/or ankle has current soft tissue and/or bone infection, appropriate antibiotics should be initiated with attention to prior intraoperative culture results and infectious disease consultation as needed. Full assessment of the index surgical procedure and determining what may have led to the postoperative complication(s) is vital for preoperative planning.

DETAILED SURGICAL TECHNIQUES WITH CLINICAL CASES

Operative management of full-thickness surgical wound dehiscence entails débridement of the wound base and margins to healthy, viable soft tissue and/or bone when necessary. Hydrosurgical devices may be utilized in these cases for more precise and deliberate soft tissue excisional débridement. If encountering postoperative abscess formation, aggressive débridement with intraoperative soft tissue and/or bone cultures to determine further antibiotic therapy is required, with staging of surgical wound closure if indicated. Larger soft tissue defects may require negative pressure wound therapy to assist with granulation tissue coverage over bone, joint, or tendon (Fig. 26.3). Likewise, exposed but stable internal fixation hardware may also benefit from a period of negative pressure wound therapy for secondary wound healing or to prepare for later definitive wound closure. Loosened and/or unstable internal fixation hardware should be removed if at the site of osteomyelitis. Large osseous and/or soft tissue defects left after aggressive débridement of osteomyelitis can be addressed with antibiotic-impregnated polymethylmethacrylate cemented beads and/or spacers (Fig. 26.4).

In open wounds that are not amenable to primary closure and once adequate wound bed preparation has been performed,

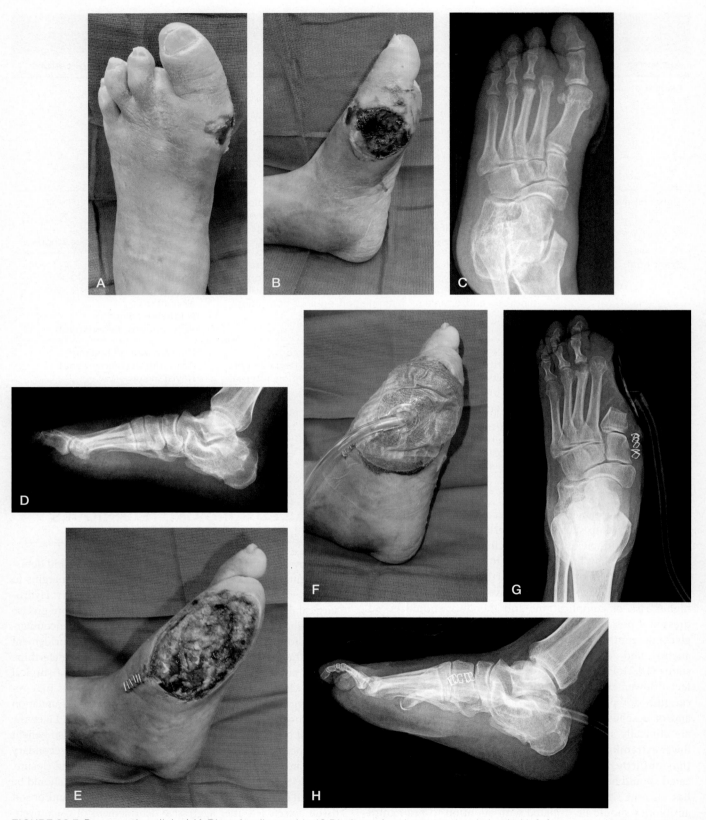

FIGURE 26.3 Preoperative clinical **(A,B)** and radiographic **(C,D)** views showing a previously healed left foot second toe amputation with a severe diabetic infection and soft tissue emphysema at the first metatarsophalangeal joint. Patient underwent an initial open partial first ray (hallux and metatarsal) amputation with excisional débridement of all nonviable tissues **(E)** being followed by a revisional partial first ray amputation and negative pressure wound therapy (NPWT) 2 days after the initial surgery **(F–H)**. *(continued)*

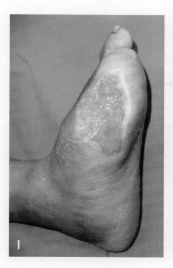
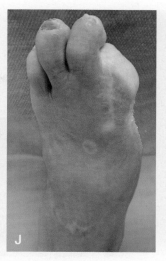
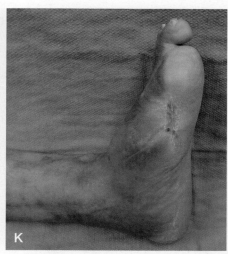

FIGURE 26.3 *(Continued)* The patient was followed closely in an outpatient and wound care specialty clinics for NPWT and local wound care dressings. Postoperative clinical outcomes at 7 weeks **(I)** and 18 weeks follow-up **(J,K)**.

dermal allografts (Figs. 26.5 and 26.6), and/or split-thickness skin grafts may be considered (Figs. 26.7 to 26.9). For more complex wound closure, options such as local flaps, pedicle flaps, or perforator flaps are also available. In cases of nonunion that have not responded to extended conservative measures such as immobilization, bracing, and/or bone stimulation, appropriate surgical excision with autogenous and/or allogenic bone grafting may be a viable option. Complications of malunion may also be addressed with corrective osteotomy and/or arthrodesis. Choice between internal or external fixation should be carefully considered in order to circumvent prior failure of fixation. Surgical off-loading with circular external fixation can also be utilized as an adjunct therapy to stabilize both soft tissue and/or osseous reconstructive procedures (Fig. 26.10).

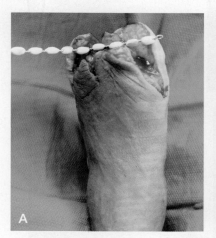
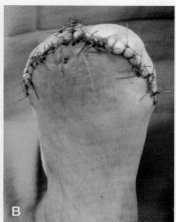
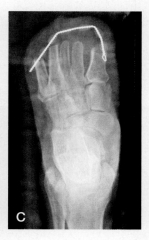

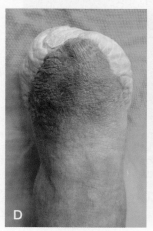
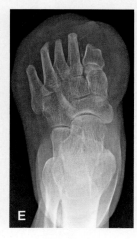

FIGURE 26.4 Intraoperative **(A,B)** and postoperative radiographic **(C)** views showing a diabetic modified left foot transmetatarsal amputation (TMA) with the insertion of antibiotic-impregnated polymethylmethacrylate (PMMA) cemented beads at the surgical site. Patient underwent removal of the retained antibiotic-impregnated PMMA cemented beads and excisional débridement 9 weeks after the modified TMA. Patient required 2 additional surgical débridements at the first metatarsal stump and subsequent wound closure. Postoperative outcomes at approximately 19 months **(D)** and 23 months follow-up **(E)**.

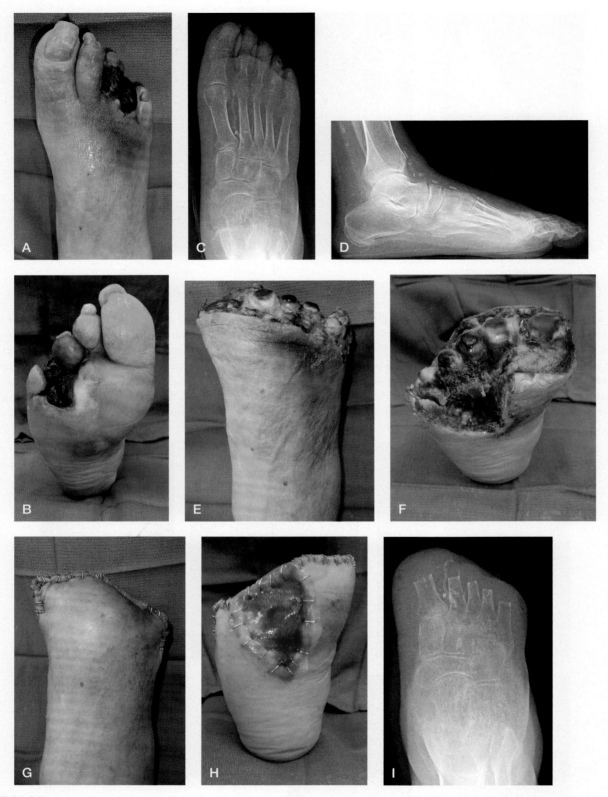

FIGURE 26.5 Preoperative clinical **(A,B)** and radiographic **(C,D)** views showing a right foot diabetic infection with gangrenous changes of the third and fourth toes as well as acute osteomyelitis of the fourth toe. Patient had a history of a percutaneous transluminal angioplasty of the anterior tibial and dorsalis pedis arteries approximately 1 month prior to forefoot amputation. Patient underwent an initial open amputation of the first, second, third, fourth, and fifth toes at the metatarsophalangeal joint articulations with excisional débridement of all nonviable tissues **(E,F)** being followed by a revisional modified transmetatarsal amputation 5 days after the initial surgery **(G,H)**. At the second staged procedure, a dermoconductive acellular dermal replacement was applied at the surgical site **(H)**. *(continued)*

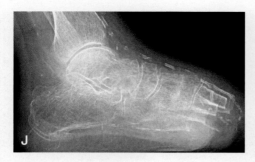

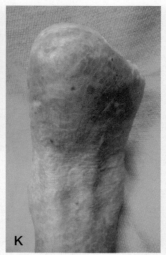

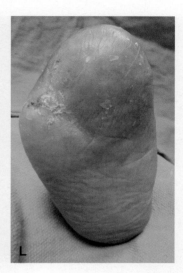

FIGURE 26.5 *(Continued)* During the post-operative course, the patient was followed closely in an outpatient and wound care specialty clinics for hyperbaric oxygen therapy and local wound care treatments. Post-operative outcomes at 3 months **(I,J)** and 11½ months follow-up **(K,L)**.

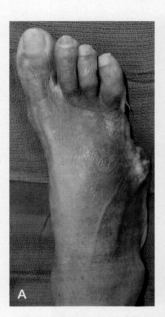

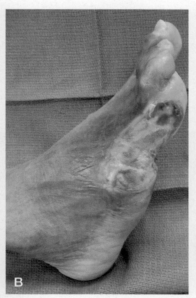

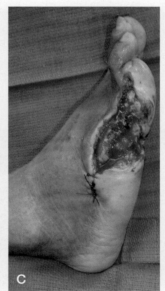

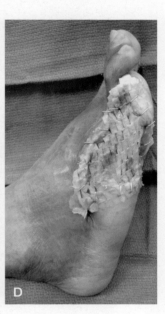

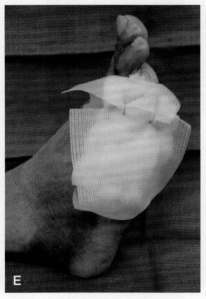

FIGURE 26.6 Preoperative clinical **(A,B)** views of a diabetic revisional right foot open partial fifth ray (toe and metatarsal) amputation with negative pressure wound therapy and chronic nonhealing fibrotic wound with residual osteomyelitis of the fifth metatarsal stump and fourth metatarsophalangeal joint. Vascular surgery consultation consisted of multiple simultaneous selective catheterization and angioplasty interventions prior to further right foot surgery. Five days after the vascular surgery procedures, patient underwent a revisional partial fifth ray amputation combined with a partial fourth ray amputation followed by an excisional débridement of all nonviable tissues, revisional partial fourth ray amputation, and application of a dermoconductive acellular dermal replacement 2 days after the revisional foot surgery **(C,D)**. Note the bolster dressing composed of a non-adherent material and sterile sponges soaked in saline applied over the dermoconductive acellular dermal replacement and secured to the recipient site with surgical staples **(E)**. *(continued)*

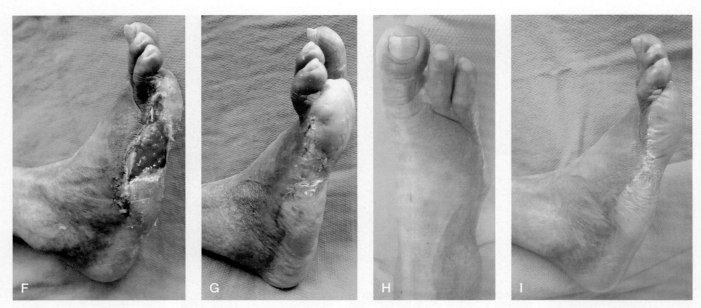

FIGURE 26.6 *(Continued)* During the postoperative course, the patient was followed closely in the outpatient clinical setting for local wound care. Postoperative clinical outcomes at 7 weeks **(F)**, 15 weeks **(G)**, and approximately 30 weeks **(H,I)** following the dermoconductive acellular dermal replacement application.

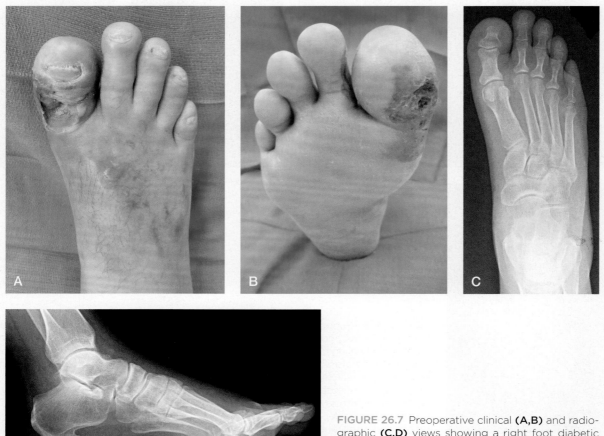

FIGURE 26.7 Preoperative clinical **(A,B)** and radiographic **(C,D)** views showing a right foot diabetic infection with extensive cellulitis after a puncture wound at the hallux (great toe) area. *(continued)*

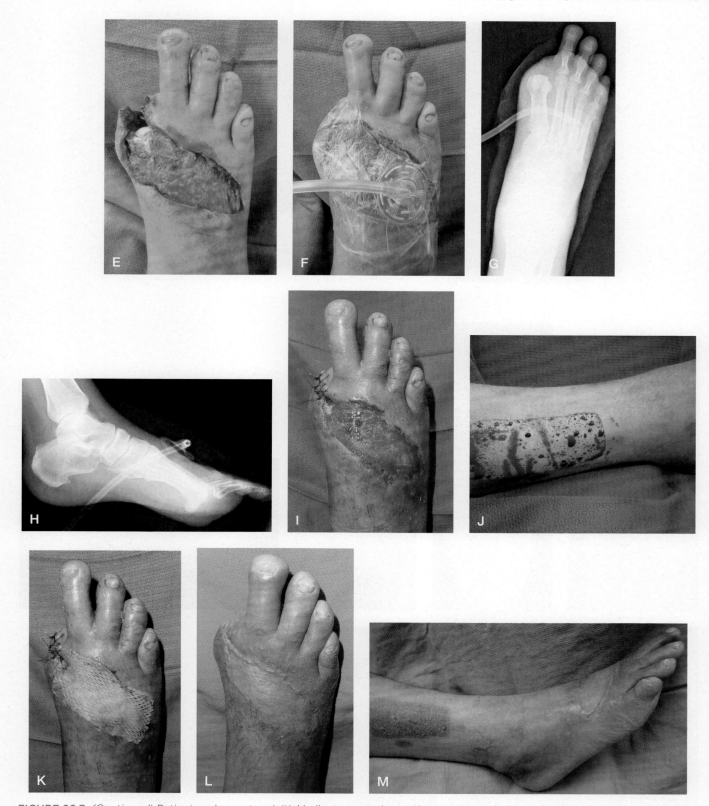

FIGURE 26.7 *(Continued)* Patient underwent an initial hallux amputation at the metatarsophalangeal joint with excisional débridement of all nonviable tissues being followed by a revisional surgical débridement 2 days after the initial surgery **(E)**. At the second staged procedure, an intraoperative negative pressure wound therapy (NPWT) device was applied to the surgical wound bed **(F–H)**. The patient was followed closely in an outpatient and wound care specialty clinics for NPWT and local wound care dressings. Five weeks later, the patient underwent hydrosurgical excisional débridement and wound bed preparation **(I)** with autogenous split-thickness skin graft (STSG) from the ipsilateral lower extremity **(J)** to the foot **(K)**. *(continued)*

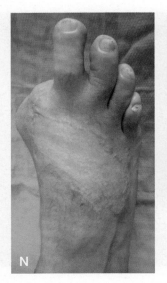

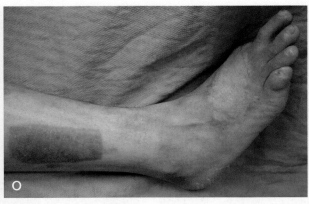

FIGURE 26.7 *(Continued)* Postoperative clinical outcomes at 2 months **(L,M)** and 7½ months **(N,O)** following the autogenous STSG application.

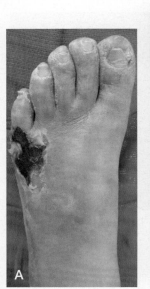

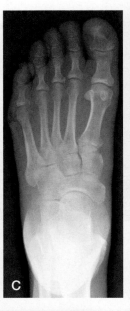

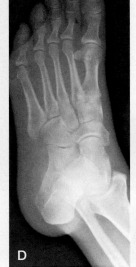

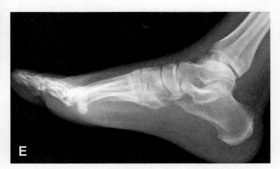

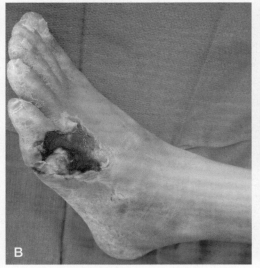

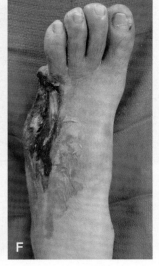

FIGURE 26.8 Preoperative clinical **(A,B)** and radiographic **(C-E)** views showing a left foot severe diabetic infection with gangrenous changes of the fifth toe as well as acute osteomyelitis of the fifth metatarsal head and associated soft tissue emphysema. *(continued)*

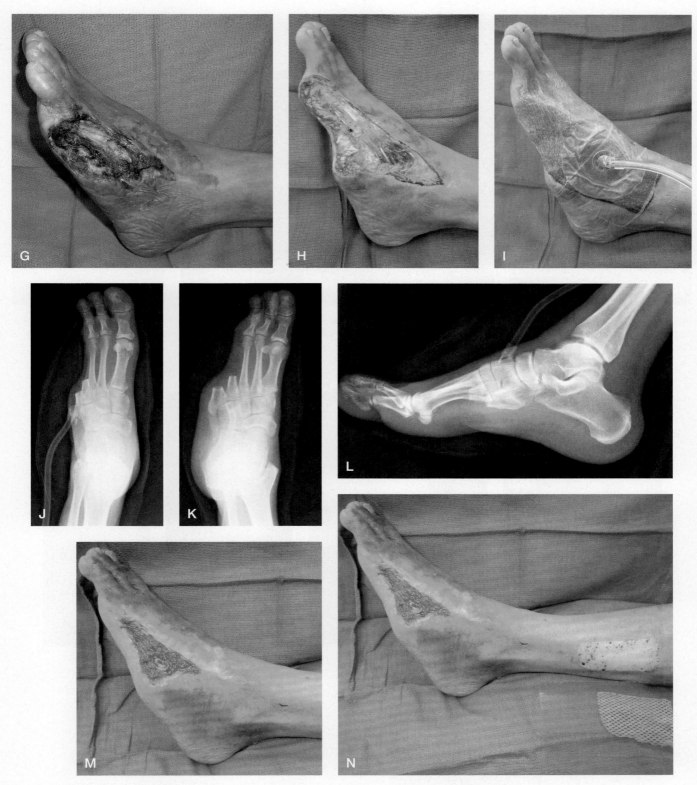

FIGURE 26.8 *(Continued)* Patient underwent an initial open partial fifth ray amputation (toe and metatarsal) with excisional débridement of all nonviable tissues followed by angioplasty and stent placement of the superficial femoral and popliteal arteries 4 days after the initial foot surgery. Five days after the initial foot surgery **(F,G)**, the patient underwent a revisional partial fifth ray amputation, partial fourth ray amputation, excisional débridement of all nonviable tissues, and application of an intraoperative negative pressure wound therapy (NPWT) device **(H–L)**. The patient was followed closely in an outpatient and wound care specialty clinics for NPWT and local wound care dressings. At approximately 3 months after the second surgical foot procedure, the patient underwent hydrosurgical excisional débridement and wound bed preparation **(M)** with autogenous split-thickness skin graft (STSG) from the ipsilateral lower extremity **(N)** to the foot **(O)**. *(continued)*

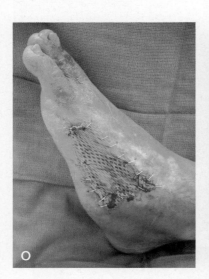
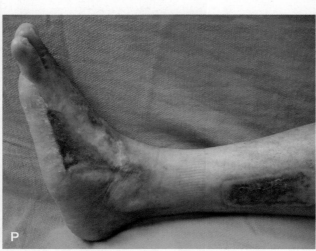
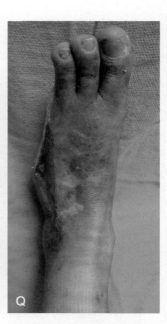

FIGURE 26.8 *(Continued)* Postoperative clinical outcomes at 13 weeks **(P,Q)** following the autogenous STSG application. In addition, the patient also underwent a revisional superficial femoral artery percutaneous transluminal angioplasty for an in-stent restenosis at 11 months after the initial vascular surgery intervention.

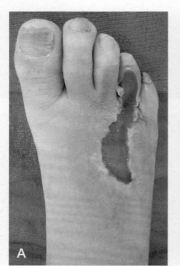
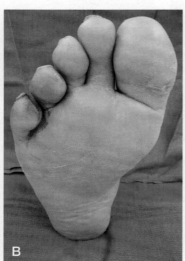
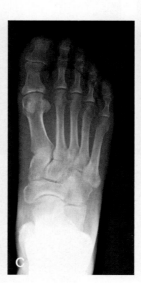
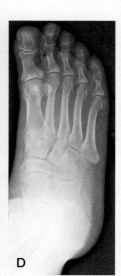

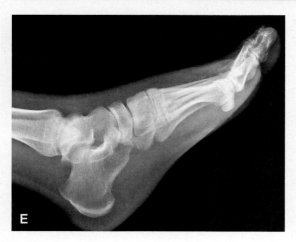

FIGURE 26.9 Preoperative clinical **(A,B)** and radiographic **(C–E)** views showing a right foot severe diabetic infection with gangrenous changes of the fourth toe, soft tissue emphysema and purulence of the fourth interspace, and extensive cellulitis. Patient underwent an initial open partial fourth and fifth ray (toe and metatarsal) amputation with excisional débridement of all nonviable tissues being followed by a revisional surgical excisional débridement and partial fourth and fifth ray amputation 2 days after the initial surgery **(F)**. *(continued)*

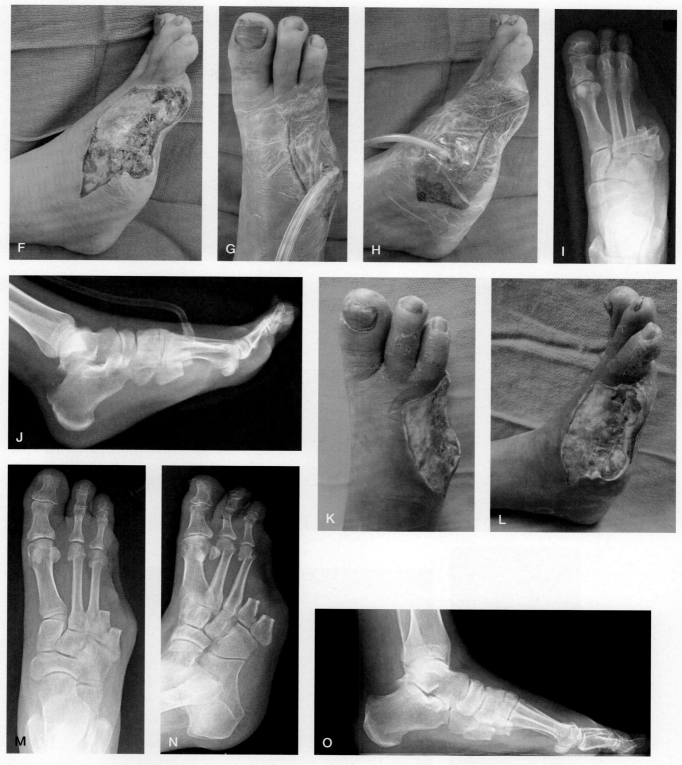

FIGURE 26.9 *(Continued)* At the second staged surgical procedure, an intraoperative negative pressure wound therapy (NPWT) device was applied to the surgical wound bed **(G–J)**. At 3½ weeks follow-up **(K,L)**, the patient had sustained asymptomatic second and third metatarsal fractures **(M–O)**. *(continued)*

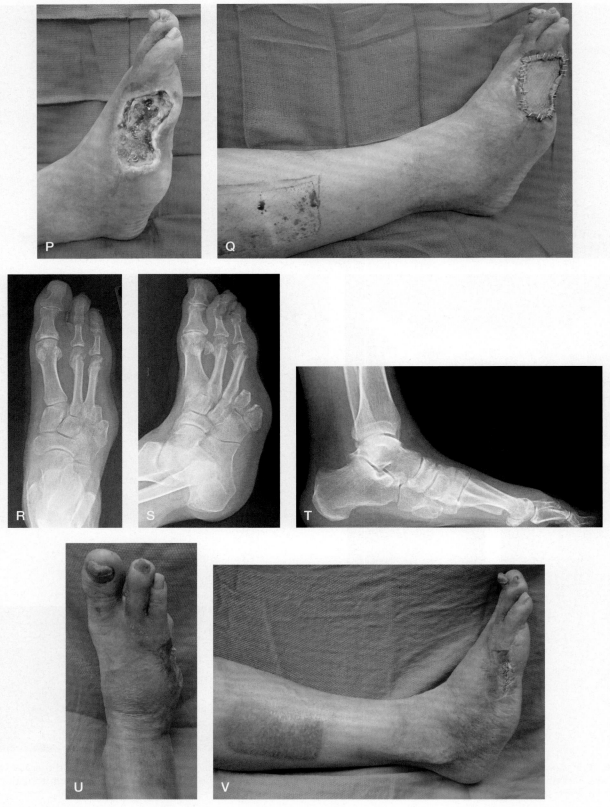

FIGURE 26.9 *(Continued)* Three months after the revisional partial foot amputation, the patient underwent hydrosurgical excisional débridement and wound bed preparation **(P)** with autogenous split-thickness skin graft (STSG) from the ipsilateral lower extremity **(Q)** to the foot. Postoperative outcomes at 16 weeks **(R–T)** and 14 months **(U,V)** following the autogenous STSG application.

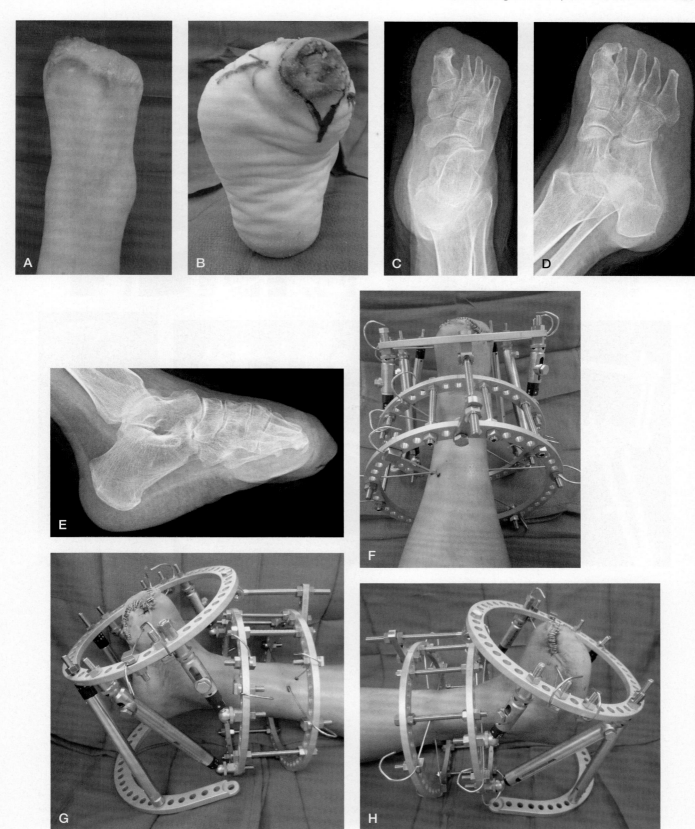

FIGURE 26.10 Preoperative clinical **(A,B)** and radiographic **(C–E)** views showing a diabetic right foot transmetatarsal amputation (TMA) with a chronic nonhealing wound and acquired equinus deformity. Patient underwent a surgical excisional débridement of all nonviable tissues, revisional TMA, local advancement rotational flap closure, and a gastrocnemius recession of the lower extremity. In addition, a circular external fixation device was utilized for a simultaneous equinus deformity correction and alignment, soft tissue and osseous stabilization of the foot to the lower extremity, and surgical off-loading **(F–L)**. *(continued)*

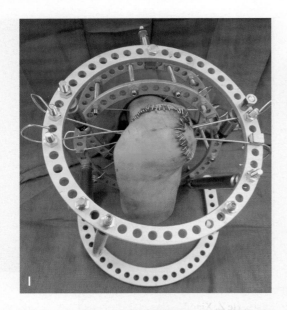

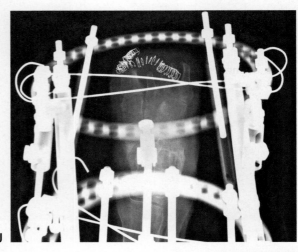

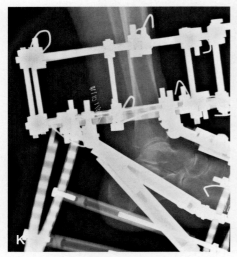

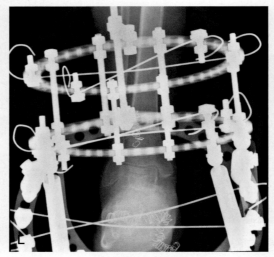

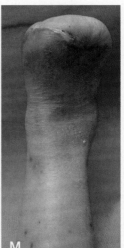

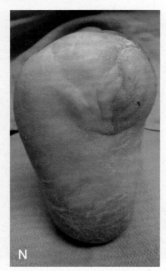

FIGURE 26.10 *(Continued)* The circular external fixation device was removed at 7 weeks postoperatively. Postoperative clinical outcomes at 14 weeks follow-up since the flap closure, equinus correction, and circular external fixation application **(M,N)**.

POSTOPERATIVE CARE

Depending on the patient's medical status and surgical procedure(s) performed to address diabetic foot or ankle complications, postoperative care may include hospitalization and/or further placement in a rehabilitation facility. Continuous medical optimization and long-term intravenous antibiotics may be required in cases of complicated osteomyelitis. Physical and occupational therapy for assistance in compliance with non–weight-bearing status and overall conditioning is also recommended for these patients. Overall, this particular patient population requires close monitoring and regular clinical follow-up with continued patient education to avoid further complications.

Conclusion

Surgeons treating patients with diabetic foot and ankle conditions are destined to encounter postoperative complications at some point. This chapter emphasizes the most commonly reported postoperative diabetic foot and ankle complex wounds with several surgical options available to address them. In carefully selected diabetic patients, skilled surgeons may use this knowledge coupled with ingenuity to help produce better outcomes.

References

1. Al-Mayahi M, Cian A, Kressmann B, et al. Associations of diabetes mellitus with orthopaedic infections. Infect Dis (Lond) 2016;48:70–73.

2. Anderson JJ, Hansen M, Rowe GP, et al. Complication rates in diabetics with first metatarsophalangeal joint arthrodesis. Diabet Foot Ankle 2014;5.

3. Barp EA, Erickson JG. Complications of tendon surgery in the foot and ankle. Clin Podiatr Med Surg 2016;33:163–175.

4. Basques BA, Miller CP, Golinvaux NS, et al. Morbidity and readmission after open reduction and internal fixation of ankle fractures are associated with preoperative patient characteristics. Clin Orthop Relat Res 2015;473:1133–1139.

5. Basques BA, Webb ML, Bohl DD, et al. Adverse events, length of stay, and readmission after surgery for tibial plateau fractures. J Orthop Trauma 2015;29:121–126.

6. Beaulieu RJ, Grimm JC, Lyu H, et al. Rates and predictors of readmission after minor lower extremity amputations. J Vasc Surg 2015;62:101–105.

7. Blotter RH, Connolly E, Wasan A, et al. Acute complications in the operative treatment of isolated ankle fractures in patients with diabetes mellitus. Foot Ankle Int 1999;20:687–694.

8. Caravaggi CM, Sganzaroli AB, Bona F, et al. Square, random fasciocutaneous plantar flaps for treating noninfected diabetic plantar ulcers: a patient series. J Foot Ankle Surg 2016;55:1100–1105.

9. Chahal J, Stephen DJ, Bulmer B, et al. Factors associated with outcome after subtalar arthrodesis. J Orthop Trauma 2006;20:555–561.

10. Choi MS, Jeon SB, Lee JH. Predictive factors for successful limb salvage surgery in diabetic foot patients. BMC Surg 2014;14:113.

11. Choi WJ, Lee JS, Lee M, et al. The impact of diabetes on the short- to mid-term outcome of total ankle replacement. Bone Joint J 2014;96:1674–1680.

12. Connizzo BK, Bhatt PR, Liechty KW, et al. Diabetes alters mechanical properties and collagen fiber re-alignment in multiple mouse tendons. Ann Biomed Eng 2014;42:1880–1888.

13. Connolly JF, Csencsitz TA. Limb threatening neuropathic complications from ankle fractures in patients with diabetes. Clin Orthop Relat Res 1998;348:212–219.

14. Cooper PS. Application of external fixators for management of Charcot deformities of the foot and ankle. Foot Ankle Clin 2002;7:207–254.

15. Costigan W, Thordarson DB, Debnath UK. Operative management of ankle fractures in patients with diabetes mellitus. Foot Ankle Int 2007;28:32–37.

16. Dalla Paola L, Brocco E, Ceccacci T, et al. Limb salvage in Charcot foot and ankle osteomyelitis: combined use single stage/double stage of arthrodesis and external fixation. Foot Ankle Int 2009;30:1065–1070.

17. DeVries JG, Berlet GC, Hyer CF. Predictive risk assessment for major amputation after tibiotalocalcaneal arthrodesis. Foot Ankle Int 2013;34:846–850.

18. Ding L, He Z, Xiao H, et al. Risk factors for postoperative wound complications of calcaneal fractures following plate fixation. Foot Ankle Int 2013;34:1238–1244.

19. Dix B, Grant-McDonald L, Catanzariti A, et al. Preoperative anemia in hindfoot and ankle arthrodesis. Foot Ankle Spec 2017;10:109–115.

20. Dodd AC, Lakomkin N, Attum B, et al. Predictors of adverse events for ankle fractures: an analysis of 6800 patients. J Foot Ankle Surg 2016;55:762–776.

21. Domek N, Dux K, Pinzur M, et al. Association between hemoglobin A1c and surgical morbidity in elective foot and ankle surgery. J Foot Ankle Surg 2016;55:939–943.

22. Ducic I, Attinger CE. Foot and ankle reconstruction: pedicled muscle flaps versus free flaps and the role of diabetes. Plast Reconstr Surg 2011;128:173–180.

23. Egemen O, Ozkaya O, Ozturk MB, et al. The biomechanical and histological effects of diabetes on tendon healing: experimental study in rats. J Hand Microsurg 2012;4:60–64.

24. Eschler A, Gradl G, Wussow A, et al. Prediction of complications in a high-risk cohort of patients undergoing corrective arthrodesis of late stage Charcot deformity based on the PEDIS score. BMC Musculoskelet Disord 2015;16:349.

25. Farber DC, Juliano PJ, Cavanagh PR, et al. Single stage correction with external fixation of the ulcerated foot in individuals with Charcot neuroarthropathy. Foot Ankle Int 2002;23:130–134.

26. Flynn JM, Rodriguez-del Rio F, Pizá PA. Closed ankle fractures in the diabetic patient. Foot Ankle Int 2000;21:311–319.

27. Folk JW, Starr AJ, Early JS. Early wound complications of operative treatment of calcaneus fractures: analysis of 190 fractures. J Orthop Trauma 1999;13:369–372.

28. Ganesh SP, Pietrobon R, Cecilio WA, et al. The impact of diabetes on patient outcomes after ankle fracture. J Bone Joint Surg Am 2005;87:1712–1718.

29. Grant WP, Garcia-Lavin SE, Sabo RT, et al. A retrospective analysis of 50 consecutive Charcot diabetic salvage reconstructions. J Foot Ankle Surg 2009;48:30–38.

30. Gvazava T, Smirnov G, Petrova V, et al. Improving the performance of small amputations in complicated forms of diabetic foot. Georgian Med News 2015;(240):7–11.

31. Holmes GB Jr, Hill N. Fractures and dislocations of the foot and ankle in diabetics associated with Charcot joint changes. Foot Ankle Int 1994;15:182–185.

32. Lanting SM, Twigg SM, Johnson NA, et al. Non-invasive lower limb small arterial measures co-segregate strongly with foot complications in people with diabetes. J Diabetes Complications 2017;31:589–593.

33. Lee YK, Park KY, Koo YT, et al. Analysis of multiple risk factors affecting the result of free flap transfer for necrotising soft tissue defects of the lower extremities in patients with type 2 diabetes mellitus. J Plast Reconstr Aesthet Surg 2014;67:624–628.

34. McCormack RG, Leith JM. Ankle fractures in diabetics. Complications of surgical management. J Bone Joint Surg Br 1998;80: 689–692.

35. Mendicino RW, Catanzariti AR, Saltrick KR, et al. Tibiotalocalcaneal arthrodesis with retrograde intramedullary nailing. J Foot Ankle Surg 2004;43:82–86.

36. Mohsenifar Z, Feridoni MJ, Bayat M, et al. Histological and biomechanical analysis of the effects of streptozotocin-induced type one diabetes mellitus on healing of tenotomised Achilles tendons in rats. Foot Ankle Surg 2014;20:186–191.

37. Myers TG, Lowery NJ, Frykberg RG, et al. Ankle and hindfoot fusions: comparison of outcomes in patients with and without diabetes. Foot Ankle Int 2012;33:20–28.

38. Nehler MR, Whitehill TA, Bowers SP, et al. Intermediate-term outcome of primary digit amputations in patients with diabetes mellitus who have forefoot sepsis requiring hospitalization and presumed adequate circulatory status. J Vasc Surg 1999;30:509–517.

39. Pinzur MS. Neutral ring fixation for high-risk nonplantigrade Charcot midfoot deformity. Foot Ankle Int 2007;28:961–966.

40. Pinzur MS, Sostak J. Surgical stabilization of nonplantigrade Charcot arthropathy of the midfoot. Am J Orthop 2007;36: 361–365.

41. Pollard J, Hamilton GA, Rush SM, et al. Mortality and morbidity after transmetatarsal amputation: retrospective review of 101 cases. J Foot Ankle Surg 2006;45:91–97.

42. Raikin SM, Kane J, Ciminiello ME. Risk factors for incision-healing complications following total ankle arthroplasty. J Bone Joint Surg Am 2010;92:2150–2155.

43. Ramanujam CL, Han D, Fowler S, et al. Impact of diabetes and comorbidities on split-thickness skin grafts for foot wounds. J Am Podiatr Med Assoc 2013;103:223–232.

44. Ramanujam CL, Han D, Zgonis T. Lower extremity amputation and mortality rates in the reconstructed diabetic Charcot foot and ankle with external fixation: data analysis of 116 patients. Foot Ankle Spec 2016;9:113–126.

45. Rensing N, Waterman BR, Frank RM, et al. Low risk for local and systemic complications after primary repair of 1626 Achilles tendon ruptures. Foot Ankle Spec 2017;10(3):216–226.

46. Sato T, Ichioka S. Ostectomy and medial plantar artery flap reconstruction for Charcot foot ulceration involving the midfoot. J Foot Ankle Surg 2016;55:628–632.

47. Schipper ON, Jiang JJ, Chen L, et al. Effect of diabetes mellitus on perioperative complications and hospital outcomes after ankle arthrodesis and total ankle arthroplasty. Foot Ankle Int 2015;36:258–267.

48. Shibuya N, Humphers JM, Fluhman BL, et al. Factors associated with nonunion, delayed union, and malunion in foot and ankle surgery in diabetic patients. J Foot Ankle Surg 2013;52:207–211.

49. Siebachmeyer M, Boddu K, Bilal A, et al. Outcome of one-stage correction of deformities of the ankle and hindfoot and fusion in Charcot neuroarthropathy using a retrograde intramedullary hindfoot arthrodesis nail. Bone Joint J 2015;97:76–82.

50. Tantigate D, Jang E, Seetharaman M, et al. Timing of antibiotic prophylaxis for preventing surgical site infections in foot and ankle surgery. Foot Ankle Int 2017;38(3):283–288.

51. Thompson RC Jr, Clohisy DR. Deformity following fracture in diabetic neuropathic osteoarthropathy. Operative management of adults who have type-I diabetes. J Bone Joint Surg Am 1993;75:1765–1773.

52. Thorud JC, Jupiter DC, Lorenzana J, et al. Reoperation and reamputation after transmetatarsal amputation: a systematic review and meta-analysis. J Foot Ankle Surg 2016;55:1007–1012.

53. White CB, Turner NS, Lee GC, et al. Open ankle fractures in patients with diabetes mellitus. Clin Orthop Relat Res 2003;414:37–44.

54. Wukich DK. Diabetes and its negative impact on outcomes in orthopaedic surgery. World J Orthop 2015;6:331–339.

55. Wukich DK, Crim BE, Frykberg RG, et al. Neuropathy and poorly controlled diabetes increase the rate of surgical site infection after foot and ankle surgery. J Bone Joint Surg Am 2014;96:832–839.

56. Younger AS, Awwad MA, Kalla TP, et al. Risk factors for failure of transmetatarsal amputation in diabetic patients: a cohort study. Foot Ankle Int 2009;30:1177–1182.

57. Zarutsky E, Rush SM, Schuberth JM. The use of circular wire external fixation in the treatment of salvage ankle arthrodesis. J Foot Ankle Surg 2005;44:22–31.

58. Zhang W, Chen E, Xue D, et al. Risk factors for wound complications of closed calcaneal fractures after surgery: a systematic review and meta-analysis. Scand J Trauma Resusc Emerg Med 2015;23:18.

59. Zou RH, Wukich DK. Outcomes of foot and ankle surgery in diabetic patients who have undergone solid organ transplantation. J Foot Ankle Surg 2015;54:577–581.

CHAPTER 27

Stepwise Approach to Diabetic Partial Foot Amputations

Troy J. Boffeli • Mark S. Goss

INTRODUCTION

Lower extremity amputation procedures are frequently performed to manage complications of diabetes mellitus including infected neuropathic ulcers, deep abscess, osteomyelitis, gangrene, necrotizing fasciitis, and Charcot neuroarthropathy. Approximately 73,000 nontraumatic lower extremity amputation procedures were performed in 2010 for diabetic patients 20 years and older (22). This comprises approximately 60% of all nontraumatic lower extremity amputations in the United States (22). An estimated 9.3% of the U.S. population has diabetes mellitus, and 8.1 million people are thought to be undiagnosed (22).

Comorbid conditions are common in diabetes mellitus–related foot disorders including peripheral arterial disease, peripheral neuropathy, and biomechanical dysfunction (23,24, 26,39). These factors predispose the diabetic patient to foot ulceration, with a lifetime risk of up to 25% (19). Lower extremity amputation is frequently required for treatment of subsequent foot infection, osteomyelitis, and gangrene. In these cases, the primary goals of amputation are prompt resolution of infection with a combined medical and surgical approach, removal of nonviable tissue to a level that is capable of healing yet hopefully preserves a functional foot, and obtainment of biopsy and culture to direct antibiotic therapy. Partial foot amputation is generally preferred over leg amputation; however, selection of the most appropriate level of amputation for a given patient is a complex decision.

When evaluating an individual diabetic patient to determine the best operative plan for amputation, several factors must be considered. Initially, it is helpful to know if the amputation will be performed in a single-stage or if subsequent operations will be necessary. In the absence of an acute soft tissue infection including abscess or cellulitis, a single-stage amputation with primary closure is generally preferred for treatment of complicated wounds, osteomyelitis, and gangrene. A staged surgical plan may be indicated if the patient is septic or if acute soft tissue infection is present. If so, the initial operation typically includes incision and drainage of abscess if present, resection of exposed or infected bone, deep bone biopsy, excision

of necrotic soft tissue, and open amputation. Serial incision and drainage procedures may be required if there is evidence of persistent soft tissue infection, with each stage being more aggressive if the patient is not showing signs of improvement. The final stage procedure is performed once the acute infection resolves and local tissues have demarcated. Staged surgery also allows vascular evaluation and intervention prior to final determination of optimal amputation level. The final stage procedure typically involves conservative revision of previous incision margins, biopsy of the proximal bone margin, excision of any residual nonviable tissue, and wound closure if possible. Adjunct procedures including tendo-Achilles lengthening are commonly performed at this time. An important consideration with staged surgery is to preplan likely flap closure options prior to making the initial stage 1 surgical incision because a poorly placed incision and drainage wound may compromise future soft tissue coverage options.

Table 27.1 details additional factors that should be considered when selecting the most appropriate level of partial foot amputation. Lower extremity perfusion at the level being considered for amputation (below-the-knee amputation versus transmetatarsal amputation [TMA] versus disarticulation at metatarsophalangeal joint) is an important factor that could potentially be modified with vascular intervention. Noninvasive arterial assessment is indicated if there is evidence of lower extremity arterial disease such as diminished pedal pulses, intermittent claudication, rest pain, dependent rubor, delayed capillary fill time, or ischemic wounds. Ideally, arterial inflow should be optimized to the level of the toes, but the most distal site of adequate perfusion for healing should be determined. An amputation level distal to this site should not be selected because there is a very high risk of complication including failure to heal the incision, recurrent infection or gangrene, and the need for repeat amputation. Direct visual assessment of tissue perfusion at the time of amputation should not be underestimated because invasive and noninvasive preoperative arterial assessment can be misleading.

The extent of tissue compromise associated with gangrene of the foot should be assessed in addition to tissue quality just proximal to the line of demarcation. Areas of gangrene should

TABLE 27.1	Considerations in Selecting Appropriate Levels of Partial Foot Amputation in Diabetic Patients

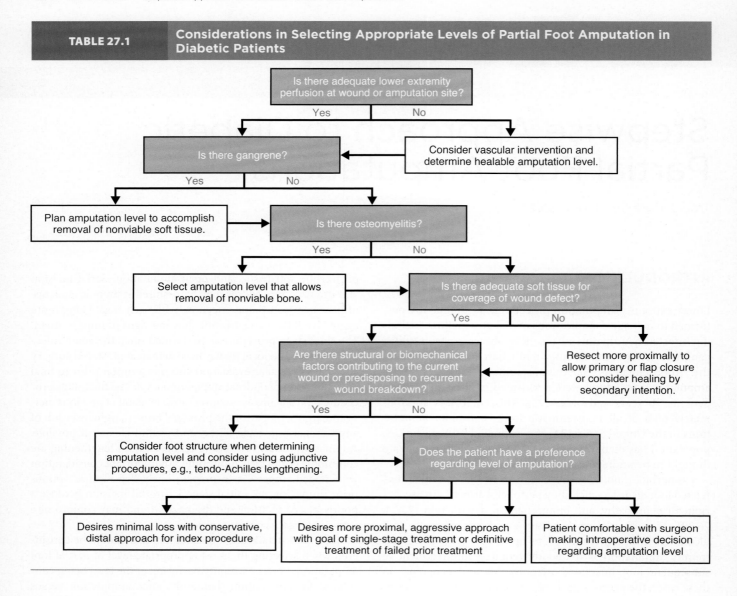

be assessed for associated infection including cellulitis, osteomyelitis, joint sepsis, gas-forming infection, and necrotizing fasciitis. These factors have implications regarding timing and extent of amputation and postamputation antibiotic needs (Fig. 27.1).

Ideally, the selected amputation level will allow adequate viable soft tissue for tension-free closure to cover local wound defects and exposed bone, although secondary healing is commonly necessary. Advanced amputation techniques such as advancement, transpositional, or rotational flap closure may be utilized if there is not adequate local soft tissue for closure. Compared to standard amputation techniques, flap closure may allow a more distal level of amputation in an effort to preserve mechanical function of the foot while achieving soft tissue coverage of the exposed bone structure.

Many diabetic patients have structural or biomechanical abnormalities that contribute to nonhealing wounds such as ankle equinus, hallux limitus, hallux valgus, hammertoe contracture, and Charcot neuroarthropathy. The ideal level of amputation would address such factors to reduce pressure points that might predispose to recurrent wound breakdown. If the amputation level alone cannot address these factors, adjunctive surgical procedures should be considered. For example, a diabetic neuropathic patient with a complicated plantar forefoot wound may have concomitant ankle equinus that should be surgically corrected (Fig. 27.2). Failure to correct the deforming forces that lead to increased focal pressure predisposes to reulceration of the amputation site (6). The timing of adjunctive procedures must be carefully considered. Performing adjunctive procedures at the time of amputation may increase the risk of surgical site infection by cross-contamination. Alternatively, adjunctive procedures may be performed in a delayed fashion allowing resolution of infection and open wounds. Adjunctive procedures may also be required to manage iatrogenic biomechanical dysfunction.

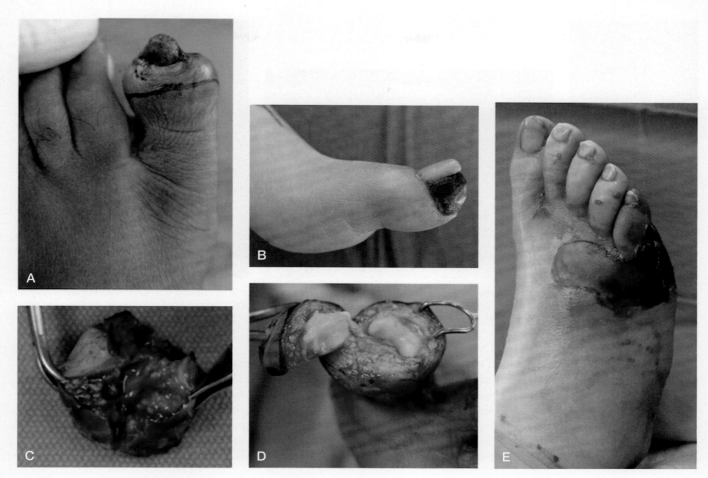

FIGURE 27.1 Localized forefoot gangrene is commonly treated with demarcation and vascular intervention if necessary. **A.** Tip of toe gangrene is amenable to autoamputation but frequently results in exposure of the distal phalanx as seen here after autoamputation of the tip of the hallux. This will not heal without surgical treatment that may include distal Syme hallux amputation or metatarsophalangeal joint disarticulation. Timely surgery once bone becomes exposed may be helpful to avoid osteomyelitis. **B–D.** Note pus within the distal phalanx at the time of back table surgical biopsy, yet no signs of infection at the interphalangeal resection site. **E.** Waiting until areas of gangrene become infected with abscess and osteomyelitis increases the likelihood of more proximal amputation. Broad areas of gangrene will require more proximal amputation, and limb loss is likely. Note cellulitis and acute infection around the areas of wet gangrene.

Amputation certainly alters the structure and biomechanical function of the foot. For example, complete fifth ray (toe and metatarsal) resection results in loss of peroneus brevis (PB) tendon function that predisposes to inversion deformity. Tendon balancing procedures are commonly necessary to maintain a plantigrade foot position that is more amenable to ambulation and bracing.

Patient preferences should also be considered when determining the most appropriate level of amputation. Determination of the ideal level of amputation for an individual patient should balance healing potential, resolution of infection, functionality of the foot, and the patient's goals of care. The patient may desire minimal loss, with a very conservative distal amputation approach or may refuse partial foot amputation altogether. Alternatively, the patient may desire a more aggressive amputation approach for management of failed prior treatment or for a single-stage treatment with

the hope of prompt healing. A candid discussion regarding the severity of the patient's condition, available treatment options, and expectations for healing and potential complications should be part of the surgical planning process. It is also helpful to determine if the patient is comfortable with the surgeon making an intraoperative decision regarding amputation level.

When attempting diabetic limb salvage, the surgeon must also consider the respective advantages and disadvantages of partial foot amputation versus proximal leg amputation. Partial foot amputation is generally thought to allow a more functional gait compared to leg amputation (21,25). If partial foot amputation is not an option due to extensive gangrene or rearfoot osteomyelitis, an alternative to proximal leg amputation is Syme amputation (Fig. 27.3). This procedure generally involves amputation of the foot with disarticulation at the ankle joint. Syme amputation is contraindicated in the absence

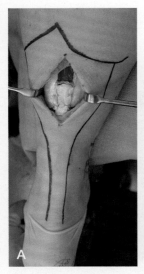
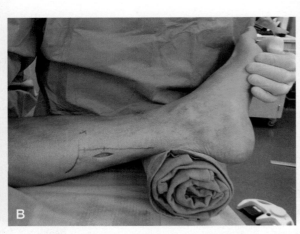
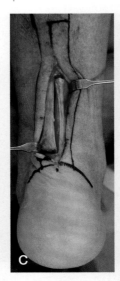
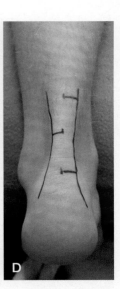

FIGURE 27.2 Posterior leg muscle lengthening is commonly necessary with partial foot amputation. Options include open tongue and groove gastrocnemius lengthening **(A)**, medial approach gastrocnemius recession **(B)**, open Z-lengthening of the Achilles tendon **(C)**, and minimally invasive triple hemisection tendo-Achilles lengthening **(D)**.

of a viable plantar heel pad, although it is commonly avoided due to concern for plantar fat pad migration and subsequent ulceration. Partial foot amputation preserves the ankle joint and, by definition, some residual foot length. Preservation of a portion of the foot may also provide some cosmetic value. A commonly held belief regarding lower extremity amputations is that ambulation involves increased energy demand with

more proximal amputation levels (31,45,46). The associated energy demand is thought to contribute to significant morbidity and mortality. However, more recent research suggests that energy demands and mechanics between some levels of partial foot amputation and transtibial amputation may not be as disparate as originally thought (27). Regarding transtibial amputations, there appears to be a higher rate of healing

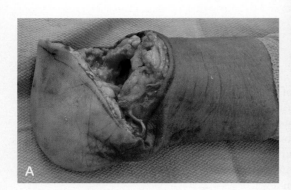
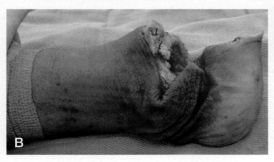
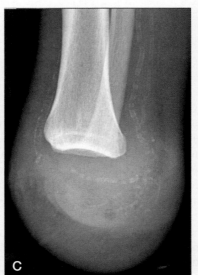
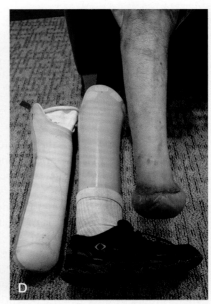

FIGURE 27.3 Syme amputation may be indicated for infected and unstable Charcot neuroarthropathy, extensive frostbite, and osteomyelitis of the calcaneus. **A,B.** Syme amputation requires intact skin on the plantar surface of the heel which is often compromised in patients requiring complete foot amputation. **C,D.** Loss of the talus and calcaneus creates substantial limb length deficit requiring lower leg prosthetic accommodation similar to below-the-knee amputation.

when compared to partial foot amputations (28,29,35,36,44). A troubling observation regarding partial foot amputations is that many are reported to have complications including dehiscence, ulceration, and the need for subsequent amputation (38,41,42). This underscores the importance of careful surgical planning and preoperative workup to select the most appropriate amputation level that will result in successful healing and prevention of wound recurrence which will allow a functional outcome for this high-risk patient population.

Each amputation level discussed in this chapter has unique considerations. However, the actual surgical technique for partial foot amputation for treatment of diabetes mellitus–related complications is generally consistent and differs from typical elective foot surgical techniques in a variety of ways (15). Amputation incisions are generally made in a full-thickness fashion and are extended down to bone without layered dissection. The tip of the scalpel enters the skin with the scalpel positioned 90 degrees to the skin surface. This 90 degree position of the scalpel should be maintained as the incision is advanced around anatomic contours. The goal of this full-depth incision technique is to avoid devitalization of soft tissues that could occur with skiving or undermining. The full-thickness flap should comprise the entire soft tissue envelope, including all tissue from skin to periosteum. However, subperiosteal dissection should not extend beyond the level of disarticulation or osteotomy in an effort to maintain local perfusion and minimize the risk of heterotopic ossification (Fig. 27.4) (12,16).

Full-thickness flaps should extend just distally enough to allow tension-free closure. If flaps are too short, closure may result in excessive tension and impaired wound healing.

However, excessive flap length can increase dead space at the amputation site and thus increase the risk of hematoma formation. A minimal-touch technique is preferred for flap manipulation because maintaining flap viability is crucial. A wide double-prong skin hook is used in deep tissue to retract the flaps, with care taken to avoid the unnecessary trauma to the wound margins that can occur with forceps. Once visualized, soft tissue and bone structures should be carefully evaluated for viability and likelihood of infection. The flexor and extensor tendon sheaths and fascial planes should be evaluated, especially in the presence of acute soft tissue infection because proximal extension of abscess can occur rapidly at these sites. Soft tissue and bone samples should also be collected for culture and pathological analysis, if appropriate. This allows confirmation of a clean proximal margin, diagnosis of osteomyelitis with microscopic pathology evaluation, and microbiology culture to direct appropriate antibiotic therapy.

Postoperative weight bearing restrictions vary with amputation level, location of incision in relation to the weight bearing surface of the foot, and use of concomitant adjunctive procedures. Appropriate rest and aggressive elevation are required to reduce operative site edema, minimize risk of hematoma, and avoid local tissue trauma associated with neuropathy. In general, limited weight bearing is tolerated with toe or partial ray amputation, provided the incision does not involve the plantar surface. More proximal levels of partial foot amputation will do poorly if weight bearing is resumed prior to healing.

The amputation levels discussed in detail include distal Syme, toe, partial ray, transmetatarsal, Lisfranc, Chopart, and partial calcanectomy.

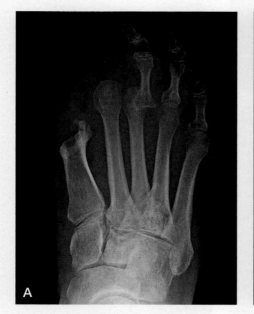
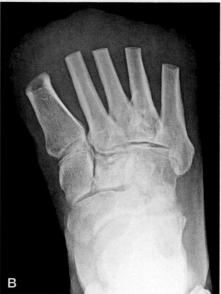

FIGURE 27.4 Heterotopic ossification (HO) is common after partial resection of long bones and can be clinically significant with reulceration and recurrent infection after partial metatarsal resection. **A.** Heterotopic bone formation is shown following partial first ray resection through the metatarsal neck. Subsequent digital amputation intentionally involved disarticulation of the second toe in an effort to avoid HO. **B.** Single-dose radiation therapy was performed at the time of conversion to transmetatarsal amputation years later which has been shown to decrease HO formation in high-risk patients (25,47).

TOE AMPUTATION

Distal Syme Amputation

Distal Syme amputation is indicated for tip of toe and nail bed wounds associated with osteomyelitis of the distal phalanx and gangrene isolated to the distal toe (Fig. 27.5). This minimal resection technique is not indicated in the setting of wounds at or proximal to the proximal interphalangeal joint (IPJ). Toe amputation is more appropriate in cases that involve extensive gangrene or proximal wounds.

Distal Syme amputation is typically performed without a tourniquet, but a Penrose drain may be placed around base of the toe for local hemostasis. Electrocautery is avoided if possible due to the fragile nature of the tuft flap, although bleeding plantar toe vessels may need spot electrocautery or suture ligation. Advancement and suturing of the flap creates a tamponade effect which is generally sufficient for hemostasis (5).

The incision design for distal Syme hallux (first toe) amputation is demonstrated in Figure 27.6. The dorsal incision is transverse at the level of the IPJ. Care is taken to place the

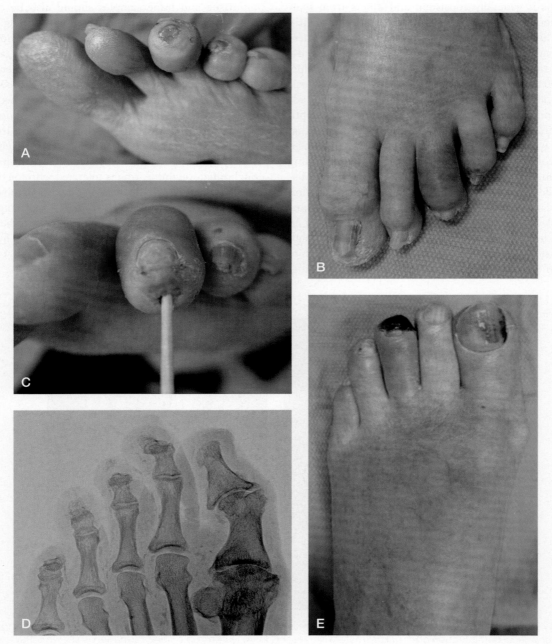

FIGURE 27.5 A. Distal Syme amputation is indicated for tip of toe ulcers with suspected osteomyelitis of the distal phalanx. **B,C.** Note tip of third toe neuropathic ulceration with toe cellulitis and positive probe to bone suggestive of osteomyelitis. **D.** Plain radiographs of the foot indicated erosive changes to the distal phalanx. **E.** Distal Syme amputation may also be indicated for tip of toe gangrene.

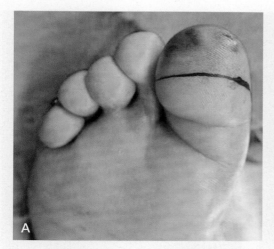
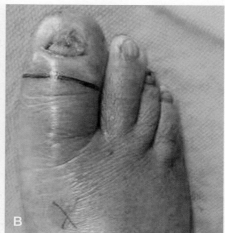
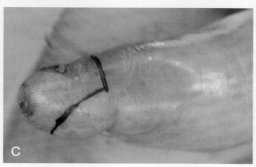

FIGURE 27.6   **A,B.** Distal Syme amputation can be performed on the first toe for complicated tip of toe ulcers associated with a long or contracted hallux. Tip of hallux gangrene and nail bed ulceration with osteomyelitis isolated to the distal phalanx are also indications for distal Syme hallux amputation. **B,C.** Note how the dorsal incision is transversely positioned over the interphalangeal joint. Closure is through an advancement flap of intact plantar tissue.

incision proximal to the nail matrix because retained matrix tissue may result in persistent nail growth. The plantar incision wraps around the tip of the hallux to create a plantar flap that will be advanced dorsally to cover the wound defect, following bone and nail bed excision. The dorsal incision is deepened directly into the IPJ allowing easy disarticulation of the distal phalanx. The plantar flap is raised off bone to preserve a thick vascular flap that can withstand weight bearing stress. The distal wound, toenail, nail matrix, and distal phalanx are then removed as one unit. The tip of the proximal phalanx is remodeled to remove bony prominence which also procures bone for proximal margin biopsy (Fig. 27.7). Separate instrumentation

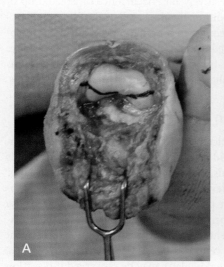
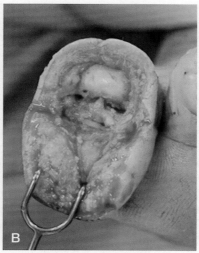
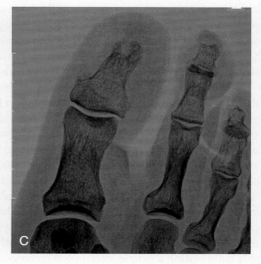

FIGURE 27.7 Distal Syme amputation on the first toe typically requires some degree of remodeling at the head of the proximal phalanx due to irregular bone structure after disarticulation at the interphalangeal joint. **A.** Note prominence of the medial and lateral condyles at the head of the proximal phalanx after interphalangeal joint disarticulation in patient shown in Figure 27.1B–D. Lines are drawn with a marker to indicate desired resection to remodel the tip of the proximal phalanx. **B.** Remodeled tip of the proximal phalanx without bone prominence. **C,D.** Before and after images that demonstrate remodeled first proximal phalanx. *(continued)*

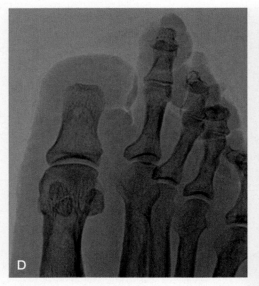

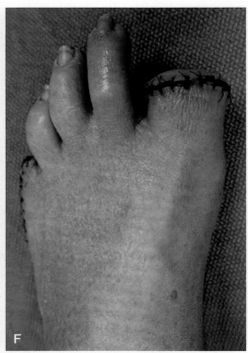

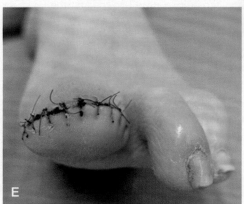

FIGURE 27.7 *(Continued)* Note erosive changes at the tip of the distal phalanx indicating osteomyelitis **(C)** and how the end of the remodeled proximal phalanx now resembles the anatomy of the tip of the distal phalanx **(D)**. **E,F.** Healing amputation site 2 weeks after surgery.

and new gloves are used to remove the IPJ sesamoid and remodel the proximal phalanx. The medial, lateral, and plantar condylar prominences are resected with a bone saw to reduce pressure and mimic distal phalanx morphology, but care is taken to avoid excessive shortening of the proximal phalanx. The plantar flap is then advanced dorsally and closed with nonabsorbable suture using a simple interrupted technique.

Distal Syme amputation of a lesser toe involves an incision that is similar to distal Syme hallux amputation (Fig. 27.8). A plantar flap is preserved, which is then advanced to cover the wound defect (5). The incision is deepened to bone using the previously described technique. As with distal Syme hallux amputation, the distal wound, toenail, nail matrix, and distal phalanx are removed. New instrumentation is used to remove the distal one-third to one-half of the middle phalanx if needed to mobilize the flap, further shorten the toe if desired, or procure proximal margin biopsy. The plantar flap is advanced dorsally and flap margins are approximated with nonabsorbable suture using a simple interrupted technique. Sutures are generally left in place for longer than 2 weeks because delayed wound healing is common in this setting. Immediate weight bearing in an open-toed surgical shoe is generally permitted following partial toe amputation.

Distal Syme amputation is not commonly performed at the fifth toe due to the relatively rare occurrence of isolated tip of fifth toe wounds. Additionally, the small size of this digit frequently necessitates complete amputation for adequate infection control and to reduce lateral prominence. The procedure can be performed for tip of fifth toe gangrene or osteomyelitis isolated to the distal phalanx associated with an ulcerated callus.

Toe Amputation

Toe amputation is typically performed for treatment of toe gangrene, proximal spread of soft tissue infection or osteomyelitis from tip of toe wounds, and complicated diabetic wounds at or proximal to the IPJ level. If infection involves the metatarsophalangeal joint, more proximal resection may be required. Toe amputation may be performed via disarticulation at the metatarsophalangeal joint; however, transverse migration of adjacent toes may occur with central toe disarticulation. To avoid this, the base of the proximal phalanx may be preserved if resection of nonviable bone and soft tissue can still be accomplished with adequate soft tissue coverage for tension-free closure. There is some debate regarding preservation of articular cartilage at the metatarsal head with metatarsophalangeal joint disarticulation.

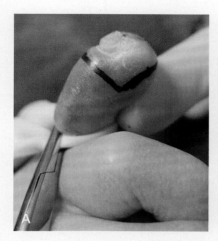
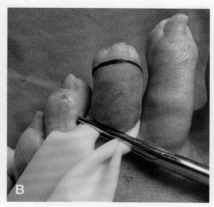
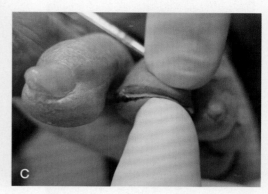

FIGURE 27.8 **A.** Incision plan for central toe distal Syme amputation with Penrose drain tourniquet at the base of the toe. **B.** The dorsal incision is transverse at the level of the distal interphalangeal joint (DIPJ) just proximal to the nail matrix. Note that the dorsal soft tissues do not contribute to flap closure. Careful incision directly to bone helps to preserve a thick plantar flap that is crucial to immediate healing and long-term survival of the flap once weight bearing is resumed. The distal phalanx is disarticulated through the DIPJ along with the neuropathic ulcer, toenail, and nail matrix. Bone biopsy is taken from the tip of the distal phalanx to include culture and pathological specimens. The distal one-third of the middle phalanx can be resected to allow proximal margin biopsy and relaxation of the soft tissues if needed for better coverage. **C.** Note how the flap easily advances to create a new tip of the toe.

Preservation of cartilage is advocated because it may act as a barrier to infection that could otherwise extend directly into the medullary canal (40). Those who advocate denuding the cartilage suggest that in the absence of synovial fluid, the cartilage is no longer viable and therefore at risk of necrosis (20,34). The authors typically address metatarsal head articular cartilage on a case-by-case basis and have not appreciated complications associated with either approach. The surgical technique is similar for amputation of each toe; however, there are unique considerations for the hallux, central toes (second, third, and fourth toes), and the fifth toe.

Hallux amputation typically involves raising full-thickness dorsal and plantar flaps (Fig. 27.9). A semi-elliptical incision is placed at the dorsal aspect of the toe and converges medially

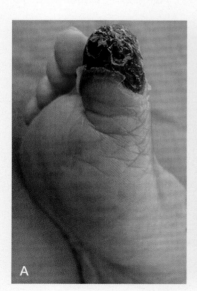
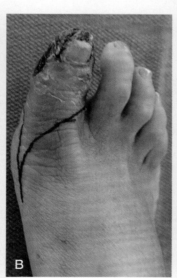
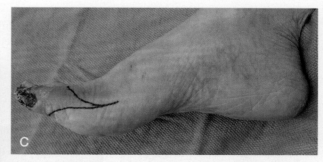
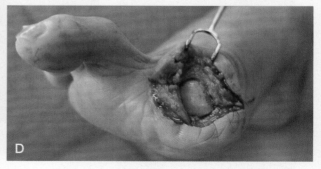

FIGURE 27.9 **A.** Hallux amputation involves resection through the base of the proximal phalanx or first metatarsophalangeal joint as shown here for hallux gangrene. **B,C.** Dorsal and plantar soft tissue flaps are preserved which allows medial convergence and proximal run out for access to the metatarsophalangeal joint. The incision can be lengthened proximally if part of the first metatarsal needs to be remodeled or removed. **D.** Removal of the exposed cartilage on the first metatarsal head is at the discretion of the surgeon. The joint capsule can be sutured over the metatarsal head for layered closure if desired.

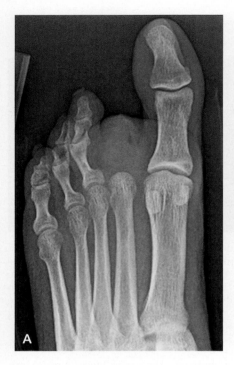

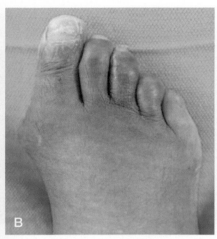

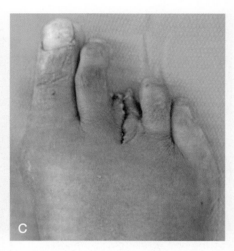

FIGURE 27.10 **A.** Central toe amputation typically involves disarticulation at the metatarsophalangeal joint, although a portion of the proximal phalanx can be preserved if desired. The traditional incision design involves medial and lateral soft tissue flaps with dorsal or plantar proximal incision run out depending on whether a plantar neuropathic ulcer is being excised. Incision design ideally preserves tissue at the base of the toe for tension-free closure. **B.** Toe gangrene oftentimes extends to the base of the toe resulting in compromised primary closure options. **C.** Open amputation with secondary healing is commonly necessary under these circumstances.

and laterally with a similarly placed semi-elliptical incision at the plantar aspect. The distal extent of each flap is typically at the midshaft of the proximal phalanx, although flap geometry may need to be modified based on the location of nonviable tissue (9). The medial incision apex should bisect the foot from dorsal to plantar and may be extended proximally if conversion to partial first ray resection becomes necessary. The incisions converge laterally in the first interdigital space at the base of the hallux.

Central toe amputation typically involves raising full-thickness medial and lateral flaps with medial and lateral

semi-elliptical incisions that converge dorsally and plantarly (Fig. 27.10). This allows proximal extension of the dorsal convergence to access the metatarsophalangeal joint for disarticulation or to convert to partial ray resection (14). If poor interdigital tissue quality or ulceration compromises the potential for medial and lateral flaps, dorsal and plantar flaps may be raised as an alternative, although this approach does not provide access for central ray amputation. Interdigital wounds or gangrene can be closed with a toe trap door flap raised from the opposite side of the toe (3). Figure 27.11 demonstrates an

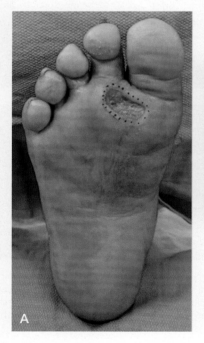

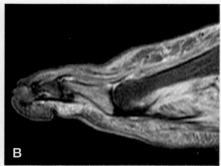

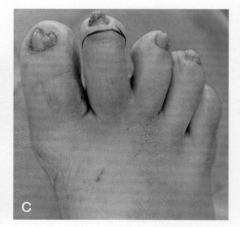

FIGURE 27.11 **A.** This patient presented with an oval-shaped wound located just distal to the first and second metatarsal heads. **B.** Magnetic resonance imaging raised suspicion for osteomyelitis within the second proximal phalanx. Standard second toe amputation incision techniques would not allow closure of the plantar wound which could be left open to heal secondarily. *(continued)*

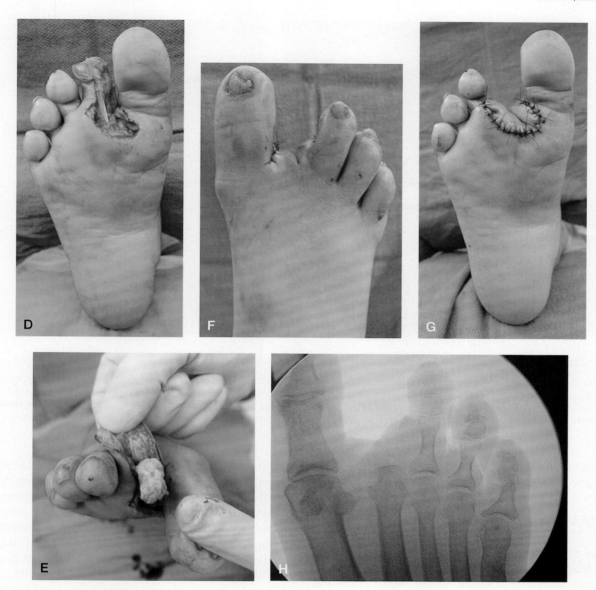

FIGURE 27.11 *(Continued)* **C–G.** Fillet of second toe flap technique was incorporated to allow plantar advancement of the dorsal toe soft tissues to achieve plantar wound coverage after toe amputation. **H.** Intraoperative imaging with disarticulation at the metatarsophalangeal joint level.

advanced toe fillet flap amputation technique that was used to treat osteomyelitis of the second proximal phalanx associated with a neuropathic ulcer located just distal to the plantar metatarsophalangeal joint area. Creativity with incision design is often needed with partial toe or foot amputation depending on the size and location of wound deficit.

Fifth toe amputation typically involves raising a dorsal and plantar flap in a full-thickness fashion, similar to hallux amputation (Fig. 27.12). Of note, fifth toe amputation frequently requires concomitant resection of the fifth metatarsal head because preservation may increase lateral prominence and predisposition to reulceration (15). The previously discussed incision plan allows proximal extension of the lateral incision convergence to allow access to the fifth metatarsal head if remodeling or resection is necessary.

Surgical technique for toe amputation involves a careful skin incision that is deepened directly to bone. Interdigital incisions are challenging because the adjacent toes are in the way. A penetrating towel clamp is used to grasp the toe for ease of manipulation. Flaps are raised from the underlying bone in a full-thickness fashion. If disarticulation is desired, dissection extends proximally to the metatarsophalangeal joint, where pericapsular structures are incised. If transphalangeal amputation is desired, an osteotomy is performed transversely through the proximal phalanx with a slight bevel, directed distal dorsal to proximal plantar to reduce prominence at the weight bearing surface. Deep closure is rarely necessary for amputation of toes. Full-thickness flaps are advanced, and wound margins are approximated with nonabsorbable suture. Sutures are typically left in place for longer

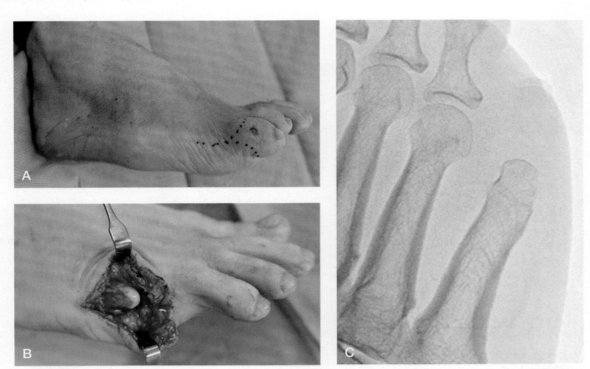

FIGURE 27.12 Incision design for fifth toe amputation typically creates dorsal and plantar flaps. **A.** Fifth toe ulceration localized to the interphalangeal joint region with secondary osteomyelitis is amenable to metatarsophalangeal joint disarticulation. **B.** Proximal extension of the incision allows remodeling of the fifth metatarsal head laterally to avoid bony prominence after metatarsophalangeal joint disarticulation. **C.** Imaging after fifth toe amputation and removal of the lateral condyle of the fifth metatarsal head.

than 2 weeks, and limited weight bearing in an open-toed surgical shoe is permitted.

PARTIAL RAY AMPUTATION

Partial ray amputation, or partial removal of a metatarsal and the associated toe, is typically performed to manage diabetic wounds complicated by gangrene, abscess, septic arthritis at the metatarsophalangeal joint, or osteomyelitis involving the distal aspect of the metatarsal. Figure 27.13 shows an example of a patient being considered for first ray amputation to treat an ulcerated bunion with secondary osteomyelitis of the first

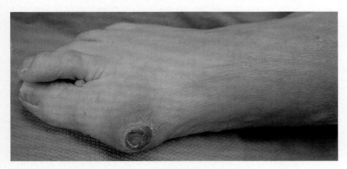

FIGURE 27.13 Medial first metatarsophalangeal joint ulceration associated with bunion deformity. Note surrounding cellulitis. Undermining of the wound margins and secondary osteomyelitis was treated with first ray amputation.

metatarsal head. Wounds are also frequently located plantar to the metatarsal heads due to excessive metatarsal length or relative metatarsal plantarflexion, but partial ray resection may also be required for proximal spread of infection from a toe wound. As with toe amputation, there are unique considerations for resection of the first ray, central rays, and the fifth ray. This procedure is frequently performed without a tourniquet. If used, the tourniquet should be released prior to closure, with hemostasis achieved using selective electrocautery or suture ties.

Partial First Ray Amputation

The traditional incision plan for first ray amputation is similar to that of hallux amputation which is designed to create dorsal and plantar flaps (Fig. 27.14). The medial convergence of the dorsal and plantar elliptical incisions is extended proximally to the mid-diaphyseal region of the first metatarsal. If the wound defect is located plantarly beneath the first metatarsal head and sesamoids, the incision plan can be modified to allow advancement of a rotational flap for adequate soft tissue coverage and immediate closure (Figs. 27.15 and 27.16).

The incision is deepened to bone with the scalpel oriented 90 degrees from the skin surface. Full-thickness flaps are raised, and the hallux is disarticulated. An osteotomy is then performed at the first metatarsal, just proximal to the distal metaphyseal flare. This approach preserves functional length of the metatarsal but reduces prominence that may result from preservation of the metaphyseal flare. Orienting the osteotomy distal dorsal

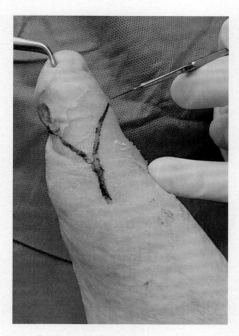

FIGURE 27.14 Traditional first ray amputation involves creation of dorsal and plantar flaps with proximal incision run out allowing excision of first toe and medially located metatarsophalangeal ulcers. A similar approach is used for fifth ray amputation associated with toe infection, gangrene, or ulcerated Tailor's bunion. Note incision technique with the scalpel plunging directly to bone followed by subperiosteal dissection to raise the flaps.

to proximal plantar minimizes plantar prominence and a slight bevel is introduced to avoid medial prominence as well.

The exposed medullary canal is then inspected. Ideally, viable cancellous bone is visualized, but there may be evidence of purulence or necrosis. In the setting of healthy cortical bone, a more proximal osteotomy is not preferred because this may compromise the structural support of the medial column. In addition, preserving cortical length allows conversion to a functional TMA level if needed at a later date. Curettage of the medullary canal is performed and a proximal biopsy sample is collected to assess for clean margin. Antibiotic-impregnated implants such as beads or cement may be used within the canal if desired. Flaps are advanced and closed with nonabsorbable sutures. Sutures are generally left in place for 3 to 6 weeks, and patients are non–weight-bearing until sutures are removed. Postoperative antibiotic therapy is frequently needed if amputation through the metatarsal does not provide a surgical cure of osteomyelitis.

Central Ray Amputation

The incision plan for central ray (second, third, or fourth ray) amputation is similar to that which is used for central toe amputation. The dorsal incision convergence is extended proximally for access to the metatarsal neck. The incision plan can be modified to allow excision of a plantar ulceration, if present, simply by extending the plantar incision convergence to circumscribe the toe wound (14). The incision is deepened to bone with the scalpel oriented 90 degrees from the skin surface.

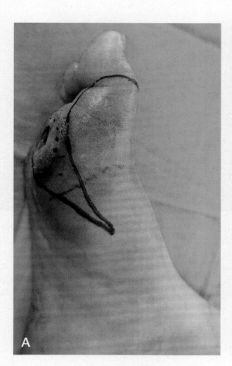
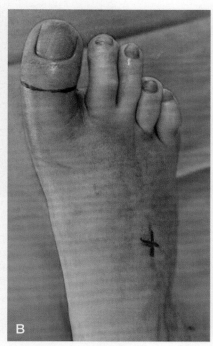
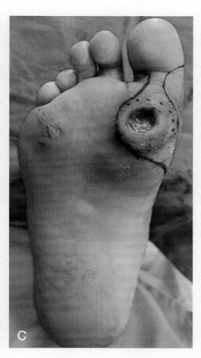

FIGURE 27.15 **A–C.** Neuropathic ulcers located plantar to the first metatarsophalangeal joint compromise the plantar flap necessary for primary closure after standard ray amputation. Advanced plastic surgical techniques are useful under these circumstances in an effort to rotate the dorsal medial soft tissues to provide plantar wound coverage. The proximal incision run out is curved away from the plantar arch and toward the medial midline of the foot which improves rotation of the flap and allows conversion to transmetatarsal amputation.

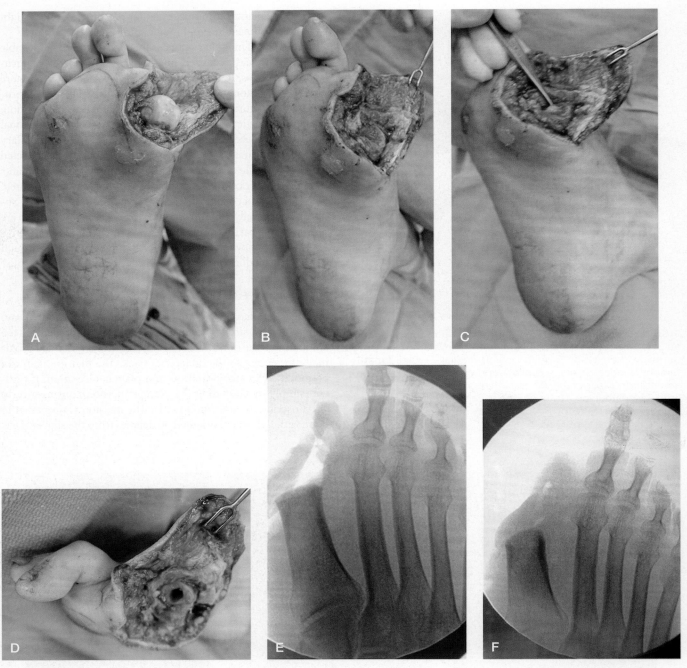

FIGURE 27.16 A. The first ray amputation flap shown in Figure 27.15 was raised full-thickness to include periosteum, neurovascular structures, and skin which allowed access for first metatarsophalangeal joint disarticulation. **B.** A bone saw was then used to resect the first metatarsal head. The flap is not native plantar tissue but is able to withstand plantar weight bearing forces because the metatarsal is shortened proximal to the flap. **C,D.** A bone curette was used here to débride the medullary canal which appeared abnormal on magnetic resonance imaging. **E.** Intraoperative imaging identified that the distal metaphyseal flare was still present. **F.** Repeat bone resection allowed removal of the distal metaphyseal flare with proper beveling of the metatarsal stump. *(continued)*

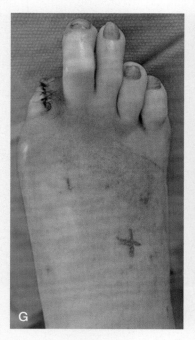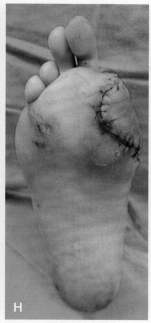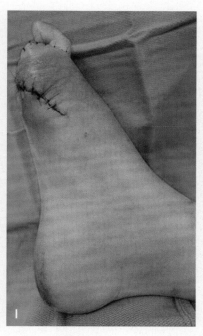

FIGURE 27.16 *(Continued)* **G–I.** Advancement and rotation of the flap in the plantar distal direction achieved complete coverage of the plantar wound defect.

Full-thickness flaps are raised, and the central toe is disarticulated at the metatarsophalangeal joint. An osteotomy is then performed at the central metatarsal, proximal to the metaphyseal flare. The osteotomy is oriented distal dorsal to proximal plantar to minimize plantar prominence. The osteotomy and removal of the capital fragment should be accomplished without unnecessary intermetatarsal dissection or periosteal elevation. As with first ray resection, the medullary canal and remaining cortical bone should be evaluated for viability with samples taken for microbiological and pathological analysis if indicated. Antibiotic-impregnated implants may also be used (Fig. 27.17). Full-thickness flaps are advanced, and wound margins are approximated with nonabsorbable suture. Sutures are generally left in place for 2 to 4 weeks, and minimal weight bearing in an open-toed surgical shoe is permitted unless a plantar wound is excised. Adequate soft tissue for tension-free closure is not always available, especially in cases involving gangrene. Secondary healing may be necessary under these less ideal circumstances.

Partial Fifth Ray Amputation

Fifth ray resection should be considered when performing fifth toe amputation even in the absence of concomitant metatarsal infection. Without the fifth toe, the fifth metatarsal head is prone to lateral prominence that predisposes to ulceration (13). Timeliness of surgical intervention for complicated fifth ray ulcers is important because early intervention may allow simple metatarsal head resection while delayed intervention allows progression of osteomyelitis (Fig. 27.18). Advanced infection with abscess, tissue necrosis, gas gangrene, or necrotizing fasciitis may require broad open amputation, increasing likelihood of poor outcome (Fig. 27.19).

The incision plan for fifth ray resection in the absence of ulceration at the plantar aspect of the fifth metatarsal head is similar to the previously discussed plan for fifth toe amputation. Dorsal and plantar flaps are created with the lateral convergence directed proximally along the lateral aspect of the fifth metatarsal. The medial convergence is deep in the fourth interdigital space at the base of the fourth toe. This incision plan allows excision of a complicated fifth toe or lateral fifth metatarsal wound and access to the metatarsal head for resection. The incision is deepened to bone with the scalpel advancing 90 degrees to the skin surface. Full-thickness flaps are raised and the fifth toe is disarticulated at the MPJ. An osteotomy is then performed at the fifth metatarsal, just proximal to the distal metaphyseal flare. The osteotomy is oriented to minimize lateral and plantar prominence. The osteotomy and removal of the capital fragment should be accomplished without any unnecessary dissection in the fourth intermetatarsal space. The medullary canal and remaining cortical bone should be evaluated for viability, with samples taken for microbiological and pathological analysis as appropriate. Full-thickness flaps are advanced, and wound margins are approximated with nonabsorbable suture. Sutures are left in place for 3 to 4 weeks, and limited heel weight bearing is permitted if a standard incision and closure are used. If a rotational flap is used to cover a plantar defect, the patient is to be non–weight-bearing until the flap heals.

Complete Fifth Ray Amputation with Peroneal Tendon Balancing

The ideal level of resection through the fifth metatarsal is variable depending on extent of infection, wound deficit, and lateral metatarsal bowing. It has been our experience that lateral

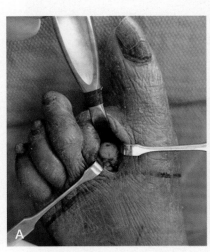
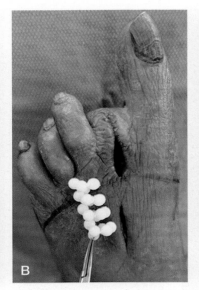
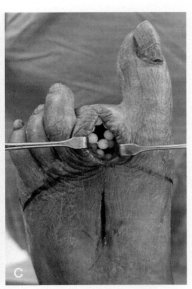

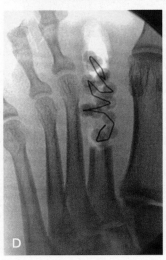

FIGURE 27.17 A. Isolated central ray amputation is a reasonable alternative to transmetatarsal amputation (TMA). Note how the transverse dorsal incision for TMA was drawn preoperatively with the intent to preserve the dorsal flap should more aggressive treatment with TMA be necessary in the short term. A more proximal counter incision was used here to allow access for midshaft metatarsal resection due to extensive osteomyelitis. **B-D.** A coiled string of antibiotic-impregnated beads were implanted in the dead space created by metatarsal resection. Coiling the beads increases the surface area and allows ease of removal through the proximal or distal incision. Staged surgery is necessary under these conditions with removal of the antibiotic beads 2 weeks later.

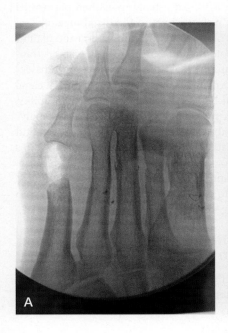
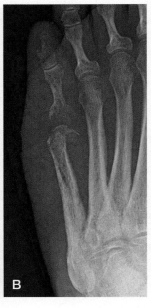

FIGURE 27.18 The decision to perform fifth metatarsal head resection versus partial fifth ray amputation is oftentimes determined by extent of bone infection, condition of the toe regarding deformity or function, viability of surrounding soft tissue, and patient preference. The fifth toe is often part of the deforming force, and metatarsal head resection can alleviate or promote contracture of the toe. **A.** Fifth metatarsal head resection was performed here for a nonhealing, uncomplicated plantar ulceration. The fifth metatarsal is likely the most tolerant of metatarsal head resection with limited likelihood of transfer lesions depending on foot structure. **B.** Alternatively, extensive osteomyelitis of the metatarsal and proximal phalanx necessitates partial or complete fifth ray amputation.

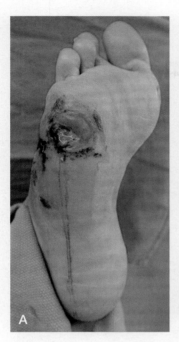
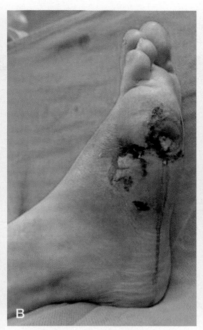
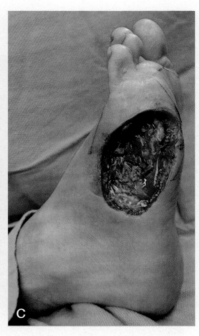

FIGURE 27.19 A,B. Fifth metatarsal head plantar neuropathic ulceration developed into gas gangrene which is a life- and limb-threatening infection that needs emergency surgery. **C.** Aggressive and broad resection to viable tissue margins is critical. This type of amputation does not follow preferred incisional approaches and preserving local flaps for coverage is typically not an option. Assessment for necrotizing fasciitis in the foot or leg is needed, and the surgeon should plan for revisional surgery in the following 2 to 3 days. Conversion to a more proximal level of amputation is an option, although adjunctive therapies like negative pressure wound therapy, muscle flaps, and skin grafts are commonly employed. The wound healed secondarily over the course of 6 months.

column reulceration is common when less than one-half of the fifth metatarsal is preserved. If partial fifth ray resection does not allow preservation of the proximal half of the metatarsal, the surgeon should consider complete amputation of the fifth ray with tendon transfer to preserve peroneal function (Fig. 27.20) (4). Figure 27.21 demonstrates an advanced approach to complete fifth ray amputation with incorporation of a rotational flap distally to close a plantar or lateral fifth metatarsophalangeal joint wound (11).

TRANSMETATARSAL AMPUTATION

TMA is indicated for management of forefoot gangrene, osteomyelitis, or irreparable distal ischemia that is not amenable to isolated toe or ray amputation. TMA should also be considered if more than 1 ray is being amputated or if there is an infected transfer ulcer secondary to prior resection of an adjacent ray (33). The general rule is that leaving only 3 metatarsal heads makes the diabetic foot prone to forefoot

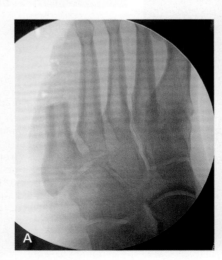
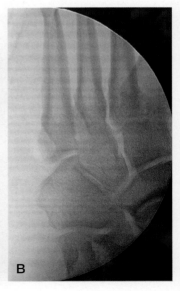

FIGURE 27.20 The decision to perform partial or complete fifth ray amputation is based on a variety of factors including location and extent of wound, extent of bone infection, failure of prior partial resection, and foot deformity including Charcot neuroarthropathy or metatarsus adductus. Cavovarus foot structure frequently leads to lateral column wounds that are hard to resolve. **A.** Note how preserving less than half of the fifth metatarsal creates lateral prominence that frequently leads to proximal transfer of tissue breakdown. **B.** Removal of the entire fifth metatarsal reduces lateral prominence although many patients require restoration of peroneal tendon function with this approach.

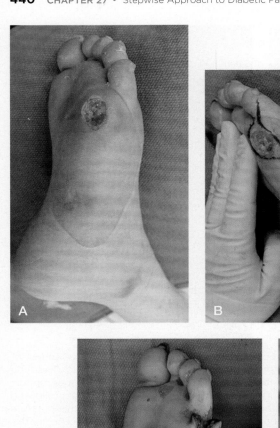

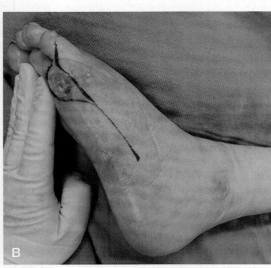

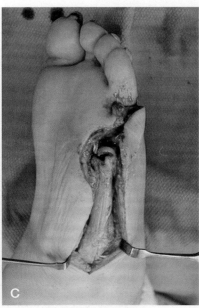

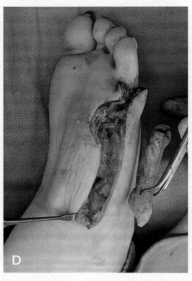

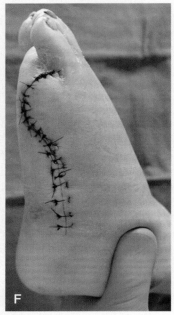

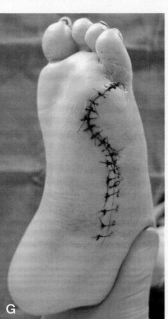

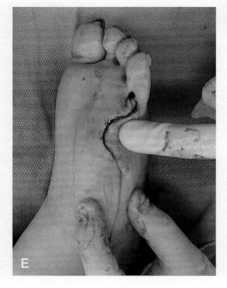

FIGURE 27.21 Recurring lateral column ulcers at the fifth metatarsal head and base on both feet were associated with neuromuscular contracture and being confined to a wheelchair. Treatment involved bilateral tendo-Achilles lengthening and complete fifth ray amputation with incorporation of rotational flaps to cover fifth metatarsophalangeal joint pressure sores. **A.** Preoperative fifth metatarsophalangeal joint wound with osteomyelitis and healed but recurring fifth metatarsal base wound. **B.** Incision plan for fifth toe fillet rotational flap and complete fifth ray amputation. Note equinus contracture at the ankle. **C.** The fifth toe was amputated after the flap was raised. Biopsy was taken from the fifth metatarsal head. Proximal dissection exposed the base of the fifth metatarsal. **D,E.** Removal of the entire fifth metatarsal (in bone clamp) creates laxity in the tissues which allows tissue mobility to cover the wound defect. Peroneal tendon transfer is common with this technique, but this patient was nonambulatory. **F,G.** Healing amputation site 2 weeks later.

reulceration (Fig. 27.22). Although this rule is based on clinical reality, no diabetic foot surgery is definitive, and the decision to convert a foot with multiple ray amputations to TMA should be determined on a case-by-case basis.

TMA may be performed with sedation and a local anesthetic block in a patient with peripheral neuropathy, but general anesthesia may be required in a sensate patient undergoing TMA for distal gangrene. A pneumatic ankle tourniquet may be used if robust perfusion is expected, which is common in diabetic patients undergoing TMA for complications of neuropathy.

Standard Transmetatarsal Amputation Procedure

The standard TMA incision plan involves transverse semi-elliptical incisions placed at the dorsal and plantar forefoot (Fig. 27.23). The flaps ideally extend just distal to the level of the metatarsophalangeal joints, but the plantar flap may be longer due to the naturally distal extent of the plantar toe sulci. The dorsal and plantar incisions converge medially and laterally, with the medial and lateral apices at the midshaft of the first and fifth metatarsals, respectively. The incision may need to be placed more proximally, depending on the location of infection and compromised tissue. Ideally, metatarsal resection is just proximal to the distal metaphyseal flare in order to preserve functional length yet allow tension-free flap closure. Location of metatarsal resection is variable and depends on location of wounds, extent of osteomyelitis, flap length, tissue loss from gangrene, and metatarsal length at prior amputation sites (18). Significant effort is made to preserve at least

the metatarsal bases because Lisfranc (tarsometatarsal) disarticulation further compromises foot function and results in potential loss of important extrinsic musculature insertions. Additionally, the surgeon must appreciate the presence of any ankle joint equinus because this may predispose an otherwise successful TMA to failure. Tendo-Achilles lengthening should be considered to reduce plantar pressures at the forefoot.

Once planned, the incision is deepened in a full-thickness fashion to the level of the metatarsal necks dorsally and metatarsophalangeal joints plantarly. The dorsal flap is retracted to permit access of a McGlamry elevator for subperiosteal dissection at each metatarsal. Subperiosteal dissection should extend proximally, just to the desired level of bone resection. An osteotomy is then performed at each metatarsal using a bone saw. As with individual ray resection, each osteotomy is placed proximal to the distal metaphyseal flare and is oriented distal dorsal to proximal plantar to avoid plantar prominence. The first and fifth metatarsals should be slightly beveled to reduce medial and lateral prominence, respectively. The goal with TMA is to recreate a native metatarsal parabola. The metatarsal heads are then carefully dissected from the associated plantar soft tissue to avoid disruption of flap perfusion and the metatarsal heads and toes are removed as 1 unit. The plantar plate apparatus associated with each metatarsal head is then dissected from the plantar flap to expose vascular tissue and debulk the flap. Any major bleeding vessels should be ligated as necessary to minimize hematoma formation. Electrocautery is used selectively to address bleeding vessels or muscle tissue. Deep sutures may be placed to reduce dead space and minimize skin tension, although this is typically not required. The use of a closed suction drain

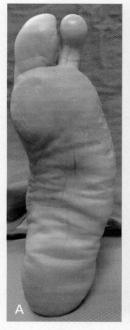 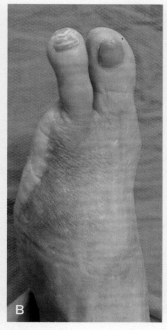 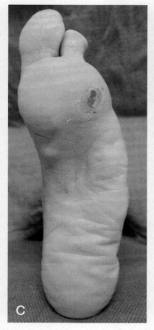 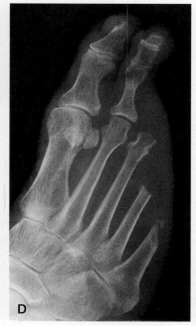

FIGURE 27.22 A,B. Multiple partial ray amputations with preservation of 2 or 3 toes typically leads to transfer neuropathic wounds at the adjacent metatarsophalangeal joints. **C,D.** Recurrent plantar breakdown occurred in this case beneath the third metatarsal head as would be expected.

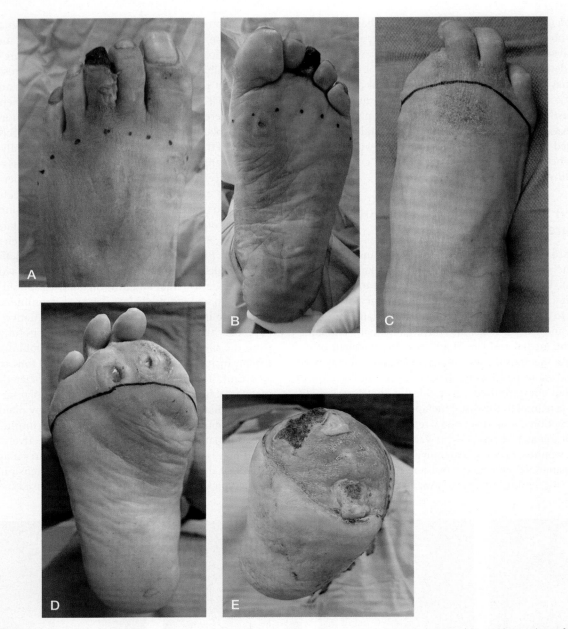

FIGURE 27.23 A,B. The standard transmetatarsal amputation incision plan requires intact plantar skin as shown here for toe gangrene and vascular insufficiency. **C,D.** Alternatively, the plantar flap can be incised more proximally if ulceration is present under the metatarsal heads. This approach typically requires more proximal bone resection to allow soft tissue coverage. **E.** Lack of primary or flap coverage requires secondary healing which is challenging over exposed bone. Note healthy granulation tissue 1 month after surgery yet persistent bone exposure which led to secondary osteomyelitis and conversion to Chopart amputation.

should be considered in the setting of robust perfusion, anticipated dead space, or perioperative anticoagulation. The ideal exit point for a drain is at the dorsal forefoot, approximately 2 cm from the incision margins and may be placed medially or laterally. The wound margins are approximated and closed with nonabsorbable suture using a simple interrupted technique. Sutures are left in place for up to 6 weeks, and patients should be non–weight-bearing until healed. At that time, the patient is fit with custom orthotic inserts and toe box filler. Shoe accommodations including high-top diabetic shoes

may improve gait. A carbon plate shoe insert may improve toe-off but increases the likelihood of pathological pressure at the metatarsal amputation site.

Angiosome-based Plantar Flap Options in Transmetatarsal Amputation

The presence of a plantar soft tissue defect associated with neuropathic ulceration, gangrene, or infection may prevent immediate closure with the standard TMA flap geometry and level of metatarsal resection. An alternative option is to perform a more proximal osseous resection to allow adequate soft tissue coverage. However, more proximal amputation levels often result in increased biomechanical dysfunction. Healing by secondary intention is appropriate in some cases, but prolonged exposure of bone may complicate healing at the amputation site (17,18).

Mobilization of angiosome-based plantar flaps is an alternative option that allows immediate closure without the need for excessive bone resection. The defect resulting from excision of a lateral forefoot defect can be covered with rotation of a medial plantar artery angiosome (MPAA) rotational flap (Fig. 27.24). Similarly, excision of a medially localized forefoot wound can be covered with a lateral plantar artery angiosome (LPAA) rotational flap (Fig. 27.25). Coverage of a central defect can be achieved with a combination of MPAA and LPAA rotational flaps (Fig. 27.26). The LPAA is more extensive than the MPAA and involves the majority of the plantar foot. The pivot points for LPAA and MPAA flaps are located at the midarch region. Rotation results in shortening of the flap so the transverse incision is placed more distally than the standard TMA plantar incision. Following excision of

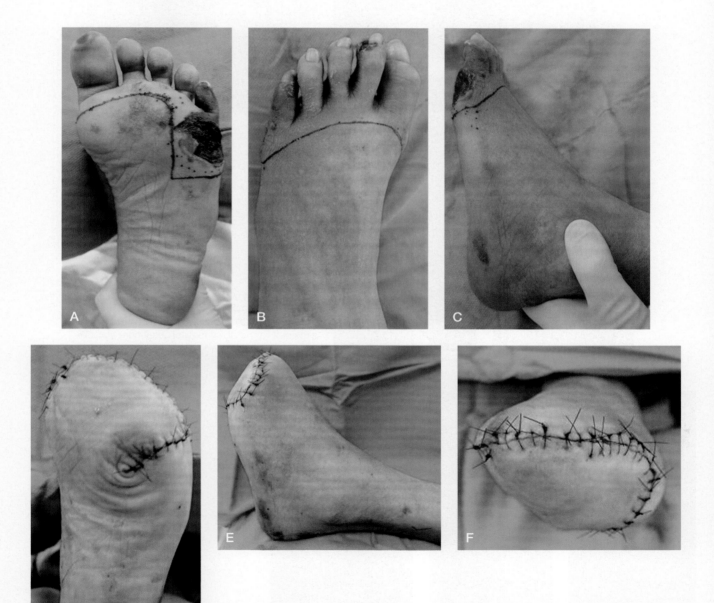

FIGURE 27.24 Compromised tissue on the distal lateral aspect of the plantar weight bearing surface may necessitate incorporation of advanced plastic surgical techniques if soft tissue coverage is to be achieved. The medial plantar artery angiosome (MPAA)–based rotational flaps allow amputation at the transmetatarsal level. **A–C.** A MPAA flap is shown here for broad gangrene of the forefoot. **D–F.** Dorsal and lateral rotation of the MPAA flap achieved complete coverage after transmetatarsal amputation (TMA). *(continued)*

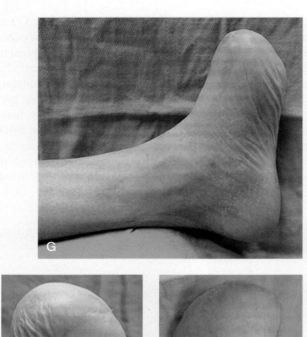

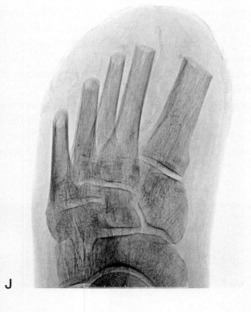

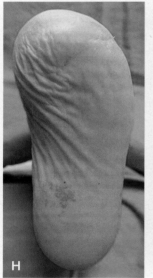

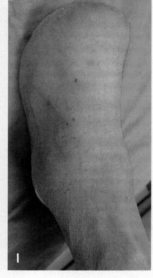

FIGURE 27.24 *(Continued)* **G-I.** Healed MPAA flap TMA at 14 weeks postoperatively with plain radiographs **(J)** showing bone resection just proximal to the distal metaphyseal flare and desired metatarsal parabola.

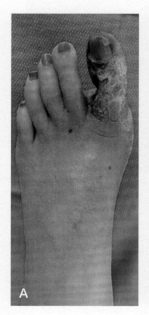

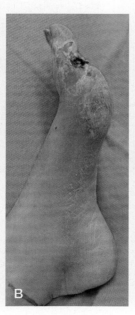

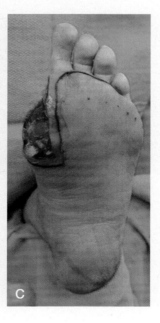

FIGURE 27.25 A,B. The lateral plantar artery angiosome (LPAA) rotational flap at the transmetatarsal amputation (TMA) level is shown here for compromised distal medial tissue associated with gangrene and infection. *(continued)*

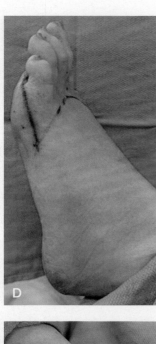

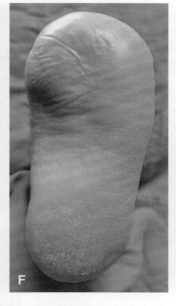

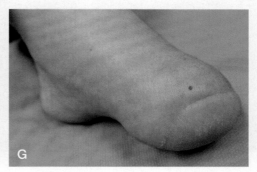

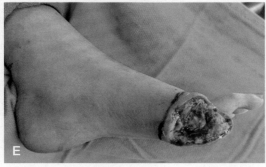

FIGURE 27.25 *(Continued)* **C–E.** Second staged surgery with LPAA incision design. Note how the first surgery open amputation specifically avoided the LPAA allowing resolution of acute infection and vascular intervention prior to TMA with flap closure. **F,G.** Healed amputation stump is without recurrent wound breakdown.

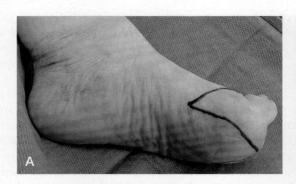

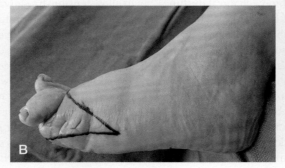

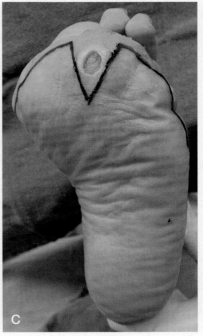

FIGURE 27.26 A–C. Combined medial and lateral plantar artery angiosome flaps are used in the "V" to "T" flap transmetatarsal amputation technique which allows wedge resection to excise a central ray neuropathic ulceration. *(continued)*

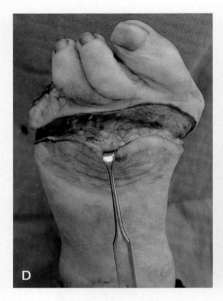
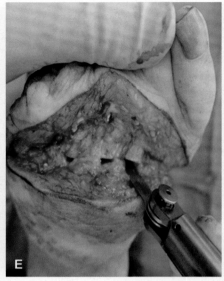
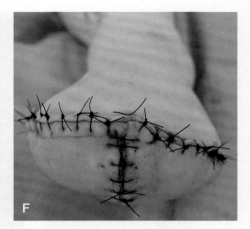
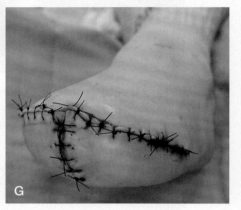

FIGURE 27.26 *(Continued)* **D,E.** Full-depth incisions are made to bone, and the dorsal flap is minimally elevated to gain access for metatarsal resection with a power saw. **F,G.** Note how the medial and lateral plantar flaps converge with the dorsal incision to form a T-shaped incision.

nonviable tissue, the dorsal flap and plantar angiosome-based flaps are raised in a full-thickness fashion with care taken to avoid damage to the associated plantar artery and proximal perforating arteries. Similar concepts may also be applied to achieve immediate soft tissue coverage with more proximal amputation levels including Lisfranc and Chopart.

LISFRANC AMPUTATION

Indications for amputation at the tarsometatarsal joint (TMTJ), or Lisfranc joint, include extensive forefoot gangrene that cannot be addressed with a TMA, and midfoot wounds complicated by osteomyelitis of a metatarsal base. Lisfranc amputation is a less desirable procedure when compared to TMA due to the significant iatrogenic biomechanical dysfunction that can result. Disarticulation at the first TMTJ at least partially disrupts the insertion of the tibialis anterior (TA) and peroneus longus (PL) tendons. Additionally, the insertion of the PB tendon is completely lost with disarticulation of the fifth TMTJ joint. This results in a significant tendon imbalance with unopposed plantarflexion and inversion forces. To achieve a plantigrade foot position that is amenable to bracing, a tendo-Achilles lengthening is frequently required and an attempt to preserve or transfer the disrupted tendon attachments should be considered. The standard Lisfranc amputation procedure is

described as follows, although LPAA and/or MPAA rotational flaps may be utilized if needed for coverage of complex plantar wounds (Fig. 27.27) (17,18).

Lisfranc amputation may be performed with sedation and a local anesthetic block in a patient with advanced peripheral neuropathy, but general anesthesia is required in a sensate patient with extensive gangrene due to vascular disease. A pneumatic ankle tourniquet may be used, especially if robust perfusion is expected.

The incision plan for Lisfranc amputation is similar to that of TMA, but the dorsal and plantar flaps are created with the goal of advancement over the exposed tarsal bones with no tension. A semi-elliptical incision is placed dorsally, approximately 2 cm distal to the TMTJ. A similar incision is placed plantarly but extends further distally than the dorsal incision to allow tension-free advancement of the plantar flap. The medial convergence is located at the middle of the medial cuneiform and the lateral convergence is at the middle of the cuboid, both at a point that bisects the foot from dorsal to plantar (18). Each incision is deepened to bone using the aforementioned technique. Following the skin incision with a scalpel, plantar dissection with electrocautery should be considered due to presence of intrinsic musculature in this area. An osteotomy is performed at the second metatarsal base to create a smooth and continuous surface across the tarsal bones. Prior to disarticulation, the PB tendon should be tagged for future

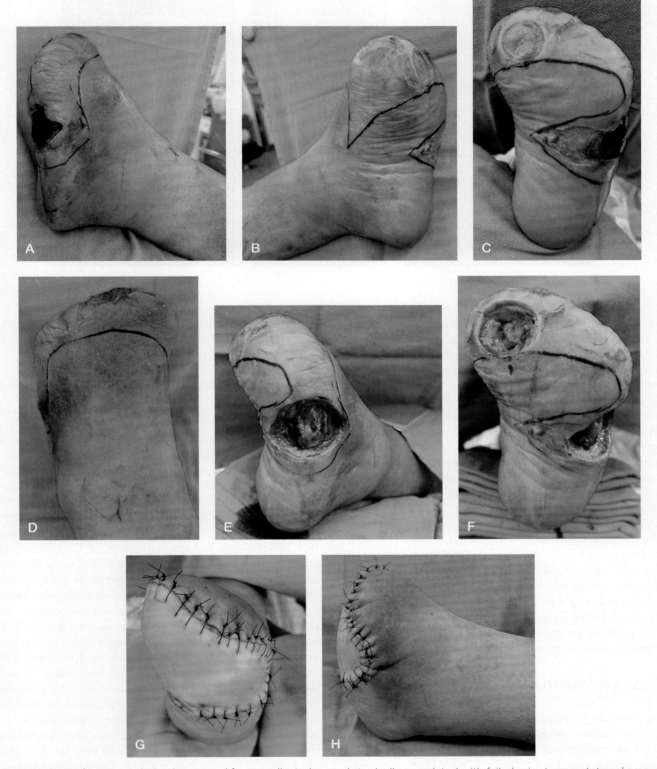

FIGURE 27.27 Lisfranc amputation is reserved for complicated wounds typically associated with failed prior transmetatarsal amputation or Charcot neuroarthropathy with midfoot ulceration. **A–D.** This patient had infected transfer ulcers beneath the first metatarsal and fifth metatarsal base on a previously healed transmetatarsal amputation (TMA) stump. A 2-staged approach allowed incision and drainage of the 2 wound areas including bone débridement and biopsy to determine if the foot could be salvaged with Lisfranc amputation. An incision for medial plantar artery angiosome (MPAA) rotational flap TMA was drawn prior to incision and drainage in an effort to preserve necessary tissues for coverage of the extensive defects. **E,F.** Clinical appearance at staged second surgery performed 3 days later during initial hospitalization. **G,H.** Our baseball flap midfoot amputation technique is shown here with rotation of the MPAA rotational flap to cover the plantar lateral wound deficit. Note how the appearance of the sutured flap resembles a baseball. *(continued)*

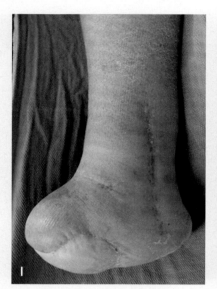
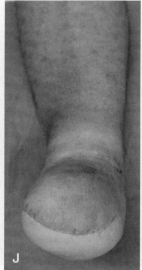
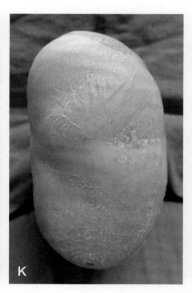

FIGURE 27.27 *(Continued)* **I–K.** Healed amputation site 6 months later.

transfer, if planned. The periarticular structures at the TMTJ are then sharply incised, thus disarticulating the foot at this level, and the forefoot is removed a single unit. Any osseous prominence at the tarsal bones should be remodeled to reduce potential for areas of increased pressure. If possible, the TA and PL tendon insertions at the medial cuneiform should be preserved to provide some opposition to the tibialis posterior and Achilles tendons. Any major bleeding vessels should be ligated as necessary to minimize hematoma formation. Deep sutures may be placed to reduce dead space and minimize skin tension, although this is typically not required. The use of a closed suction drain should be considered in the setting of robust perfusion, anticipated dead space, or perioperative anticoagulation. The wound margins are apposed and closed with nonabsorbable suture using a simple interrupted technique. The flaps may be remodeled if needed to allow better apposition. Sutures are typically left in place for 4 to 6 weeks. Patients are strictly non–weight-bearing for 6 weeks to allow adequate healing. Once weight bearing is resumed, a custom ankle foot orthosis or partial foot prosthesis should be considered due to the potential for equinovarus contracture and the limited propulsion available from a short stump.

CHOPART AMPUTATION

Indications for transtarsal or Chopart amputation include extensive midfoot gangrene that cannot be addressed with a Lisfranc amputation and midfoot wounds complicated by osteomyelitis of a tarsal bone. As with Lisfranc amputation, iatrogenic loss of TA, PL, and PB tendons predispose to contracture and instability. Due to the biomechanical and prosthetic challenges that may arise postoperatively, this procedure is typically reserved for those who refuse a proximal leg amputation and those who will primarily use their stump for transfers and limited ambulation. The standard Chopart

amputation procedure is described as follows, although LPAA and/or MPAA rotational flaps may be utilized if needed for coverage of complex plantar wounds (10).

Standard Chopart Amputation Procedure

Semi-elliptical transverse incisions are placed dorsally and plantarly over the TMTJ. Incisions extend proximally to converge medially and laterally at the level of the midtarsal joint (Fig. 27.28). Flap geometry may require modification to allow adequate coverage and apposition with minimal tension in the setting of compromised local tissue. The incision is deepened in a full-thickness fashion. The TA and PB tendons are identified, dissected from their insertions, and tagged for possible transfer. The dorsal and plantar flaps are raised in a full-thickness fashion to the level of the talonavicular and calcaneocuboid joints, which are then sharply disarticulated. The distal segment of the foot is then removed as 1 unit. Once exposed, the anterior aspect of the calcaneus should be evaluated for areas of prominence and remodeled if necessary. Adjunctive tendon balancing procedures include TA tendon transfer to the talar neck, tendo-Achilles lengthening, and PB transfer to the anterior calcaneus. These procedures may be performed at the time of the amputation or may be staged if there is concern for persistent infection. Bleeding vessels should be ligated as necessary to minimize blood loss and hematoma formation. Electrocautery is selectively used to address any minor bleeding vessels in cases of peripheral arterial disease and gangrene. It can also be used for deep plantar dissection if circulation is intact. The flaps are advanced with minimal handling and closed with nonabsorbable suture. Deep closure is typically not needed, but use of a closed suction drain should be considered. Sutures are left in place for up to 6 weeks. Six to 8 weeks of strict non–weight-bearing is to be expected for full healing. A partial foot prosthetic device is preferred in an effort to maximize function and balance.

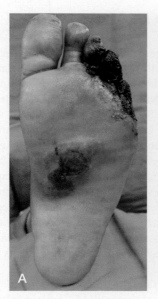
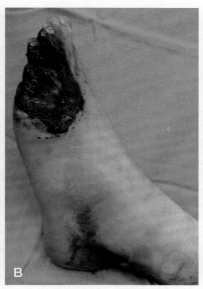
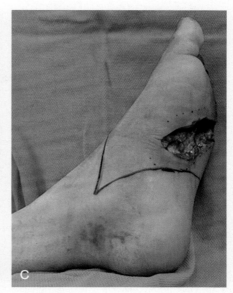

FIGURE 27.28 A,B. Chopart amputation for gangrene, vascular compromise, osteomyelitis, and abscess. **C.** Dorsal and plantar incision design is shown with medial and lateral midline apex.

Modified Chopart Amputation Procedure

Chopart amputation is associated with poor outcome due to excessive weight bearing along the distal aspect of the plantar calcaneus. Loss of calcaneal inclination is expected after amputation of the forefoot and the majority of weight bearing stress will be on the anterior aspect of the calcaneus.

Our preferred procedure with bone resection modifications is described in Figure 27.29. We prefer to maintain the navicular and remodel the anterior calcaneus in an effort to balance the foot and minimize lateral wound breakdown (10). Surgical technique and postoperative appearance are described in Figure 27.30.

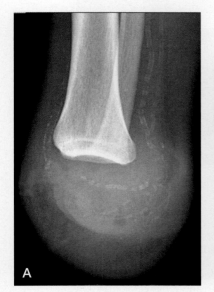
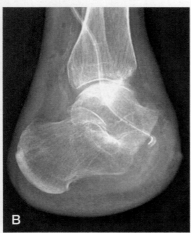
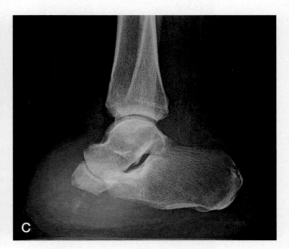

FIGURE 27.29 A. Plain radiographs are shown to compare levels of bone resection with Syme amputation, standard Chopart amputation **(B)**, and modified Chopart amputation **(C)**. Chopart amputation preserves the overall length of the limb compared with Syme amputation; however, weight bearing is on a small surface area of the calcaneus which predisposes to recurrent stump breakdown. Our modified Chopart amputation technique preserves the navicular in an effort to maintain some weight bearing along the medial column because the talar head is not likely to bear weight after midtarsal joint disarticulation. The distal weight bearing surface of the calcaneus is also remodeled to minimize plantar lateral prominence. Note how the modified Chopart amputation stump lays flat on the ground with maximum plantarflexion through the ankle joint. This modified technique attempts to balance equal weight in front of and behind the functional portion of the talar dome. *(continued)*

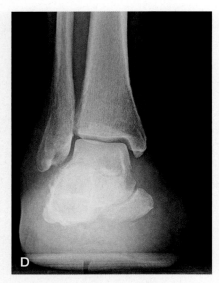

FIGURE 27.29 *(Continued)* **D.** Weight bearing plain radiograph after modified Chopart amputation demonstrates balanced pressure between the preserved navicular and remodeled anterior calcaneus.

PARTIAL CALCANECTOMY

Partial calcanectomy is generally viewed as a last resort option for limb salvage in the setting of a heel wound associated with necrosis and osteomyelitis of the calcaneus. Complicated decubitus heel wounds with secondary calcaneal osteomyelitis and tissue necrosis create challenges associated with the large wound deficit (Fig. 27.31). The structural and functional importance of the calcaneus in addition to the likely presence of locally devitalized soft tissue are factors to consider when determining the viability of this limb salvage approach (Fig. 27.32). In many cases, the extent of calcaneal necrosis and lack of viable soft tissue for closure make a proximal leg amputation the most appropriate choice. This procedure is typically reserved for those with osteomyelitis limited to the calcaneus, adequate local soft tissue for closure, and for patients who are minimally ambulatory.

Figure 27.33 demonstrates the traditional technique without flap closure. Flap closure of the wound is sometimes necessary with flap geometry and ideal donor site dictated by the extent and location of the decubitus wound (7,8). The procedure is

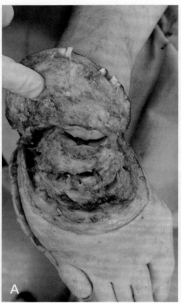

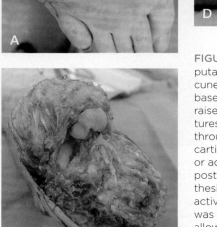

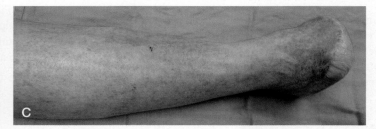

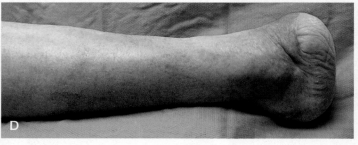

FIGURE 27.30 **A.** The surgical technique for modified Chopart amputation involves raising the dorsal flap to gain access for naviculocuneiform disarticulation *(finger pointing)*. Note how the metatarsal bases and cuneiforms are skeletonized confirming that the flap was raised full-thickness including the periosteum and all vascular structures. **B.** A large plantar flap is shown here after disarticulation through the naviculocuneiform and calcaneocuboid joints. Intact cartilage can be removed if there is concern about nidus for infection or adherence of the flap. **C.** Healed Chopart amputation at 6 months postoperatively, with return to full ambulation in a partial foot prosthesis 6 weeks after surgery without need for rehabilitation. **D.** Note active dorsiflexion even though no tendon transfers or lengthening was performed. The anterior tendons form scar tissue adhesions that allow active dorsiflexion, yet this is ineffective at maintaining calcaneal inclination which is why the navicular is preserved. This patient is able to ambulate in the home without the prosthesis.

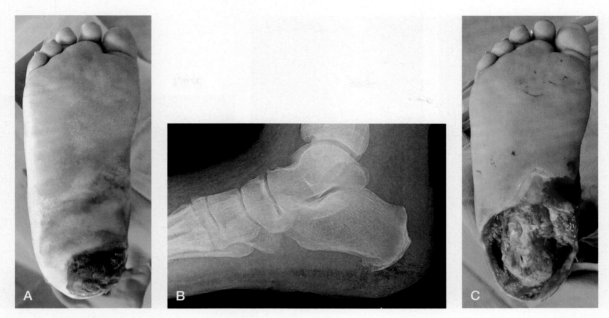

FIGURE 27.31 Partial calcanectomy may not be a feasible option in patients with extensive soft tissue necrosis surrounding the heel. **A.** Acute necrosis of soft tissue is shown with secondary infection associated with chronic decubitus heel ulceration. **B.** Plain radiograph indicates gas gangrene. **C.** Emergency incision and drainage was performed with wide resection of the necrotic tissue. Note broad exposure of the calcaneus with limited options for soft tissue coverage after even complete calcanectomy. Guillotine amputation was necessary 2 days later with delayed conversion to below-the-knee amputation after the acute infection resolved.

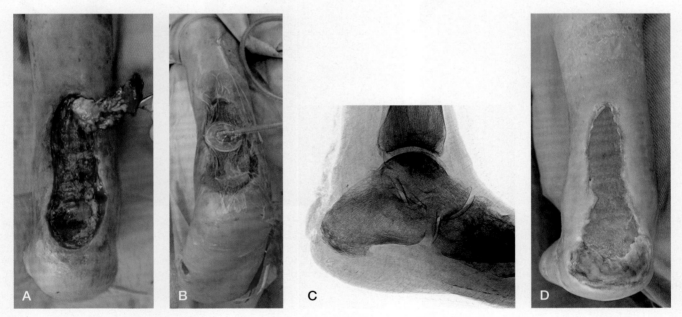

FIGURE 27.32 A. Decubitus heel ulceration resulted in exposure and necrosis of the Achilles tendon *(in forceps)*. Secondary infection of the calcaneus developed while waiting for tissue demarcation. The calcaneus is seen at the distal extent of the wound which was discolored, necrotic, filled with purulence, and lacked intact cortical structure. **B.** Broad wound débridement, complete excision of the Achilles tendon, partial calcanectomy, and application of negative pressure wound therapy (NPWT). **C.** An attempt was made to preserve the plantar weight bearing surface of the heel. **D.** Note healthy granulation tissue after 6 weeks of NPWT, however, with progressive necrosis of the skin and subcutaneous tissue at the distal extent of the wound. This area likely suffered ongoing decubitus pressure which required resection and secondary healing prior to split-thickness skin grafting.

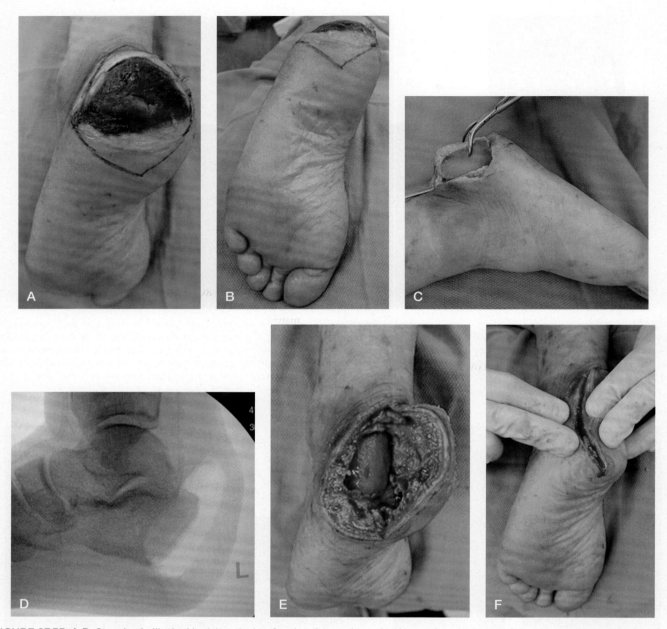

FIGURE 27.33 A,B. Standard elliptical incision design for decubitus ulceration located at the apex of the heel. **C.** Removal of a large section of the calcaneal tuberosity allows mobility of the medial and lateral soft tissues for designed primary closure. **D.** Remodeling of the superior, inferior, medial, and lateral edges of the calcaneal tuberosity minimizes pressure points associated with weight bearing and decubitus pressure when walking, lying in bed, or sitting in a wheelchair. **E.** The tuberosity is frequently viable despite osteomyelitis. Note healthy-appearing cancellous bone with intact bone bleeding and viable wound margins. **F.** Advancement of the medial and lateral tissues frequently allows primary closure.

performed in the prone position and a pneumatic ankle tourniquet may be used but is not required. The heel wound is excised in a full-thickness fashion with the scalpel entering the skin at a 90 degree angle and following the contour of the heel. If the procedure is to be staged, flap closure and calcanectomy may be delayed until acute infection has resolved. Soft tissue is raised off the calcaneus with care taken to avoid injury to the medial neurovascular structures. An osteotomy guide pin is placed in the calcaneus at the anticipated angle of resection which is then evaluated with intraoperative fluoroscopy. The osteotomy

should be placed such that nonviable bone is removed, and there is no focal prominence in areas likely to receive sustained pressure, including the posterior heel when lying in the supine position. Extensive removal of bone promotes tension-free flap closure because wide resection of bone introduces soft tissue laxity. A sagittal saw is typically used to start the osteotomy, using the radiographically confirmed guide pin position as a reference. An osteotome may be used to complete the osteotomy because it is likely to exit deep within plantar soft tissue. Following removal of the calcaneal fragment, the exposed calcaneal surfaces are evaluated for rough edges or areas of prominence and remodeled as necessary. Nonabsorbable sutures are used for closure and are removed in approximately 6 weeks. The operative extremity should be non–weight-bearing for approximately 6 weeks, with care taken to off-load the heel at all times, including while prone in bed. Loss of Achilles tendon function and calcaneal height requires use of an accommodative rigid ankle foot orthosis to allow the operative extremity to serve as a stable support.

ADJUNCTIVE THERAPIES

Persistent and recurrent wounds associated with diabetic partial foot amputation can be complex and challenging to heal, especially if immediate wound closure is not attainable. There are many adjunctive therapies that can be utilized to improve healing potential in conjunction with careful surgical planning and execution. Negative pressure wound therapy is commonly used and has been shown to promote granulation tissue and reduce time to complete wound closure when compared to standard moist wound therapy options (1,2,32). Split-thickness skin grafts can also be used to promote healing (37,47). Split-thickness skin grafts must be placed over viable granular tissue and may be used in conjunction with platelet-rich plasma and negative pressure wound therapy. For wounds that have not responded to standard treatments, hyperbaric oxygen therapy has been shown to be beneficial for long-term healing (30,43).

Conclusion

Lower extremity amputation procedures are frequently performed to manage complications of diabetes mellitus including infected neuropathic ulcers, deep abscess, osteomyelitis, gangrene, necrotizing fasciitis, and Charcot neuroarthropathy. There are many treatment options available for salvage of the diabetic foot, including various levels of partial foot amputations and adjunctive procedures. The most appropriate procedure should be selected on a case-by-case basis; however, the stepwise approach we describe can serve as a guide to decision making. The primary goals of amputation are prompt resolution of infection with a combined medical and surgical approach, removal of nonviable tissue to a level that is functional and capable of healing, and obtainment of biopsy and culture to direct antibiotic therapy. Long-term success requires a detailed evaluation of the patient's biomechanical and functional needs and the healing potential with the implementation of a carefully selected and performed amputation plan. A multidisciplinary approach including the added expertise of the foot and ankle surgical team helps to optimize treatment outcomes for the high-risk diabetic population.

References

1. Armstrong DG, Lavery LA. Negative pressure wound therapy after partial diabetic foot amputation: a multicentre, randomised controlled trial. Lancet 2005;366:1704–1710.

2. Blume PA, Walters J, Payne W, et al. Comparison of negative pressure wound therapy using vacuum-assisted closure with advanced moist wound therapy in the treatment of diabetic foot ulcers: a multicenter randomized controlled trial. Diabetes Care 2008;31:631–636.

3. Boffeli TJ, Abben KW. Acral fibrokeratoma of the foot treated with excision and trap door flap closure: a case report. J Foot Ankle Surg 2014;53:449–452.

4. Boffeli TJ, Abben KW. Complete fifth ray amputation with peroneal tendon transfer—a staged surgical protocol. J Foot Ankle Surg 2012;51:696–701.

5. Boffeli TJ, Abben KW, Hyllengren SB. In-office distal Symes lesser toe amputation: a safe, reliable, and cost-effective treatment of diabetes-related tip of toe ulcers complicated by osteomyelitis. J Foot Ankle Surg 2014;53:720–726.

6. Boffeli TJ, Bean JK, Natwick JR. Biomechanical abnormalities and ulcers of the great toe in patients with diabetes. J Foot Ankle Surg 2002;41:359–364.

7. Boffeli TJ, Collier RC. Near total calcanectomy with rotational flap closure of large decubitus heel ulcerations complicated by calcaneal osteomyelitis. J Foot Ankle Surg 2013;52:107–112.

8. Boffeli TJ, Collier RC. Osteomyelitis of the calcaneus. In: Boffeli TJ, ed. Osteomyelitis of the foot and ankle: medical and surgical management. Cham, Switzerland: Springer International Publishing, 2015:297–323.

9. Boffeli TJ, Hyllengren SB, Peterson MC. First ray osteomyelitis. In: Boffeli TJ, ed. Osteomyelitis of the foot and ankle: medical and surgical management. Cham, Switzerland: Springer International Publishing, 2015:167–196.

10. Boffeli TJ, Mahoney KJ. Chopart's amputation for osteomyelitis of the midfoot. In: Boffeli TJ, ed. Osteomyelitis of the foot and ankle: medical and surgical management. Cham, Switzerland: Springer International Publishing, 2015:283–296.

11. Boffeli TJ, Peterson MC. Rotational flap closure of first and fifth metatarsal head plantar ulcers: adjunctive procedure when performing first or fifth ray amputation. J Foot Ankle Surg 2013;52:263–270.

12. Boffeli TJ, Pfannenstein RR, Thompson JC. Radiation therapy for recurrent heterotopic ossification prophylaxis after partial metatarsal amputation. J Foot Ankle Surg 2015;54:345–349.

13. Boffeli TJ, Tabatt JA, Abben KW. Fifth ray osteomyelitis. In: Boffeli TJ, ed. Osteomyelitis of the foot and ankle: medical and surgical management. Cham, Switzerland: Springer International Publishing, 2015:229–251.

14. Boffeli TJ, Thompson JC. Central metatarsal osteomyelitis. In: Boffeli TJ, ed. Osteomyelitis of the foot and ankle: medical and surgical management. Cham, Switzerland: Springer International Publishing, 2015:217–228.

15. Boffeli TJ, Thompson JC. Partial foot amputations for salvage of the diabetic lower extremity. Clin Podiatric Med Surg 2014;31:103–126.

16. Boffeli TJ, Thompson JC, Waverly BJ, et al. Incidence and clinical significance of heterotopic ossification after partial ray resection. J Foot Ankle Surg 2016;55:714–719.

17. Boffeli TJ, Waverly BJ. Medial and lateral plantar artery angiosome rotational flaps for transmetatarsal and Lisfranc amputation in patients with compromised plantar tissue. J Foot Ankle Surg 2015;55:351–361.

18. Boffeli TJ, Waverly BJ. Transmetatarsal and Lisfranc amputation. In: Boffeli TJ , ed. Osteomyelitis of the foot and ankle: medical and surgical management. Cham, Switzerland: Springer International Publishing, 2015:253–282.

19. Boulton AJ, Armstrong DG, Albert SF, et al. Comprehensive foot examination and risk assessment: a report of the Task Force of the Foot Care Interest Group of the American Diabetes Association, with endorsement by the American Association of Clinical Endocrinologists. Diabetes Care 2008;31:1679–1685.

20. Bowker JH. Partial foot amputations and disarticulations. Foot Ankle Clin 1997;2:153–170.

21. Brown ML, Tang W, Patel A, et al. Partial foot amputation in patients with diabetic foot ulcers. Foot Ankle Int 2012;33:707–716.

22. Centers for Disease Control and Prevention. National diabetes statistics report. Available at: http://www.cdc.gov/diabetes/data/statistics/2014statisticsreport.html. Published 2014. Accessed November 11, 2015.

23. Clark N, Sheehan P, Edmonds M, et al. Peripheral arterial disease in people with diabetes. Diabetes Care 2003;26:3333–3341.

24. Davis WA, Norman PE, Bruce DG, et al. Predictors, consequences and costs of diabetes-related lower extremity amputation complicating type 2 diabetes: the Fremantle Diabetes Study. Diabetologia 2006;49:2634–2641.

25. DeCotiis MA. Lisfranc and Chopart amputations. Clin Podiatr Med Surg 2005;22:385–393.

26. Frykberg RG, Zgonis T, Armstrong DG, et al. Diabetic foot disorders. A clinical practice guideline (2006 revision). J Foot Ankle Surg 2006;45(5 suppl):S1–S66.

27. Göktepe AS, Cakir B, Yilmaz B, et al. Energy expenditure of walking with prostheses: comparison of three amputation levels. Prosthet Orthot Int 2010;34:31–36.

28. Keagy BA, Schwartz JA, Kotb M, et al. Lower extremity amputation: the control series. J Vasc Surg 1986;4:321–326.

29. Landry GJ, Silverman DA, Liem TK, et al. Predictors of healing and functional outcome following transmetatarsal amputations. Arch Surg 2011;146:1005–1009.

30. Löndahl M, Katzman P, Nilsson A, et al. Hyperbaric oxygen therapy facilitates healing of chronic foot ulcers in patients with diabetes. Diabetes Care 2010;33:998–1003.

31. Marks RM, Long JT, Exten EL. Gait abnormality following amputation in diabetic patients. Foot Ankle Clin 2010;15:501–507.

32. Mendonca DA, Cosker T, Makwana NK. Vacuum-assisted closure to aid wound healing in foot and ankle surgery. Foot Ankle Int 2005;26:761–766.

33. Miller JD, Zhubrak M, Giovinco NA, et al. The too few toes principle: a formula for limb-sparing low-level amputation planning. Wound Med 2014;4:37–41.

34. Moore JC, Jolly GP. Soft tissue considerations in partial foot amputations. Clin Podiatr Med Surg 2000;17:631–648.

35. Nehler MR, Coll JR, Hiatt WR, et al. Functional outcome in a contemporary series of major lower extremity amputations. J Vasc Surg 2003;38:7–14.

36. Nguyen TH, Gordon IL, Whalen D, et al. Transmetatarsal amputation: predictors of healing. Am Surg 2006;72:973–977.

37. Picard F, Hersant B, Bosc R, et al. The growing evidence for the use of platelet-rich plasma on diabetic chronic wounds: a review and a proposal for a new standard care. Wound Repair Regen 2015;23:638–643.

38. Pollard J, Hamilton GA, Rush SM, et al. Mortality and morbidity after transmetatarsal amputation: retrospective review of 101 cases. J Foot Ankle Surg 2006;45:91–97.

39. Reiber GE, Vileikyte LO, Boyko ED, et al. Causal pathways for incident lower-extremity ulcers in patients with diabetes from two settings. Diabetes Care 1999;22:157–162.

40. Rosen RC. Digital amputations. Clin Podiatr Med Surg 2005;22:343–363.

41. Sage R, Pinzur MS, Cronin R, et al. Complications following midfoot amputation in neuropathic and dysvascular feet. J Am Pod Med Assoc 1989;79:277–280.

42. Santi M, Thoma BJ, Chambers RB. Survivorship of healed partial foot amputations in dysvascular patients. Clin Orthop Relat Res 1993;292:245–249.

43. Thom SR. Hyperbaric oxygen: its mechanisms and efficacy. Plast Reconstr Surg 2011;127(suppl 1):131–141.

44. Thomas SR, Perkins JM, Magee TR, et al. Transmetatarsal amputation: an 8-year experience. Ann R Coll Surg Engl 2001;83:164–166.

45. Ward KH, Meyers MC. Exercise performance of lower-extremity amputees. Sports Med 1995;20:207–214.

46. Waters RL, Perry J, Antonelli D, et al. Energy cost of walking of amputees: the influence of level of amputation. J Bone Joint Surg Am 1976;58:42–46.

47. Zgonis T, Stapleton JJ, Roukis TS. Advanced plastic surgery techniques for soft tissue coverage of the diabetic foot. Clin Podiatr Med Surg 2007;24:547–568.

CHAPTER 28

Tendon Balancing and Osseous Procedures for Diabetic Foot Amputations

Devin C. Simonson • Andrew D. Elliott • Thomas S. Roukis

INTRODUCTION

Partial foot amputation is largely considered an undesired end point when treating limb-threatening conditions of the diabetic lower extremity. Although all reasonable attempts to preserve a patient's foot should be considered, the functionality of the limb and likelihood of recurrent ulceration or infection must be assessed.

INDICATIONS/CONTRAINDICATIONS

Even though early toe amputation in the diabetic patient has been shown to be cost-effective in the short term, the natural history of toe amputations does not provide a predictably durable outcome over the long term (1,7). In some cases, a well-balanced partial forefoot or midfoot amputation will provide the patient a more functional extremity that will better maintain their independence than a salvage procedure (1,7,8). Unfortunately, performing an isolated partial forefoot or midfoot amputation does not guarantee a functional, durable limb. In the diabetic neuropathic patient, ulcerations result from excessive, repeated pressure and shear on a concentrated area of the foot. Diabetic neuropathic patients with deformity and a history of ulceration have a 36 times greater risk for reulceration than the general population. Equinovarus deformity is a widely recognized complication of transmetatarsal and Chopart amputations. This often leads to recurrent ulceration and more proximal amputation (1–8).

Transmetatarsal amputation is most commonly indicated when gangrene or soft tissue necrosis has occurred in 2 or more toes or when 2 or more ray (toe and metatarsal) resections are necessary. Other indications include open traumatic injury of the forefoot or significant forefoot deformity with chronic pain or recurrent ulceration (Fig. 28.1) (6). Chopart amputation is indicated when the metatarsal or tarsal bones have severe deformity or infection that would preclude the ability to perform a transmetatarsal amputation but when the plantar heel pad anatomy is undisturbed (Fig. 28.2) (8). Transmetatarsal

and Chopart amputations have been employed with varying degrees of success since first being formally evaluated in the later part of the 19th century and early part of the 20th century. Although the surgical approach has evolved from an open amputation with protracted periods of bed rest and wound packing followed by skin grafting to a single-stage procedure with primary closure of a thick plantar flap, it is interesting to note that the overall success rate has not improved. Failure rates for transmetatarsal and Chopart amputations have been reported from 17% to 50% (6,8). In looking critically at these complications, the majority can be traced back to 3 etiologies: (a) patient noncompliance, (b) patient medical comorbidities, and (c) unaddressed patient pedal deformity (6,8). Great care should be taken to evaluate the patient and address these potential etiologies for failure preoperatively and throughout the recovery course. A well-done primary below-the-knee amputation through clean tissue planes is preferred in a patient who is unable or unwilling to proceed through the lengthy involved recovery required for limb salvage surgery, including transmetatarsal and Chopart amputations. However, cardiac demand, energy expenditure, and mortality rates have been shown to be decreased with partial foot amputations compared to below-the-knee and above-the-knee amputations making partial foot amputations preferable when appropriate (8).

PREOPERATIVE CONSIDERATIONS

Deciding on the appropriate amputation level for an individual patient is based on multiple considerations, including vascular supply, available soft tissue coverage, lower extremity deformities, and/or history of previous surgery. An ankle-brachial index of ≤0.45 is generally considered incompatible with healing, whereas transcutaneous oxygen tension of ≥30 mmHg or greater indicates, but does not guarantee, the potential to heal. More recently, toe pressure of ≤30 mmHg has also demonstrated a low healing potential. When a patient's arterial supply is in question, a vascular surgeon or endovascular specialist should

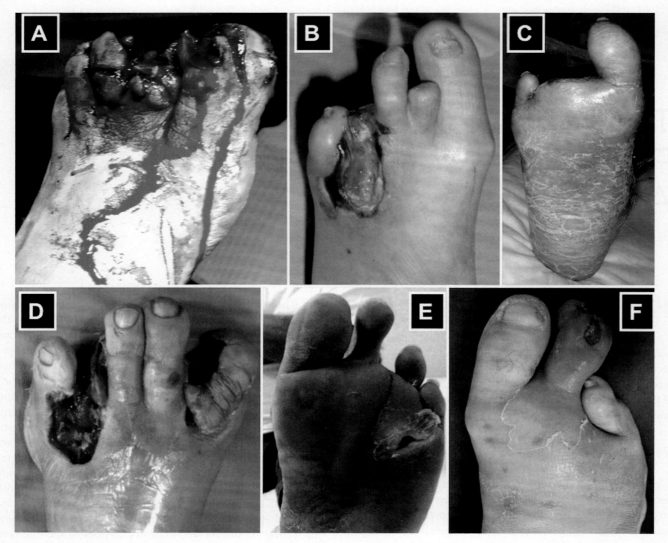

FIGURE 28.1 Clinical photographs demonstrating multiple open fractures **(A)**, residual forefoot deformity following toe and metatarsal amputations **(B)**, residual forefoot with multiple amputations of the second, third, and fourth toes **(C)**, open amputation of the medial and lateral forefoot **(D)**, transfer ulceration at the plantar fourth metatarsal head following third ray amputation **(E)**, and osteomyelitis of the second toe following third and fourth toe amputation **(F)**. Each of these situations is amenable to a well-performed and balanced transmetatarsal amputation.

be consulted to determine if revascularization procedures are indicated. The partial foot amputation must be performed at a level with adequate perfusion to heal and working closely with a vascular surgeon is strongly recommended (1,6,8,10,12).

Large open wounds on the dorsal or plantar foot must be excised prior to definitive closure of an amputation. These findings may necessitate more proximal amputation if adequate soft tissue is not available for coverage, especially of the plantar tissues. Although primary closure is preferred, alternate methods of wound closure can be utilized if necessary. Skin grafts are generally thought to be a poor choice for coverage on weight bearing areas but can be utilized in non-weight-bearing areas of the foot for wound closure. Local flap coverage of plantar wounds may be possible depending on the size of the defect, mobility of the regional tissue, and adequacy of arterial supply. Free flaps have been described but are less than ideal. They can leave excessive bulk that is difficult to fit in a shoe or

brace and prone to breakdown from the shear forces between the native and transferred tissue. Performing the amputation at a level in which primary closure can be performed will avoid the additional incisions and potential vascular compromise associated with alternate wound coverage techniques and may ultimately lead to a more functional and durable result (12).

Equinovarus deformity seen after transmetatarsal and Chopart amputations performed without proper balancing often results in ulceration at the plantar-lateral aspect of the stump. Following transmetatarsal and Chopart amputation, the foot is reduced in length leading to overpowering by the gastrocnemius-soleus complex, and the transverse arch of the foot is structurally aligned in varus due to the loss of the metatarsal heads and tarsal contents. Therefore, the foot automatically assumes an equinovarus posture. When left unaddressed, the equinus deformity will worsen due to the elimination of extensor digitorum longus and extensor hallucis longus

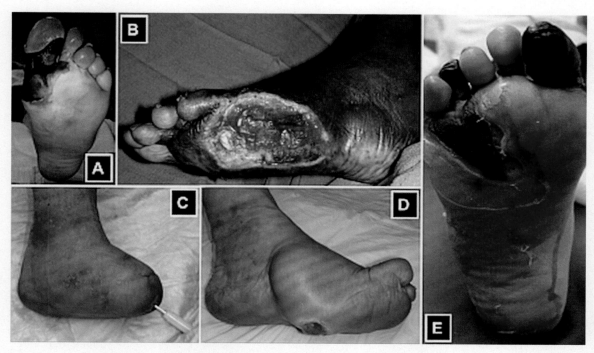

FIGURE 28.2 Clinical photographs demonstrating necrosis of the entire medial forefoot **(A)**, chronic wound with osteomyelitis of the lateral forefoot **(B)**, failed transmetatarsal amputation with osteomyelitis of the medial forefoot (note the culture swab extending along the medial column into the hindfoot) **(C)**, ulcerated Charcot neuroarthropathy of a midfoot deformity with abscess **(D)**, and necrosis of the hallux and central-lateral forefoot **(E)**. Each of these situations is amenable to a well-performed and balanced Chopart amputation.

muscle function postoperatively in transmetatarsal amputations or the tibialis anterior and peroneus brevis in Chopart amputations. The loss of these muscle attachments causes an imbalance between the posterior compartment and the anterior compartment resulting in plantarflexion at the ankle joint. Likewise, the varus deformity will worsen if left unaddressed secondary to the loss of intrinsic muscle function and disruption of the insertion of the plantar fascia. This causes subtalar joint imbalance and increased inversion pull of the tibialis anterior and deep posterior muscles which overpower the eversion strength of the peroneus brevis muscle in transmetatarsal amputations and loss of all lateral restraint in Chopart amputations. Therefore, when performing amputations, the surgeon must evaluate the patient's global foot structure and determine the etiology of the initial problem and what potential deformities may occur postoperatively. The amputation must be performed at the most distal level compatible with healing and wound closure. If each of the patient's deformities and potential deforming forces can be surgically addressed, the likelihood of recurrent ulceration should be reduced because proper balancing of the residual stump will generally provide a durable, stable, and functional foot (3,4,5,9,10,12).

SURGICAL TECHNIQUE

Transmetatarsal Amputation

Transmetatarsal amputation begins with the patient positioned in the supine position on the operating room table with a well-padded bolster placed beneath the ipsilateral buttock

to control physiologic external rotation of the lower limb. The procedure is most commonly performed under general anesthesia with popliteal and saphenous peripheral nerve block because tendo-Achilles lengthening or gastrocnemius recession that accompanies transmetatarsal amputations requires anesthesia of the lower leg. Local regional anesthesia is contraindicated in the presence of active infection or gangrene in the field to be infiltrated. The use of a tourniquet is avoided in the presence of peripheral arterial disease but is routinely employed in patients without vascular compromise to decrease the time necessary to complete the procedure, improve visualization of the anatomy, and limit acute blood loss.

Each of the toes should be grasped with a towel clamp through the distal interphalangeal joint (Fig. 28.3) in order to both facilitate dissection by employing the clamp as a "toggle" to move the toe as well as limit handling of the infected necrotic tissue by the surgical team which maintains an aseptic surgical field. The toes are plantarflexed as a unit that makes the dorsal aspect of the metatarsal heads prominent at the distal forefoot (Fig. 28.4A). The initial incision extends from the medial aspect of the first metatarsal head across each of the central metatarsal heads and culminates over the lateral aspect of the fifth metatarsal head. The surgical knife is carried through the subcutaneous tissues into the underlying metatarsophalangeal joints with care taken to deepen the knife into the intermetatarsal spaces as it is advanced from one joint to the next (Fig. 28.4B). This technique maintains a full-thickness dorsal skin flap and speeds dissection (Fig. 28.4C). Next, the toes are dorsiflexed as a unit, and the second incision extends from the medial incision across the plantar forefoot to connect with the lateral incision coursing

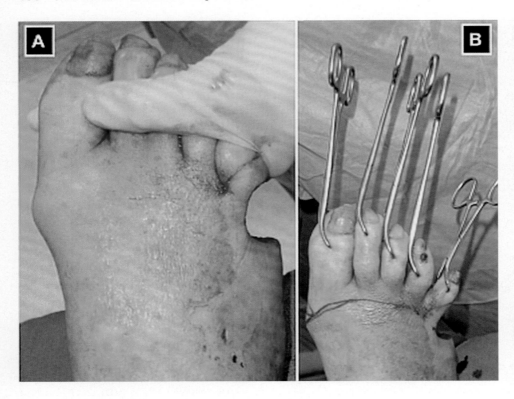

FIGURE 28.3 Clinical photographs demonstrating the incorrect (A) and correct (B) way to grasp the toes during transmetatarsal amputation.

along the junction between the plantar toe skin and forefoot fat padding (Fig. 28.5). In the presence of medial (Fig. 28.6), plantar (Fig. 28.7), or lateral (Fig. 28.8) forefoot ulceration, the incision is modified to include the ulceration in the resected tissue. The surgical knife is then carried from the base of the exposed proximal phalanges proximally to the level of the metatarsophalangeal joints just superficial to the flexor tendons and plantar plates. This allows the plantar flap to remain full-thickness that in turn maintains vascular supply. The forefoot is then disarticulated at the joint level by severing the remaining

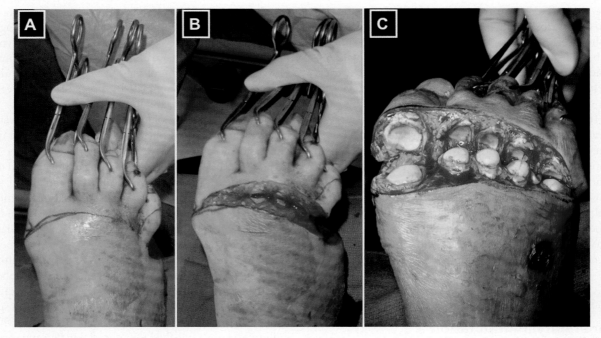

FIGURE 28.4 Clinical photographs demonstrating the surgeon grasping the towel clamps in the nondominant hand (A) followed by incision across the forefoot at the metatarsophalangeal joint level (B). With proper attention to detail, a single pass of the surgical knife will cleanly incise the metatarsophalangeal joints (C).

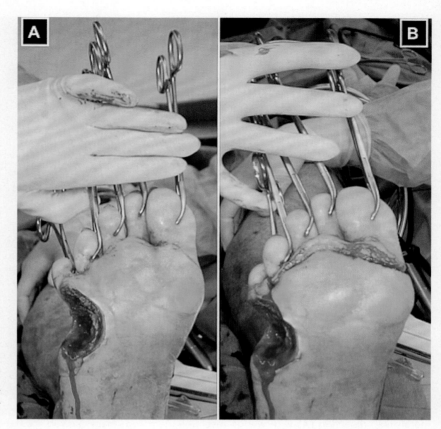

FIGURE 28.5 Clinical photographs demonstrating dorsiflexion of the toes **(A)** followed by full-thickness incision at the digital sulcus level **(B)**.

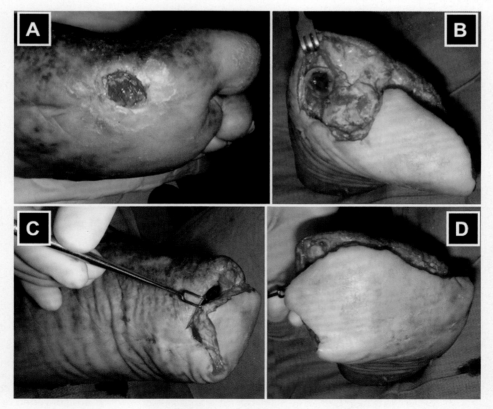

FIGURE 28.6 Clinical photographs demonstrating a full-thickness ulceration, underlying osteomyelitis and deformed forefoot **(A)**. The ulceration and first ray (toe and metatarsal) have been resected leaving a full-thickness plantar flap **(B)** that can easily be rotated medially to cover the resultant defect as demonstrated in pictures **(C)** and **(D)**.

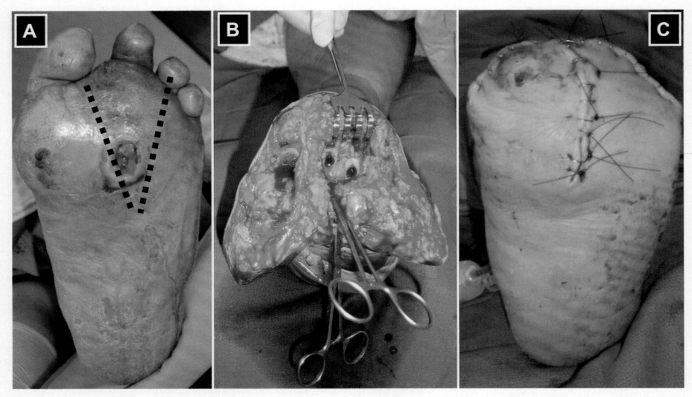

FIGURE 28.7 Clinical photographs demonstrating transfer ulceration to the second metatarsal head following third ray (toe and metatarsal) resection **(A)** with wedge resection identified *(black hashed lines)*. Following resection of the forefoot, the resultant medial and lateral plantar flaps are demonstrated **(B)** followed by layered closure **(C)**.

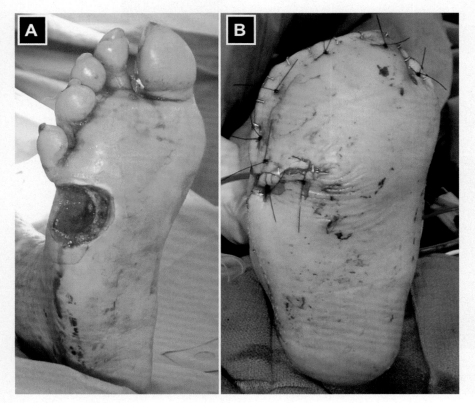

FIGURE 28.8 Clinical photographs following resection of the fourth and fifth metatarsals and resultant soft tissue defect **(A)**, which was converted to a transmetatarsal amputation using a medially based full-thickness flap that has been rotated to cover the lateral defect **(B)**.

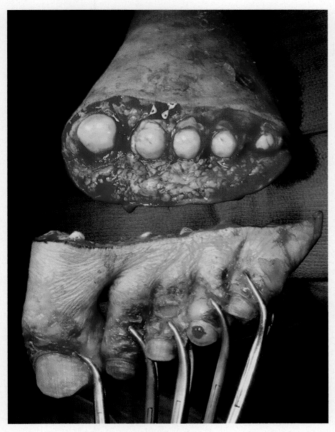

FIGURE 28.9 Clinical photograph after disarticulation of the toes from the metatarsophalangeal joints demonstrating well-perfused and full-thickness soft tissues retained in the residual forefoot.

capsular and ligamentous connections (Fig. 28.9). The capsule and periosteal tissues overlying the dorsal, medial, and lateral aspect of the first metatarsal are freed with a surgical knife followed by placement of a large key elevator or, alternatively, a narrow osteotome which is advanced along the dorsal surface of the metatarsal until the proximal extent of subperiosteal dissection and the elevator is lifted dorsally. This technique frees the metatarsal about its dorsal aspect in atraumatic fashion and preserves the intrinsic muscles and adipose tissue within the intermetatarsal spaces where the metatarsal arteries and veins travel. This preserves the vascular flow to the plantar tissues and minimizes the potential for ischemic compromise. The same process is then performed for the second through fifth metatarsals (Fig. 28.10). Once the metatarsals have been freed, a medium-width, long-length saw blade is passed from dorsal to plantar at the desired level of resection with care taken to bevel the distal ends of the metatarsals. The first and fifth metatarsal should be resected obliquely as shown in the illustrations (Fig. 28.11). The proximal part of the first metatarsal shaft is left to enhance the weight bearing area and retain the insertion of tibialis anterior and peroneus longus tendons. The peroneus brevis tendon insertion is preserved at the base of the fifth metatarsal. The residual metatarsal parabola should be evaluated under intraoperative image intensification and adjusted until appropriate (Fig. 28.12). The most commonly employed formula is when the residual first and second metatarsals are of equal length or when the second metatarsal is slightly longer than the first and the remaining metatarsals gradually taper as they progress laterally. Following resection of the metatarsals, the plantar plates of the metatarsophalangeal joints are grasped with a metallic clamp from distal to proximal (Fig. 28.13A) and

FIGURE 28.10 Clinical photographs demonstrating use of a periosteal elevator along the shaft of the second metatarsal **(A)** that is advanced to the level of resection and then elevated under controlled force to strip the dorsal soft tissues from the metatarsal yet maintain the vascular structures within the adjacent intermetatarsal spaces **(B)**.

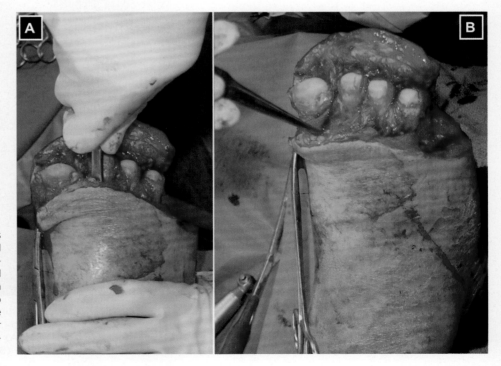

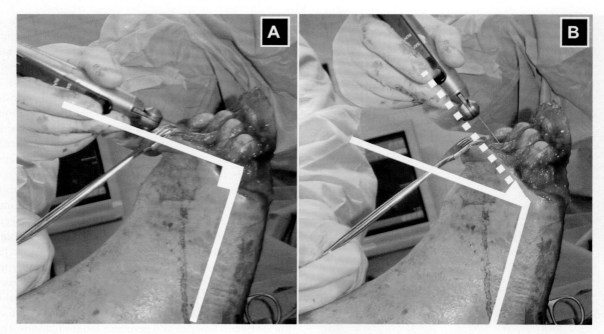

FIGURE 28.11 Clinical photographs demonstrating incorrect **(A)** and correct **(B)** sagittal plane orientation for resection of the metatarsals during transmetatarsal amputation.

circumferentially released of adjacent soft tissues with stout scissors (Fig. 28.13B). Care should be taken to avoid iatrogenic injury to the arteries and veins coursing through the intermetatarsal spaces at the level of the proximal edge of the plantar plates to preserve the vascular flow to the plantar flap. The long and short flexor tendons are grasped with a metallic clamp, retracted distally with the foot plantarflexed, and transected with stout scissors with the retained tendons recoiling within the foot. At the completion of resection of the toes, metatarsals,

plantar plates, and flexor tendons (Fig. 28.14), the residual foot should reveal a proper metatarsal parabola with completely retained intrinsic muscle and adipose tissue within the intermetatarsal spaces as well as full-thickness and well-vascularized plantar flap (Fig. 28.15).

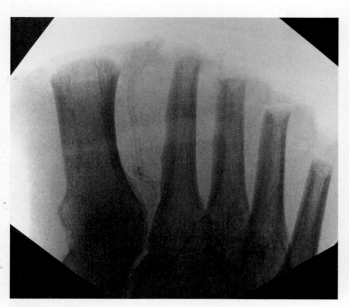

FIGURE 28.12 Intraoperative image intensification anteroposterior view demonstrating proper metatarsal parabola following transmetatarsal amputation.

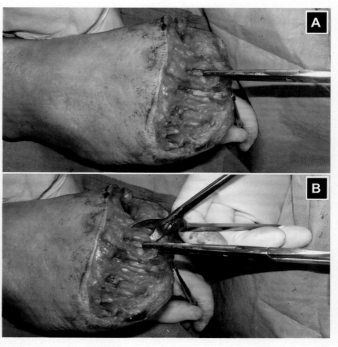

FIGURE 28.13 Clinical photographs demonstrating use of a metallic clamp to grasp the plantar plate of the second metatarsophalangeal joint **(A)** followed by use of a stout scissors to resect the plantar plate **(B)**.

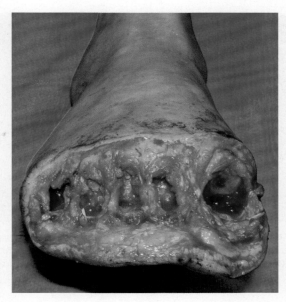

FIGURE 28.15 Clinical photograph demonstrating residual fore-foot following transmetatarsal amputation with well-perfused and full-thickness soft tissues and preserved vascular structures within the intermetatarsal spaces.

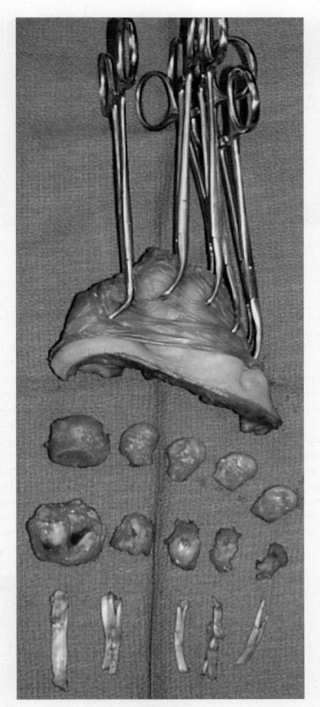

FIGURE 28.14 Clinical photograph demonstrating, from top to bottom, resected toes affixed with sharp towel clamps, metatarsal heads, plantar plates, and flexor tendons following transmetatarsal amputation.

The surgical site is then copiously irrigated with sterile saline or bacitracin-infused saline under pulsatile lavage. At this point, cultures may be obtained. Identifying the arteries and veins within the dorsal and plantar flaps and clamping them with a hemostat for several minutes achieves hemostasis. This is followed by either application of electrocautery or

suture ligatures to the exposed vessel ends. Finally, the exposed distal ends of the residual metatarsals are cauterized with electrocautery to limit both bleeding from the exposed medullary canals and potential for ectopic bone growth over time (Fig. 28.16). A suction drain is placed within the surgical site with the deep portion sutured to the skin with a half-buried horizontal mattress suture, and the exit site is stapled or sutured to the skin in order to limit potential for migration and loss of suction. The deep tissues are approximated with buried absorbable sutures, and the skin edges are then approximated with widely spaced nonabsorbable sutures in vertical mattress fashion interposed by metallic skin staples (Fig. 28.17).

If insufficient soft tissue is present to allow for tension-free primary closure of a transmetatarsal amputation, 1 of 3 options exists: (a) cover the soft tissue defect with a split-thickness skin graft (Fig. 28.18), (b) advance adjacent soft tissues to cover the defect (Fig. 28.19), or (c) convert to a Chopart amputation.

Tendon Balancing Following Transmetatarsal Amputation

Due to muscle contractures, the residual foot after a transmetatarsal amputation is often in an equinovarus posture. To address the equinus contracture, a percutaneous tendo-Achilles lengthening or open gastrocnemius recession is routinely performed (10,13). Additional tendon or osseous balancing is required to address or prevent varus deformity. The following techniques to balance transmetatarsal amputations will be discussed: (a) peroneus brevis to peroneus longus tendon transfer, (b) flexor hallucis longus and extensor digitorum longus transfers, (c) split tibialis anterior tendon

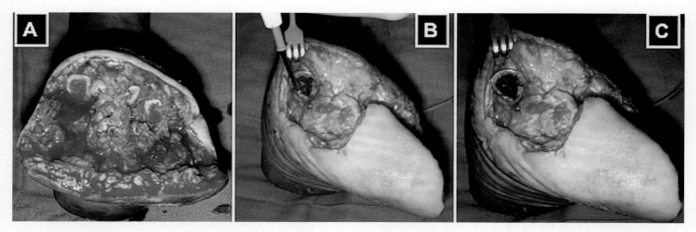

FIGURE 28.16 Clinical photographs following transmetatarsal amputation demonstrating bleeding medullary canal and periosteal tissues for each metatarsal **(A)**. Application of electrocautery to the metatarsal canal and periosteum **(B)** readily achieves hemostasis **(C)** and has the added benefit of limiting ectopic regrowth of bone from the residual metatarsal.

transfer, (d) tibialis posterior and tibialis anterior recessions, and (e) intramedullary screw fixation.

Peroneus Brevis to Peroneus Longus Tendon Transfer

After a transmetatarsal amputation, transfer of the peroneus brevis to the peroneus longus tendon effectively plantarflexes the first ray while simultaneously everting the forefoot, thereby correcting the forefoot varus deformity. This can be performed either distally in the foot or proximal in the lateral lower leg. Performing this procedure in the lower leg is favored in patients with less severe deformities. When the transfer is performed at the level of the foot, it can afford more robust correction, albeit with greater

dissection and risk of devitalizing the lateral aspect of the residual foot (9).

When this transfer is performed in the foot, the incision is mapped out at the midpoint between the posterior edge of the distal tip of the lateral malleolus and the dorsal edge of the posterior aspect of the fifth metatarsal base and is approximately 3 cm in length (Fig. 28.20A). The skin is incised approximately 1 cm in depth exposing the underlying peroneal retinaculum that should be visible at the base of the incision. The peroneal retinaculum is incised in line with the skin incision allowing visualization of the peroneus brevis tendon inferiorly and the peroneus longus tendon superiorly (Fig. 28.20B). Review of the vascular anatomy to this region reveals a rich interconnection between the lateral calcaneal, lateral malleolar, and lateral tarsal artery. The lateral malleolar artery courses deep to the peroneal

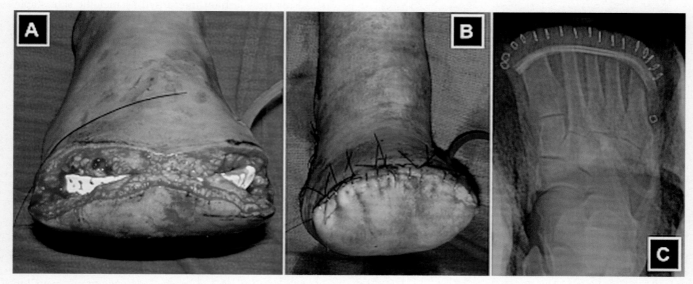

FIGURE 28.17 Clinical photographs following hemostasis demonstrating a fully perforated silicone drain sutured and stapled in place **(A)** followed by layered closure of the soft tissues **(B)**. Postoperative anteroposterior radiograph demonstrating proper metatarsal parabola and placement of the silicone drain **(C)**.

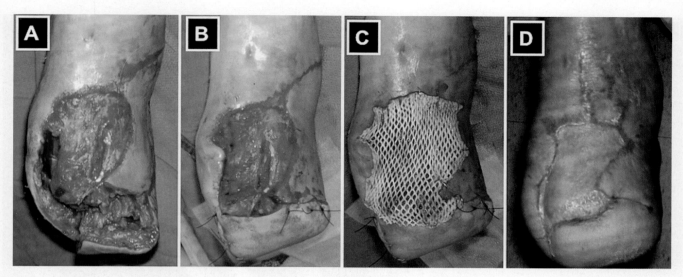

FIGURE 28.18 Clinical photographs demonstrating transmetatarsal amputation with insufficient plantar lateral tissues to cover an extensive dorsal and medial defect **(A)**. The plantar lateral flap was utilized to cover the weight bearing portion of the residual metatarsals **(B)**, and the dorsal defect was covered with a split-thickness skin graft **(C)** that allowed for successful limb salvage **(D)**.

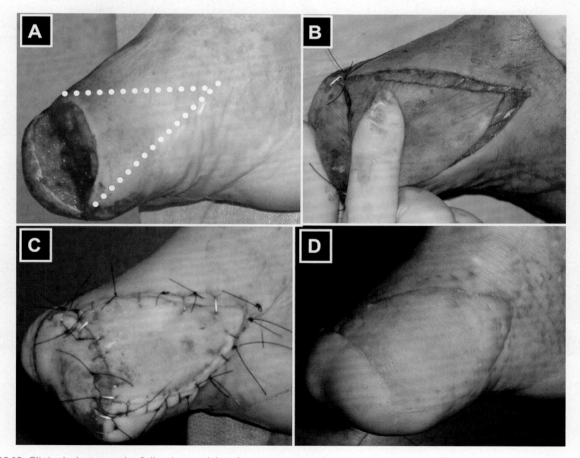

FIGURE 28.19 Clinical photographs following revisional transmetatarsal amputation with insufficient tissues to cover an extensive medial soft tissue defect **(A)** demonstrating V-Y advancement flap along the medial forefoot/midfoot *(white hashed lines)*. The medially based V-Y advancement flap has been raised and advanced **(B)** to cover the soft tissue defect without tension **(C)** and provide stable coverage **(D)** allowing preservation of the length of the residual foot.

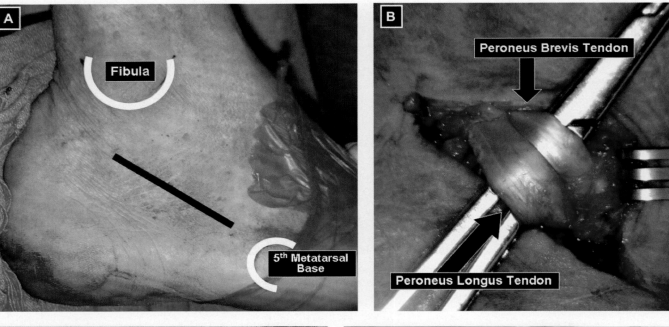

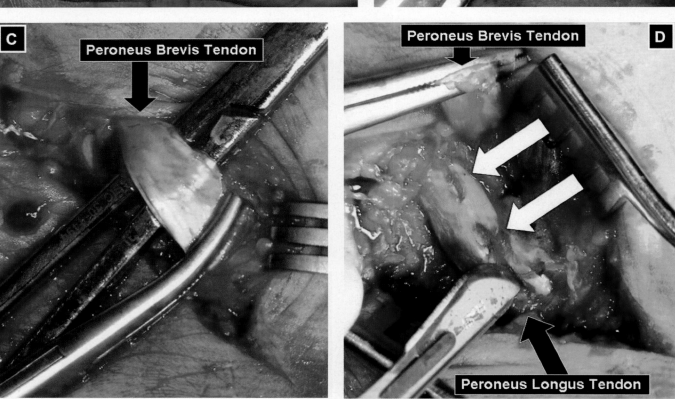

FIGURE 28.20 Clinical photographs of the operative landmarks and surgical incision for the peroneus brevis to longus tendon transfer **(A)**. The peroneus brevis and longus tendons are exposed after incision of the peroneal retinaculum **(B)**. The peroneus brevis tendon has been clamped distally and transected **(C)**. The peroneus longus tendon has been "scored" with electrocautery at the location of the proposed tenotomy incisions **(D)**. *(continued)*

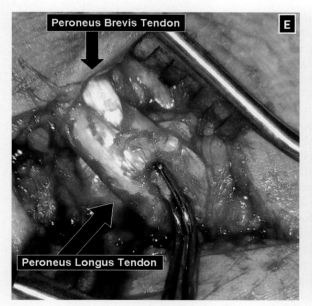
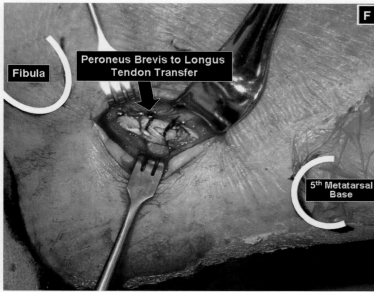

FIGURE 28.20 *(Continued)* A 90-degree clamp is brought from deep to superficial through the proximal peroneus longus tenotomy incision, and the peroneus brevis to longus tendon transfer has been completed **(E)** followed by placement of heavy gauge sutures within the conjoined tendon transfer **(F)**.

tendons against the lateral surface of the calcaneus and therefore is not injured with proper dissection. The intertendinous portion of the peroneal retinaculum is excised to facilitate the transfer. A clamp is placed about the peroneus brevis tendon adjacent to its insertion. The peroneus brevis tendon is then transected distal to the clamp and retrieved from the surgical site (Fig. 28.20C). Electrocautery is utilized to mark the location of 2 longitudinal tenotomy incisions in the peroneus longus tendon through which the peroneus brevis tendon will be weaved. Two stab incisions are performed (Fig. 28.20D), and then a 90-degree clamp is placed from deep to superficial to advance the peroneus brevis tendon through the peroneus longus tendon at the proximal tenotomy site. A second 90-degree clamp is placed from superficial to deep through the distal tenotomy incision and used to advance the peroneus brevis through this incision site (Fig. 28.20E). Distal tension is applied to the peroneus brevis tendon with the forefoot held with the residual first metatarsal plantarflexed and the midfoot/hindfoot in eversion, thereby correcting the forefoot varus deformity. With the foot held in corrected position and distal tension placed on the transferred peroneus brevis tendon, heavy gauge nonabsorbable suture is placed in a figure-of-eight locking pattern at the proximal and distal tenotomy sites incorporating both the peroneus brevis and peroneus longus tendons in each area (Fig. 28.20F). The surgical site is irrigated, and skin closure is performed with widely spaced nonabsorbable sutures in vertical mattress fashion interposed by skin staples.

To perform the transfer in the lower leg, proper incision is paramount. This is done through the following sequence of marking topographic anatomic landmarks on the lateral aspect of the lower leg. First, the lateral aspect of the knee joint and the distal edge of the lateral malleolus are marked. Next, the lateral aspect of the lower leg is divided into thirds between these 2 anatomic markers. The first incision is placed just proximal to the junction of the middle and distal one-third of the lateral aspect of the lower leg, 1 cm to the posteriormost edge of the fibula. The incision is deepened through the subcutaneous tissues and deep fascia of the lower leg exposing the peroneus longus tendon, which is mobilized posteriorly, thereby exposing the peroneus brevis tendon. To ensure the correct tendons have been identified, it is acceptable to tug on each tendon and verify proper action in the foot. The peroneus brevis tendon is then transected and secured via side-to-side anastomosis to the peroneus longus tendon with robust nonabsorbable suture. Care is taken to hold the foot in the corrected position, and proper tension is placed on the tendons prior to securing with suture. This often requires a skilled assistant to properly achieve.

Potential complications associated with these procedures include tendon rupture, infection, and nonhealing of the incision site. The distal procedure is contraindicated in the dysvascular foot due to a significantly increased risk of wound dehiscence with placement of additional incisions on the foot. Postoperative care consists of non–weight-bearing in a well-padded plaster splint for 4 to 6 weeks postoperatively, or longer, dependent on the rate of incision healing at both the tendon transfer site and the amputation stump.

Flexor Hallucis Longus and Extensor Digitorum Longus Tendon Transfers

In situations where additional incisions about the hindfoot are contraindicated, the use of readily available and traditionally expendable extrinsic foot tendons to balance the transmetatarsal amputation represents a viable option. Specifically, transfer of the flexor hallucis longus tendon to the residual first metatarsal in conjunction with transfer of the extensor digitorum

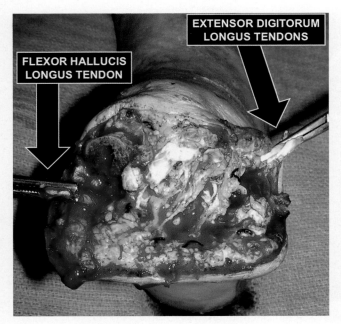

FIGURE 28.21 Intraoperative axial photograph of a transmetatarsal amputation demonstrating harvest of the flexor hallucis longus and extensor digitorum longus tendons that are shown held in metallic clamp.

longus tendon to the residual fourth metatarsal allows for dynamic reduction of forefoot varus through plantarflexion of the medial column along with dorsiflexion of the lateral column during gait, respectively (4).

The transmetatarsal amputation is performed as mentioned earlier except that the flexor hallucis longus and extensor digitorum longus tendons are identified, freed of surrounding soft tissue restraints, and clamped for transfer (Fig. 28.21). A drill hole between 6 and 8 mm in diameter is placed through the dorsal aspect of the residual first metatarsal approximately 10 mm proximal to the distal edge. The drill hole is angled to exit at the junction between the plantar cortex and medullary canal at the distal end of the residual first metatarsal. Just proximal to the drill hole at the dorsal cortex, a 1 mm drill hole is placed through the proximal cortex only and is used to accept a small suture anchor. The flexor hallucis longus tendon is passed from plantar-distal through the drill hole to exit dorsally, and the medial forefoot is plantarflexed to balance the medial aspect of the residual forefoot. With the foot held in this corrected position, the flexor hallucis longus tendon is tensioned by drawing it proximally, and a running locking suture is weaved through the tendon using the suture needle attached to the suture anchor (Fig. 28.22). Once properly tensioned and secured, the suture is tied and the alignment verified. Next, a 1 mm drill hole is placed approximately 10 mm from the distal edge of the residual fourth metatarsal through the dorsal cortex, and a suture anchor is placed as described earlier. With the lateral forefoot simultaneously dorsiflexed and everted, the extensor digitorum longus tendon slips are placed under distal traction and secured to the residual fourth metatarsal as described earlier (Fig. 28.23). At the completion of the tendon transfers, the overall alignment to the residual forefoot is evaluated which should demonstrate an even frontal plane metatarsal position, free of forefoot varus deformity, as well as secure tendon transfers. Any excess length of the transferred tendons can be resected or secured to surrounding soft tissue structures with additional sutures. Layered skin closure as described earlier is performed over a suction drain. This approach is advantageous in situations where additional incisions on the foot or

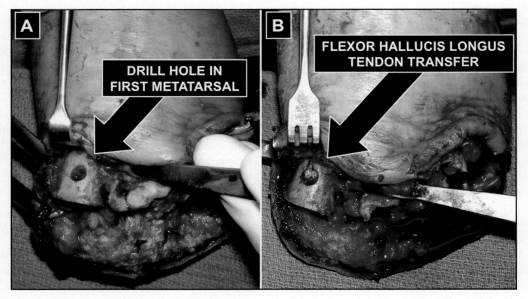

FIGURE 28.22 Intraoperative photographs of the dorsal aspect of the residual forefoot following transmetatarsal amputation demonstrating the drill hole through the residual first metatarsal **(A)** through which the flexor hallucis longus tendon has been transferred and secured with the small suture anchor **(B)**.

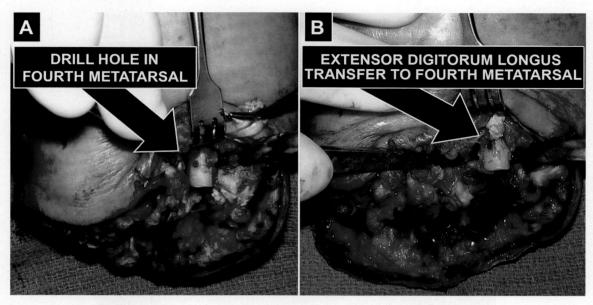

FIGURE 28.23 Intraoperative photographs of the dorsal aspect of the residual forefoot following transmetatarsal amputation demonstrating the drill hole through the residual fourth metatarsal **(A)** into which the small suture anchor has been placed to allow secure transfer of the extensor digitorum longus tendon **(B)**.

delivery of internal fixation could result in wound healing or infectious problems.

Potential complications in addition to those associated with transmetatarsal amputation include necrosis of the tendon ends leading to infection, over- or undercorrection of the forefoot varus deformity, and rupture or loss of the transferred tendons from the bone interface.

Split Tibialis Anterior Tendon Transfer

Split tibialis anterior tendon transfer is a powerful procedure to correct forefoot varus after transmetatarsal amputation (Fig. 28.24A). However, this procedure requires 3 incisions and may be contraindicated in patients who have undergone peripheral arterial bypass surgery secondary to the potential for disrupting or compressing the bypass site which can lead to dorsal soft tissue necrosis. Additionally, split tibialis anterior tendon transfer requires prolonged immobilization in order to allow for osseous ingrowth of the tendon transfer to the midfoot under proper tension (12).

The procedure is performed upon completion of the amputation and after wound closure. The tibialis anterior tendon is identified just proximal to the superior extensor retinaculum adjacent to the lateral edge of the anterior tibial crest (Fig. 28.24B). A 1.5 cm vertical incision is placed at this location and carried down through the subcutaneous tissues until the sheath of the tibialis anterior tendon is encountered. The sheath is incised in line with the skin incision, and the tibialis anterior tendon is retrieved into the surgical field with a large vessel loop. The foot is plantarflexed and everted while simultaneously pulling on the vessel loop in a proximal direction. This allows identification

of the terminal insertion of the tibialis anterior tendon at the medial aspect of the first tarsal-metatarsal articulation. A second 1.5 cm incision is placed directly over the terminal insertion of the tibialis anterior tendon (Fig. 28.24B), and the lateral one-half of the tendon is secured with heavy gauge nonabsorbable suture in a locking fashion followed by transection of the lateral one-half of the tendon. Once completed, the lateral one-half of the tendon should separate from the medial one-half with gentle traction. This should be performed carefully because there is slight torsion to the tibialis anterior tendon that must be respected in order to limit potential for iatrogenic rupture or isolation of a diminutive tendon slip for transfer. A curved metallic clamp is placed through the proximal incision until it grasps the suture secured in the tendon. The metallic clamp is carefully withdrawn proximally which effectively "splits" the tendon into a retained medial one-half and working lateral one-half intended for transfer. If any difficulty is encountered, umbilical tape should be used to gently separate the tendon rather than repeated manipulation or forced traction which could avulse the tendon from its proximal or distal attachments. Finally, a third 1.5 cm incision placed over the base of the fourth metatarsal (Fig. 28.24B) and the underlying bone is freed of periosteum and roughened with a metallic rasp. A metallic soft tissue anchor is placed into the base of the fourth metatarsal, and the lateral one-half of the tibialis anterior tendon is transferred deep to the superior and inferior extensor retinaculum with the use of a large curved metallic clamp. The clamp is initially placed through the distal incision, the suture in the lateral one-half of the tibialis anterior tendon is grasped, and then the clamp is withdrawn through the distal incision over the fourth metatarsal base.

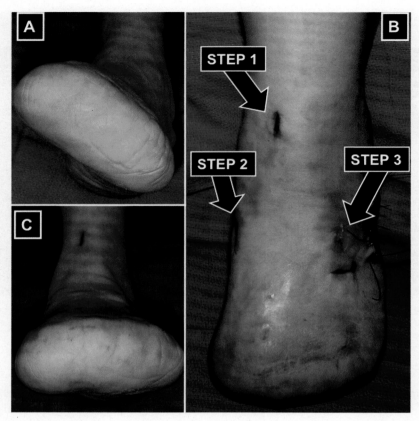

FIGURE 28.24 Clinical photographs demonstrating a varus deformity following transmetatarsal amputation **(A)** that has been corrected with a 3-incision split tibialis anterior tendon transfer **(B)** ensuring that the foot has been slightly overcorrected **(C)** because over time, some loss of correction will occur.

With the foot held in full dorsiflexion and eversion, the lateral one-half of the tibialis anterior tendon is placed under maximum tension and secured to the fourth metatarsal base with the sutures included in the suture anchor system. Any residual tendon can be further secured to the surrounding soft tissues to afford additional reinforcement. Alternatively, the residual portion of tendon can be resected to minimize the presence of dysvascular tissue in the surgical field. Other methods of tendon–bone attachment such as an interference screw can be employed if desired by the surgeon. Layered skin closure is performed using a combination of widely spaced nonabsorbable sutures in vertical mattress fashion interposed by skin staples. At the completion of the transfer, the residual foot should assume neutral to slightly overcorrected alignment (Fig. 28.24C).

Potential complications associated with this procedure include tendon rupture, infection, compression of the anterior tibial or dorsalis pedis arteries by the transferred portion of tendon, and nonhealing of the incision sites. The procedure is contraindicated in the dysvascular foot due to a significantly increased risk of wound dehiscence and compression of the anterior vasculature. Postoperative care consists of non–weight-bearing in a well-padded plaster splint for 4 to 6 weeks postoperatively, or longer, dependent on the

rate of incision healing at both the tendon transfer site and the amputation stump.

Tibialis Posterior Recession

A less invasive, albeit less powerful, way to correct residual varus contracture is to weaken the deforming muscles through recessions in the lower leg. This location allows for minimal dissection in a more vascularized area leading to more predictable healing.

The technique involves stressing the ankle in eversion, and if the ankle cannot achieve slight eversion (i.e., between 5 and 10 degrees) alignment, then a tibialis posterior recession is performed. The proper location for the tibialis posterior recession is determined by first marking the medial aspect of the knee joint and the distal edge of the medial malleolus. Next, the medial aspect of the lower leg is divided into thirds between these 2 anatomic markers. The incision is placed just distal to the junction of the middle and distal one-thirds of the lower leg at the posterior edge of the tibia. The tibialis posterior lies directly posterior to the medial-posterior aspect of the tibia at this level in the lower leg. The incision is deepened through the subcutaneous tissues and deep fascia of the lower leg, exposing the posterior aspect of the tibia. The tibialis posterior muscle is easily identified at the posterior aspect of the tibia at this level. The musculotendinous junction of the tibialis posterior is identified, and the tendon is transected within the muscle belly with the use of electrocautery while the foot is simultaneously dorsiflexed and everted until the varus contracture is corrected, thus completing the recession. Closure of the tissues ensues in layers. Postoperative care is similar to the aforementioned procedures.

Tibialis Anterior Recession

This technique offers similar advantages to the tibialis posterior recession, although applicable when the tibialis anterior is determined to be the deforming force. The procedure, like all others listed, is typically performed under general anesthesia without use of tourniquet. An incision is made along the course of the tibialis anterior tendon beginning just distal to the ankle joint to just proximal to its insertion on the medial cuneiform. The dissection is carried through the deeper tissue layers until the tibialis anterior tendon sheath is identified. The sheath is then opened, revealing the tendon within which is freed from the sheath and exposed with a tongue depressor or malleable retractor. A sagittal plane Z lengthening is then performed. The distance between the proximal and distal incisions in the tendon substance should be approximately 4 to 5 cm. After these incisions are made, the foot is plantarflexed allowing the 2 segments of the tendon to translate on one another resulting in desired lengthening. The segments are then sutured together in a side-to-side or end-to-end fashion with nonabsorbable suture. The tendon sheath can be repaired using an absorbable suture or left unrepaired. Postoperative care is similar to the aforementioned procedures (2).

Intramedullary Screw Fixation

Intramedullary screw fixation is indicated for balancing of the residual forefoot after transmetatarsal amputation in patients with peripheral arterial disease who have a high-risk of wound dehiscence and in whom additional incisions should be avoided. The procedure can be performed through the amputation incision site and therefore does not add additional wound healing risk to the patient. This technique must only be utilized when the surgical sites reveal no cardinal signs of infection or necrotic tissue. The procedure is performed upon completion of the amputation and prior to wound closure. An assistant holds the foot in corrected position with the medial column plantarflexed and the forefoot in eversion to create a plantigrade residual foot (Fig. 28.25).

A guidewire for a large-diameter cannulated screw is then placed through the medullary canal of the exposed first metatarsal and driven across the articulations of the medial column into the talus with care taken to avoid inadvertent penetration of the ankle joint, especially medially. The position is verified by intraoperative image intensification visualization. Once the position is deemed appropriate, an appropriate length 7.5 mm cannulated threaded head screw is advanced through the medial column until the head of the screw engages the subchondral bone of the first metatarsal (Fig. 28.26). Drilling over the guidewire is not recommended prior to screw insertion because it will reduce screw purchase and stability. If the screw head is prominent, the abductor hallucis muscle is used to cover the end of the bone in order to protect the hardware from direct exposure in the case of wound dehiscence (Fig. 28.27). The end result should be a stable and well-aligned forefoot. Layered skin closure is performed using a combination of widely spaced nonabsorbable

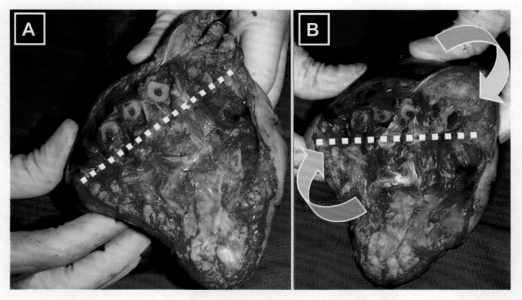

FIGURE 28.25 Clinical photographs demonstrating an inverted forefoot following transmetatarsal amputation **(A)** and the final position following manual positioning of the medial column in plantarflexion and the forefoot in slight eversion **(B)** prior to guidewire insertion.

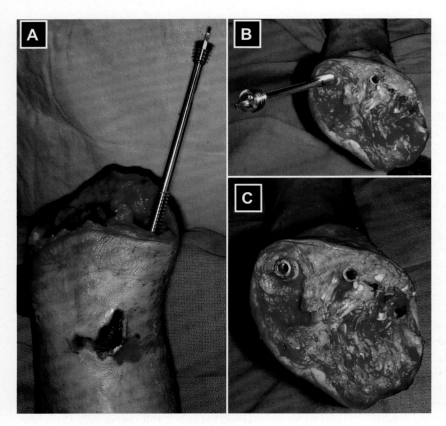

FIGURE 28.26 Clinical photographs **(A,B)** following transmetatarsal amputation demonstrating insertion of a guidewire and threaded head screw along the medial column of the residual foot. Clinical photograph following full insertion of the threaded head screw within the first metatarsal **(C)**.

sutures in vertical mattress fashion interposed by skin staples over a suction drain as described earlier.

The use of an intramedullary screw across the medial column can maintain a stable, functional transmetatarsal amputation and obviate the need to perform a tendon transfer, thereby reducing the number of incisions, the risk of dehiscence, and the potential for postoperative infection in this high-risk patient population (11).

Potential complications of the procedure include distal migration of the screw, especially if a nonthreaded head screw is employed (Fig. 28.28), infection which could seed the retained hardware and spread along the cannulated portion of the screw into the hindfoot as well as iatrogenic fracture of the involved bones. Patients will have a stiff midfoot and hindfoot postoperatively; therefore, the hardware should only be placed

after it has been verified that the foot is being held in fully corrected position.

SURGICAL TECHNIQUE

Chopart Amputation

Chopart amputation begins with the patient positioned in the supine position on the operating room table with a well-padded bolster placed beneath the ipsilateral buttock to control physiologic external rotation of the lower limb. This procedure is most commonly performed under general anesthesia with added popliteal and saphenous peripheral nerve block, as tendon procedures described elsewhere in this textbook are often needed with Chopart amputations. Local regional anesthesia

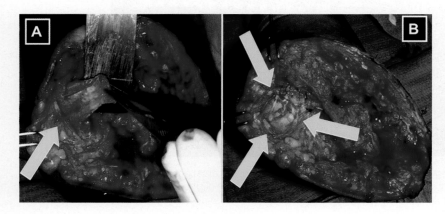

FIGURE 28.27 Clinical photograph demonstrating freeing of the abductor hallucis muscle from its fascial attachments medially, with care taken to preserve the musculocutaneous arterial branches plantar-medial at the level of the proximal aspect of the first metatarsal **(A)**. The abductor hallucis muscle has been transposed over the first metatarsal stump to cover the head of the implanted screw within the medial column of the residual foot **(B)**.

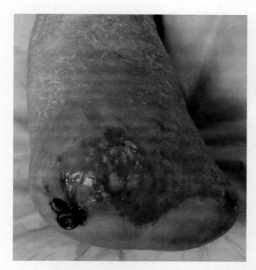

FIGURE 28.28 Clinical photograph demonstrating distal migration of a nonthreaded head screw through the distal soft tissue envelope.

is contraindicated in the presence of active infection or gangrene in the field to be infiltrated. Tourniquet use is avoided in the presence of peripheral arterial disease but is routinely employed in patients without vascular compromise to decrease the time necessary to complete the procedure, improve visualization of the anatomy, and limit acute blood loss in the high-risk patient.

The dorsal incision is centered over the midtarsal joint and extends from the inferior aspect of the navicular tuberosity medially to the inferior aspect of the cuboid laterally. The plantar incision extends distally to the junction of the proximal and middle one-thirds of the metatarsals with horizontal incisions connecting the dorsal and plantar incisions along the medial and lateral aspects of the foot (Fig. 28.29). Any ulceration should be excised with 1 cm margins of healthy tissue to limit potential for retention of infected or necrotic tissue in the plantar flap. The toes or residual forefoot are grasped with towel clamps as

described for performing transmetatarsal amputation. The dorsal incision is incised through the skin, superficial and deep fascia with intervening tendons being transected under tension and allowed to recoil proximally. The dorsalis pedis artery and vein centrally and lateral tarsal artery and vein laterally are clamped and coagulated with electrocautery or ligated with suture. The medial and lateral incisions are then carried down to the level of the underlying abductor hallucis and abductor digiti minimi muscles starting proximally and coursing distally. The plantar incision is performed with care taken to ensure that the intrinsic layer of muscles is included within the plantar flap. The flexor hallucis longus and flexor digitorum longus tendons are resected under tension and allowed to recoil proximally. The medial plantar artery between the flexor hallucis longus and flexor digitorum brevis as well as the lateral plantar artery between the flexor digiti minimi and flexor digitorum brevis are clamped and coagulated as described earlier. Next, the periosteum is elevated from the underlying osseous structures with electrocautery by first incising the tarsal-metatarsal joints from medial to lateral such that the only remaining tissues are the plantar ligaments. Using electrocautery, the plantar ligaments of the tarsal-metatarsal joints are incised under distal traction placed on the towel clamps. Once the plantar ligaments are incised, each metatarsal is elevated in a dorsal-distal direction with care taken to clamp both the tibialis anterior tendon at its insertion and the peroneus brevis tendon at its insertion and to preserve the peroneus longus as it courses from lateral to medial. The peroneus longus is more commonly used for transfer than the peroneus brevis due to the additional length that is available. The metatarsals are removed in a "skeletonized" fashion in order to preserve the intrinsic musculature and intermetatarsal spaces through which the vasculature supplying the plantar flap course (Fig. 28.30). Once the dissection is completed, the forefoot is

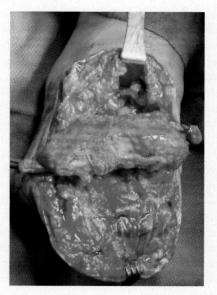

FIGURE 28.30 Clinical photograph following resection of the metatarsals and elevation of full-thickness dorsal and plantar soft tissue flaps for a Chopart amputation demonstrating the contents of the tarsal bones.

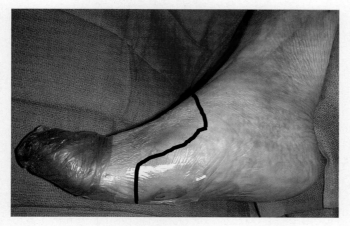

FIGURE 28.29 Clinical photograph of the medial foot demonstrating outline of the surgical incision for a Chopart amputation.

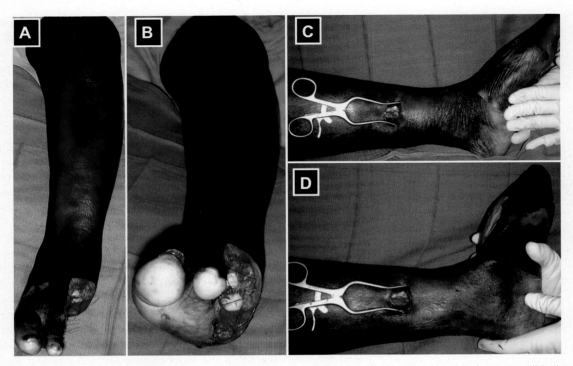

FIGURE 28.31 Clinical photographs **(A,B)** following resection of the lateral forefoot for deep abscess and osteomyelitis demonstrating a varus foot posture. Medial view of the lower leg and foot demonstrating exposure of the tibialis posterior musculotendinous junction **(C)** that has been incised, thereby allowing correction of the varus contracture **(D)** to allow for completion of a Chopart amputation.

transferred from the operative field. Attention is then directed to the cuneiforms that can usually be resected as a unit using the same technique described earlier with electrocautery. The navicular and cuboid are resected in a similar fashion with care taken to resect the tibialis posterior tendon medially such that it visibly retracts proximally into the tarsal canal. Several small insertion points within the tissues surrounding the navicular can exist, and if left behind, these could interfere with proper balancing or predispose to development of a varus deformity of the foot. Occasionally, it is necessary to perform a tibialis posterior recession in the lower one-third of the leg in order to correct a persistent or latent varus contracture (Fig. 28.31). The end result should be a resected forefoot in toto and skeletonized tarsal and midtarsal osseous contents (Fig. 28.32). The residual foot should have the tibialis anterior and peroneus longus (most commonly) or peroneus brevis tendon secured within metallic clamps and clean healthy, well-perfused soft tissues throughout the operative site (Fig. 28.33). The articular cartilage should be resected from the head of the talus. The anterior one-third of the calcaneus should be resected slightly posterior to the talar head resection that approximates the anterior neck of the calcaneus. This creates a broad surface for the soft tissue flaps to adhere postoperatively. It has been suggested that this technique limits potential for migration of the flap and reduce flap breakdown.

The next step involves transfer of the tibialis anterior and peroneus brevis or longus tendon when the peroneus brevis tendon is not available. This may be done in one of the following ways: (a) transfer the tibialis anterior and either peroneal tendon into one another, (b) transfer to either the talus or calca-

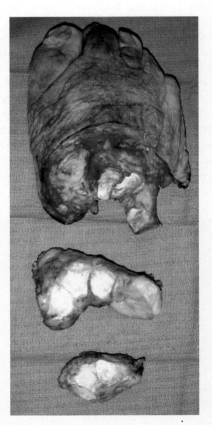

FIGURE 28.32 Clinical photograph demonstrating, from top to bottom, resected toes and metatarsals, cuneiforms and cuboid, and navicular following Chopart amputation.

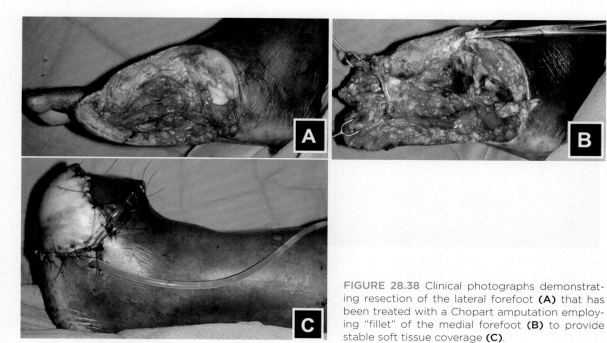

FIGURE 28.38 Clinical photographs demonstrating resection of the lateral forefoot **(A)** that has been treated with a Chopart amputation employing "fillet" of the medial forefoot **(B)** to provide stable soft tissue coverage **(C)**.

situations, it is important to allow the soft tissues to fully incorporate with the underlying osseous structures and become firm/nonmobile such that prosthetic bracing will be able to maintain a viable limb without excessive risk of junctional incision breakdown. Finally, in situations where the patient is moribund or when there is no ability to perform tendon transfer to balance the Chopart amputation, a tibiotalocalcaneal arthrodesis should be considered. This has been shown to be a viable alternative to below-the-knee amputation and easier to fashion with a prosthetic brace (Fig. 28.40) (1).

Potential complications associated with this procedure include tendon rupture, infection, and nonhealing of the incision site. The procedure is contraindicated in the dysvascular foot unless direct inline arterial flow is present to the posterior tibial artery to supply the entirety of the plantar flap because no communication of significance exists between the anterior, peroneal, and posterior tibial arteries following Chopart amputation. Additionally, an intact plantar heel pad must exist to support weight bearing within a properly fashioned and consistently utilized prosthetic brace. Late development of an equinocavovarus foot posture is possible but should be rarely encountered with proper balancing of the Chopart amputation. If a significant contracture exists, then soft tissue tendon balancing consisting of selective lengthening or transfer should be considered, or a tibiotalocalcaneal arthrodesis is performed. Any ectopic bone formation that

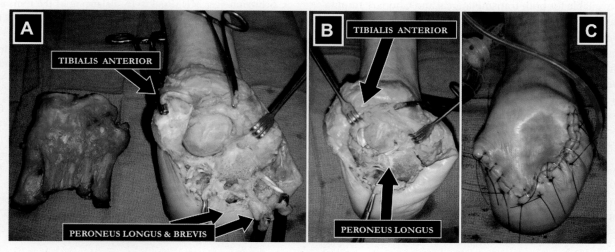

FIGURE 28.39 Clinical photographs demonstrating resection of the residual forefoot and identification of the tibialis anterior and peroneus brevis and longus tendons **(A)** that have been utilized for balancing a Chopart amputation **(B)** and covered with a dorsal soft tissue flap **(C)**. Note that the weight bearing portion of the heel pad has been preserved, thereby allowing use of the dorsal skin for coverage and protection of the residual lower extremity in a properly fitted brace.

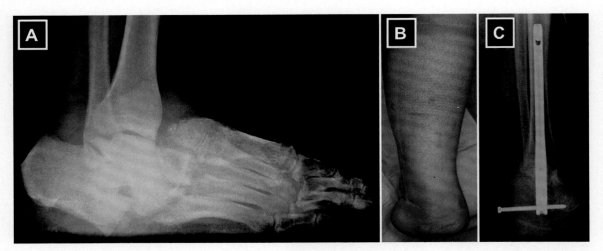

FIGURE 28.40 Lateral weight bearing radiograph demonstrating a severe midfoot Charcot neuroarthropathy in a moribund, medically ill patient with proximal migration of the tibialis anterior tendon that was determined intraoperatively to be nonusable **(A)** that has been treated with a Chopart amputation **(B)** balanced with a tibiotalocalcaneal arthrodesis using an intramedullary locked nail **(C)**.

results in ulceration or interferes with bracing should be resected. Postoperative care consists of non–weight-bearing in a well-padded plaster splint for 4 to 6 weeks postoperatively, or longer, depending on the rate of incision healing at both the tendon transfer site and the amputation stump or if tibiotalocalcaneal arthrodesis has been performed.

CLINICAL TIPS AND PEARLS

1. Transmetatarsal and Chopart amputations are valuable procedures when performed for proper indications, the soft tissue and osseous structures have been adequately débrided of necrotic or infected tissues, and tendon or osseous balancing is performed.

2. A number of soft tissue and osseous balancing procedures are available for both transmetatarsal and Chopart amputations, and each has its own risk of complications. Surgeon experience is integral to achieving a good outcome.

3. Close follow-up and daily patient use of protective shoe gear/bracing is essential to the maintenance of a durable lower extremity capable of withstanding the repeated shear and stress associated with ambulation following transmetatarsal and Chopart amputations.

References

1. Andersen CA, Roukis TS. The diabetic foot. Surg Clin North Am 2007;87:1149–1177.

2. Garwood CS, Steinberg JS. Soft tissue balancing after partial foot amputations. Clin Podiatr Med Surg 2016;33:99–111.

3. Roukis TS. Extra-articular ankle stabilization: a case series. Foot Ankle Spec 2010;3:125–128.

4. Roukis TS. Flexor hallucis longus and extensor digitorum longus tendon transfers for balancing the foot following transmetatarsal amputation. J Foot Ankle Surg 2009;48:398–401.

5. Roukis TS. Tibialis posterior recession. J Foot Ankle Surg 2009;48:402–404.

6. Roukis TS, Singh N, Andersen CA. Preserving functional capacity as opposed to tissue preservation in the diabetic patient: a single institution experience. Foot Ankle Spec 2010;3:177–183.

7. Roukis TS, Stapleton J, Zgonis T. Addressing psychosocial aspects of care for patients with diabetes undergoing limb salvage surgery. Clin Podiatr Med Surg 2007;24:601–610.

8. Schade VL, Roukis TS, Yan J. Factors associated with successful Chopart amputation in patients with diabetes: a systematic review. Foot Ankle Spec 2010;3:278–284.

9. Schweinberger MH, Roukis TS. Balancing of the transmetatarsal amputation with peroneus brevis to peroneus longus tendon transfer. J Foot Ankle Surg 2007;46:510–514.

10. Schweinberger MH, Roukis TS. Extraarticular immobilization for protection of percutaneous tendo-Achilles lengthening following transmetatarsal amputation and peripheral arterial bypass surgery. J Foot Ankle Surg 2008;47:169–171.

11. Schweinberger MH, Roukis TS. Intramedullary screw fixation for balancing of the dysvascular foot following transmetatarsal amputation. J Foot Ankle Surg 2008;47:594–597.

12. Schweinberger MH, Roukis TS. Soft-tissue and osseous techniques to balance forefoot and midfoot amputations. Clin Podiatr Med Surg 2008;25:623–639.

13. Schweinberger MH, Roukis TS. Surgical correction of soft-tissue ankle equinus contracture. Clin Podiatr Med Surg 2008;25:571–585.

CHAPTER 29

Surgical Off-loading Reconstructive Procedures for the Diabetic Foot and Ankle

Crystal L. Ramanujam • Thomas Zgonis

INTRODUCTION

As reconstructive surgical options for the many clinical manifestations of the diabetic foot and ankle have continued to expand, the importance of off-loading has remained a vital component of wound and bone healing. Although traditional conservative off-loading devices including bracing, splinting, and casting, may provide varying degrees of immobilization, surgical off-loading through the use of external fixation has demonstrated levels of advanced protection and stability for the preservation of soft tissue and osseous reconstructions in certain clinical settings.

LITERATURE REVIEW AND CLINICAL OUTCOMES

External fixation has long been used for extremity trauma, finding a significant role in skeletal stabilization and management of extensive soft tissue injuries. Whereas the orthoplastic approach has been applied to the treatment of severe extremity trauma with combined fractures and soft tissue injuries, the combination of circular external fixation with plastic surgical wound closure with or without osseous correction in the diabetic foot has contributed to the development of the podoplastic approach. Circular external fixation fulfills the basic principles of off-loading including rigid stability that minimizes shear movements, providing elevation of the extremity and removing any direct pressure to the flap closure techniques (11). Because excessive motion creates shearing forces that can compromise flap and/or vascular anastomosis, the use of external fixation enhances the survival rates of soft tissue reconstruction through deliberate control of ankle motion. Reduction of tension at the wound margins and traction treatment may further stimulate wound healing. Although internal fixation often requires more considerable soft tissue dissection, circular external fixation invokes less iatrogenic trauma on the soft tissues through the use of smooth transosseous wires (4). Additionally, circular external fixation is ideal for maintaining bone and joint

alignment in situations where extensive bone resection is necessary such as in diabetic Charcot neuroarthropathy deformity correction and/or osteomyelitis. Furthermore, circular external fixation can be designed to provide compression in arthrodesis procedures when osseous realignment is necessary for reconstruction of the lower extremity. This type of external fixation can be used for the podoplastic approach and has been particularly useful in the treatment of diabetic Charcot neuroarthropathy in the presence of open wounds and/or osteomyelitis (12).

Literature regarding surgical off-loading for the diabetic foot and ankle is steadily increasing. Several single-case reports have been published in support of circular external fixation combined with soft tissue reconstruction for the diabetic foot using various plastic surgical techniques: local advancement flaps (2,9), medial plantar artery flap (13), muscle flaps (1,3,8), and reverse sural artery neurofasciocutaneous flap (10). Many of these reports also included osseous corrective procedures. Large or high-level studies providing reliable long-term outcomes are lacking. In 2008, Clemens et al. (4) retrospectively analyzed the use of multiplanar external fixation in 12 patients to off-load wounds on weight bearing surfaces of the foot after soft tissue reconstructions, resulting in an 83% overall limb salvage rate. In 2012, Pinzur et al. (7) demonstrated 95.7% limb salvage in 68 diabetic patients using a single-staged resection of osteomyelitis, acute correction of Charcot neuroarthropathy deformity with circular external fixation, and parenteral culture-specific antibiotic therapy. In 2016, Hegewald et al. (6) provided results of the use of combined internal and external fixation for diabetic Charcot neuroarthropathy reconstruction in 22 patients, demonstrating limb salvage in 90.91% of their studied population. Later in 2016, Dalla Paola et al. (5) reported 100% healing in 18 diabetic patients with heel wounds who underwent partial calcanectomy, application of negative pressure wound therapy (NPWT) with dermal substitute, split-thickness skin grafting and circular external fixation for hindfoot stabilization and off-loading. Although the current body of scientific evidence is limited for surgical off-loading with circular external fixation, the existing information demonstrates relative success for these diabetic foot and ankle reconstructive procedures when performed on the carefully selected patient within a multidisciplinary health care setting. Additional higher levels of evidence-based research with longer clinical outcomes are necessary to further enhance treatment protocols in the diabetic population.

INDICATIONS AND CONTRAINDICATIONS

Indications for surgical off-loading circular external fixation in the diabetic foot and ankle are patient-specific and highly dependent on the individual clinical scenario. This modality serves for protection of soft tissue and/or osseous reconstructions that are not conducive to conventional conservative lower extremity off-loading with casts or splints. The unique anatomical contours of the lower extremity already pose significant challenges when it comes to diabetic reconstruction, not to mention further impositions created by conservative options for off-loading. Typical casts or splints are difficult to properly construct and place with regard to certain complex surgical procedures. Furthermore, elevation of the lower extremity with external fixation decreases compartmental pressures within the lower extremity while also eliminating increased pressures in the extremity secondary to direct contact on the surgical site from foam elevators or pillows. Circular external fixation allows direct visualization and easy access to wounds and/or flaps for meticulous postoperative management. Common applications of surgical off-loading circular external fixation in the diabetic foot and ankle include, but are not limited to, the treatment of wounds at weight bearing or decubitus surfaces, variety of plastic reconstructive procedures for definitive wound closure throughout the lower extremity, selective bone resection for osteomyelitis, partial foot amputations, exostectomies, osteotomies, isolated or multilevel arthrodeses, equinus correction, free tissue transfer, and/or a combination of the aforementioned techniques.

Contraindications for surgical off-loading circular external fixation include poor bone quality or pathology that cannot support half pin/wire fixation, retained internal fixation that does not allow for half pin/wire placement, patient's inability to tolerate external fixation with regard to the device itself or cooperation with postoperative care and non–weight-bearing status. Surgical off-loading circular external fixation may not be used in patients with poor lower extremity vascular status that has not been properly addressed prior to reconstructive procedures. This method of surgical off-loading should be reserved for surgeons with specific training and extensive experience with external fixation. Furthermore, surgeons should have the proper resources to support the laborious perioperative care involved with surgical off-loading.

PREOPERATIVE CONSIDERATIONS

Patient selection is critical to the overall successful use of surgical off-loading circular external fixation with concomitant soft tissue and/or osseous reconstruction. Complete preoperative history and physical examination are vital to determining the most appropriate surgical plan for these patients, including review of all prior lower extremity surgeries. Ideally, chronic hyperglycemia should be addressed prior to reconstructive surgical procedures because this will likely interfere with wound and/or osseous healing. A multidisciplinary team approach with an interest in the management of the diabetic patient should be utilized for preoperative optimization, which may include involvement of internists, endocrinologists, nephrologists, cardiologists, infectious disease specialists, vascular surgeons, plastic surgeons, nursing staff, wound care specialists, physical therapists, and nutritionists.

Common medical comorbidities of diabetes mellitus, particularly cardiovascular disease, peripheral arterial disease, peripheral neuropathy, and nephropathy, should be addressed. Preoperative evaluation from a medical imaging standpoint should begin with plain radiographs and then proceed with appropriate selection of advanced modalities such as magnetic resonance imaging, computed tomography, and nuclear imaging based on the clinically suspected foot and ankle pathology. Deformity evaluation, especially those associated with diabetic Charcot neuroarthropathy, is key to deciding whether osseous and/or other adjunctive soft tissue procedures are necessary for functional correction.

Preoperative vascular evaluation of the lower extremities should begin with noninvasive arterial testing including ankle-brachial index, toe-brachial index, Doppler waveforms, and pulse volume recordings to determine whether a vascular surgical consultation is warranted to optimize perfusion to the affected site. This assessment is critical in diabetic patients being considered for plastic surgical procedures because additional diagnostic tools such as angiography and vein mapping may be used in further surgical planning.

Formal surgical débridement of infected wounds with appropriate antibiotic therapy is assigned based on intraoperative cultures and followed by performance of staged reconstruction when indicated. Osseous reconstructive procedures such as exostectomies, osteotomies, and arthrodesis should be performed in the absence of infected bone and soft tissue. For the management of open wounds in the presence of deformity, surgeons should carefully choose surgical wound closure technique(s) and osseous correction(s) that complement one another rather than hinder each other. Additionally, placement of half pins/wires involved with the surgical off-loading circular external fixation should be carefully considered so as not to compromise the wound closure technique(s) involved. Finally, once the surgical plan has been formulated, the patient should be educated in detail regarding the extensive perioperative course, emphasizing the possibility of complications and providing realistic expectations.

SURGICAL TECHNIQUE WITH CLINICAL CASE PRESENTATIONS

Although there have been various designs described for external fixation applied to the diabetic foot and ankle, the basic construct for surgical off-loading circular external fixation will be initially described, followed by clinical cases illustrating surgical off-loading as an adjunct to specific soft tissue and/or osseous reconstructive procedures.

The application of surgical off-loading circular external fixation proceeds in a new sterile field after the conclusion of the soft tissue and/or osseous reconstructive procedures. It is recommended that the application of circular external fixation is performed at the end of the associated reconstructive procedure(s) and after any tourniquet use has been deflated and surgical wound closure has been achieved. The use of C-arm intraoperative fluoroscopy may also be utilized if necessary during the half pin/wire insertion for proper placement and alignment of the circular external fixation device.

Most commonly, 2 tibial circular rings connected by threaded rods form a *tibial block* which is placed 10 to 15 cm proximal to the ankle joint with adequate alignment to the lower extremity and space to permit postoperative edema. The tibial block is secured to the lower extremity with 2 transosseous wires attached to each circular ring of the tibial block. Following appropriate tightening and tensioning (value ranging between 110 and 130 kg of force) wire fixation techniques, the tibial block is then checked for stability and for additional insertion of smooth transosseous wires and/or half pins if necessary. The ends of the transosseous wires are then cut and bent appropriately for protection.

Attention is then directed to the foot region of where the previous soft tissue and/or osseous reconstructions were performed. An additional circular ring is then added to the foot and secured with 2 transosseous wires that are manually tightened to the circular ring. At that time, the foot can be manipulated and positioned in the desired anatomic alignment depending on the previous reconstructive procedure(s) performed. Multiple medial and lateral ankle hinges or struts are then incorporated between the tibial block and foot circular ring and secured into place. The hinges are used to correct, align, and stabilize the foot to the lower extremity in the desired anatomic position. The ends of the foot transosseous wires are then cut and bent appropriately for protection. Additional external fixation support can be applied by connecting the foot circular ring to the tibial block if necessary.

After completion of the circular external fixation device and performance of any compression wire fixation techniques, attention is then directed to the plantar aspect of the foot for the surgical off-loading. A kickstand apparatus is applied via distally carbon fiber bars which are inserted on the medial and lateral aspects of the device and secured posteriorly with a carbon fiber bar and bar-to-clamp devices. Special attention is given to the plantar aspect of the calcaneus, making sure that it is appropriately off-loaded and protected from any weight bearing surfaces. Finally, the entire circular external fixation system is checked for stability and proper lower extremity alignment (Fig. 29.1).

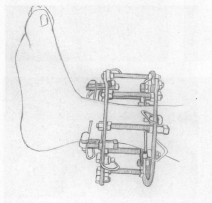

A

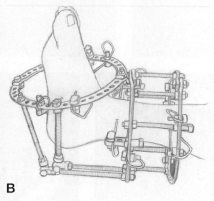

B

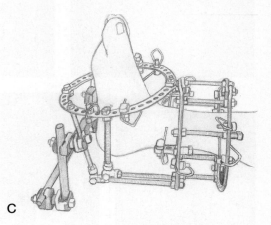

C

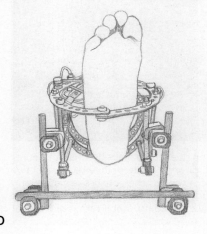

D

FIGURE 29.1 A. Schematic illustration showing 2 tibial circular rings connected by threaded rods forming the tibial block which is placed approximately 10 to 15 cm proximal to the ankle joint. The tibial block is secured to the lower extremity with 2 transosseous wires attached to each circular ring of the tibial block. **B.** An additional circular ring is then added to the foot and secured with 2 transosseous wires that are manually tightened to the circular ring. The foot can then be manipulated and positioned in the desired anatomic alignment depending on the previous reconstructive procedure(s) performed. Multiple medial and lateral ankle hinges or struts are then incorporated between the tibial block and foot circular ring and secured into place. The hinges are used to correct, align, and stabilize the foot to the lower extremity in the desired anatomic position. **C,D.** Finally, a kickstand apparatus is then applied via distally carbon fiber bars which are inserted on the medial and lateral aspects of the device and secured posteriorly with a carbon fiber bar and bar-to-clamp devices.

Surgical Off-loading for Flap Closure with or without Osseous Reconstruction

For chronic plantar foot wounds with stable diabetic Charcot neuroarthropathy deformity involving the midfoot/hindfoot, an initial surgical débridement may be performed to excise the wound of nonviable tissue including bursa formation, and deep soft tissue and/or bone cultures are obtained. Once infection is ruled out, the next surgical stage of reconstruction consists of excision of the soft tissue defect in a geometrical pattern that is suitable for the flap design and definitive closure. The designed flap can be raised in either fasciocutaneous, muscle, or based on a major neurovascular pedicle and rotated to the previously excised full-thickness ulceration and/or osteomyelitic defect. Through loupe magnification, careful dissection is performed and any osseous prominences and/or infected areas are resected, ensuring resection does not destabilize the existing joints. After deflation of any tourniquet use, hemostasis is achieved and the raised flap is then inset with minimal handling and without tension at the recipient site. The remaining defect at the donor site is closed with autogenous split-thickness skin graft, allogenic skin graft, or primarily if feasible. Application of the surgical off-loading circular external fixation device is then performed as it was described previously, ensuring that half pin or transosseous wire placement does not compromise the flap closure (Figs. 29.2 to 29.5).

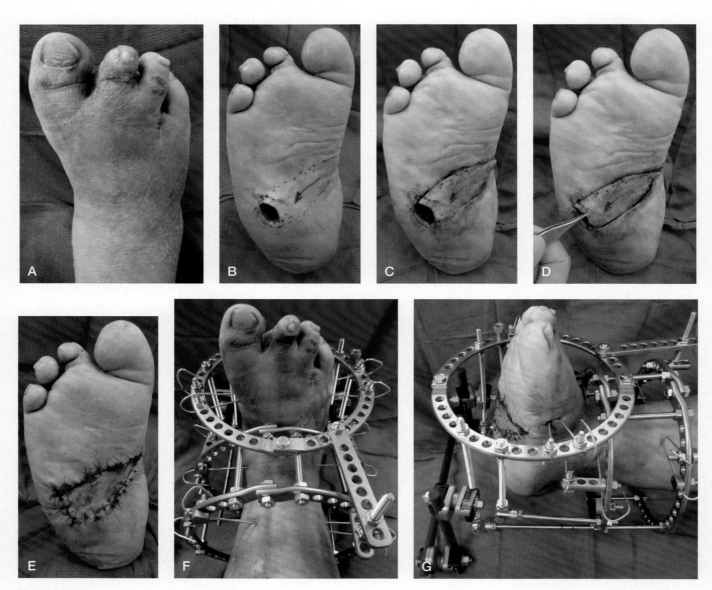

FIGURE 29.2 Intraoperative pictures **(A,B)** of a right foot chronic plantar centrolateral ulceration of a stable diabetic Charcot neuroarthropathy excised in full-thickness. Patient underwent an initial surgical débridement 2 days prior to the definitive reconstructive procedure. Picture **(C)** shows the raised local random transposition flap ready for advancement toward the soft tissue defect and after a gastrocnemius recession was performed for equinus correction **(D)**. Any tourniquet use is deflated before insetting of the raised flap to the recipient site **(E)**. The circular external fixator provided simultaneous surgical off-loading, stabilization of the foot to the lower extremity, and correction of the equinus deformity **(F–I)**. *(continued)*

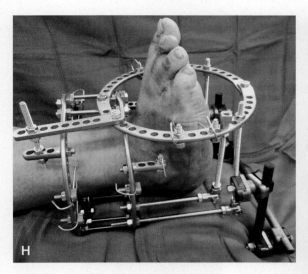

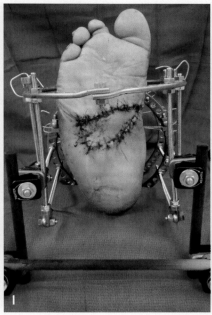

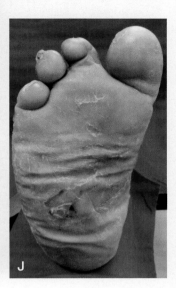

FIGURE 29.2 *(Continued)* The surgical off-loading circular external fixation device was removed at approximately 5 weeks with a clinical outcome at 14 weeks after the external fixation removal **(J)**.

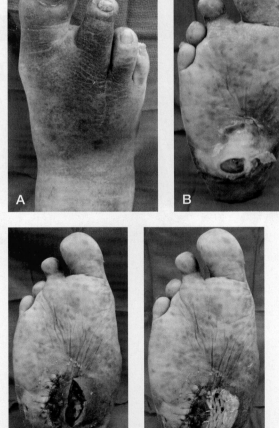

FIGURE 29.3 Intraoperative pictures **(A,B)** of a right foot chronic plantar central ulceration after surgical débridement of a stable diabetic Charcot neuroarthropathy excised in full-thickness at the initial surgery **(C)**. The patient returned to the operative room 2 days after the initial surgery for a revisional surgical débridement, double rhomboid advancement flap closure **(D–F)**, and surgical off-loading with a circular external fixator **(G–M)**. *(continued)*

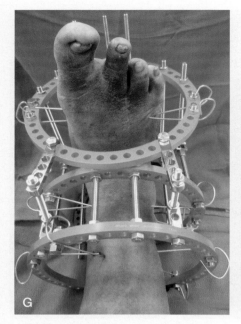

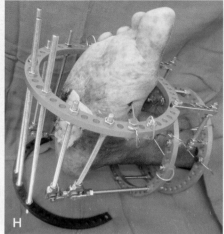

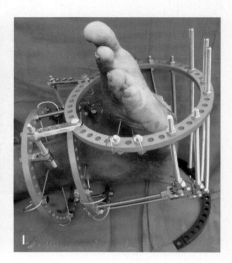

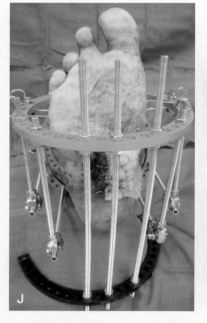

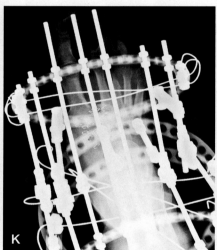

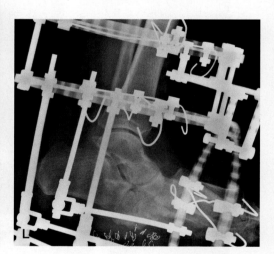

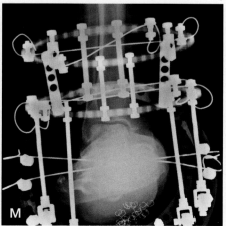

FIGURE 29.3 *(Continued)* Note that the donor site at the flap closure was covered with a dermoconductive acellular dermal replacement in a non–weight-bearing area of the foot **(F)**. The circular external fixator provided simultaneous surgical off-loading, stabilization of the foot to the lower extremity, and correction of the equinus deformity **(G–M)**. *(continued)*

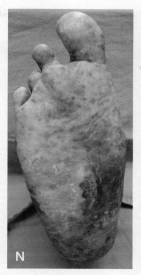
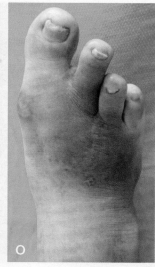
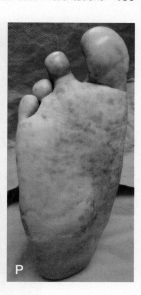

FIGURE 29.3 *(Continued)* The surgical off-loading circular external fixation device was removed at approximately 7 weeks postoperatively. Clinical outcomes at approximately 3.5 months **(N)** and 12 months **(O,P)** after the flap closure.

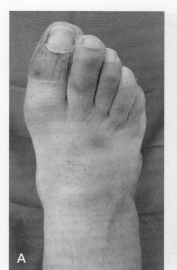
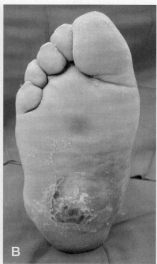
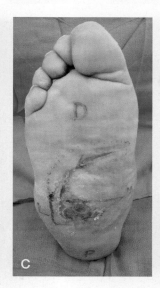
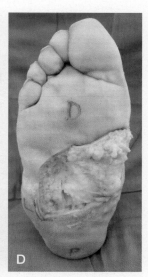

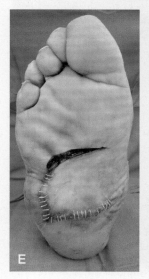
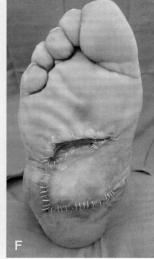

FIGURE 29.4 Intraoperative pictures **(A,B)** of a right foot chronic plantar centrolateral ulceration of a stable diabetic Charcot neuroarthropathy excised in full-thickness and in a triangular fashion **(C)**. Picture **(D)** shows the raised local rotational advancement flap toward the laterally oriented base of the excised triangular soft tissue defect **(D)**. Note the exposure of this direct approach for the simultaneous plantar exostectomy that was performed on this patient **(D)**. Any tourniquet use is deflated before insetting of the raised flap to the recipient site **(E)**. Note that the donor site at the flap closure was covered with a dermoconductive acellular dermal replacement in a non–weight-bearing area of the foot **(F)**. *(continued)*

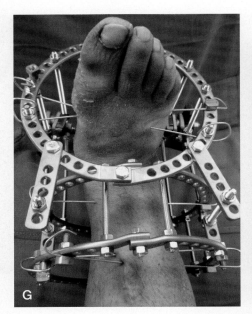

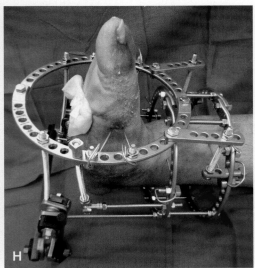

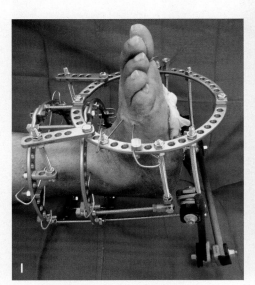

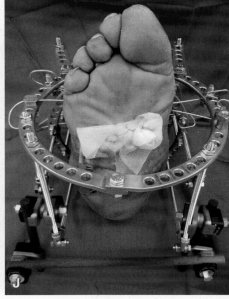

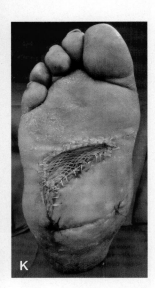

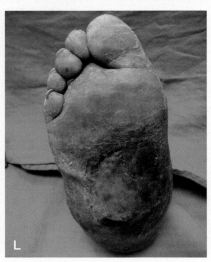

FIGURE 29.4 *(Continued)* The circular external fixator provided simultaneous surgical off-loading, stabilization of the foot to the lower extremity, and correction of the equinus deformity **(G–J)**. The surgical off-loading circular external fixation device was removed at approximately 6.5 weeks postoperatively where an autogenous split-thickness skin graft was harvested from the ipsilateral lateral aspect of the leg and placed over the previous granular surgical site created from the dermoconductive acellular dermal replacement at the flap donor site **(K)**. **L.** Clinical outcome at approximately 5 months after the flap closure.

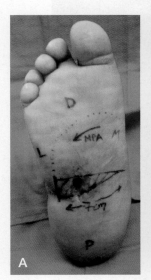
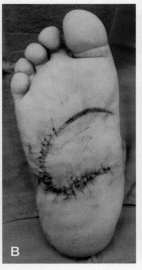
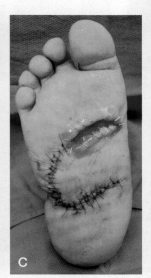
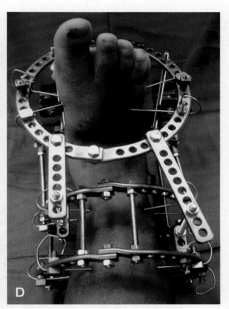
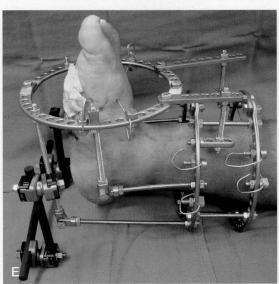
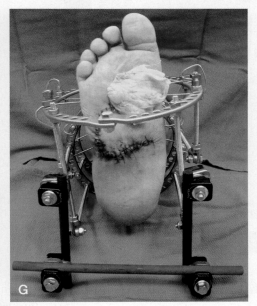
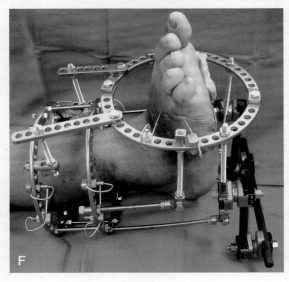

FIGURE 29.5 Intraoperative picture **(A)** of a right foot chronic plantar centrolateral ulceration after multiple surgical débridements of a stable diabetic Charcot neuroarthropathy with concomitant osteomyelitis excised in full-thickness and in a triangular fashion. The patient returned to the operative room 2 days after the initial surgery for a revisional surgical débridement, local rotational advancement flap closure **(B,C)** and surgical off-loading with a circular external fixator **(D–J)**. *(continued)*

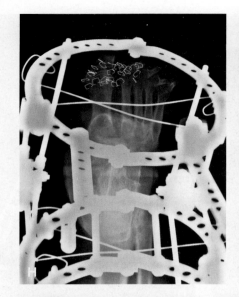
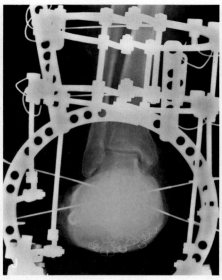
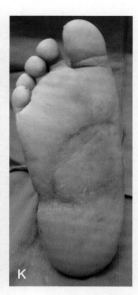

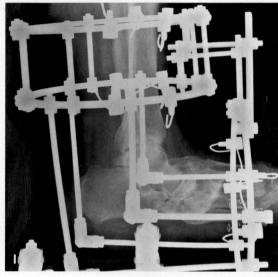

FIGURE 29.5 *(Continued)* Note the raised local rotational advancement flap toward the laterally oriented base of the excised triangular soft tissue defect followed by a dermoconductive acellular dermal replacement in the donor non–weight-bearing area of the foot **(B,C)**. The circular external fixator provided simultaneous surgical off-loading, stabilization of the foot to the lower extremity, and correction of the equinus deformity **(D–J)**. The surgical off-loading circular external fixation device was removed at approximately 7.5 weeks postoperatively. **K.** Clinical outcome at approximately 7 months after the flap closure.

Surgical Off-loading for Flap Closure and Equinus Correction

Equinus contracture of the lower extremity associated with diabetic Charcot neuroarthropathy can be surgically addressed through percutaneous or open tendo-Achilles lengthening versus gastrocnemius recession. Prior to definitive osseous reconstruction, surgical correction of equinus may facilitate reduction and/or manipulation of the diabetic Charcot neuroarthropathy deformity. A gastrocnemius recession is performed through separation of the gastrocnemius from the soleus just proximal to the gastrocnemius–soleus aponeurosis and allows the transected gastrocnemius tendon to retract proximally. This technique allows a controlled soft tissue release with decreased risk of either overlengthening or Achilles tendon rupture. The appropriate joints are then placed in realignment through arthrodesis with application of circular external fixation providing compression and maintaining the equinus correction. The kickstand apparatus is then applied to the circular external fixation for surgical off-loading.

In addition, equinus correction of the lower extremity may also need to be addressed when performing a flap closure with or without any osseous reconstruction. Surgical off-loading circular fixation can provide simultaneous maintenance of the equinus correction while stabilizing and aligning the lower extremity in the desired anatomic position (Fig. 29.6).

DISCUSSION

Combined internal and external fixation methods for surgical reconstruction of the diabetic Charcot foot neuroarthropathy may also be indicated in the absence of ulcerations, septic arthritis, and/or osteomyelitis. In these cases, multiple-joint arthrodesis is performed with the use of internal fixation and the addition of circular external fixation can provide further stabilization, compression, and surgical off-loading when necessary.

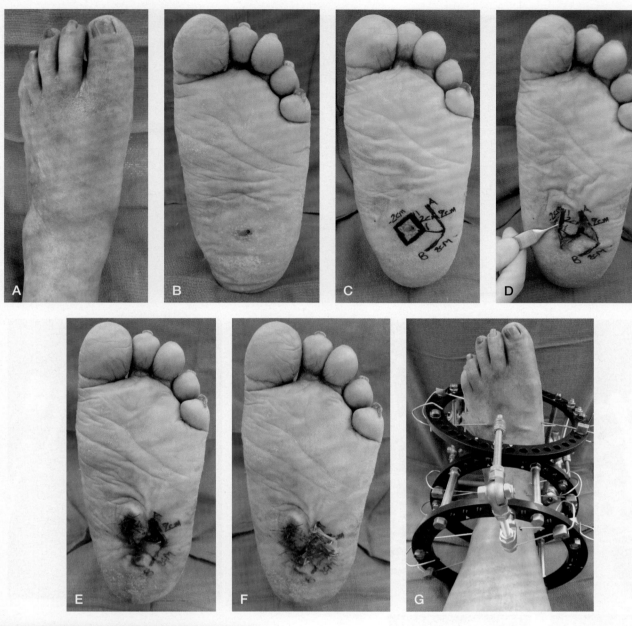

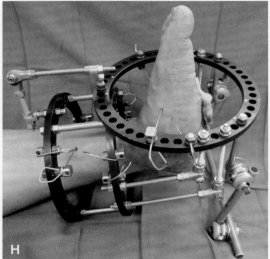

FIGURE 29.6 Intraoperative pictures **(A,B)** of a left foot chronic plantar central ulceration of a stable diabetic Charcot neuroarthropathy excised in full-thickness rhomboid fashion **(C)** and prior to an open gastrocnemius recession of the lower extremity for a single-stage reconstruction. Picture **(C)** shows the versatility of the rhomboid flap that can create 4 different donor sites to cover the original defect. A single rhomboid advancement flap of exactly the same shape and size of the defect was raised and advanced into the recipient site **(D,E)**. Note that the donor site at the flap closure was covered with a dermoconductive acellular dermal replacement in a non–weight-bearing area of the foot **(F)**. The circular external fixator provided simultaneous surgical off-loading, stabilization of the foot to the lower extremity, and correction of the equinus deformity **(G–M)**. *(continued)*

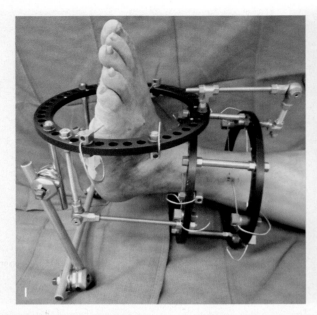

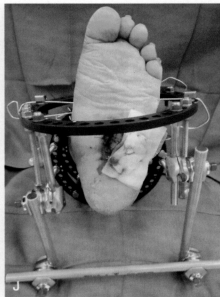

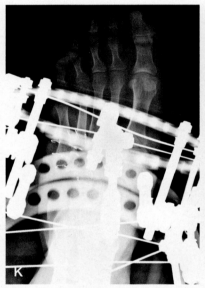

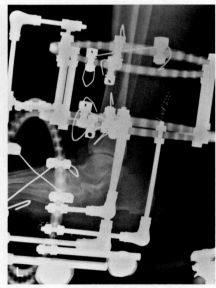

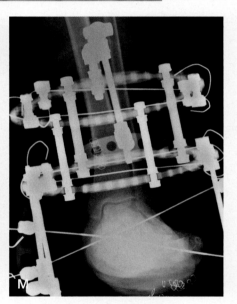

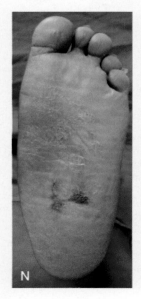

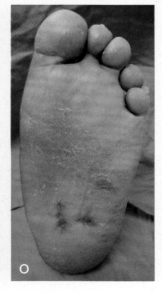

FIGURE 29.6 *(Continued)* The surgical off-loading circular external fixation device was removed at approximately 7 weeks postoperatively where an autogenous split-thickness skin graft was harvested from the ipsilateral lateral aspect of the leg and placed on the original and rhomboid flap donor sites. Clinical outcomes at approximately 6 months **(N)** and 8 months **(O)** after the flap closure.

Similarly, surgical off-loading with circular external fixation can also be implemented for cases with large soft tissue and osseous defects that are not ready for definitive wound closure and/or osseous reconstruction. Due to the presence of a large osseous defect from prior resection of osteomyelitis, antibiotic-impregnated cement beads on cerclage wire or spacers are carefully fashioned and placed into the void, providing a temporary stabilization of the adjacent tissues while simultaneously delivering local antibiotic therapy. The wounds can then be closed primarily when feasible or NPWT can be applied and changed subsequently throughout the postoperative period. The surgical off-loading circular external fixation is applied to the lower extremity accordingly and assists in the management of lower extremity stabilization, postoperative wound care, and preparation for the definitive surgical procedure.

Some of the main advantages of surgical off-loading with circular external fixation include rigid stability that minimizes shear movements, providing elevation of the lower extremity, allowing access for wound/flap care and delivering compression to augment osseous and soft tissue reconstruction while maintaining the equinus correction.

Management of diabetic patients undergoing the podoplastic approach utilizing circular external fixation is best carried out in a multidisciplinary health care setting. The diabetic patient must be educated regarding the extensive perioperative course, emphasizing the possibility of complications and providing realistic patient and family expectations. Preoperative planning encompasses thorough medical optimization and detailed options for the soft tissue and/or osseous reconstruction, with staging of procedures as needed. For the management of open wounds in the presence of deformity, surgeons should carefully choose surgical wound closure technique(s) and osseous correction(s) that complement one another with soft tissue and skeletal reconstruction. Placement of half pins/wires involved with the surgical off-loading external fixation should be carefully considered so as not to compromise the wound closure technique(s) involved.

Finally, surgical off-loading circular external fixation should be reserved for surgeons with specific training and extensive experience with external fixation, as complications with this method may be encountered in the complex diabetic population.

POSTOPERATIVE CARE

These patients are most commonly managed in the hospital setting for the first postoperative week. Duration of hospital stay is directly proportional to the extent of surgical reconstruction performed. Intravenous antibiotic therapy is provided for the remainder of the hospital stay based on intraoperative cultures if available. For major flap reconstruction, flap viability is monitored closely in the first 48 hours postoperatively. Physical therapy and rehabilitation is gradually provided, beginning with simple transfer training and upper body strengthening followed by progressive non–weight-bearing status of the affected lower extremity with use of an assistive device. Following discharge from the hospital, these patients are typically followed in the outpatient clinic setting at 1- to 2-week intervals where the flap closure is assessed and serial radiographs are taken to evaluate positioning of the external fixation along with healing of the osseous reconstruction. Appropriate surgical wound, flap, and half pin/wire care is performed as indicated and based on the given reconstructive procedures. If NPWT was utilized for a deep wound, this dressing is replaced 3 times a week until adequate granulation tissue has formed allowing definitive wound closure. In contrast, if NPWT was placed to secure a skin graft or flap, this modality is removed at 5 to 7 days postoperatively and replaced with sterile dressings. When bolster-type dressings are utilized to secure grafts, they are left intact approximately 2 to 4 weeks postoperatively.

Circular external fixation applied solely for surgical off-loading is typically removed at 6 to 10 weeks postoperatively. Longer duration of circular external fixation is often necessary for simultaneous soft tissue and osseous reconstructive procedures. Further immobilization after removal of the external fixation device by using casts or splints is usually followed by gradual assisted weight bearing in modified braces, and finally, ambulation is maintained through accommodative shoe gear with or without assistive bracing. Patients should be properly educated in the preoperative period regarding the prolonged recovery associated with these types of reconstructive procedures.

COMPLICATIONS

Early and/or late postoperative complications in this high-risk diabetic patient population are possible, and therefore, these procedures may be performed by experienced reconstructive surgeons who are prepared for the technical demands involved with circular external fixation and plastic reconstruction. Complications related to the surgical off-loading circular external fixation may usually be related to technical errors in application or poor patient selection. When using surgical off-loading circular external fixation, risk of complications related specifically to plastic surgical reconstructive procedures are theoretically reduced because this technique allows easy access to the site for frequent monitoring, flap surveillance, and care. However, complications following plastic surgical reconstruction may manifest such as wound dehiscence flap ischemia or necrosis, infection, venous congestion, and reulceration. Protection of the contralateral lower extremity should also be employed during the postoperative period due to elevated risk of injury.

Conclusion

Surgical off-loading circular external fixation is a versatile technique that can be modified for a variety of indications in the diabetic foot and ankle and can be performed in combination with several soft tissue and osseous reconstructive procedures. This method provides immediate surgical off-loading, skeletal and soft tissue stabilization, compression, and access for wound/flap care. Although these techniques show promising initial short-term results regarding the podoplastic approach for diabetic foot and ankle reconstruction, future higher powered, long-term studies are necessary to fully assess its efficacy in this challenging patient population.

References

1. Belczyk R, Ramanujam CL, Capobianco CM, et al. Combined midfoot arthrodesis, muscle flap coverage, and circular external fixation for the chronic ulcerated Charcot deformity. Foot Ankle Spec 2010;3:40–44.

2. Belczyk R, Stapleton JJ, Zgonis T. A case report of a double advancement flap closure combined with an Ilizarov technique for the chronic plantar forefoot ulceration. Int J Low Extrem Wounds 2009;8:31–36.

3. Capobianco CM, Zgonis T. Abductor hallucis muscle flap and staged medial column arthrodesis for the chronic ulcerated Charcot foot with concomitant osteomyelitis. Foot Ankle Spec 2010;3:269–273.

4. Clemens MW, Parikh P, Hall MM, et al. External fixators as an adjunct to wound healing. Foot Ankle Clin 2008;13:145–156.

5. Dalla Paola L, Carone A, Boscarino G, et al. Combination of open subtotal calcanectomy and stabilization with external fixation as limb salvage procedure in hindfoot-infected diabetic foot ulcers. Int J Low Extrem Wounds 2016;15:332–337.

6. Hegewald KW, Wilder ML, Chappell TM, et al. Combined internal and external fixation for diabetic Charcot reconstruction: a retrospective case series. J Foot Ankle Surg 2016;55:619–627.

7. Pinzur MS, Gil J, Belmares J. Treatment of osteomyelitis in Charcot foot with single-stage resection of infection, correction of deformity, and maintenance with ring fixation. Foot Ankle Int 2012;33:1069–1074.

8. Ramanujam CL, Facaros Z, Zgonis T. Abductor hallucis muscle flap with circular external fixation for Charcot foot osteomyelitis: a case report. Diabet Foot Ankle 2011;2.

9. Ramanujam CL, Facaros Z, Zgonis T. External fixation for surgical off-loading of diabetic soft tissue reconstruction. Clin Podiatr Med Surg 2011;28:211–216.

10. Ramanujam CL, Zgonis T. Primary arthrodesis and sural artery flap coverage for subtalar joint osteomyelitis in a diabetic patient. Clin Podiatr Med Surg 2011;28:421–427.

11. Sagebien CA, Rodriguez ED, Turen CH. The soft-tissue frame. Plast Reconstr Surg 2007;119:2137–2140.

12. Short DJ, Zgonis T. Circular external fixation as a primary or adjunctive therapy for the podoplastic approach of the diabetic Charcot foot. Clin Podiatr Med Surg 2017;34:93–98.

13. Zgonis T, Roukis TS, Stapleton JJ, et al. Combined lateral column arthrodesis, medial plantar artery flap, and circular external fixation for Charcot midfoot collapse with chronic plantar ulceration. Adv Skin Wound Care 2008;21:521–525.

CHAPTER 30

Postoperative Therapeutic Footwear and Rehabilitation for the Reconstructed and Amputee Patient with Diabetes Mellitus

Armin Koller

INTRODUCTION

Optimization of glycemic control assists in the improvement of wound healing, decreasing symptoms of peripheral neuropathy and lowering the rate of predominantly microvascular complications (i.e., diabetic retinopathy and nephropathy) (1,12). Frequent physician visits are necessary to verify that a blood glucose level is within the normal range. The clinical lower extremity examination consists of inspecting the skin integrity, skeletal deformities, vascular pathology, signs of peripheral neuropathy and in particular for loss of protective sensation. Diabetic foot care is an essential part of the preventive measures. Removal of any hyperkeratotic or preulcerative foot lesions might be of necessity in order to reduce any local pressure that will lead into a deep infection. Patients with diabetes mellitus need to be educated on how to properly examine their feet and wear the appropriate shoe gear (Table 30.1) (7).

In the diabetic population with related complications, rehabilitation comprehends a broad range of preventive and therapeutic measures (Table 30.2). On the other hand, not every patient with diabetes mellitus needs to wear orthopedic shoes with custom-made inserts for even pressure distribution. In the presence of loss of protective sensation or considerable peripheral arterial disease, the term *diabetic foot syndrome* is justified, and the diagnosis should not be made from the detection of an ulceration. Foot deformities can lead to areas of high (plantar) pressure, thereby increasing the risk of ulceration. Structural deformities such as a clubfoot with elevated pressure under the lateral aspect of the foot and functional deformities such as a hallux rigidus with elevated pressure under the great toe have to be taken into consideration when calculating the risk of ulceration formation (17).

In the diabetic population with a history of a healed ulceration, the risk of developing a new ulceration is further increased (25). Mechanical factors contributing to an increase

risk of new ulceration formation include partial foot amputations and Charcot neuroarthropathy (CN). The latter with a potential accumulation of risk factors like peripheral neuropathy, deformity, joint stiffness, sharp bony prominences, and thin soft tissue should be regarded as one of the highest risks of ulceration development in the patient with diabetes mellitus (5). However, the diagnosis of CN of the foot and ankle comprehends a variety of conditions. CN foot deformities that are in the reconstructive phase (Eichenholtz stage III) (Table 30.3) and primarily affecting the Lisfranc joint (Sanders type 2) (Table 30.4) without deformity during the CN process can be fitted with an off-the-shelf shoe with a stiffened outer sole plus custom-molded or premolded insole. An active CN foot (Eichenholtz stage I or II), on the contrary, with concomitant instability or high-grade deformity needs further immobilization in a cast or an orthosis unless reconstructive surgery is indicated (29).

Partial foot amputations reduce the foot contact area, whether performed as a transversal, longitudinal, or internal pedal amputation. The smaller the support surface, the higher the plantar foot pressure, which is one of the most important factors causing ulcerations when it exceeds a critical threshold. A common problem of partial foot amputations is tendon imbalance leading to additional foot and ankle deformities. Although a satisfactory operative technique can guard against tendon imbalance in many cases, the remaining clinical scenarios pose a serious problem to the pedorthist secondary to the deformity progression and very high pressure over bony prominences (24).

RISK STRATIFICATION

Many countries have developed risk stratification systems for the diabetic foot syndrome. The International Working Group on the Diabetic Foot (IWGDF) proposes a risk categorization

---

TABLE 30.1

Recommendations for Foot Care in Patients with Diabetes Mellitus

Check their shoes and socks on a regular basis.

Check for foreign objects in shoes before putting them on.

Check for rough areas inside shoes.

Wear proper fitting shoes and socks that have no seams or darning.

Look at feet daily and check for cuts, scratches, or blisters.

Use a mirror or have another person check the feet in case of impaired vision.

Cut nails straight across and have corns and calluses cut by a health care provider.

Pay special attention to feet in case of loss of protective sensation.

Wash and dry feet daily (and gently between each toe).

Do not use water with temperature >37°C (98.6°F), neither use heating pads on feet.

Use a moisturizer for dry skin (but not between the toes) and do not soak feet.

Do not use chemical agents or plasters to remove corns and calluses neither strong antiseptics on feet.

Avoid barefoot walking indoors or outdoors and wearing of shoes without socks.

TABLE 30.3

Modified Staging System of Diabetic Charcot Neuroarthropathy (10)

Stage I (developmental phase):

Stage IA: Foot swollen and warm. No deformity, no osseous changes on conventional radiographs. Bone bruise on magnetic resonance imaging

Stage IB: Soft tissue inflammation and edema, joint fragmentation, osseous dislocation

Stage II (coalescent phase):

Reduction of edema, bone callus proliferation, and fracture consolidation

Stage III (reconstructive phase):

Stabilization of the foot skeleton by osseous ankylosis and hypertrophic proliferation

---

COMPONENTS OF ORTHOPEDIC FOOTWEAR

Although the footwear recommendations in Table 30.7 relate to off-the-shelf shoes designed for diabetic patients, custom-made shoes offer numerous adaptations to foot deformities and pathologies. The different components of orthopedic footwear can be assigned to 2 functions: the first function is to modulate plantar pressure and ground reaction forces, and the second function is to provide stability or adapt to a structural deformity. However, some of the components could fulfill both functions.

Inlays or Plantar Orthoses

Inlays belong to the first group. Total contact casting, multiple-density removable inlays that are directly molded to the patient's foot or a model made after a footprint, a foam impression, or a fiberglass cast, can reduce plantar pressure peaks. Evenly soft insoles without any supporting elements have an inferior effect on pressure relief. Areas of the sole of the foot that are covered with robust skin and tissue with sufficient weight bearing capacity need to be exposed to higher pressure in order to relieve vulnerable areas. Excavations filled with

---

system with 4 levels (Table 30.5). This rather basic classification has proven its applicability to function as a tool to prevent foot complications related to diabetes mellitus (27). On the other hand, no detailed information is given about protective or therapeutic footwear.

The more comprehensive classification system by the University of Texas Health Science Center (UTHSC) in San Antonio, Texas (Table 30.6), includes additional pathology like infection and CN, but it also cannot be used as a guide for prescription form for orthopedic shoes like all the other classification systems (19).

The prescribing physician must have detailed knowledge about the different types of shoes and orthoses and their components. Although conditions like peripheral neuropathy or history of an ulcer can be treated with shoes in a rather uniform manner, pathologies like partial foot amputations and CN require individual considerations concerning therapeutic footwear (Table 30.7).

TABLE 30.2

Rehabilitation Measures in Patients with Diabetes Mellitus and Related Complications

Glycemic control	Foot care
Walking aids	Custom-made orthopedic shoes
Patient education	Regular physician visits
Preventive shoes	Prostheses and orthoses

TABLE 30.4

Sanders Classification of Diabetic Neuropathic Osteoarthropathy (30)

Type 1: Metatarsophalangeal joints

Type 2: Lisfranc joint

Type 3: Chopart joint

Type 4: Ankle and subtalar joints

Type 5: Calcaneus

TABLE 30.5

IWGDF Diabetic Foot Risk Categorization

Category	Risk Profile	Check-up Frequency
1	No sensory neuropathy	Once a year
2	Sensory neuropathy	Once every 6 months
3	Sensory neuropathy, signs of peripheral arterial disease and/or foot deformities	Once every 3 months
4	Previous ulceration	Once every 1–3 months

IWGDF, international working group on the diabetic foot.

compressible material serve for additional relief under bony prominences. The stiffness and viscoelastic properties of the inlay material are under debate. Too soft and thin materials bear the risk of a bottoming-out effect, which reduces the material's ability to distribute force (20). Soft and flexible inlays and shoes may increase shear forces due to increased adhesion during forward movement of the foot within the shoe. The material should resist permanent deformation from repeated shear and compression after long-term use (6). Therefore, semirigid materials are recommended to fulfill both criteria of pressure reduction and durability.

On the other hand, material stiffness may have unexpected effects on the diabetic foot. Gefen et al. (11) developed a finite element (FE) model of the plantar tissue under the second ray (toe and metatarsal) of the foot, suggesting a positive

TABLE 30.6

UTHSC Diabetic Foot Risk Categorization

Category	Possible Treatment (with regard to shoes)
0: No pathology	Possible shoe accommodations
1: Neuropathy, no deformity	Possible therapeutic footwear
2: Neuropathy with deformity	Pedorthic/orthotist consultation for possible molded/extra depth shoe accommodation
3: History of pathology	Pedorthic/orthotist consultation for molded/extra depth shoe accommodation
4A: Neuropathic wound	
4B: Acute Charcot neuroarthropathy joint	
5: Infected diabetic foot	
6: Ischemic lower extremity	

UTHSC, University of Texas Health Science Center (San Antonio)

TABLE 30.7

Footwear Recommendations for Preventive Shoes in Patients with Diabetes Mellitus

The shoe should:
Match the shape of the foot and fit snugly without being too tight
Have a deep enough toe box to accommodate forefoot shape and deformities
Have a well-fitted heel counter that will keep the foot in place together with a secure fastening mechanism
Have means of closure such that can be handled by the patient
Have a wide sole to provide sufficient stability
Have a heel height that does not exceed 1 in.
Have a removable insole and a shock absorbent midsole
Have an upper made of leather or comparable material to allow for breathability, durability, and hygiene
Have a 0.6 in gap between the tip of the big toe and the toe box
Allow for modifications of upper and sole
Have a smooth inside lining free from seams or wrinkles

feedback mechanism of diffusion of ulcerations in the diabetic foot, where the lesion is spreading from deep muscles to the skin surface by an evolving mechanical stress wave. With a soft insole material, FE simulations for an uninjured diabetic foot suggested compression within the plantar musculature that was about 1.25-fold greater than compression with a stiffer insole. Also, the soft insole produced shear stresses on muscle tissue that were about 1.3-fold greater in comparison to the stiffer insole (11). As long as deep internal tissue stresses cannot be measured routinely, quality management of protective insoles can only rely on plantar pressure measurements.

Apart from the discussion on viscoelastic material properties, the shape of the inlay should not be underestimated because molded orthoses are more effective than nonmolded orthoses in reducing plantar pressure (21). The feasibility of regular disinfection of the inlays must be guaranteed without altering surface qualities and moisture should not lead to cracks and hardening of the inlay because it happens with drying leather. Basic recommendations for therapeutic shoe inserts for patients with diabetes mellitus have been summarized by Medicare (Table 30.8).

Rocker Bottom Soles

Stiffened rocker bottoms are also effective in reducing plantar pressure in the area of the metatarsal heads. When relief of metatarsal heads is intended, the pivot point of the rocker bottom profile needs to be proximal of the metatarsal heads (14). One mechanism for pressure reduction is the acceleration of the center of pressure (progression of the gait line), so that the rather high forces during toe-off bear down the

TABLE 30.8

Medicare Criteria for Custom-fabricated Shoe Inserts for Patients with Diabetes Mellitus

1. The therapeutic shoe insert for diabetic patients is a total contact, custom-fabricated, multiple-density removable inlay that is molded to a model of the individual's foot so that it conforms to the plantar surface and makes total contact with the foot, including the arch.

2. The insert must retain its shape during use for the life of the insert.

3. A custom-fabricated device is made from materials that do not have predefined trim lines for heel cup height, arch height and length, or toe shape.

4. The base layer of the device must be of a sufficient thickness and durometer to maintain its shape during use (e.g., at least 3/16 in. of Shore A 35 material or higher).

5. The base layer is allowed to be thinner in the custom-fabricated device because appropriate arch fill or other additional material will be layered up individually to maintain shape and achieve total contact.

6. The central portion of the base layer of the heel may be thinner (but at least 1/16 in.) to allow for greater pressure reduction.

7. The specified thickness of the lateral portions of the base layer must extend from the heel through the distal metatarsals and may be absent at the toes.

8. The top layer of the device may be of a lower durometer and must also be heat moldable.

9. The materials used should be suitable with regard to the individual's condition.

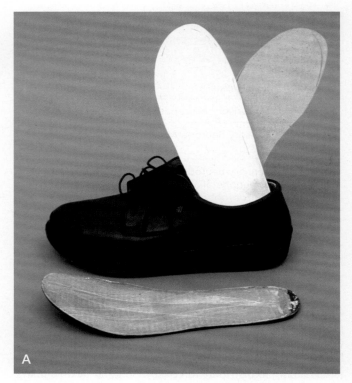

A

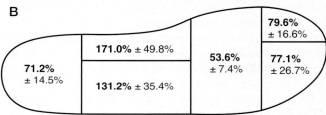

B

FIGURE 30.1 **A.** Combination of custom-made full-contact inlays and stiffened outsole with pivot point proximal of the metatarsal heads. **B.** Medium-pressure relief (10 healthy volunteers walking at self-selected speed in low shoes of the same manufacturer) at different foot areas relative to shoes without rocker bottom soles and with flat cork inlay (9).

area of the metatarsal heads for a shorter period of time. The other mechanism is restriction of hyperextension in the metatarsophalangeal joints, which otherwise exposes the metatarsal heads to a high pressure. Peak pressure relief in the area of the metatarsal heads is as effective as by means of inlays, but in contrast, its efficacy decreases with lower walking speed (9). However, patients with diabetic neuropathy should not be encouraged to walk faster because peak pressure is expected to increase with higher walking speed and stride length (26).

The effects of these different pressure-relieving methods are additive so that an inlay should always be combined with a stiffened rocker bottom for optimum pressure relief. Under the metatarsal heads, where the majority of plantar ulcerations occur, the combination of both methods is twice as efficacious as each single measure alone and can amount to some 50% peak pressure reduction in comparison with shoes with flat cork inlays and without rocker bottom soles (9) (Fig. 30.1).

A stiffened rocker bottom (Fig. 30.2) also contributes to stabilization of the foot structure, protecting the tarsal and metatarsophalangeal joints from bending and torque forces. Besides pressure reduction in a particular area of the foot, a stiffened outsole serves for deformity correction and immobilization of the foot in the shoe. In addition, molded inlays should always

be combined with stiffened rocker bottoms for pressure relief under the metatarsal heads.

Cushioned Heel

Besides alleviation of impact force during heel strike, a cushioned heel acts like a posterior rocker and thereby displaces the center of pressure anteriorly. In cases of thin or fragile skin under the calcaneal tuberosity, a cushioned heel can redirect impact forces toward a more robust tissue under the anterior calcaneus. In cases of a mild foot drop deformity, the cushioned heel diminishes dropping of the foot at the heel contact. An exaggerated anterior rocker and cushioned heel (posterior rocker) narrow the contact area substantially, thereby interfering with postural stability. Please note that optimum pressure distribution has to be weighed against stance and gait stability.

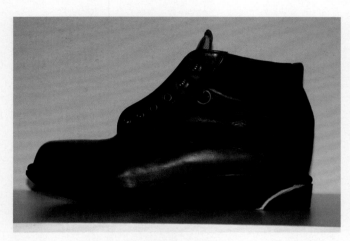

FIGURE 30.2 Stiffened rocker bottom with pivot point proximal of the metatarsal heads. The cushioned heel is marked on the shoe.

Shoe Height and Reinforced Leg

Stability in terms of resistance against deforming forces and adaptation to an already existing foot deformity, the second function of shoe components, can only be achieved by means of a high shoe. Shoe height may vary from bottine (ankle-high) shoes to high shoes with a leg extending above the ankle joint. The proper degree of flexibility of the leg depends on outsole flexibility. Because diabetic feet after partial amputation or surgical reconstruction are ideally protected by a stiffened outsole, a high leg should also be stiff in order to prevent wrinkling of the shoe and friction between the foot and the shoe (8).

Shoe height and reinforcing elements of the leg are chosen according to which movement of the foot needs to be restricted. If the ankle joint is stable and offers a reasonable range of motion, restriction of pronation and supination may be sufficient by means of medial and lateral reinforcing elements (Fig. 30.3) within the leg, and the shoe height is about 6.5 in. This type of shoe is lighter than a high (8.5 in.) and completely stiff shoe and facilitates roll-off and stepping on the gas which is an important aspect with respect to the common walking disability of many diabetic patients with foot problems. Additionally, the reinforcing elements can be fabricated as an integral part of the inlay (Fig. 30.4). If the ankle joint demonstrates considerable instability or deformity in the sagittal plane, a high shoe is inevitable, and the leg has to be reinforced at the medial, lateral, and dorsal aspect of the shoe.

Shoe Tongue and Closure

The 3-point principle is applied if maximal fixation of the shoe in the foot is mandatory. In addition to leg and outsole, the shoe tongue is also stiffened (8). If all 3 components of the shoe are stiff and the patient has a stiff foot, donning and doffing a shoe can be quite a challenge despite a wide opening. The effectiveness of a stiffened shoe tongue with regard to immobilization of the foot depends on the

patient's ability to close the shoe. The required strong and high closure method is worthless if the patient or a helping person cannot handle it. Hook-and-loop fastener, buckles, lacing, or a combination of different closure systems are some modifications that allow for the use of orthopedic shoes by diabetic patients unable to use the original closure due to bony deformity of the foot, dysfunction of their hands, or motion limitations. The risk of noncompliance increases considerably, unless self-dependent donning and doffing the shoe is ascertained.

Flared Heel or Sole

A sole flare improves stability by widening the base of support of the shoe. A medial flare resists eversion, whereas a lateral flare resists inversion of the foot. A heel flare is also applied either medially or laterally and improves sagittal alignment in cases of varus or valgus deformity of the hindfoot.

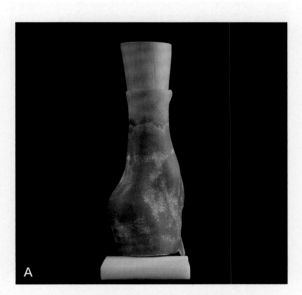

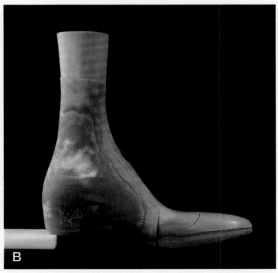

FIGURE 30.3 **A,B.** Reinforcement of a high shoe leg.

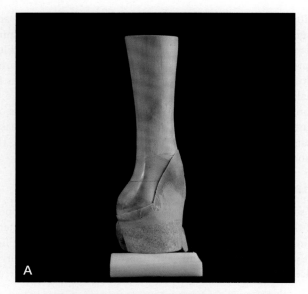

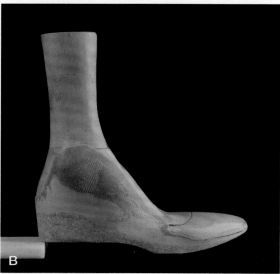

FIGURE 30.4 **A,B.** Medial reinforcement as integral part of the inlay in order to counterbalance hindfoot valgus.

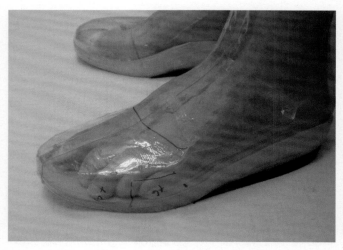

FIGURE 30.5 Loaded foot with check shoe. Areas of insufficient clearance are marked.

POSTOPERATIVE ORTHOSES, DEVICES, AND THERAPEUTIC FOOTWEAR FOR THE DIABETIC PATIENT WITH CHARCOT NEUROARTHROPATHY RECONSTRUCTION

Lower extremity amputations and CN are the most demanding and challenging problems with regard to conservative treatment with shoes or orthoses. CN foot and ankle deformities that can be fitted with an off-the-shelf shoe are exceptions because in most cases, the CN process leads to deformities that require a custom-made shoe. An active CN process needs treatment with rigid fixation in an orthosis or a total contact cast, and CN feet after operative reconstructions will also have to be protected from excessive loading or from bending and torque forces by means of postoperative orthotic management.

After reconstructive CN foot and ankle surgery, weight bearing of the lower extremity has to be restricted so that the performed arthrodesis can be achieved. Internal osteosynthesis may require postoperative non–weight-bearing for some weeks, followed by partial or full weight bearing for several months. External fixation surgery for the management of CN also needs orthoses for follow-up treatment for even a longer time, but a distinction has to be made between midfoot and hindfoot/ankle surgery. Reconstructions in the area of the midfoot have to be protected against external forces, whereas axial loading may be necessary to improve bony or fibrous arthrodesis in the area of the hindfoot/ankle (17). Prefabricated walkers or custom-made orthoses with different designs are available to fulfill distinct demands concerning after surgical treatment.

The utilization of a total contact cast after surgical reconstruction of the diabetic CN foot and/or ankle deformity may be utilized with extreme caution. The total contact cast is made of plaster of Paris or fiberglass by the physician or a cast

Check Shoe

An orthopedic check shoe is not a part of the shoe but a transparent flexible plastic shoe formed over a patient's foot last. When placed on the patient's foot, the check shoe allows for visualization of the distribution and magnitude of skin loading as revealed in tissue blanching and blushing. The diabetic neuropathic patient cannot give an accurate feedback on pressure within the shoe, and therefore, this device is rather helpful for optimum shoe fit and avoidance of pressure sores. When the test is performed with the patient standing on their inlays, the amount of clearance afforded between the shoe and the foot in vulnerable regions can be recognized (Fig. 30.5). Similarly, the check shoe is a valuable tool to minimize the risk of pressure sores within custom-made orthopedic shoes.

technician, so that it is cheap in fabrication and immediately available. The foot and lower leg have to be wrapped in cotton wool or a comparable padding, and bony prominences are separately protected from high pressure by local pads. Frequent replacements of the total contact cast may be necessary due to regression of swelling which lead to increasing patient costs and are very time-consuming. Although the total contact cast has been the "golden standard" for the treatment of neuropathic plantar ulcerations (2), it cannot be recommended unreservedly for the treatment of CN feet and in particular after reconstructive surgery, when weight bearing is intended. Mechanical stability and restriction of movements of the foot and ankle joints are better controlled by custom-made orthoses. Walking in a total contact cast may therefore have a higher risk of inadequate immobilization of the osteosynthesis or the arthrodesis joints after removal of the external fixation.

Similar to the total contact cast, a prefabricated diabetic walker (DW) is also available immediately if it can be stored. Mechanical stability decreases with use, depending on the model. In principle, the DW is an off-the-shelf total contact cast, and therefore, some authors even lock it with cable fixers to prevent its removal by the patient, thereby trying to enforce compliance. Irremovable devices have proven to be as safe and effective as a total contact cast for the treatment of diabetic neuropathic ulcerations (28). However, with regard to CN, the DW has little scope for modifications; its shape is designed to enclose a foot with some swelling but not with considerable deformity. Because CN feet mostly retain at least some degree of deformity after surgery, the DW is not the orthosis of choice after reconstructive foot and ankle

surgery in diabetic patients with polyneuropathy. Recent developments could ensure a more precise embedding of the foot in a prefabricated DW by using chambers filled with Styrofoam granules for fixation of the foot and lower leg (Fig. 30.6A). After evacuating the chambers, the cushioning material becomes stiff and maintains its shape until air is filled in again. The same method is used for adjustments after edema regression or tissue atrophy. Even if a CN foot with a marked deformity is not a suitable subject to be treated with such a DW, the assumed more rigid fixation of the foot in comparison to a DW with air chambers could offer an advantage in the orthotic treatment of the initial stage of the disease, when a skeletal deformity is not yet present, or after reconstructive surgery, if the foot is well-aligned after the operation (see Fig. 30.6B,C).

The Charcot restraint orthotic walker (CROW) fits more precisely than a total contact cast or a DW because it is made over a positive model. The CROW device is durable and allows for good control of edema. Load transmission on lower leg depends on the way of fastening the device. High pressure on soft tissues thereby enforces their atrophy, which can lead to worse fit of the orthosis and undesirable motions in the area of the osteosynthesis or the arthrodesis joints. Provided that the CROW is applied correctly and examined regularly, it is a useful tool for mobilization of the patient but immobilization of the CN joint(s) (Fig. 30.7) (4,23).

Frame orthosis (FO), as it is built in the author's institution, follows the CN neurotraumatic theory and provides attention on joint immobilization. Based on this principle, FO is a consistent derivative of the CROW device. The CN neurotraumatic theory asserts that the loss of neurogenic joint

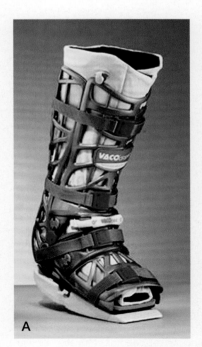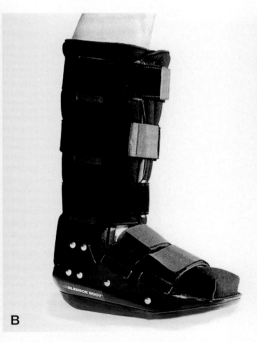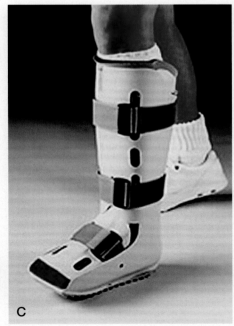

FIGURE 30.6 Diabetic walkers of various manufacturers. **A.** Vacuum cushion molded device. **B.** Bledsoe. **C.** Aircast.

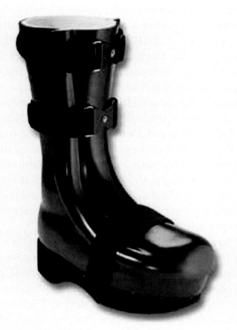

FIGURE 30.7 Charcot restraint orthotic walker (CROW) (Langer, Inc., Deer Park, NY).

control with repetitive stress leads to the initiation of an inflammatory response that results in destruction of cartilage and bone. The inflammatory model proposes that an initial traumatic event, even a minor one, would suffice to trigger an inflammatory cascade through increased expression of proinflammatory cytokines. Hence, it appears to be logic that orthoses for the treatment of CN feet have to be targeted

at protection from joint movements by means of restricting bending and torque forces instead of vertical unweighting as it is exerted in the treatment of diabetic neuropathic plantar ulcerations.

With the FO application (Fig. 30.8), full axial load is used to facilitate the joint arthrodesis after external fixation surgery and removal, particularly with CN of the hindfoot/ankle. Depending on the surgeon's demands, the FO can also be constructed with an additional infracondylar or infrapatellar support. The rigid 3-dimensional fixation of the foot serves for the reduction of shearing forces. An important feature is a pretibial shell form-locking with the triangular shape of the tibia in order to eliminate lower leg rotary motion because this is forwarded via the subtalar joint to the midtarsal joints. The FO with rear entrance and a solid heel holder wedges the lower leg from the tibial head to heel so that the fastener around the calf is no longer the factor determining suspension in this orthosis. Additionally, the foot is fixed through a tongue from synthetic leather. A relatively thin pad appears to be more suitable to control motion of the foot because stability is more important than soft padding. Vulnerable bony prominences have to be protected against high pressure (18).

Manufacturing of the FO starts with cast taking of the foot in the corrected position. Particularly, if the ankle joint is still flexible, exact adjustment of the foot is the key step in the production of the author's orthotic device because the vector of plantar forces is determined by this. Before suction molding of the interim orthosis that is made of polyethylene terephthalate glycol (PETG), a relatively thin soft pad made of 6 mm nonperforated ethylene vinyl acetate is wrapped around the foot and ankle of the model. As a clear transparent material, PETG allows identification of pressure marks and modification of the

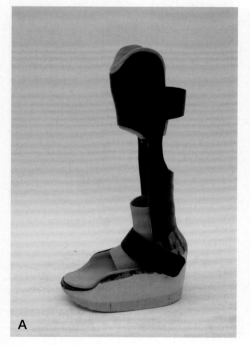
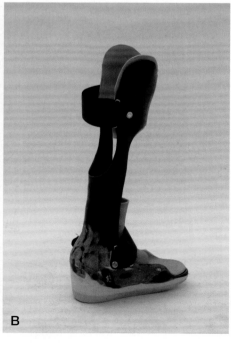

FIGURE 30.8 **A,B.** Frame orthosis. (Courtesy of the Department of Technical Orthopaedics, Münster University Hospital, Germany.)

orthosis using a hot air gun. Finally, the interim orthosis is reinforced with carbon fibers. The final orthosis is made from epoxy casting resin and is fitted after edema regression. The rocker bottom is foamed from polyurethane and individually ground during dynamic gait analysis. In addition to an anterior and posterior rocker bar, the plateau of the sole is important for safe standing and stance phase stability. The comfortable rear and front cutouts make the orthosis lightweight, with concomitant stability.

Custom-made shoes are fitted following orthotic treatment. A high shoe (about 8.5 in.) with a reinforced leg in combination with a stiffened rocker bottom sole is prescribed. A medially or laterally flared heel or sole is necessary in cases of malalignment of the foot in the frontal plane. If the foot is well-aligned in the sagittal and frontal plane, the following shoe after wear out of the first pair can be constructed with a shorter leg (about 6.5 in.), but still, a mediolateral stabilization of the rearfoot is recommended. When only the midfoot is involved (Sanders types 2 and 3), this type of shoe is an alternative to the aforementioned high shoe (arthrodesis boot). A rigid rocker bottom sole with cushioned heel serves for protection of the foot structure. The patient with a diabetic foot syndrome is in need of at least 2 pair of shoes, unless he or she is not able to walk outside the house. The shoes worn at day have to dry out overnight in order to avoid hygienic problems. It should be kept in mind that the foot has to be protected by means of custom-made shoes also in the house, where many of the patients spend most of their time during the day. Hence, orthopedic house shoes may be even more important than outdoor shoes. Low shoes without any stabilization of the ankle cannot be recommended, even though a very compliant patient with a minimally deformed CN foot might be able to wear them without notable complications.

REHABILITATION AFTER EXTERNAL FIXATION SURGERY FOR DIABETIC CHARCOT NEUROARTHROPATHY

After removal of the external fixation device, the subsequent plaster cast and edema reduction treatment for 2 to 3 days is followed by fitting of an interim orthosis. Because most of the diabetic patients with polyneuropathy are not able to reduce weight loading of the foot in a controlled manner with the help of crutches, full weight bearing is allowed immediately, but time is limited to 15 to 30 minutes at the beginning. Unless problems such as ulcerations, pain, or swelling develop, the duration of weight bearing is continuously increasing slowly. The axial compression leads to compaction of the osseous structures of the hindfoot/ankle (Fig. 30.9). This can require a correction of the interim orthosis. After an extended period of full weight bearing, it is occasionally detectable on plain radiographs that the distance between the bone fragments has declined.

The final resin-casted orthosis is fabricated after 3 to 5 months, as soon as constant volume conditions of the soft tissue can be resumed. Orthotic treatment is continued after external fixation surgery for 9 to 12 months because the risk of recurrent foot and ankle malalignments is higher after a short postoperative orthotic care. If a considerable deformity of the foot does not exist, custom-made orthopedic shoes can be fitted. A smooth transition from orthoses to shoes should be preferred. A fixing shoe with rolling sole (high shoe with stiffened leg) is initially worn for not more than 15 to 30 minutes per day. Unless skin lesions or a new episode of CN occur, ambulation time in shoes may increase. In summary, orthotic treatment after external fixation surgery of CN feet is an integral part of the treatment concept and therefore requires close teamwork between the surgeon and orthopedic technicians.

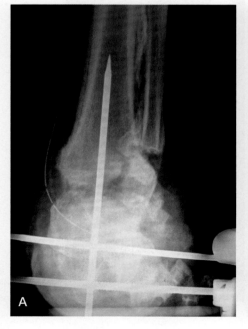
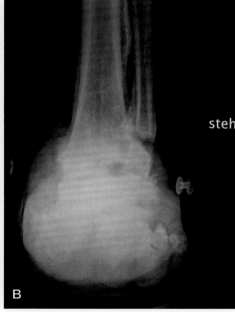

FIGURE 30.9 Charcot neuroarthropathy of the foot after reconstructive surgery with external fixation. **A.** An osseous gap between the distal tibia and foot is noted. **B.** Tibia impacting the foot under axial load within frame orthosis.

REHABILITATION AFTER INTERNAL FIXATION SURGERY FOR DIABETIC CHARCOT NEUROARTHROPATHY

After osteosynthetic stabilization of non-CN fractures in diabetic patients with peripheral polyneuropathy, the non–weight-bearing time has to be twofold in comparison to patients without peripheral polyneuropathy. The reason for the prolonged immobilization is not just the incidence of impaired fracture healing commonly encountered in patients with diabetic neuropathy. It is the risk of an acute CN process to be provoked by the operation or the preceding trauma (16,22). If postoperative weight bearing starts too early, the following inflammatory process (Eichenholtz stage I) with joint fragmentation and osseous dislocation destabilizes the retained osteosynthesis of the CN foot and/or ankle. Continual walking in the absence of pain leads to movements of the retained internal fixation hardware against the foot structure. Broken hardware and destructed bone is one of the worst clinical scenarios for the reconstructive surgeon (Fig. 30.10). The same problems may also occur after reconstructive surgery of pre-existing CN feet with screws, plates, or intramedullary nails.

Prevention of an acute CN process is achieved by non–weight-bearing, casting, and bracing. After several weeks of non–weight-bearing in a cast, mobilization in an orthosis or a cast starts with partial weight bearing. On average, full loading of the foot is allowed 2 or 3 months after the operation. Protection of the foot with bracing or casting is necessary for 6 to 12 months, before custom-made shoes can be fitted.

Despite differences with regard to the postoperative orthotic treatments, it is obvious that considerable time of non–weight-bearing is important to avoid the aforementioned problems.

In contrast to external fixation surgery, axial loading of the hindfoot/ankle in order to facilitate the joint arthrodesis is not indicated. Bracing or casting is rather targeted at additional rigid external fixation of the foot. The required postoperative duration of casting and immobilization also depends on the location and type of arthrodesis. In general, the hindfoot/ankle has to bear more stress than the midfoot, which can be protected easier from bending forces by a device with a rigid lever extending to the tibial tuberosity. Walking with a well-fitted orthosis is not usually harmful but can even improve the rate of osseous healing (33).

Lastly, an important point to mention is that the surgeon is able to follow and examine the reconstructed diabetic CN patients on a regular basis over a longer time. In contrast to standardized procedures like after total hip or knee replacement, each diabetic patient needs a rather individualized rehabilitation strategy depending on clinical and radiographic examinations every 6 weeks within the first half year and at least every 3 months thereafter.

POSTOPERATIVE ORTHOSES, DEVICES, AND THERAPEUTIC FOOTWEAR FOR THE AMPUTEE PATIENT WITH DIABETES MELLITUS

Amputations eventually shorten the foot and lead to a substantial loss of weight bearing areas on the diabetic neuropathic patient. To overcome the consequent problems with postural instability and increase of load on the remaining tissue, ray (toe and metatarsal) amputations or inner pedal amputations are at the surgeon's discretion. These kind of operative procedures only make sense if the fitting of orthopedic

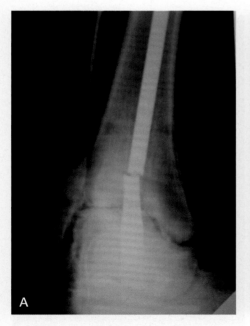
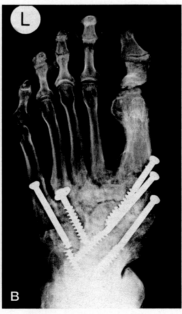

FIGURE 30.10 **A,B.** Examples of broken retained osteosynthesis due to improper postoperative treatment.

shoes or prostheses can be guaranteed. In addition, adequate shoes can only be provided under the precondition that the foot stump allows for weight bearing and does not show larger axial deviations.

The postoperative device, regardless of whether built as a foot orthosis in a standard shoe, a custom-made shoe or prosthesis covering the complete lower leg has to compensate for the loss of weight bearing area. Load transmission to the ground while walking requires a reliable connection of the residual foot with the prosthesis without any so-called "stump-pseudoarthrosis." Axial deviations are difficult to compensate with prosthetic modifications; therefore, operative corrections should be considered.

A snug fit of the stump with the prosthesis can only be achieved by a total surface contact of the residual foot. For amputations at the Lisfranc joint or more distal, it is desirable to avoid a support proximal to the ankle joint. Chopart stumps need to be stabilized by fixing the ankle joint with the aim to prevent excessive pressure at the stump end. A high prosthetic socket is particularly advisable if there are additional factors interfering with postural stability. Some of those negative factors include contralateral amputations, postural sway due to peripheral polyneuropathy, weak knee extensor muscles, or axial deviations of the stump.

Toe Amputations

Toe fillers are contraindicated in the presence of peripheral arterial disease. Adjacent toes tend to close the gap caused by the amputated one between them, although there is no vital necessity to prevent this natural mechanism. Cosmetic replacement of several toes does not result in any improvement of stance or gait. Loss of the great toe leads to overloading of the adjacent rays with the risk of plantar ulcerations or metatarsal fatigue fractures. In these cases, the shoe should have a stiffened rocker sole. The optimal position of the rocker axis is slightly proximal of the metatarsal heads, whereas the inlay has an internal metatarsal support.

Ray (Toe and Metatarsal) Amputations

Unlike metatarsal resections, ray amputations may result in a considerable reduction of the weight bearing plantar surface, depending on the extent of the forefoot segments removed. Medial or lateral ray amputations may affect mediolateral instability with additional pressure problems. Amputations of the fifth ray with disarticulation at the fifth metatarsocuboid joint are crucial because of the risk of detaching the peroneus brevis tendon, sometimes leading to a progressive supination deformity. Custom-made multilayer multidensity insoles are appropriate for even pressure distribution under the remainder of the foot. In cases of first ray amputation, the molded insole needs to support the medial border of the foot. A boot-type shoe is recommended in order to provide mediolateral stability, which can be further improved by a reinforced heel counter. Central ray resections are usually less problematic, and the foot is easy to fit in shoes with minor modifications and a molded insole.

Transmetatarsal and Lisfranc Amputations

Amputations at the transmetatarsal (TMA) and Lisfranc level allow for wearing a shoe, whether off-the-shelf or custom-made, whereas a custom-fitted or custom-molded foot orthosis may be used as a replacement or substitute for missing parts of the foot. The end of the stump has to be in close contact with the foot orthosis in order to avoid friction forces. Additionally, the stump end is protected by a rigid cap which extends to the plantar surface. The hardness of the forefoot filler greatly influences the gait pattern. A soft material eases roll-off but reduces stance stability (the functional weight bearing area is smaller). Kinking at toe-off increases the risk of pressure ulcers at the stump end. On contrary, a hard material or a long stiff sole exerts a knee stabilizing moment during gait. The rigid lever reduces the risk of pressure ulcers at the distal end of the stump. Sliding out of the heel has to be prevented by an exact anatomic fit of the foot orthosis. TMA and Lisfranc amputations proceed through the apex of the foot arch, so that the stump end shows a pretended supination. Pronation movement in the subtalar joint only enables partial correction, so that a foot orthosis with a medial wedge and a lateral shell-like rim is necessary.

A heel clamp prosthesis is a partial foot prosthesis whose suspension is provided by a posterior "clamp." The sole is reinforced by carbon fibers and acrylic resin, and a nylon belt strengthens the heel clamp (3). Donning and doffing the prosthesis is more difficult in comparison to a foot orthosis with forefoot filler. Pressure on the non–weight-bearing soft tissue is generally higher in the area of the heel clamp, and therefore, this type of prosthesis may be harmful for an amputee who lost parts of his foot due to peripheral neuropathy or peripheral arterial disease. Hidden in a sock, the heel clamp (Bellman) prosthesis is rather modest in appearance (Fig. 30.11).

A silicone forefoot prosthesis offers possibly the best cosmetic restoration. Its flexibility provides adaptation to different heel heights to some degree. Just like the heel clamp prosthesis, the design of the silicon prosthesis is geared to wear it in a standard shoe. The fixation of the prosthesis onto the stump is ensured by surface adhesion and full contact fit. Prior to the fabrication of the definitive prosthesis, a trial prosthesis serves for testing by the patient and taking notes of necessary adjustments. The durable silicone of the definitive prosthesis makes further modifications impossible, so an inconstant stump volume or pressure ulcerations are a contraindication for this type of device. Further points of criticism are the rather heavy weight of the silicone material and the high price, so this type of prosthesis is not covered by most of the health insurances. Although the silicone prosthesis may offer high functionality in a traumatic amputee, the device deserves the same skepticism as the heel clamp prosthesis when a diabetic amputee with sensory neuropathy or peripheral arterial disease is involved.

Rearfoot Amputations

The shock-absorbing capacity of the heel pad together with a full-thickness sole skin provide an end-bearing rearfoot stump

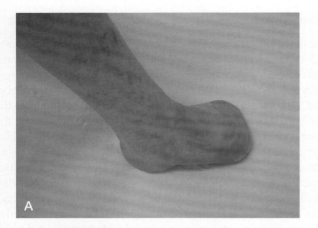

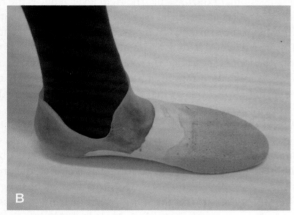

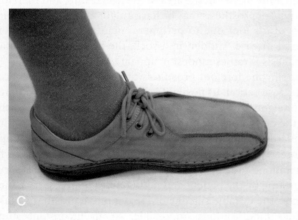

FIGURE 30.11 **A.** Lisfranc stump. **B.** Bellman prosthesis. **C.** Prosthesis with shoe.

despite its markedly reduced support surface. In the absence of deformities, plantar bony prominences, or skin grafts, no support at the tibial head is necessary. Any proximal support would rather impair venous and lymphatic circulation (edema) and implicate a potential risk of skin lesions. The pear-shaped rearfoot stumps bear a challenge for an appealing prosthetic cosmesis.

As a rule, prostheses for rearfoot stumps in diabetic amputees have a high shaft extending to the tibial tuberosity, thereby fixing the ankle joint. Embedding with dorsiflexion

and pronation helps to counter the disposition of the stump to develop equinus or supination deformity due to tendon imbalance. As an exception, stumps following the amputation lines of Bona-Jaeger and Chopart may facilitate the fitting of footwear as described for the more distal amputations under the precondition that the stump has no deformity in any plane. The prosthetist may also abandon the high shaft if the diabetic patient has very limited walking capacity. Balance disorders as a result of diabetic polyneuropathy or contralateral amputation should also be excluded in this case.

The high shaft prosthesis for Bona-Jaeger and Chopart stumps has a socket design similar to the mentioned FO with a pretibial shell, heel holder, and rear entrance. The rigid lever arm eliminates peak forces during heel strike and toe-off. The construction is lightweight and makes the use of a standard shoe possible, unless the stump is too bulky. If the stump has a rather cylindrical shape or if the ankle joint is no longer present (Pirogoff and Syme stump), the prosthetic shaft consists of an inner soft socket and a container made of casting resin or carbon fibers (Fig. 30.12).

A low-level prosthetic foot serves for leg length compensation after a Pirogoff (1 to 1.5 in.) or Syme (2 to 3 in.) amputation. Modern carbon feet act like a spring ("energy storing") and help to decrease energy consumption while walking. Sagittal alignment requires 1 to 2 in. lateral displacement of the prosthetic foot (Table 30.9).

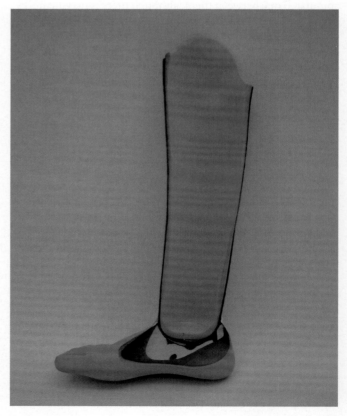

FIGURE 30.12 Cut through Syme prosthesis with inner soft socket.

TABLE 30.9
When to Prescribe a High Shaft/Socket in Cases of Diabetic Partial Foot Amputations
High-grade mobility or labor
Deformity of the stump
Skin graft in weight bearing areas
Balance disorder (polyneuropathy, impaired vision)
Contralateral amputation
Pirogoff and Syme amputation

Inner Foot Amputations

Resections of a single metatarsal bone are well-established procedures in the treatment of osteomyelitis. This procedure can be extended to all 5 metatarsal bones as an alternative to a forefoot amputation. Inner Lisfranc or even Chopart amputations are also possible as well as en block resections of all tarsal bones without any osteosynthesis. With shrinkage of the soft tissue, the foot shortens and stabilizes. In contrast to a "classical" amputation, the supporting area of the foot is larger, the tendons do not retract, and the diabetic patient does not sense that he or she is amputated. As an exception, wearing of standard shoes with custom-made molded insoles plus stiffened rocker bottom sole is possible in cases of an inner TMA. As a rule, inner amputations at the TMA or Lisfranc level require custom-made high shoes with a heel counter extended above the ankle joint, and the strengthened leg of the shoe has a minimal length of 6 in. (Fig. 30.13). The shoe also has a stiffened rocker bottom sole and a cushioned heel. The same type of footwear is prescribed for en block resections of all tarsal bones. Internal Chopart amputations result in a foot that is very short but plantigrade. In a rather obese patient, additional footwear modifications such as a higher leg (8.5 in.) or an extended and stiffened tongue may be necessary in order to share load during toe-off.

Calcanectomy

Ulcerations and infections of the bone are indications for resections of the calcaneus. Depending on the extent of tissue damage, partial resection or total calcanectomy is performed. In cases of a partial calcaneal resection, the function of the foot depends on the preservation of the Achilles tendon attachment. If the Achilles tendon is fully intact, a foot orthosis serves for compensation of the heel defect with loss of foot height and length. If the skin has been thinned out and lost its viscoelastic capacity, the orthosis needs to be soft in the area of the heel. The heel section of the shoe has to be adapted to the altered outer shape, and the shoe should have a boot form to prevent slip of the heel during toe-off.

Detachment of the Achilles tendon weakens plantarflexion and supination substantially so that additional modifications of the shoe are necessary. In a normal foot, the pull of the Achilles tendon effects a varus position of the calcaneus during heel lift. By this mechanism, the midtarsal joints are locked so that the foot can work as a rigid and effective lever during toe-off. The shoe has to compensate for the biomechanical foot alterations. A reinforced and extended heel counter is recommended as well as a flared heel allowing for a wider base to control the distribution of body weight to the foot and its gravitational center. The lever function of the foot is re-established with the help of a stiffened outsole.

After total calcanectomy, custom-made orthopedic shoes are prescribed routinely. Weight bearing in the area of the rearfoot is problematic so that the material of the foot orthosis needs to be extra soft under the talus. As a consequence, the transmission of ground reaction force happens anteriorly to the axis of the ankle joint. The lacking counter pull of the Achilles tendon results in dorsiflexion, adding unwanted load to the area of the rearfoot. Hence, the supporting area of the inlay has to be extended posteriorly. If exaggerated ankle dorsiflexion cannot be controlled by this measure, the shoe must have a long and reinforced leg, if required in combination with a cushioned and strengthened shoe tongue.

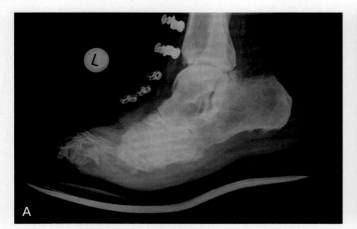
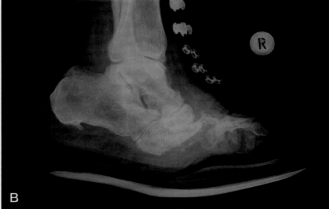

FIGURE 30.13 Plain radiographs of both feet of a patient within high orthopedic shoes with stiffened rocker bottom. **A.** Inner transmetatarsal amputation on the left foot. **B.** Inner Lisfranc amputation on the right foot.

Transtibial Amputation

Depending on the amputation level, the weight bearing capacity differs significantly. Long stumps (distal half of the tibia) have a forceful lever arm but limited weight bearing capacity due to the small diameter of the long bones at the resection level in combination with poor muscle coverage. In the presence of peripheral arterial disease, a more proximal amputation level (proximal third of the tibia) is recommended. The cutting plane lies within the transition zone between tubular and cancellous bone. With further shortening of the stump, weight bearing capacity increases, but contact surface and lever arm decrease. Transtibial amputations in diabetic patients most often result in a medium length or short stump.

Basically, 2 different prosthetic designs are available: (a) A prosthesis with joints and a thigh lacer offers maximum mediolateral or anteroposterior stability in cases of knee joint instability and provides prevention of genu recurvatum. If partial unloading of the residual lower extremity is necessary due to skin problems, the thigh corset provides some degree of shared weight bearing. The tight-fitting corset may lead to thigh muscle atrophy and distal edema. Joints and corset add considerable weight to the prosthesis. Even joint centers located at the best result in movements between leg and prosthesis. Knee flexion >90 degrees is hardly possible. Further disadvantages are the unappealing cosmesis, the longer fabrication time, and the higher price in comparison to a short prosthesis. (b) A full contact short prostheses have become the standard device for transtibial amputees recently. The design of the laminated or molded plastic socket is patellar tendon bearing or has a condyle bearing. A model of the patient's stump is used to achieve a total contact fit. Most often, the outer hard socket is supplemented with an inner soft socket in order to add comfort and protection from excessive impact or shear forces. Patients with peripheral arterial disease or peripheral neuropathy, bony prominences, and scarred skin, benefit from a soft socket.

Suspension during the swing phase of gait is provided by different technical measures. The socket either has a supracondylar suspension or a supracondylar suprapatellar suspension with extended medial, lateral, and anterior walls for additional knee stability. Further suspension aids are suprapatellar cuffs or belts, removable medial brims or wedges, and suspension sleeves. A different suspension technique is implemented by the silicone suction socket or Icelandic roll-on silicone socket. This type of short prosthesis uses a prefabricated or custom-made silicone liner. The inherent suction capabilities of the silicone against the skin and a distal shuttle lock mechanism provide improved suspension. Shear forces due to socket pistoning are reduced by the liner. Originally, the liner was used strictly to provide suspension, whereas further developments have yielded other materials like polyurethane or liner with increased wall thickness to add comfort and cushion.

REHABILITATION AFTER AMPUTATION IN PATIENTS WITH DIABETES MELLITUS

The goal of the postsurgical phase is mobilization of the amputee patient in a controlled manner under physiotherapeutic guidance in order to prevent joint contractures and reduce stump edema (31). Control of edema is very important for the healing process and makes earlier prosthetic fitting possible (32). Stump dressings should be performed only by trained and skilled physiotherapists, nurses, and/or physicians. In particular, partial foot stumps in a patient with peripheral arterial disease with thin and vulnerable skin are prone to pressure necrosis. Padding with cotton wool keeps the foot stump warm and protects bony prominences against pressure sores. Elastic bandages or stockinettes should enclose the complete lower leg for optimum edema control. In cases of a transtibial amputation, the distal half of the thigh has to be included as well. If the dressing is not retained properly, circular strangulation may affect the opposite of what was intended. Silicone liners can also be used for volume control and for shaping of a below-the-knee amputation stump (15). They offer equal compression independent of personnel and are simple to disinfect. With decrease of volume, another silicone liner with a smaller diameter has to be applied for continued shaping of the residual lower extremity.

Immediate postoperative prostheses (IPOP) can help to reduce pain and swelling after amputation and support mobilization of the amputee. The IPOP is applied after the surgical wound has stabilized, usually in the second or third postsurgical week. Excessive weight bearing soon after the operation has to be avoided to prevent damage to the wound site. Further benefits of the IPOP are improvement of balance and safety during transfers and protection of the wound site from trauma. The IPOP should be used under supervision of an experienced rehabilitation team.

Although hospitals for acute cases typically focus on treatment of impairment, the social and environmental consequences of impairment are better managed by a well-coordinated multidisciplinary team in a rehabilitation center (13). Before transferring the diabetic amputee to a respective center, a decision has to be made of whether or not the patient is a suitable candidate for prosthetic fitting. In addition, rehabilitation is equally indispensable for those patients who do not want a functional prosthesis or who are technically impossible to fit. In such cases, a basic prosthesis can aid transfer between wheelchair and bed or a cosmetic device can augment the patients' self-respect.

Conclusion

The diabetic patient with multiple comorbidities, in particular coronary arterial disease, may be medically unsuitable for prosthetic fitting, similar to older or more disabled patients. The selection of patients to whom a functional prosthesis may not be supplied is not a pleasant but a demanding task for the physician concerned with this problem.

References

1. American Diabetes Association. Consensus development conference on diabetic foot wound care: 7–8 April 1999, Boston, Massachusetts. Diabetes Care 1999;22:1354–1360.

2. Armstrong DG, Stacpoole-Shea S. Total contact casts and removable cast walkers. Mitigation of plantar heel pressure. J Am Podiatr Med Assoc 1999;89:50–53.

3. Bellmann D. Ein neuer Vorfußprothesentyp. Medizinisch-Orthopaedische Technik 1985;105:21–22.

4. Boninger ML, Leonard JA Jr. Use of bivalved ankle-foot orthosis in neuropathic foot and ankle lesions. J Rehabil Res Dev 1996;33:16–22.

5. Boyko EJ, Ahroni JH, Stensel V, et al. A prospective study of risk factors for diabetic foot ulcer. The Seattle diabetic foot study. Diabetes Care 1999;22:1036–1042.

6. Brodsky JW, Kourosh S, Stills M, et al. Objective evaluation of insert material for diabetic and athletic footwear. Foot Ankle 1988;9:111–116.

7. Cavanagh PR, Lipsky A, Bradbury AW, et al. Treatment for diabetic foot ulcers. Lancet 2005;366:1725–1735.

8. Dahmen R, Haspels R, Koomen B, et al. Therapeutic footwear for the neuropathic foot: an algorithm. Diabetes Care 2001;24:705–709.

9. Drerup B, Wetz HH, Kolling C, et al. Der Einfluß der Fußbettung und Schuhzurichtung auf die plantare Druckverteilung. Medizinisch-Orthopaedische Technik 2000;120:84–90.

10. Eichenholtz SN. Charcot joints. Springfield, IL: Charles C. Thomas, 1966.

11. Gefen A, Gefen N, Linder-Ganz E, et al. In vivo muscle stiffening under bone compression promotes deep pressure sores. J Biomech Eng 2005;127:512–524.

12. Guyton GP, Saltzman CL. The diabetic foot: basic mechanisms of disease. Instr Course Lect 2002;51:169–181.

13. Ham R, Regan JM, Roberts VC. Evaluation of introducing the team approach to the care of the amputee: the Dulwich study. Prosthet Orthot Int 1987;11:25–30.

14. Janisse DJ. Prescription insoles and footwear. Clin Podiatr Med Surg 1995;12:41–61.

15. Johannesson A, Larsson GU, Oberg T. From major amputation to prosthetic outcome: a prospective study of 190 patients in a defined population. Prosthet Orthot Int 2004;28:9–21.

16. Johnson JE. Surgical treatment of neuropathic arthropathy of the foot and ankle. Instr Course Lect 1999;48:269–277.

17. Koller A, Hafkemeyer U, Fiedler R, et al. Reconstructive foot surgery in cases of diabetic-neuropathic osteoarthropathy [in German]. Orthopade 2004;33:983–991.

18. Koller A, Meissner SA, Podella M, et al. Orthotic management of Charcot feet after external fixation surgery. Clin Podiatr Med Surg 2007;24:583–599.

19. Lavery LA, Armstrong DG, Harkless LB. Classification of diabetic foot wounds. J Foot Ankle Surg 1996;35:528–531.

20. Lemmon D, Shiang TY, Hashmi A, et al. The effect of insoles in therapeutic footwear—a finite element approach. J Biomech 1997;30:615–620.

21. Lord M, Hosein R. Pressure redistribution by molded inserts in diabetic footwear: a pilot study. J Rehabil Res Dev 1994;31:214–221.

22. Marks RM. Complications of foot and ankle surgery in patients with diabetes. Clin Orthop Relat Res 2001;391:153–161.

23. Morgan JM, Biehl WC III, Wagner FW Jr. Management of neuropathic arthropathy with the Charcot restraint orthotic walker. Clin Orthop Relat Res 1993;296:58–63.

24. Mueller MJ, Sinacore DR. Rehabilitation factors following transmetatarsal amputation. Phys Ther 1994;74:1027–1033.

25. Murray HJ, Young MJ, Hollis S, et al. The association between callus formation, high pressures and neuropathy in diabetic foot ulceration. Diabet Med 1996;13:979–992.

26. Perry J. Gait analysis: normal and pathological function. Thorofare, NJ: Slack, 1992.

27. Peters EJ, Lavery LA. Effectiveness of the diabetic foot risk classification system of the International Working Group on the Diabetic Foot. Diabetes Care 2001;24:1442–1447.

28. Piaggesi A, Macchiarini S, Rizzo L, et al. An off-the-shelf instant contact casting device for the management of diabetic foot ulcers: a randomized prospective trial versus traditional fiberglass cast. Diabetes Care 2007;30:586–590.

29. Rajbhandari SM, Jenkins RC, Davies C, et al. Charcot neuroarthropathy in diabetes mellitus. Diabetologia 2002;45:1085–1096.

30. Sanders LJ, Frykberg RG. Diabetic neuropathic osteoarthropathy: the Charcot foot. In: Frykberg RG, ed. The high risk foot in diabetes mellitus. New York: Churchill Livingstone, 1993:297–336.

31. van Ross E, Larner S. Rehabilitation after amputation. In: Boulton AJM, Connor H, Cavanagh PR, eds. The foot in diabetics. 3rd ed. New York: John Wiley & Sons, 2000:309–321.

32. van Velzen AD, Nederhand MJ, Emmelot CH, et al. Early treatment of trans-tibial amputees: retrospective analysis of early fitting and elastic bandaging. Prosthet Orthot Int 2005;29:3–12.

33. Warren G, Nade S. The care of neuropathic limbs: a practical manual. Pearl River, NY: Parthenon, 1999.

Index

Page numbers in italic refer to figures; page numbers followed by *t* refer to tables.